THE
PRACTICE ENVIRONMENT
OF NURSING

Issues & Trends

THE PRACTICE ENVIRONMENT OF NURSING

Issues & Trends

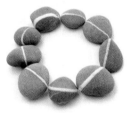

KARIN A. POLIFKO
PhD, RN, NEA-BC
Vice President, Operations and Academic Affairs
Remington Colleges
Heathrow, Florida

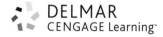
DELMAR
CENGAGE Learning™

Australia • Canada • Mexico • Singapore • Spain • United Kingdom • United States

DELMAR
CENGAGE Learning

The Practice Environment of Nursing: Issues and Trends, First Edition
Karin A. Polifko

Vice President, Career and Professional Editorial: Dave Garza

Director of Learning Solutions: Matt Kane

Executive Editor: Maureen Rosener

Managing Editor: Marah Bellegarde

Senior Product Manager: Juliet Steiner

Editorial Assistant: Samantha Miller

Vice President, Career and Professional Marketing: Jennifer Ann Baker

Executive Marketing Manager: Wendy Mapstone

Senior Marketing Manager: Michele McTighe

Marketing Coordinator: Scott Chrysler

Production Director: Carolyn Miller

Production Manager: Andrew Crouth

Content Project Manager: Anne Sherman

Senior Art Director: Jack Pendleton

Technology Project Manager: Mary Colleen Liburdi

Production Technology Analyst: Christopher Catalina

Library of Congress Control Number: 2009922774

ISBN-13: 978-1-4283-1792-5
ISBN-10: 1-4283-1792-9

Delmar
5 Maxwell Drive
Clifton Park, NY 12065-2919
USA

Cengage Learning products are represented in Canada by Nelson Education, Ltd.

For your lifelong learning solutions, visit **delmar.cengage.com**.
Visit our corporate website at **cengage.com**.

Notice to the Reader

Publisher does not warrant or guarantee any of the products described herein or perform any independent analysis in connection with any of the product information contained herein. Publisher does not assume, and expressly disclaims, any obligation to obtain and include information other than that provided to it by the manufacturer. The reader is expressly warned to consider and adopt all safety precautions that might be indicated by the activities described herein and to avoid all potential hazards. By following the instructions contained herein, the reader willingly assumes all risks in connection with such instructions. The publisher makes no representations or warranties of any kind, including but not limited to, the warranties of fitness for particular purpose or merchantability, nor are any such representations implied with respect to the material set forth herein, and the publisher takes no responsibility with respect to such material. The publisher shall not be liable for any special, consequential, or exemplary damages resulting, in whole or part, from the readers' use of, or reliance upon, this material.

Printed in Canada
1 2 3 4 5 6 7 12 11 10 09

Dedication

To my family.

CONTENTS

SECTION 3: TRANSITION AND GROWTH

PREFACE

Nursing is continually evolving as a profession and discipline. Students today can no longer rely on rituals or the "this is how we have always done it" approach and remain respected and valued members of the health care team. Ever the life-long learners, nurses need information about evolving issues such as policy development, insurance, and health disparities, as well as other pertinent issues that both directly and indirectly affect their patient care.

Like the larger health care delivery model, the field of nursing continues to change, resulting in a need for nursing education to provide the baseline for essential information necessary not only to function within the profession but to share and impart knowledge to a variety of consumers and customers. There are so many issues involved in the increasingly complex system of health care in the United States, including social, political, cultural and, especially as of late, financial, that to practice nursing effectively requires broad knowledge in a myriad of subjects outside the profession. Further, there is a continued clinical and faculty nursing shortage that affects not only clinical decision making but also the educational system that develops future practitioners. Information sources continue to grow exponentially, necessitating informed and thoughtful dissection and dissemination of materials. As we prepare graduates, we need to keep in mind that one cannot master all information as a generalist, so we need to provide our students the tools to critically think, question, and, it is hoped, arrive at outcomes that support best-practice outcomes.

The primary purpose of *The Practice Environment of Nursing: Issues and Trends* is to provide the student with tools to begin thoughtful discussions and problem solving within the social context, rather than the clinical arena, in which one practices nursing. The intended audience is any registered nurse student, whether enrolled as a second-degree, as a generic baccalaureate, or as a returning RN student. The book can be used as a primary textbook in the final semester for students as they turn their learning attention to the environment that drives clinical-practice decision making, or it can be used to augment learning experiences throughout the curriculum.

Organization

The Practice Environment of Nursing: Issues and Trends is written in a manner that encourages the students and the instructor to become engaged in an active discussion, whether it is in a traditional classroom or an online classroom. This book, with the contributions of expert clinicians, administrators, and educators in their respective fields, is based upon many years of experience as to what is needed for the successful transition from graduate to registered nurse. First and foremost, the book focuses on the necessary knowledge of a new graduate, regardless of where the new graduate chooses employment, be it in an acute care setting, a public health department, or an assisted living facility. *The Practice Environment of Nursing: Issues and Trends* offers relevant concept discussions for graduates to apply in their first professional role as a registered nurse. This book supports discussion and critical thinking through the following:

- The book engages the reader with interactive questions in the form of Case Scenarios, Internet Exercises, and Writing Exercises.
- Chapter Case Scenarios may be used individually or as a group assignment to foster either individual writing skills or group discussion and problem solving.
- There is extensive use of application in the clinical setting, allowing a student to immediately visualize a variety of situations with nurses' potential responses.
- Guided questions are placed throughout the chapters to encourage continuing dialogue, thoughtful discussion, and, oftentimes, classroom debate.

The Practice Environment of Nursing: Issues and Trends is organized into three sections:

Section 1: Past to Present in the Profession

Section 1 presents the background information of the nursing profession and offers viewpoints on key issues surrounding the field, including an introduction to entry-into-practice issues. A unique feature of this book is the inclusion of the origins of medicine and several of the allied health professions that have an influence on nursing care delivery.

Workforce issues, whether it be the aging workforce, generational differences, or mandatory overtime, are addressed as part of the environment in which nursing exists. Likewise, a critical issue affecting the vast majority of nursing colleges and schools, the lack of qualified faculty members, is addressed by a nurse educator. This section ends with a review of the newest nursing specialties to intrigue and expand the student's perspective on the breadth and depth of the nursing field.

Section 2: The Environment That Influences Nursing Care

Section 2 is a review of the factors that have influenced patient-care delivery to assist the student in understanding the current practice environment. Topics of health policy, political influences, and the use of outcomes to drive access and quality in terms of practice decisions frame this chapter. A thorough discussion of health care economics and the health care insurance industry is presented from the perspective of a health care executive, assisting the student in understanding the complicated implications of finance on health care delivery. The section on information access in health care is written by a medical librarian. The final chapter discusses the duty, under OSHA, of employers to provide a safe and healthful workplace, with an in-depth questionnaire for the graduate to use with prospective employers to ascertain critical safety measures in the workplace.

Section 3: Transition and Growth

Section 3 focuses on the student in the transition to the role of graduate nurse. Test-taking strategies, including specifics regarding the NCLEX, GRE, and certification exams, are reviewed in depth, offering numerous hints and tips for success. A mentoring chapter assists the graduate in asking decisive questions to prospective employers about their preceptorships, including how to work toward successful relationships between the mentor and mentee. A chapter on transitioning from student to new employee speaks to pertinent workforce issues that cause many new graduates stress—and how to deal with these issues instead of avoiding them. A known nurse lobbyist speaks to advocacy in the public arena, offering suggestions for graduates on ways not only to support their patients and their families but how to be part of the larger nursing workforce in promoting health care for all. Finally, the culminating chapter logically discusses present-day forces that continue to shape the environment in which nurses practice, pulling together the various thoughts and writings throughout the book to create the larger picture of the practice of nursing within the U.S. health care system.

Features

Each chapter contains the following features to enhance learning in a variety of methods:

- Learning Objectives: Listed at the beginning of each chapter, these help organize the course and illuminate the main concepts in each chapter.
- Key Terms: These terms, with accompanying definitions in the end-of-book glossary, help the reader determine which critical terms are necessary to understand the material.
- Case Scenarios: Each chapter has at least two case scenarios, taken from real-life experiences of the contributors, which encourage the reader to critically think and debate. While there are usually no distinct right or wrong answers, case scenarios offer the opportunity to provide supportive evidence for responses.
- Writing Exercises: Each chapter has at least two writing exercises that can be used to practice critical thinking and writing skills while evaluating the reader's understanding of the topic at hand.
- Internet Exercises: Each chapter has at least two Internet exercises that can be used to evaluate the reader's ability to locate accurate and appropriate information using a stable Web site.

Teaching and Learning Package

The supplement package for *The Practice Environment of Nursing: Issues and Trends* was created to achieve two goals:

1. To assist students in learning the information and concepts essential to bridging the gap to professional nursing practice.
2. To assist instructors in planning and implementing their programs for the most efficient use of time and resources.

Instructor Resources (ISBN 10: 1-4283-1793-7/ISBN 13: 978-1-4283-1793-2)

The Instructor's Resource to Accompany The Practice Environment of Nursing: Issues and Trends is an all-inclusive electronic product with instructor slides created in PowerPoint, a computerized test bank created in ExamView, and an instructor's manual.

Instructor Slides Created in PowerPoint

More than 300 slides are available and designed to support and facilitate lecture and classroom instruction.

Computerized Test Bank in ExamView

This computerized test bank holds more than 450 questions organized by chapter, geared toward the text content, and written following the NCLEX format. Each answer is accompanied by a rationale explaining right and wrong choices, is coded by cognitive level, and is linked to related content in the text through relevant chapter headings. Using the ExamView platform, instructors can use the questions as provided or modify and add questions as needed to generate tests that meet their specific instructional needs.

Instructor's Manual

Provided electronically to allow for individual customization, this instructor's manual is organized by chapter and includes:

- Strategies for stimulating class discussion
- Answers/rationales for Internet exercises
- Answers/rationales for written exercises
- Answers and intended responses to the case study questions
- Additional Internet activities, writing exercises, and assignments

Online Companion (ISBN 10: 1-4283-1794-5/ISBN 13: 978-1-4283-1794-9)

Free to students and instructors, the *Online Companion to Accompany The Practice Environment of Nursing: Issues and Trends* is an excellent source of additional study materials and instructional resources. Students can find links to Web sites discussed in the book, learning activities, additional case studies, and additional online resources. Instructors will have online, password-protected access to all the resources found in the instructor resource, including the computerized test bank, instructor's manual, and instructor slides created in PowerPoint. For free access to the online companion, visit us online at:

http://www.delmarlearning.com/companions/index.asp?isbn=1428317929.

ACKNOWLEDGMENTS

The completion of this project could not have been successful without the many friends and colleagues who so willingly agreed to contribute their areas of expertise to this book. I am thrilled that we had so many different colleagues offering their expertise, ranging from nurse executives in practice, to specialists in industry, to nursing deans and senior faculty members. While many will not be adequately recognized for their contributions by their respective organizations, students will benefit greatly from the many pearls of wisdom found throughout this book.

A final heartfelt thank you goes to my husband, Jay, who has filled in for me many times as a deadline was approaching, always willingly and without complaint.

ABOUT THE AUTHOR

Karin A. Polifko's career has spanned both the academic and service fields of health care. Currently Vice President, Operations and Academic Affairs, at Remington Colleges, Dr. Polifko is instrumental in the strategic planning, business development, and establishment of academic programs for Remington Colleges' nursing initiatives. Along with teaching appointments and experience at the undergraduate, graduate, and doctoral levels, she has held academic positions as the Associate Dean for Academic and Student Affairs at the University of Florida's College of Nursing and Chair of Nursing and Graduate Director at Christopher Newport University in Virginia.

Dr. Polifko has extensive administrative experience in a variety of health care settings, in the roles of Vice President of System Development and Research, Administrative Director, Director of Nursing, Nurse Manager, and Clinical Nurse Specialist. Her consulting projects include nursing program development, accreditation preparation, organizational change assessment and evaluation, outcomes systems management, and leadership assessment. Her first textbook, *Case Applications in Nursing Leadership and Management,* was published in 2004, and her second textbook, *Concepts of the Nursing Profession*, was published in 2006. She is the author of multiple book chapters that focus on leadership and management topics.

Dr. Polifko received her Bachelor of Science in Nursing from the University of North Carolina, Charlotte, her Master of Science in Nursing from the University of Pennsylvania, and her Doctorate in Public Administration and a certificate in Advanced Policy Analysis from Old Dominion University. She is nationally certified as a Nurse Administrator, Advanced, from the American Nurses Credentialing Center.

LIST OF CONTRIBUTORS

Carol J. Bickford, PhD, RN-BC
Senior Policy Fellow,
Department of Nursing Practice & Policy
American Nurses Association

Rebecca Bowers-Lanier, EdD, MPH, RN
Legislative Consultant
Macaulay & Burtch, P.C.

Amy Barlow Britt, MS, RN, CEN
Instructor
Riverside School of Health Careers

Maureen C. Creegan, EdD, RN
Director and Professor, Division of Nursing
Dominican College

Sheryl L. Curtis, MSN, ARNP
Clinical Assistant Professor
University of Florida, College of Nursing

Sharron E. Guillett, PhD, RN
Associate Professor, BSN Program
School of Health Professionals
Marymount University

K. Alberta McCaleb, DSN, RN
Administrative Director
UAB Center for Nursing Excellence
University of Alabama Health System,
University of Alabama School of Nursing,
University of Alabama at Birmingham

Nancy Nivison Menzel, PhD, RN, PHCNS-BC, COHN-S, CNE
Associate Professor
University of Nevada School of Nursing

Rosemary E. S. Mortimer, MS Ed, MS, RN
Instructor
Johns Hopkins University
School of Nursing

Donna Bridgman Musser, PhD, RN
Assistant Professor of Nursing
University of Central Arkansas

Pamela Patterson, MSN, RN
Nurse Manager, RN Intern Program
University of Alabama Hospital

Mary Jo Regan-Kubinski, PhD, RN
Dean and Professor Division of
Nursing and Health Professions
Indiana University South Bend

Cathleen M. Schulz, PhD, RN, CNE, FAAN
Dean and Professor
Harding University

Pamela Sherwill-Navarro, MLS, AHIP
College of Nursing Librarian
Remington College of Nursing

Cynthia D. Sofhauser, PhD, MSN, RN, AHN-BC
Associate Professor
Indiana University South
Bend School of Nursing

Amy Spurlock, PhD, RN
Associate Professor
Troy University

Ruth Stearns, BA
Education Specialist
Remington Colleges

Sheila Cox Sullivan, PhD, RN, CNE
Associate Chief Nurse/Research
Central Arkansas Veterans Healthcare System

Aileen Wehren, EdD
Vice President, Systems Administration
Porter-Starke Services, Inc.

Kathleen M. White, PhD, RN, CEA-BC
Director, Masters and Doctor of
Nursing Practice Programs
The Johns Hopkins University
School of Nursing

Barbara G. Williams, PhD, RN
Chairperson and Professor,
Department of Nursing
University of Central Arkansas

Lillian Wise, DNS, RN
Professor and Coordinator,
RN to BSN/MSN Track
Troy University

Nancy L. York, PhD, RN
Assistant Professor of Nursing
University of Nevada, Las Vegas

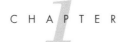

C H A P T E R

THE CURRENT STATE OF THE NURSING DISCIPLINE

CYNTHIA D. SOFHAUSER

PhD, MSN, RN, AHN-BC, Associate Professor, Indiana University South Bend School of Nursing

There is nothing new under the sun, but there are lots of old things we don't know.

–Ambrose Bierce

LEARNING OBJECTIVES

At the completion of the chapter, the learner should be able to do the following:

1. Analyze the factors germane to the discourse regarding the professional status of the nursing discipline.
2. Review the difficulties encountered when defining nursing practice.
3. Outline the various levels of educational preparation, both undergraduate and graduate, available to the nurse.
4. Describe the changes shaping the educational preparation of the nurse.
5. Discuss technological advances impacting the profession of nursing and the challenges they pose.
6. Explore the impact of current and impending nursing shortages on the discipline of nursing.

KEY TERMS

Certification
Clinical Simulation
Core Competencies
Discipline
Entry-Level Preparation

Essentials for Baccalaureate
   Nursing Education
Globalization
Integrative Health Care
Nursing Informatics

Nursing Shortage
Nursing Theory
Online Learning
Profession
Synergy Model for Patient Care

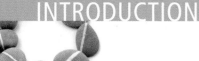

INTRODUCTION

Ambrose Bierce's satirical remark at the beginning of this chapter illuminates the fact that, although an excellent teacher, experience has its limits. Despite history and the experiences it provides, there is still much to be learned. This holds true when considering the issues faced by the **discipline** of nursing. Members of the discipline express their frustration as their **profession** continues to struggle with several age-old questions, present concerns, and emerging issues. Scholars persist in their debate over the professional and scientific status of the discipline. Is nursing a profession or merely a vocation? Is the discipline a science or an art? The relevancy of theory, particularly nursing theory, to grassroots practice is hotly debated in theoretical journals that encourage such discourse. Future nurses continue to be prepared in a variety of ways, leading to different levels of academic preparation but ultimately the same license. Future predictions of a worsening nursing shortage provide challenges for all those involved in health care. Despite predictions to the contrary, practitioners of the discipline continue to be primarily employed in acute-care settings. There they are faced with an ever-aging population fraught with a myriad of chronic health issues. The "good" nurse struggles in this environment to practice holistically, carving out the independent practice that initially drew them to the profession. The explosion of technology relative to advances in medicine challenges even the most informed nurse. Advances in informatics hold the promise of more nursing time spent with the patient and less time with the computerized chart. The basic issues facing the discipline are not necessarily new, but the solutions demand new ways of thinking and reacting.

THE DISCIPLINE DEFINED

The discipline of nursing continues to struggle with the notion of status, both as a science and a profession. The debate regarding whether the discipline is indeed a science is discussed widely in literature generated by those concerned with the question, i.e., philosophers and nurse theorists. The reader is encouraged to consult Winters and Ballou (2004) for an excellent example of this discourse. Is the discipline of nursing a profession? This is an age-old question that continues to be debated in most nursing literature in one form or another. The question of professional status is not unique to the discipline of nursing. It is a question asked by a number of practitioners of various fields. The last century witnessed many scholars who outlined the prerequisites necessary for a discipline to achieve before professional status could be claimed. This was believed to be necessary, in part, to make the argument for college-level preparation of practitioners of a profession. As members of the discipline of nursing interact and collaborate with others from related health care fields, resolving issues relative to the status of the discipline is imperative.

Perhaps the real question is not whether the discipline is or is not a profession, but rather by whose standard is the discipline of nursing to be measured? Webster's defines discipline as "a branch of knowledge" (*Webster's Online Dictionary*, 2008). In other words, a discipline is simply a body of knowledge. In combining two definitions of the term, profession is defined as the body of people in a learned occupation requiring special education (*Webster's Online Dictionary*,

2008). Nursing, at least as defined by Webster, is most certainly a discipline and a profession. Yet, the idea of being a profession means more than this simple definition implies. Most scholars interested in such discourse would probably agree that a profession is a group of individuals, educated in like manner, who are dedicated to a common cause, striving toward a common goal, and guided by a prescribed code of ethics and behaviors. However, despite all the rhetoric surrounding the issue, professional status is not something that can be bestowed upon a discipline by some accrediting body of scholars or even members of the discipline itself; but rather, it is a designation that must be earned through definition of practice.

<table>
<tr><td>Writing
Exercise
1-1</td><td>In writing, defend the following statement: The discipline of nursing is a profession.</td></tr>
</table>

If definition of practice is a necessary prerequisite for professional status, then the question becomes "What is nursing?" Theorists may argue that a particular concept defines the uniqueness of the profession. Researchers carve out a niche for the discipline by defining ubiquitous problems unique to the nurse as they care for patients in a variety of settings. Academics tout that nurses are best defined by their unique problem-solving approaches in a clinical situation, dubbed "clinical thinking." And still the question remains, "What is nursing?" At this juncture in the discussion, it is important to note that others are moving the discipline forward by asking a more specific question. For some, it is not just about defining nursing, but defining "stellar nursing care" (Curley, 2007, p. 1), as well as the expected patient and system outcomes that result. Curley believes this to be such an important issue that she is urging for universal clarity by the discipline as a definition is formulated.

To reiterate, inherent in the declaration that one is practicing as a professional is the notion that one's practice can be clearly defined. The discipline of nursing is struggling with the professional status issue partly because most practicing nurses struggle when asked to define their practice. Nurses struggle with their own identity in the health care arena primarily due to the holistic nature of their practice. Perhaps this is due in part to the reason that much of what nurses do is not unique to the profession. Since nurses deal with a patient's holistic response to an illness, at any given moment a nurse may be called upon to be many things to many people; the nurse may function as diagnostician, dietician, respiratory therapist, physical therapist, chaplain, pharmacist, social worker, etc. Furthermore, since nurses are the frontline caregivers, they are expected to carry out the plan of care initiated by other members of the health care team. This blurs the line between the role of the nurse and the roles of other members of the health care team (Figure 1-1). There is no other profession in health care in which so much is demanded of the practitioner. The knowledge base of the nurse is both broad and deep to ensure quality and safety, and the nurse's skill set is diverse.

Figure 1-1

The role of the nurse frequently overlaps with other members of the health care team.

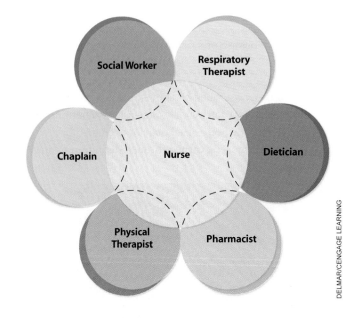

DELMAR/CENGAGE LEARNING

The development of ancillary health care roles has emerged out of this ambiguity, along with the realization that the nurse simply cannot "do it all." The lines between disciplines are often blurred in health care settings where the patients and their problems are many and the workers are few. Could this ambiguity cause erosion of nursing practice? Some might argue that as nurses perform more and more tasks once considered belonging to the purview of medicine, they lose sight of their independent practice. That is, they function less from a holistic standpoint. Unfortunately, this is occurring at a time when the antecedents of most diseases are found to have holistic roots. The "cause" of disease goes far beyond the physiologic. Mind and body are not separate entities after all. **Integrative health care**, where Western allopathic methods are blended with traditional, non-western-based ideas and therapies, is the health care delivery model of the future, and the nurse must be ready. Consumer health care needs dictate that the nurse practice from an informed, holistic standpoint; the problems are much too complex otherwise.

Further complicating the profession's identity is the fact that "what is nursing?" looks different in different health care settings. Nurses establish relationships with and care for patients wherever they may be. Practicing nurses do not fret over the question "what is nursing?" but rather are focused on the question "what is it that the patient needs from me?" Silva (1999), in downplaying the importance of a definition, states, "Nursing will be best remembered not for what nurses defined but for what nurses did or failed to do" (p. 222). She goes on to say that service is the cornerstone of any profession's contract with society and preceded the science of that discipline. Hence, the question asked by the practicing nurse—what is it that the patient needs from me?—takes on paramount importance and cannot be answered in a singular manner; the answer varies based on patient needs and the context in which care occurs. The essence of what it means to be a nurse, a caring nature with a focus on holistic healing, does not change. Yet all that surrounds this essence, the context of nursing care, does change and is further defined by technology, social values, science, and economics. Therefore, the health care consumer's needs are variable, rooted in the context of the moment and dependent on the setting. For example, the nursing-care needs of students and their parents in a school system are vastly different from the needs of a critically ill patient, surrounded by overly attentive loved ones in a critical-care setting. Is it any wonder the discipline struggles with the definition of nursing practice?

For many nurses a clearer understanding of what nursing really is and what nurses really do is found when they leave the hospital and practice in other care settings. Oftentimes, in the structured health care setting, the focus of nursing care is too strictly defined by the physician and institutional policies and procedures. Patient-care needs as defined by the patient are not fully appreciated or assessed. However, in the home and various community settings, patients are in complete control; their needs are clearly defined by them and take precedence over everything else.

The idea that patient-defined needs drive nursing care is not a new one. In fact, the belief that patient characteristics drive nurse competencies is the fundamental premise of the **Synergy Model for Patient Care** of the American Association of Critical-Care Nurses (AACN). The Synergy Model provides a framework for describing a patient-nurse relationship and acknowledges that nursing care, based on the needs of patients and their significant others, is of primary importance (Curley, 2007). Better patient outcomes result when patient characteristics and nurse competencies are in synergy. Although originally designed to direct nursing care in critical-care settings, the model has gained wide acceptance in all nursing-care settings.

Perhaps more than any other health care discipline, nursing is adaptable. Other health care practitioners practice via well-prescribed roles, and when they do not want to do what needs to be done for the sake of the patient, the nurse takes over. This adaptability has endeared the profession to the public, but has most certainly made it more difficult for the profession to define what it is exactly and precisely what a nurse does. So the question remains, what does a nurse do that no other health care worker does (Figure 1-2)? The answer is, quite simply, whatever

Figure 1-2
What does a nurse do that no other health care worker does?

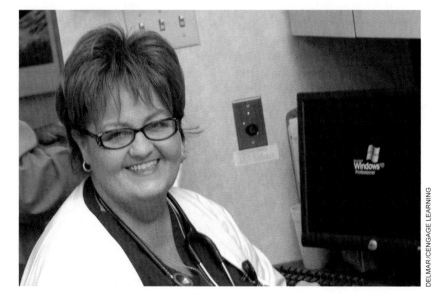

DELMAR/CENGAGE LEARNING

the patient needs for the nurse to do. Whether this fact is enough to bestow professional status to those who practice nursing is a question that is relevant only to those outside of the profession. Nurses know they are professionals and define themselves as such.

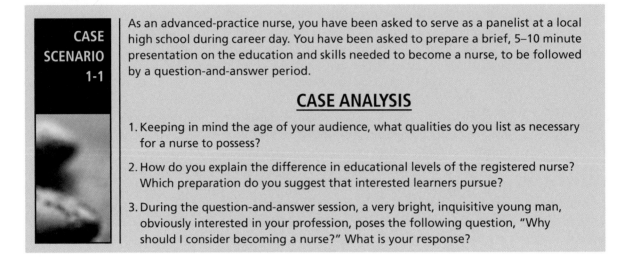

CASE SCENARIO 1-1

As an advanced-practice nurse, you have been asked to serve as a panelist at a local high school during career day. You have been asked to prepare a brief, 5–10 minute presentation on the education and skills needed to become a nurse, to be followed by a question-and-answer period.

CASE ANALYSIS

1. Keeping in mind the age of your audience, what qualities do you list as necessary for a nurse to possess?

2. How do you explain the difference in educational levels of the registered nurse? Which preparation do you suggest that interested learners pursue?

3. During the question-and-answer session, a very bright, inquisitive young man, obviously interested in your profession, poses the following question, "Why should I consider becoming a nurse?" What is your response?

THEORY: THE FOUNDATION OF PRACTICE AND RESEARCH

Mention the phrase "nursing theory," and many in nursing practice shudder. **Nursing theory** is the use of theory unique to the discipline and is used to explain, guide, and direct nursing-care activities. The relevancy and necessity of nursing theory has been questioned and hotly debated by nurses since its inception. Nursing students, at both undergraduate and graduate levels, are taught theory in the classroom and the importance of focus and use in practice, often without carryover into the clinical setting. Hence, few nurses practice from a well-defined theoretical base.

The intricate relationship between theory and research, the dependency of one on the other, is taught early on in nursing education. The development of nursing science is dependent upon this reciprocal relationship; theory drives research and research drives theory. Nowhere is this more apparent than at the doctoral level of education. Theory drives research at the doctoral level of educational preparation, as soon-to-be nurse scientists develop programs of research couched in nursing and/or other relevant theories. Through research, theory is further defined and refined. Consequently, the knowledge base of the discipline of nursing is advanced when this process occurs; knowledge is built upon knowledge.

However, many nurse researchers removed from the academic environment engage in relevant clinical research without having thought through the research problem guided by a prescribed theory. At best, a vague theoretical or conceptual framework provides some guidance in

Figure 1-3
Nursing theory
should drive
nursing practice
and research.

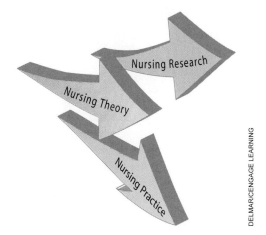

DELMAR/CENGAGE LEARNING

the formulation and clarification of the research problem. At worst, the theoretical framework is chosen after the research project is complete, oftentimes at the urging of journal editors who desire to print research reports driven by nursing theory. This begs the question as to whether a theoretical research performed by nurses is truly nursing research. How can a body of knowledge be built by a discipline with research not defined by theory important to the discipline? A theoretical base should drive practice and research, not vice versa (Figure 1-3). If scholars and researchers value nursing theory as central to the development of the discipline, why isn't nursing practice and research theory based?

Some of the lack of momentum where nursing theory is concerned has to do with nursing scholars themselves and their discourse. The terms paradigm, conceptual model, grand theory, mid-range theory, and practice theory are often ill defined in nursing literature. When defined, definitions by different scholars are often contradictory, leaving even the most conscientious nurse confused and frustrated. Debate ensues as to which paradigm should guide the development of nursing science, empiricist or interpretive (Monti & Tingen, 1999). To further the confusion, consensus on a universal theory for nursing, or even the need for consensus, is far from a reality, with many theorists touting their theory as the one theory for nursing. Theory testing/refining research, with its own convoluted language, is usually the purview of graduate students with little carry-over into the clinical setting. Unfortunately, the interventions that flow from a particular theoretical framework are rarely tested by researchers other than those wed to the theory. Consequently, theory development and theory-driven practice occur in a vacuum. Nursing science cannot be advanced with this type of silo thinking.

It is critical to remember that nurses do not work in isolation as they provide health care; they work in partnership with other health team members on a daily basis (Figure 1-4). The discipline's ability to come to terms with issues related to nursing theory can assist in defining nursing practice and solving nursing problems. Silva (1999) points out that nurses need to be able to articulate the theoretical bases of the discipline in order to work successfully with scholars from other disciplines. Theory has the potential to move the discipline beyond the task-oriented definition of nursing prescribed by those outside the discipline.

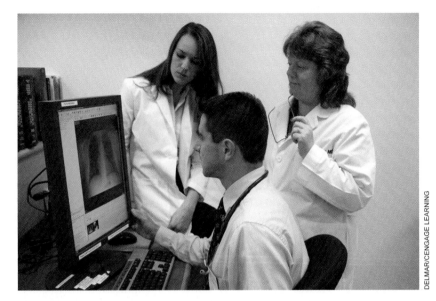

Figure 1-4
In working with other health team members, nurses must be able to articulate the theoretical basis of the nursing discipline.

DELMAR/CENGAGE LEARNING

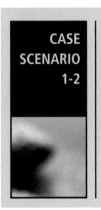

CASE SCENARIO 1-2

You are attending your nursing school 15-year reunion. In catching up with an old classmate, you tell her that you have your doctorate in nursing. She replies, "Oh no, you're not one of those people interested in theory are you? Just what the world needs, another nursing theory!"

CASE ANALYSIS

1. What beliefs about nursing in general are likely behind your friend's comments?

2. What beliefs about theory in particular must be addressed as you respond?

3. How would you go about explaining the relevancy of theory to nursing practice and research?

ENTRY INTO PRACTICE

Multiple **entry-level preparations** still exist within the discipline despite professional organizations touting the baccalaureate-prepared nurse as the "true professional." There are many educational routes to becoming a registered nurse (Figure 1-5). The interested learner can enroll in a university/college baccalaureate or associate degree program or any one of the remaining fifty-one hospital-based programs leading to a diploma degree in nursing (*NLNAC Directory of Accredited Programs*, 2008). Others pursue more nontraditional routes, first becoming a licensed practical nurse, and then entering a completion program in a vocational-technical setting. Some enter programs armed with a bachelor's degree in a non-nursing field, graduating with either a baccalaureate degree or a master's degree in nursing. Many such second-degree programs are

Figure 1-5

There are many pathways to becoming a registered nurse.

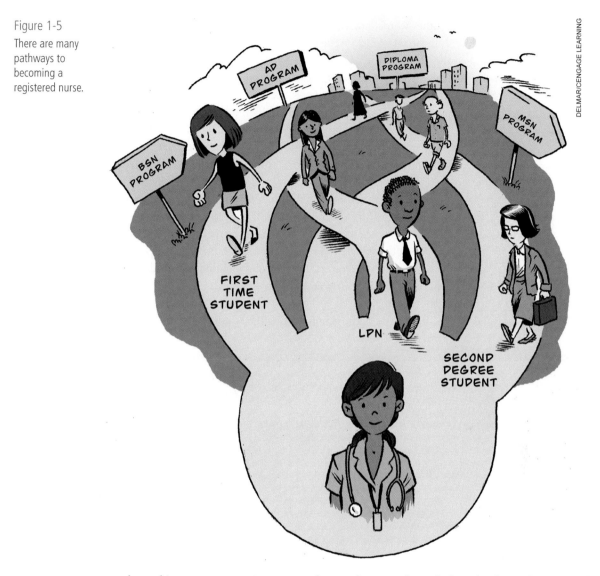

DELMAR/CENGAGE LEARNING

accelerated in nature, garnering a very select student population believed to be resilient enough to withstand the rigors of an intense curriculum.

Although associate and diploma levels of preparation provide a more expedient route to a nursing license, graduates of these programs are simply not prepared to face the issues they encounter in today's complex health care settings. As an aging population lives longer, they are often challenged with a myriad of chronic illnesses. As a result, patient care is much more complex, with "sicker" patients admitted to acute-care settings, remarkably increasing patient acuity levels. This demands the best entry-level practitioner available. The well-prepared nurse's education must be broad and liberal in nature, with sufficient depth provided in sciences needed to understand complex physical processes involved in normal and pathological conditions. Since the definition of what nursing is changes in any given patient situation, the nurse must have the background to address the patient's immediate needs, whether physiological, psychological, emotional, or spiritual. In other words, nothing short of a holistic, baccalaureate education can properly prepare the professional nurse for the world of patient care. Groundbreaking research has demonstrated the utility of the baccalaureate-prepared nurse at the bedside, with lower thirty-day mortality rates associated with hospitals that have a higher percentage of baccalaureate-prepared nurses (Aiken, Clarke, Cheung, Sloane, & Silber, 2003; Tourangeau, et. al., 2007).

The apparent gains in workforce numbers achieved by faster routes of educational preparation also fuel the growing shortage in nursing educators. Federal data indicate that baccalaureate-prepared nurses are four times more likely to pursue graduate degrees in nursing, degrees needed to teach in all academic settings (AACN, 2007). These facts help underscore why the greatest demand is for nurses prepared at the baccalaureate and graduate levels. With the shortage of nurse educators reaching crisis proportions, it should come as no surprise that the federal government is calling for baccalaureate preparation for at least two-thirds of the nursing workforce (HRSA report, 2002).

The importance of baccalaureate preparation for the registered nurse is not only recognized at the federal level, but the state level as well. Some states, e.g., New York and New Jersey, are proposing legislation that would require associate- and diploma-prepared registered nurses to obtain a baccalaureate degree within 10 years of initial licensure. The requirement would be waived for nurses already practicing, as well as those in nursing schools or on waiting lists for entry into an RN program. The license of those not meeting the requirement would be put on "hold."

Internet Exercise 1-1	Locate the following Web site: http://www.nln.org

1. What are the National League for Nursing (NLN) documents entitled "Position Statements"?

2. Locate the Position Statement, *Transforming Nursing Education*. When was it approved and by whom?

3. Under the section entitled "call to action," what do the authors suggest should be the role of the federal government in nursing education?

4. What recommendations are offered for faculty whose expertise is in nursing education?

Not all support the baccalaureate degree as the point of entry into practice. The National League for Nursing (NLN), in their Reflection and Dialogue series, is tackling the point-of-entry issue. In September 2007, the league initiated an online dialogue on the academic and professional progression of nurses, beginning with input from the NLN Board of Governors. Essentially, the NLN is suggesting a transformation of the dialogue to one in which progression within the profession is discussed and debated, rather than the point of entry into nursing practice. Nurse educators, public policy and workforce experts, health care organization representatives, and all interested parties are invited to comment. This stance makes sense given the fact that the NLN supports multiple levels of entry into nursing practice.

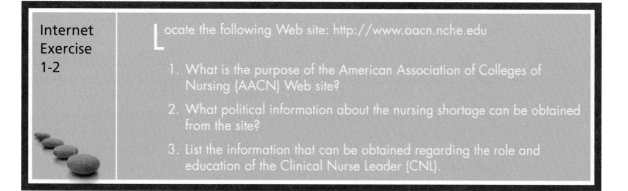

PRACTITIONER EDUCATIONAL PREPARATION

The discipline of nursing is responsive to the ever-changing health care needs of consumers. To that end, the American Association of Colleges of Nursing (AACN) is revisiting the expected competencies for graduates of a baccalaureate nursing program. The **Essentials for Baccalaureate Nursing Education** was revised in 2008 to more closely reflect current practice expectations. The Essentials document provides a framework for the education of baccalaureate-prepared nurses. This document is available for review and final comments at http://www.aacn.nche.edu. A link to the document is provided on the AACN homepage. Deans and directors from AACN member institutions, faculty, practice partners, and representatives of other health care and education organizations are invited to comment on the draft. The opportunity for stakeholders to review and provide feedback on the Essentials document is critical to the consensus process.

In the Essentials document the AACN reaffirms their position that the baccalaureate degree is the minimal level required for entry into professional nursing practice. All other nursing education builds on this baccalaureate, generalist degree. Their preferred vision of nursing education, in addition to the generalist baccalaureate degree, calls for the advanced generalist degree, and advanced specialty nursing education. The advanced generalist degree is obtained through master's programs offering the Clinical Nurse Leader (CNL) designation. Advanced specialty nursing education occurs at the doctoral level in doctorate-of-nursing-practice (DNP) or research-focused degree programs, i.e., PhD, DNS, and DNSc.

Internet
Exercise
1-2

Locate the following Web site: http://www.aacn.nche.edu

1. What is the purpose of the American Association of Colleges of Nursing (AACN) Web site?

2. What political information about the nursing shortage can be obtained from the site?

3. List the information that can be obtained regarding the role and education of the Clinical Nurse Leader (CNL).

Advanced Clinical Practice

Having espoused the baccalaureate degree as the point of entry into professional nursing practice, the AACN moved on to advanced nursing preparation. In 2004 the AACN made the decision to replace the master's degree with the DNP as the level of preparation needed for advanced clinical nursing practice by 2015. The DNP program is designed to prepare clinical leaders who will focus on multidisciplinary practice initiatives on a variety of key health care-delivery issues. Needless to say, this decision has created much turmoil and change within the profession. In response to this decree, there are currently 92 documented DNP programs in existence across the United States, with another 102 schools of nursing contemplating the DNP (AACN, 2009). Future debate will be focused on the fate of those with a DNP degree in academic settings. The DNP was initially conceptualized as the terminal degree for the clinician; the terminal degree for the academic is the PhD. The differences in preparation for scholarship activities between the two degrees will provide fertile ground for discourse as the definition of the scholarship of those with a DNP in the academic setting is explored.

Certification

Certification in one's chosen nursing specialty has become more popular within nursing ranks and is viewed by many as the mark of a true professional. Board certification is a mechanism for verification of knowledge and experience beyond the educational degree. It is typically granted after meeting specified eligibility requirements and passing a quantitative examination. Several professional nursing organizations offer certification in a variety of areas for the practicing nurse. For example, the American Nurses Credentialing Center (ANCC), a subsidiary of the American Nurses Association, provides basic certification in 19 nursing specialties for the registered nurse, boasting over 250,000 nurses certified since 1990 (ANCC, 2008). Additionally, advanced certifications are available in various specialties for the nurse practitioner, clinical nurse specialist, or nursing executive. Although the world's largest organization offering certification, the ANCC is not the only organization that certifies registered nurses. Others include the National League for Nursing (NLN), which began offering certification for nurse educators in 2005, and the AACN, which offers certification for the clinical nurse leader.

Nurse Educator Preparation

The notion of how the advanced-practice nurse is to be educated must be considered in tandem with the educational requirements of nurse educators. In a draft position statement posted online and circulated to AACN members prior to their 2008 spring annual meeting, the preferred vision of the professoriate was detailed (AACN, 2008). Of particular note in this statement is the affirmation that doctoral graduates who will be involved in the academic role must have preparation in educational methods and pedagogies. This requirement will do little, at least early on, to alleviate the looming crisis of nursing educator shortages, as those in many current doctoral programs are not receiving this necessary curricular content. No such requirements are articulated for those pursuing advanced clinical degrees, i.e., a master's degree or DNP. Yet the minimal expectation for clinical instruction is clinically focused graduate preparation. Additionally, for those pursuing a master's degree in nursing education, it would seem that the AACN does not envision a role in academia for them. This is particularly troublesome since schools of nursing have resurrected this degree to prepare nurses for primarily teaching roles in the academic setting.

Nursing Education

The issue of degrees and titles is but one facet of the educational-preparation issue. The question remains, what is the best way to prepare a nurse for the practice environment? The need for the practicing nurse to know more, about more, proves a daunting challenge for the nurse educator. Concepts relative to integrative health, geriatrics, genetics, bioinformatics, disaster-relief nursing, and safety initiatives, to name but a few, are promoted by groups inside and outside the discipline as critical components of a sound nursing curriculum. **Core competencies** for all health clinicians have been outlined by the Committee on the Health Professions Summit (2003) and serve as a guide for curricular development as well. These core competencies denote the critical behaviors of a health care provider. Therefore, the nurse is expected to be a team player who utilizes informatics effortlessly and engages in patient-centered care from an evidence-based position, all the while striving to enhance the quality of the care given. Employers in all settings desire an applicant who is assertive, analytical, and well versed in the issues surrounding evidence-based practice.

Writing
Exercise
1-3

In what ways has the changing face of technology impacted the discipline of nursing? Include in your answer considerations relative to nursing education, nursing practice, and nursing research.

Clinical Simulation

Despite predictions to the contrary, the majority of nurses continue to practice in acute-care, hospital-based settings, and future projected needs reflect this fact (HRSA, 2002). Providing students with a rich learning experience in a clinical setting that fosters the development of critical-thinking skills is a challenge for the most experienced nurse educator. The idea of providing students with structured, laboratory-created, **clinical simulation** experiences was born out of this necessity. A clinical simulation is a contrived clinical scenario performed in a structured, safe learning environment that enables the student to participate in patient care decision making and intervention. Clinical simulation involves creating a real-life, safe environment where students are free to make decisions and learn from their mistakes without the fear of doing harm to an acutely ill individual. Scenarios are carefully constructed by faculty to mimic problems nurses encounter in the hospital clinical setting. Although clinical simulation can take a more primitive form with the use of static mannequins or students posing as patients and concerned significant others, many schools have purchased advanced computerized models capable of mimicking vital human functions. These high-tech "patients" can speak, breathe, exhibit vital signs, express symptoms, etc. A debriefing session after the simulation experience is facilitated by the instructor(s) as students reflect on the events. It is important to note that clinical simulations can be created for any nursing situation and focus on a variety of nursing skills, e.g., assessment, interpersonal communication skills, leadership issues, etc.

Emerging research on clinical simulation education is quite promising; students learn a lot, and not only those participating directly in the simulation, but also those designated to be observers. Jeffries (2005) cites a number of outcomes associated with clinical simulations: increased knowledge retention, enhanced skill performance, learner satisfaction, critical thinking, and increased self-confidence and improved clinical judgment. Results are so impressive that several state boards of nursing have permitted a percentage of the student's clinical education to be obtained through clinical simulation experiences. Research is ongoing as nurse educators are involved in multi-site studies to further evaluate the use of clinical simulation as a teaching technique.

Online Learning

The idea of teaching from afar has been around for decades, but is now being interpreted in a manner quite different than in the past. Distance instruction and learning has taken on different meanings as universities have developed computer-course delivery systems. **Online learning**, distance instruction and learning via the Internet, is a more precise description of what is occurring. For many in nursing education, the bricks-and-mortar classroom has given way to the virtual classroom experience. The trend in academia is to move to distance education via online instruction. Professors are strongly encouraged to develop online courses in hopes of reaching more students in order to maintain enrollment numbers, and because it is believed that this is what the average learner wants. This is especially true for BSN completion programs and graduate education in nursing. Portions of classes, entire classes, and entire programs of study can be accessed via the personal computer. Of course, learning via cyberspace is fraught with its own set of problems, not the least of which involves the learner feeling disengaged with the professor and others in the course or program. Additionally, simply because a course or program of study can be put online doesn't mean that it should be. Although online programs achieve certification via accrediting bodies, assessment of outcomes via distance education programs lags far behind the opportunities for such instruction. The profession needs to engage in rigorous review of curricula in order to determine the appropriateness of online education.

It seems paradoxical that, at a time in the history of the discipline when the value of the relationship between the nurse and patient is being underscored, the current trends in nursing education appear to be pulling the learner away from the bedside. A question for the future will be, "How far can the nursing student get from the patient bedside and still learn what is nursing?" It is critical

Figure 1-6
Globalization is
the foundation
of addressing
diversity.

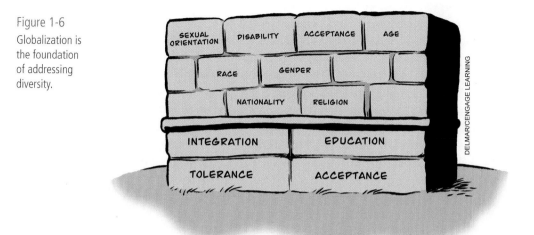

that the proverbial baby not be thrown out with the bath water. Safety in patient care is critical, and educational models that enable students to learn to practice safely are valuable. However, if the humanness of the discipline is sacrificed in the meantime, what has the discipline really gained?

Globalization

The **globalization** of the nursing curriculum is occurring in hopes of producing a more culturally-astute nurse. Globalization refers to the process of cultural integration, education, tolerance, and acceptance (Figure 1-6). As the United States becomes a more culturally diverse society due to immigration, schools of nursing are desperately attempting to recruit a more culturally diverse student body. This is being encouraged with the hope that a more diverse workforce will be better equipped to meet the needs of an increasingly diverse patient group. However, the question of whether a culturally diverse nursing workforce is a necessary antecedent to the cultural competency of those practicing the discipline has been assumed but not addressed. It is also imperative to note that globalization is but one facet of the larger concept of diversity. When the concept of diversity is incorporated into nursing-school curricula, issues related to disability, age, gender, and/or sexual orientation are also included.

TECHNOLOGY IN NURSING

Technology is changing the face of health care and, subsequently, the discipline of nursing. **Nursing informatics**, a general term describing the technological advances in the computerization of patient-care information, is a term that was foreign to nurses only a few short years ago. Now, it is a topic of presentation and discussion at almost every educator and practitioner conference.

Whether involved in nursing education, practice, or research, nurses are faced with countless changes when it comes to the way they work and communicate. Those working in academia are bombarded with electronic messages, from within and without the workplace, touting the latest book, journal, online program, or computerized gadget to enhance student learning. The practicing nurse deals on a daily basis with patients exposed to various innovative diagnostic and surgical procedures and the special care needed afterwards. Computerized charting systems are no longer futuristic ideations of informatics wizards; they are the way nurses communicate with all members of the health care team. The concept of caring for patients across vast distances is a reality via advanced visual and auditory communication systems. Nurse researchers uses multiple technologies in their quest for data, which must then be coded and entered into statistical programs for translation and analysis. Regardless of the environment of the nurse, computerized hand-held devices, i.e., personal digital assistants (PDAs) bring the information world of the Internet to the fingertips of the educator, practitioner, or researcher.

Technology is certainly not lacking in the majority of health care settings. What proves problematic is the lack of support for access and training in the use of technology on a day-to-day basis. Perhaps a lack of initiative and the proper attitude on the part of the nurse also comes into play. Colleagues in academia jest as they allude to the need to apply for a sabbatical leave to learn how to use the technology in their offices, classrooms, and available via the Internet. Nurses in patient-care areas express frustration with cumbersome computer systems that often increase the amount of time spent charting as the nurse delves into the multiple windows that appear in the act of charting a simple task. Portable computers designed to enable the nurse to chart at the bedside immediately after performing care sit dormant in hallway corridors. Technology is costly and the support, both human and material, needed to make it work effectively is costlier still. Regardless of the problems, nurses must take leadership roles in dealing with the problems that technological advances bring to the discipline. Clark (2008) is emphatic in stating that nurses need to embrace technology and learn to work with it for the benefits of themselves and their patients. She goes on further to say that if nurses don't do this, then others will make the decisions about how it is to be used.

THE NURSING SHORTAGE

A snapshot of nursing today would not be complete without a review of the **nursing shortage**. A nursing shortage occurs when the demand for registered nurses exceeds the supply, whether at the bedside or in nursing education. The discipline of nursing has most certainly experienced its share of shortages. However, the current and impending shortages are like no other, garnering federal attention. The National Advisory Council on Nurse Education and Practice (NACNEP) of the U.S. Department of Health and Human Services was formed in response to the impending crisis. In three yearly reports (NACNEP 2001, 2002, 2003), the scope of the nursing shortage was explored and chronicled in detail and has provided valuable data for those inside and outside the discipline striving to make an impact.

In order to meet the projected increased demand for nurses, federal data suggest that schools of nursing must increase the number of graduates by 90%, as shown in Figure 1-7 (HRSA, 2006; AACN, 2007). Unfortunately, despite increases in enrollment rates and graduations, schools of nursing are falling far short of this target. According to the AACN 2008–2009 Enrollment and Graduations in Baccalaureate and Graduate Programs in Nursing survey, enrollments in entry-level baccalaureate programs increased by 2.2% from 2008–2009, the seventh consecutive year of growth (AACN, 2008). Clearly, interest in the nursing profession remains strong. However, many seeking entry into the profession cannot be accommodated due to faculty short-ages and lack of resources. In 2008, survey data reveal that 49,498 qualified applicants were turned away from entry-level baccalaureate programs (AACN, 2007). The primary barriers continue to be insufficient faculty, clinical placement sites, and classroom space. Copies of the AACN 2008–2009 survey may be obtained online for a fee at http://www.aacn.nche.edu. Click on the tab on the left side of the homepage entitled "Data Center." A scroll-down menu will reveal the appropriate link, AACN Data Reports.

Full-Time Equivalent Supply Implication of Changes in Projected Number of New Graduates from U.S. Nursing Programs[3]

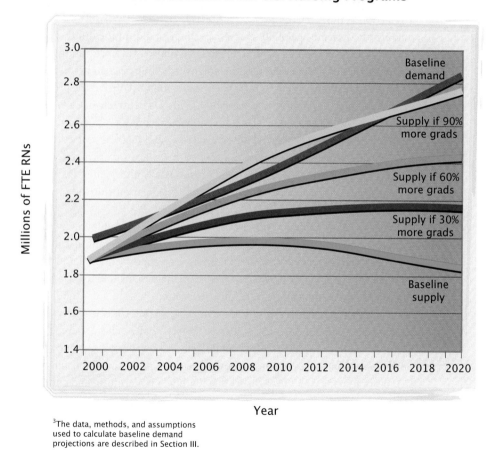

[3]The data, methods, and assumptions used to calculate baseline demand projections are described in Section III.

Figure 1-7

FTE Supply Implications of Changes in Projected Number of New Graduates from U.S. Nursing Programs. Figure courtesy of Health Resources and Services Administration (HRSA), Bureau of Health Professions (2002, July). *(National Center for Health Workforce Analysis. Projected Supply, Demand, and Shortages of Registered Nurses: 2000–2020. Washington DC: Author. Retrieved from http://www.ahca.org/research/rnsupply_demand.pdf.)*

The projected growth in supply is expected to reach a peak by 2011, with declines noted after that as the number of nurses leaving the profession exceeds the number entering. If projected trends continue, by the year 2020, the shortage of registered nurses is expected to grow to 29% (HRSA, 2002). Different sources have interpreted this percentage to mean a shortfall of approximately 800,000 to 1 million registered nurses. Incidentally, the shortage is not evenly distributed across states, with some states experiencing far greater shortages than 29%. This is due to an expected demand of 40%, with an expected growth in supply of only 6%. There are several factors driving the demand for nurses: an overall increase in the U.S. population, an increase in the elderly population, and medical advances. Various factors are behind the shortage: a declining number of graduates, aging of the registered nurse workforce, declines in earnings, and career alternatives for prospective students.

There are over half a million nurses not employed in nursing, with little known about this population (HRSA, 2002). What is known is that over 69% of those nurses not employed in nursing are over the age of 50. Nurses are often single-minded in their approach to a career in nursing, and schools often do little to alter this approach. Most training occurs in the acute-care setting, giving the impression that the only worthwhile place to practice is an acute-care setting. Although speculative, the idea that older nurses might return to the profession if positions other than those in acute-care settings were highlighted is definitely one needing exploration.

Actual earnings have enjoyed a steady increase, while "real" earnings—the amount available after inflation—have remained flat since 1991, due to the effects of inflation (HRSA, 2002). Additionally, wage increases tend to occur early in the nurse's career, with little opportunity for advancement after a certain point. As a result, staff nurses often leave the bedside, furthering their education for other career opportunities inside or outside the profession with more lucrative compensation.

The demand for nurses will continue to grow in all employment settings. The number of nurses practicing in hospitals is projected to remain constant at roughly 62% through 2020 (HRSA, 2002). Extended-care settings will see an increase in demand from 8% in 2000 to 10% in 2020, while home health will experience an increase from 6.5% to 9% (HRSA, 2002). Despite the intense focus on acute-care clinical education in academia, the fact remains that roughly 40% of nurses practice in settings other than a hospital. Unfortunately, this is a little-known fact to those interested in pursuing a nursing degree. Many believe there is only one kind of nurse, a hospital-based nurse. Perhaps potential learners shy away from nursing because they erroneously believe that in order to be a nurse one must practice in a hospital setting. Unfortunately, schools of nursing do little to dispel this myth when recruiting and educating future nurses.

CONCLUSIONS

The discipline of nursing has made great strides in defining nursing practice and building nursing knowledge through scientific modes of inquiry, thereby producing a highly educated, critical-thinking professional. Nurses have proven to be absolutely necessary to the health and well being of the patient; the health care system could not function without them. Nurse pioneer and theorist, Virginia Henderson, when asked if the world could get along without nurses replied that the world could not get along without nurses any more than it could get along without mothers (Garey, 1988). Because of nursing's inherent usefulness and necessity it is critical that the discipline continue to grow, question, and seek answers about the nature of its purpose and place in health care. In the midst of this process of inquiry and discovery, the discipline must guard and cherish what nurses do, carefully evaluating the impact of internal and external forces on that key relationship between the patient and the nurse. For it is the nurse who knows that the essence of what it means to be human is constant; technology is fleeting, and it is the nurse who will see to it that the humanness of the patient is not sacrificed to the technology of the moment.

SUMMARY

This chapter outlines the current issues facing the discipline of nursing. The concern regarding how the discipline of nursing should be defined was explored and discussed. The utility of nursing theory for the practicing nursing as well as the nurse researcher was established. Issues related to entry into basic nursing practice, educational preparation of the advanced practice nurse, and nurse educator preparation were addressed. The changes in nursing curricula and modes of didactic and clinical instruction and learning were highlighted. Challenges facing the profession relative to the nursing shortage and changes within health care delivery systems were reviewed.

The difficulty lies, not in the new ideas, but in escaping the old ones, which ramify, for those brought up as most of us have been, into every corner of our minds.

–John Maynard Keynes

REFERENCES

AIKEN, L. H., Clarke, S. P., Cheung, R. B., Sloane, D. M., & Silber, J. H. (2003). Educational levels of hospital nurses and surgical patient mortality. *Journal of the American Medical Association, 290,* 1617–1623.

AMERICAN ASSOCIATION OF COLLEGES OF NURSING. (2009, May 1). *Doctorate of nursing practice (DNP) programs.* Retrieved May 1, 2009, from http://www.aacn.nche.edu/DNP/DNPProgramList.htm

AMERICAN ASSOCIATION OF COLLEGES OF NURSING. (2008, February 15). *The essentials for baccalaureate education for professional nursing practice.* Retrieved May 1, 2009, from http://www.aacn.nche.edu/Education/pdf

AMERICAN ASSOCIATION OF COLLEGES OF NURSING. (2008, February 19). *Draft position statement: The preferred vision of the professoriate in baccalaureate and graduate nursing programs.* Retrieved

February 19, 2008, from http://www.aacn.nche.edu/Media/pdf/PSFaculty2-19-08.pdf

AMERICAN ASSOCIATION OF COLLEGES OF NURSING. (2007, December 3). *2008–2009 enrollment and graduations in baccalaureate and graduate programs in nursing.* Retrieved May 1, 2009, from http://www.aacn.nche.edu/IDS

AMERICAN NURSES CREDENTIALING CENTER. (2008, August 14). *Certification.* Retrieved August 14, 2008, from http://www.nursecredentialing.org/certification.aspx

CLARK, J. (2008). Embrace new technology or others will end up deciding how we use it. *Nursing Standard, 22*(17), 32.

COMMITTEE ON THE HEALTH PROFESSIONS EDUCATION SUMMIT BOARD ON HEALTH CARE SERVICES. (2003). In A. C. Greiner, & E. Knebel, (Eds.), *Health professions education: A bridge to quality. Institute of Medicine of the National Academies.* Washington, DC: The National Academies Press.

CURLEY, M. (2007). *Synergy: The unique relationship between nurses and patients.* Indianapolis: Sigma Theta Tau International.

GAREY, D. (Director). (1988). *Sentimental women need not apply: A history of the American nurse* [videotape]. United States: Florentine Films.

HEALTH RESOURCES AND SERVICES ADMINISTRATION (HRSA), BUREAU OF HEALTH PROFESSIONS. (2002, July). *National center for health workforce analysis. Projected supply, demand, and shortages of registered nurses: 2000–2020.* Retrieved February 19, 2008, from http://www.ahca.org/research/rnsupply_demand.pdf

HEALTH RESOURCES AND SERVICES ADMINISTRATION (HRSA). (2006). What is behind HRSA's projected supply, demand, and shortage of registered nurses? Retrieved August 14, 2008, from http://www.bhpr.hrsa.gov/healthworkforce/reports/behindrnprojections/index.htm

JEFFRIES, P. (2005). A framework for designing, implementing, and evaluating: Simulations used as teaching strategies in nursing. *Nursing Education Perspectives, 26*, 96–103.

MONTI, E. J., & Tingen, M. (1999). Multiple paradigms of nursing science. *Advances in Nursing Science, 21*(4), 64–80.

NATIONAL ADVISORY COUNCIL ON NURSE EDUCATION AND PRACTICE. (2001, November). *First report to the secretary of health and human services and the Congress.* Washington, DC: U.S. Department of Health and Human Services. Retrieved July 18, 2008, from http://bhpr.hrsa.gov/nursing/NACNEP/reports/first/1.htm

NATIONAL ADVISORY COUNCIL ON NURSE EDUCATION AND PRACTICE. (2002, November). *Second report to the secretary of health and human services and the Congress.* Washington, DC: U.S. Department of Health and Human Services. Retrieved February 12, 2008, from http://bhpr.hrsa.gov/nursing/NACNEP/reports/second/1.htm

NATIONAL ADVISORY COUNCIL ON NURSE EDUCATION AND PRACTICE. (2003, November). *Third report to the secretary of health and human services and the Congress.* Washington, DC: U.S. Department of Health and Human Services. Retrieved December 3, 2008, from http://bhpr.hrsa.gov/nursing/NACNEP/re/third/1.htm

NATIONAL LEAGUE FOR NURSING. (2007, September). *Reflection and dialogue: Academic/professional progression in nursing.* Retrieved January 10, 2008, from http://www.nln.org/aboutnln/reflection_dialogue/refl_dial_2.htm

NATIONAL LEAGUE FOR NURSING. (2007). *NLNAC Directory of Accredited Nursing Programs 2007–2008.* New York: Author.

SILVA, M. C. (1999). The state of nursing science: Reconceptualizing for the 21st century. *Nursing Science Quarterly, 12*, 221–226.

TOURANGEAU, A. E., Doran, D. M., Hall, L., Pallas, L., Pringle, D., Tu, J. V., & Cranley, L. A. (2007). Impact of hospital nursing care on 30 day mortality for acute medical patients. *Journal of Advanced Nursing, 57*, 32–44.

WEBSTER'S ONLINE DICTIONARY. (2008, March 10). http://www.websters-online-dictionary.org

WINTERS, J., & Ballou, K. (2004). The idea of nursing science. *Journal of Advanced Nursing, 45*, 533–535.

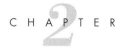

C H A P T E R 2

EVOLUTION OF THE MEDICAL AND ALLIED HEALTH PROFESSIONS

RUTH STEARNS
BA, Education Specialist, Remington Colleges

Coming together is a beginning. Keeping together is progress. Working together is success.

–Henry Ford

LEARNING OBJECTIVES

At the completion of the chapter, the learner should be able to do the following:
1. Describe the progression of medical care from ancient times to the present.
2. Define the function of essential allied health professions.
3. Explain the origin of today's allied health professions.
4. Discuss important issues in allied health today.
5. Identify the likely changes allied health professions will undergo in the future.

KEY TERMS

Allied Health
Allopathy
American Medical
    Association
Antisepsis
Apothecary
Asepsis
Black Death
Dermatologists
Doulas
Family Medicine
Galen
Girolamo Fracastoro

Health Care
    Administrators
Hippocrates
Ignaz Semmelweis
Imhotep
International Pharmaceutical
    Federation
Internists
JAMA
Library at Alexandria
Mentor
Miasmatists
Obstetrician

Ophthalmologists
Opticians
Optometrists
Osteopathy
Otolaryngology
Patients' Bill of Rights
Pediatricians
Pharmacist
Podiatry
Posology
Residency
Sanitary Commission
Trepanation

THE QUEST FOR HEALTH BEGINS

With the realization that they could warm themselves with fire, build tools from sticks and stones, and work together to achieve common goals, early humans began to understand that they could improve the way they feel by changing their environment to suit their needs. This was the beginning of a very long process of investigation, innovation, and sharing of ideas that eventually led to today's health professions.

Although ancient humans are assumed to have used a wide variety of methods to improve their physical wellbeing, their success rate was rather mixed. Predators and the elements became less and less of a threat to humans as their technological development progressed, but the changes in nutrition and disease prevalence as human society developed made life more difficult in some ways. Indeed, as Table 2-1 suggests, although the lifespan of humans increased steadily as they began to gain a greater understanding of the human body and what affects it positively and otherwise, progress toward overall health (as represented in this case by average adult stature and pelvic inlet depth) was slow (Angel, 1984).

Well before **Hippocrates** composed his oath (Figure 2-1), an Egyptian chancellor, high priest, and court physician called **Imhotep** was already making progress in both the fields of medicine and architecture around 2980 BC. He is sometimes credited, among other things, for pioneering the Egyptian art of embalming. More importantly, his writing contains an attitude of "rational empiricism" that helped propel the Greek physician's discoveries hundreds of years later (Kucharski & Todd, 2003). Temples dedicated to Imhotep, whose legacy included a very active funeral cult, have been discovered with plaster casts of human body parts, suggesting symbolic requests for healing from a god whom one temple inscription called "the greatest physician with skillful fingers" (Risse, 1986, pp. 622–624).

It is difficult to construct a perfect picture of the ancient history of medical knowledge for various reasons. The **Library at Alexandria** in Egypt, a former wonder of the world, is said to have contained volumes of Greek medical literature now lost. This consolidation of information from around the known world attracted early physicians and philosophers from countries across Europe and Asia. The Great Library became a center for investigation into anatomy, development of medical terminology, scientific inquiry, and debate. Most importantly, it contained texts from the far reaches of Europe, Asia, and Africa that were collected in one location and translated into Greek. The Library at Alexandria provided a vast amount of information and a single location for learned minds to congregate and interact. This doubtlessly assisted the development of the foundations of medical theory, until its fiery destruction in 48 BC (Hajar, 2000).

Despite this significant loss of printed material, as Vivian Nutton (2004) says in her book *Ancient Medicines*, "much of Greek and Roman medicine never made it into writing at all" (p. 128). Their cultures restricted literacy to the upper society members only. Medical knowledge could be passed through the masses much more efficiently by word of mouth. Specific skills such as bone-setting and the harvesting of healing herbs were seldom committed to writing. Where details on the step-by-step processes of basic medical procedures may be lacking for this time period, the anatomical discoveries in the period were much better preserved. The Greek physicians Erasistratus and Herophilus are particularly well known anatomists who were among the first to discover the interior structures of the body (Nutton, 2004).

Table 2-1 Health & Longevity of Ancient Peoples

Dates	Median Lifespan (yrs)		Average Adult Stature	
	Male	Female	Male (ft/in)	Female (ft/in)
30000 to 9000 BC	35.4	30.0	5'9.7"	5'5.6"
9000 to 7000 BC	33.5	31.3	5'7.9"	5'2.9"
5000 to 3000 BC	33.1	29.2	5'3.5"	5'0.7"
3000 to 2000 BC	33.6	29.4	5'5.4"	5'0.2"
2000 BC	36.5	31.4	5'5.4"	5'0.4"
Circa 1450 BC	35.9	36.1	5'7.9"	5'3.0"
1450 to 1150 BC	39.6	32.6	5'5.7"	5'0.8"
1150 to 650 BC	39.0	30.9	5'5.6"	5'1.1"
650 to 300 BC	44.1	36.8	5'7.1"	5'1.5"
300 BC to AD 120	41.9	38.0	5'7.7"	5'1.6"
AD 120 to 600	38.8	34.2	5'6.6"	5'2.2"
Medieval Greece	37.7	31.1	5'6.7"	5'1.8"
AD 1400 to 1800	33.9	28.5	5'7.8"	5'2.2"
AD 1800 to 1920	40.0	38.4	5'7.0"	5'2.0"
"Modern U.S. White"	71.0	78.5	5'8.6"	5'4.3"

(Data from Angel, 1984)

Figure 2-1

Hippocrates, the Father of Medicine, recorded some of the earliest medical observations on various conditions, as well as making great progress toward the eventual scientific approach to medicine.

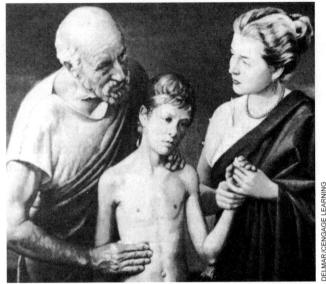

Some concepts are simply too important not to immortalize on paper, however. The Greek physician and philosopher that we are most grateful to for ignoring convention was Hippocrates, the Father of Medicine. In a time when illness was assumed to be caused by angry spirits, and religion and medicine were generally one and the same, Hippocrates consistently wrote volumes of work attributing human ailments not to human failings, but to natural causes. He emphasized the difference between belief that something is true, and knowledge supported by the proof of truth (Downs, 2004). Hippocrates even advocated basic cleanliness as a preventative measure against disease, long before asepsis was considered important to successful treatment of disease and injury.

Additionally, Hippocrates is also generally assumed to have written the oath that bears his name. Although it is often printed in copies of one of his major works, *Hippocratic Corpus*, some scholars argue that the oath was instead written by contemporaries of Hippocrates, the Pythagoreans, because some of the tenets described in the code contradict other works that bear his name (Rotham, Kiceluk, & Marcus, 1995). However it came about, the Hippocratic oath is still taken today by graduates of medical schools around the world. In speaking the words, new doctors swear to respect their teachers, do no harm to patients, let specialists handle duties they are trained to perform, engage in morally appropriate behavior, and teach medical skills and practices only to those intending to become doctors themselves.

Greece was conquered by the Romans in 149 BC, meaning that the influential anatomist and medical theorist **Galen** was born a Roman citizen 20 years later. Rome had outlawed the use of cadavers for dissection; however, using only animal bodies and his experiences as a physician at a temple and a gladiator school, Galen made some amazing innovations in medicine. He performed groundbreaking surgical procedures, treated psychosomatic illnesses, and wrote medical literature that was relied upon for hundreds of years after his death (Conrad, 1995).

The trade of medical knowledge among the Greeks, Romans, Indians, Egyptians, and other Middle Eastern groups was becoming so common in the mid-800s that the information

Internet Exercise 2-1	Locate the Web site of the National Human Genome Research Institute: http://www.genome.gov.

Locate the Web site of the National Human Genome Research Institute: http://www.genome.gov.

1. How does the study of genetics today compare to the study of anatomy two thousand years ago?

2. What was the Human Genome Project?

3. What genetic discovery do you find most exciting? What are you still waiting for researchers to discover?

4. How might you get involved in human genome research?

needed to be recorded in a better way than on a small number of books and scrolls. One of the main authors who set about the task of cataloging this information in an organized way was Abu al-Hasan Ali ibn Sahl Rabban al-Tabari, a Persian doctor and medical theorist who wrote the first encyclopedia of medicine. He combined knowledge from medical experts on three continents to create the multi-volume Arabic text *Firdous al-Hikmah* (Paradise of Wisdom), which was translated into several languages and spread across the world, enhancing the global understanding of the treatment of injury, infection, and disease (Prioreschi, 2001).

After the Greeks' astounding bursts of insight into the human body, development in the field of medicine was slowed by barbarians and the onset of the Dark Ages. The Middle Ages were also largely uneventful for medical development in Europe (Santos-Saachi & Jahn, 2001), although onset of the **Black Death** gave the continent an opportunity to work out some of the intricacies of contagious diseases. The Black Death was a pandemic of the Bubonic plague that swept Europe and Asia during the mid-1300s. It caused the demise of an estimated 30% of Europe and Asia's population. Due to the catastrophically contagious nature of the disease, newcomers wishing to enter some European cities, particularly Venice, Italy, were required to spend days in a restricted area. This was called quarantine, which was a major step toward curbing the spread of contagious diseases in Europe's already overcrowded cities (Kelly, 2005).

In the mid-1500s, understanding of disease was revolutionized when the Italian **Girolamo Fracastoro** theorized that disease was caused by invisible "spores" that infected the body. This was the foundation of modern germ theory. Not only did he construct this theory, but he differentiated between illness caused by "spore" contamination and illness caused by poison, and he constructed a basic concept of contagion (Krebs, 1999).

These advances did not go over well to begin with. Many physicians and medical experts at the time were **miasmatists**, who believed that medical maladies were caused by impure air. Removal of refuse, washing of hands, and generally sanitary practices did not catch on for some time, because people assumed that if the filth couldn't be smelled, then it could not harm human health. Even Florence Nightingale, perhaps the most famous nurse in history, was of the firm belief that the best treatment was to provide patients with fresh air (Nightingale, 1863; Lundy & Janes, 2005). The widely held Christian belief that God visited fevers and pestilence as punishment for sins did not further scientific development in this case either. Contributing to both the miasmatist and Christian believers' scorn of germ theory was a class-discriminatory view of health that implied that the poor were sick more often than the rich because the poor deserved to be sick (Collins, 2006).

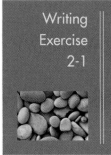

Writing Exercise 2-1

The medical field has sometimes been slow to adapt to better methods and practices because medical professionals felt that the way they have always done things is efficient enough. Have your views of the medical profession changed recently based on new information about health care? What information persuaded you to change your mind? For this exercise, explain how your understanding of modern health care developed and how new information has influenced your view of the health care professions.

DOCTORS UNITE: THE CREATION OF THE AMERICAN MEDICAL ASSOCIATION

A century ago, the idea of an organization of doctors working together to improve the quality and delivery of medical care would have been almost laughable. In the late 1800s, when care of the injured and ill was still mainly delivered by families in their homes, there were no particular rules governing who could be called a doctor. People who referred to themselves as doctors frequently provided medical care on the side, in addition to a full-time job.

These early physicians did, however, earn payment for their work. Because it was not difficult to become a doctor, there was a substantial amount of competition for doctors, particularly in major urban areas. At this time doctors were fighting desperately to draw business to their offices, while at the same time attempting to wrest control of their trade from the many specialists, such as surgeons and apothecaries, providing similar services to those provided by the physicians (Starr, 1982). Apothecaries collected various substances and combined them into mixtures to cure specific ailments, which they sold to physicians, or more often directly to patients. With this kind of pressure looming over the medical community, their choices were to outbid themselves into irrelevance by attempting to offer lower prices and more extravagant services to compete with each other, or to form an organization of doctors to set fees and standards for the profession.

Education of American Physicians

One of the first issues that physicians would have to learn to agree upon was a major point of contention: the requirements for licensure and education of new doctors. Initially, young men (new doctors were still mostly men at this time) became doctors by going through an apprenticeship.

This idea was originally developed in Europe, and the American medical community sought to replicate the system in the New World as a way of assuring quality in medical care through experiential learning.

For most of history, up until around 1800 (and slightly beyond, for surgeons and apothecaries), apprenticeship was seen as the easiest and most effective method of training new physicians. Independent study of medical texts was also generally required, but until governments and medical associations began to require it, there was very little demand for formal schooling by professional medical educators. The beneficial nature of hands-on experience, along with the added benefit of restricting entrance to the medical profession to people of doctors' choosing (Digby, 1994), kept the practice going well beyond the point at which serious doubts of its usefulness as an educational practice were raised by the medical community.

The actual information acquired by prospective doctors during their apprenticeship varied widely. The length of apprenticeships could be anywhere between two and twelve years, depending on the country, the state, the specialization, and the local physicians' preference. Some were expected to teach themselves by reading medical literature (Starr, 1982), others were only observers of the craft, although most were expected to administer at least some treatments themselves. However, depending on the location of their apprenticeship, potential doctors could sometimes acquire quite a lot of medical experience during their apprenticeship period, as was the case of one Thomas Barnes of Wigton, United Kingdom:

> Having chosen medicine as his career, he became an apprentice of the late Dr. Joshua Riggs of Wigton, at that time the only medical practitioner in the district. The office of a doctor's apprentice was no sinecure in those days, commencing his work at six in the morning and continuing uninterruptedly until ten at night, and often later. There were neither druggists, veterinary surgeons, nor dentists in Wigton, and the doctor's apprentice was expected to take the place of all three—to prepare and dispense medicine for men, women, and children, horses, cows, and dogs, to extract teeth, to supply coffee and pepper; and, in addition, he had to look after the doctor's horses and keep his books (Edinburgh Medical Journal, 1872, p. 1142).

Because he lived in the UK during the mid- and late 1800s, Thomas Barnes was also expected to obtain a medical degree from a reputable university after his apprenticeship, but this was not generally the case in the United States for some time.

Had Dr. Barnes had his apprenticeship in a more urban setting, he might have spent it working in the wards of charity hospitals. These were often used as learning environments for budding physicians, and he would have had the opportunity to perform human dissections in addition to his care of live patients. Even here, of course, his apprenticeship experience would only be as good as the person to whom he was apprenticed. Apprenticeships were finally abolished in England by the Medical Act of 1858, and the United States eventually followed suit (Digby, 1994).

Formal education was not always necessary during the developmental period of American medicine, but it was certainly always available. The late 1700s and early 1800s saw a steady increase in the number of American medical schools, many of which promised a quick path to a medical degree which, as it turned out, would provide little benefit to graduates. Because physicians were not making a great deal of money during this time, the schools couldn't charge

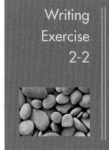
a significant tuition fee, and thus what medical education was provided wasn't particularly preparatory for the students' future careers.

Modern education for doctors is substantially more challenging than ever before. College students who want to pursue a medical career must first achieve a bachelor's degree, usually in biology or in a premed major. In the U.S., students must then attend a four-year medical school accredited by the American Medical Association or the Liaison Committee for Medical Education. Once accepted, students must pass the first two parts of the three-part United States Medical Licensing Examination (USMLE) before graduation to earn their Doctor of Medicine (or MD) degree (Hawkins, 1985). The number of first-time medical-school applicants in the U.S. is currently on an upswing from a recent low of approximately 25,000 applicants in 2002. By 2015, the number of first-time medical-school applicants is predicted to grow to 34,000 (Garrison, Matthew, & Jones, 2007).

Graduation does not end the process, however—a year of internship and the third part of the USMLE stand between new MDs and general practice. Many new doctors wish to specialize further, and to do this they must participate in a **residency** at a hospital or clinic, during which time resident physicians care for patients in their specialty fields under the observation of more experienced staff members. A residency differs from an apprenticeship, in that a residency is more comprehensive than the apprenticeship method of assigning new physicians to assist single doctors in their daily tasks. Instead, specific conditions must be met during the residency for the experience to qualify resident physicians to challenge the examination for board certification in their chosen specialties. Some examples of specialty fields that require a residency experience before MDs are eligible for board certification in the subject are pediatric medicine, radiology, anesthesiology, internal medicine, and surgery, which is discussed at greater length later in this chapter.

The board governing residents' chosen specialties grants approval to physicians at the completion of their residency. There are a total of 24 such boards, all under the American Board of Medical Specialties. These govern the major specialties and subspecialties of physicians, of which the following are some in which doctors may choose to practice.

Internal Medicine

Internal Medicine is the most commonly chosen specialty for physicians, and it focuses on diagnosis and nonsurgical treatment of adults. Forty-two percent of primary-care specialists and subspecialists are **internists**, or doctors who specialize in internal medicine (American Medical

Association, 2007, p. 275). The American Board of Internal Medicine has been responsible for certifying qualified physicians in internal medicine since 1936. After completing a fellowship, internists may acquire board certification in a subspecialty of internal medicine such as cardiology, pulmonology, infectious disease, or endocrinology.

Dermatology

The American Board of Dermatology is the nationally recognized board in charge of certification of **dermatologists,** or doctors who have chosen to specialize in the diagnosis and treatment of skin ailments. According to the American Academy of Dermatology, the residencies required to become dermatologists are the most competitive of all medical specialties. Formal residency training for dermatology normally lasts three years, like other residency training programs, and culminates in challenging the board examination. Subspecialties of dermatology include dermatopathology, pediatric dermatology, and clinical and laboratory dermatological immunology.

Pediatrics

Another competitive specialization is pediatrics, which is governed by the American Board of Pediatrics. **Pediatricians** account for over 20% of the specialist physician population (American Medical Association, 2007, p. 275) and are specially trained to care for infants, children, and teenagers. In many ways, the career of a generalist pediatrician is similar to that of a generalist internist. Pediatricians often encounter a standard selection of common childhood ailments, such as ear infections, asthma, and gastroenteritis, rather than a series of afflictions in specific parts of the body as other specialists work with regularly. Pediatricians may diagnose mental or physical developmental difficulties, such as autism, attention deficit/hyperactivity disorder (ADHD), and cerebral palsy. However, growing human bodies, particularly those of very young children, present different challenges in treatment than do those of adults.

There are numerous subspecialty certifications available to qualified pediatricians, including pediatric critical care, neonatal-perinatal medicine, and developmental-behavioral pediatrics. Pediatricians may also choose to get additional certification in medical toxicology, sports medicine, or one of several other certificate options to further narrow their area of expertise.

Family Medicine

The specialization in family medicine is one of the more recently developed certifications. In the late 1960s, physicians were becoming less interested in going into general practice because specialists had a higher income. To solve that problem, the American Board of Family Medicine developed a **family medicine** specialization, with the understanding that family medicine training would encompass the following:

1. first-contact care
2. continuous care
3. comprehensive care

4. personal care

5. family care

6. competency in scientific general medicine.

These tenets, laid out by the first executive director of the board, Dr. Nicholas J. Piscano, provide an in-depth study of a generalist approach to health care (American Board of Family Medicine, 2007).

Obstetrics

Another family-related specialist is the **obstetrician**, a medical doctor who specializes in the care of pregnant women. Obstetricians often receive referrals from women's family physicians when it seems that they are in for a difficult or complicated pregnancy. However, many obstetricians also become gynecologists so that they can provide care for the entire reproductive system, and their regular gynecological patients may return for obstetric care during pregnancy (Rooks, 1999).

It is important to be able to differentiate obstetricians and midwives. Both are qualified to help women give birth and provide prenatal and postpartum care. However, midwives often take a more osteopathic approach to the process and may practice with largely informal training only (although a more comprehensive education is required for nurse midwives), whereas obstetricians are generally trained in the allopathic tradition of medicine and have earned an MD. Obstetricians are also trained in obstetric surgery, which is not a procedure that midwives are qualified to perform. For this reason, midwives generally work with low-risk patients, while obstetricians are well qualified to deal with the more difficult cases.

Ophthalmology

Of the sensory organs, few are more complicated, sensitive, and vital than the eyes. For that reason, there is an entire field of medical care devoted to them, with three major levels of education and care. These medical professionals can be identified by the prefix ophth-, which refers to eyes, and are known as ophthalmologists, optometrists, and opticians. The science of ophthalmology flourished earliest in ancient Egypt and Mesopotamia, because eye problems were so common there. Today, ophthalmology is a popular specialty, as the hours are generally reasonable and compensation is reasonable as well.

The essential difference between the three major types of ophthalmology professionals is education and the nature of their college degrees. **Ophthalmologists** are either Doctors of Medicine (MDs) or Doctors of Osteopathic Medicine (DOs) who specialize in the treatment of eyes. Ophthalmologists attend medical school and complete an internship in general medicine after graduation. Once this is completed, future ophthalmologists complete a three-year residency program to gain supervised ophthalmology experience. Some ophthalmologists choose to specialize on a single part of the eye or a common eye condition, which requires an additional fellowship focusing on that topic. After all of that schooling, ophthalmologists are qualified to check vision, prescribe corrective lenses, and diagnose and treat medical conditions affecting the eyes. U.S. physicians, including surgeons specializing in ophthalmology, are certified and governed by the American Board of Ophthalmology.

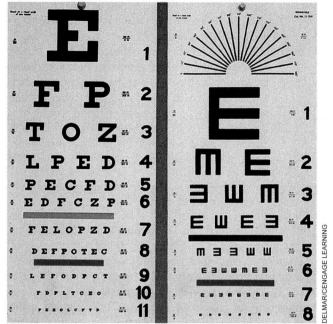

Figure 2-2
The Snellen Chart is an eye chart used by eye-care professionals to measure visual acuity. The numbers on the right are the testing distance / the smallest text correctly read by people with normal vision.

DELMAR/CENGAGE LEARNING

Surgery

Humans have been trying to understand the inner workings of the human body for thousands of years, and an inside view has been insightful to many budding anatomists. Beyond the need for knowledge, it has also been a long-standing assumption that cutting into the body can be beneficial to health. For example, there is preserved evidence of **trepanation**, the use of a drill or other instrument to make a hole in the skull to expose a small part of the brain, at archaeological sites dated at around 6500 BC. Instructions for this procedure have been found in collections of ancient Greek, Roman, and Egyptian medicine, and Europe during the Renaissance period for treatment of mental disorders.

Some of the oldest documented records of surgical treatment of disease and illness come from India, circa 500 BC. *Sushruta Samhita*, or the collection of the author, Sushruta, was a text describing over 120 surgical instruments, 300 surgical procedures, and a classification of human surgery into 8 categories. This was the result of a long and mostly oral tradition of surgical medicine in India. In addition to the lifesaving surgical information, Samhita may have recorded instructions for early procedures in cosmetic surgery in the *Sushruta Samhita* (Prioreschi, 2001).

Although surgery has saved many, many lives over the years and has been a logical part of medical treatment for ages, there were grave challenges to successful surgical treatment early on. Not all surgeons concentrated solely on their craft—some were barbers or hunters on the side. Patients frequently died because of poorly controlled hemorrhaging or complications from infection after their original health problem was cured. The lack of safe and effective anesthesia made it a traumatic procedure for patients and doctors alike.

Extensive bleeding was originally treated, somewhat ineffectively, with cauterization where possible. In the 16th century, the development of the ligature by Ambrose Pare allowed attending physicians to stop bleeding by closing off severed blood vessels. Today, tourniquets serve a similar purpose in emergencies, and surgical tourniquets are applied during surgical procedures to reduce blood loss during treatment.

Without effective anesthesia, a good surgeon was judged by the thorough removal of whatever internal ailment was harming the patient, and by the speed with which the procedure was conducted. Patients were conscious throughout the procedure and doubtless remembered their experience to the end of their days (which in many cases were not numerous despite surgical treatment).

Today, the level of consciousness deprivation can be more closely controlled by anesthesiologists, and the level is adjusted by procedure. Anesthesiologists preparing patients for major surgery may select general anesthesia, defined as "[D]rug-induced loss of consciousness during which patients are not arousable, even by painful stimulation" (American Society of Anesthesiologists, 2004, p. 1). General anesthesia is so thoroughly incapacitating that patients often cannot breathe without assistance. For much milder procedures, patients may be placed under minimal sedation, or anxiolysis, defined as "[D]rug-induced state during which patients respond normally to verbal commands" (American Society of Anesthesiologists, 2004, p. 1). This has become a popular level for such procedures as wisdom teeth removal, which is made easier by having a responsive patient who is also not pained by the extraction procedure.

The development of proper asepsis dramatically increased the success rates of surgical procedures, but it didn't begin to develop until the mid-1800s. This was the time at which the Vienna, Italy, native and famous obstetrician **Ignaz Semmelweis** identified the source of the person-to-person transmission of puerperal infection, which was the hands of the surgeons treating them and, somewhat more understandably, the leeches with which patients were occasionally treated (Carter & Carter, 2005). Later, discoveries by Louis Pasteur (Figure 2-3) (after whom the process

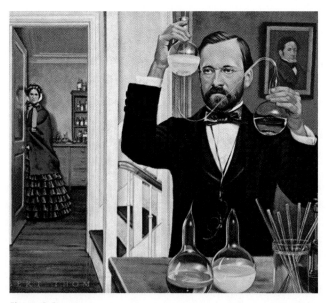

Figure 2-3

Louis Pasteur, the Father of Microbiology, studied and developed vaccines to prevent a wide range of communicable diseases. Pasteurization is the process of heating liquids to a temperature that is lethal to disease-causing microorganisms. *(Courtesy of Parke-Davis and Company, copyright 1957.)*

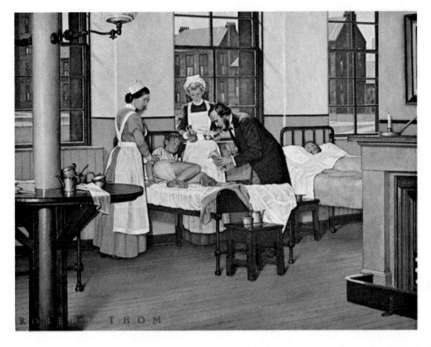

Figure 2-4

Joseph Lister, the Father of Sterile Surgery, used carbolic acid as an antiseptic in the operating room. *(Courtesy of Parke-Davis and Company, copyright 1957.)*

of pasteurization was named—he is responsible for a continued supply of fresh dairy products that do not go bad as quickly as they would naturally) and Joseph Lister (of whom one can think fondly while using Listerine mouthwash) (Figure 2-4) introduced the use of carbolic acid as an antiseptic and reduced surgical infections rates.

Although **asepsis** and **antisepsis** sound the same, and ideally lead to a clean operating environment in which patients live longer, the method implied by the two terms differs. Antisepsis refers to the use of antiseptics, which kill germs and bacteria chemically. Asepsis, by contrast, refers to preventive measures taken to stop harmful microbes from coming anywhere near sensitive patients who could succumb to infection. Lawson Tait was the main proponent of asepsis, an appreciation he gained while caring for his many obstetric and gynecologic patients, and his concepts on cleanliness are still valid today (Shepherd, 1986).

Although many surgeons today practice general surgery, there are also specialties that surgeons may pursue. Orthopedic surgery is one of the most commonly selected specialties, and involves care of the musculoskeletal system. Specialists in neurological surgery treat the brain, spinal cord, and other parts of the nervous system, and cardiovascular surgeons specialize in heart and blood vessel surgery, as one might expect. Lesser known are surgeons that specialize in **otolaryngology**, which involves medical care focusing on the ears, nose, and throat. Perhaps the best-publicized specialized surgeons are plastic or reconstructive surgeons, whose work is designed to improve the physical appearance of their patients (Bureau of Labor Statistics, 2007).

Approaches to Medicine and Surgery

The traditional Western approach to medicine is called **allopathy** (Figure 2-5), and involves "treating illness by counteracting the symptoms of illness" (Weil, 2004, p. 121). This is a focused

Figure 2-5

Allopathy is a focused approach to medical care that utilizes scientifically proven pharmaceuticals, up-to-date technology, and treatment techniques to alleviate the symptoms and effects of a medical condition. *(Courtesy of the Centers for Disease Control and Prevention. Photo credit James Gathany, 2006.)*

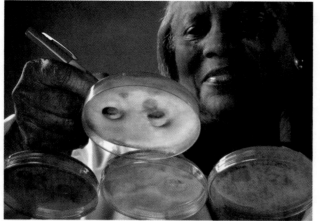

approach to medical care that utilizes scientifically proven pharmaceuticals, up-to-date technology, and treatment techniques to alleviate the symptoms and effects of a medical condition. The official view of this approach is that health is the absence of disease. This is a relatively recently formalized approach—it is approximately 200 years old. Allopathic medicine is very effective with acute conditions, as it treats the problem directly and aims for the most comprehensive physical cure in the shortest amount of time possible (DeLaune & Ladner, 2002).

Although most physicians maintain a traditional treatment approach to the ailments of the human body, there are alternative ways to go about medical treatment. One of these is called **osteopathy**. This approach to medical care, formalized in the United States by Andrew Stills in the late 1800s, emphasizes health and wellness of the musculoskeletal system, and a combination of mental and physical wellness. Although it was met with a great deal of skepticism at the time, it attained a gradual following as a result of Stills's publicity efforts, and is still a viable approach today. This is sometimes categorized as "complementary" or "alternative" medicine. Despite this, Doctors of Osteopathy are fully recognized in the United States (Gevitz, 2004).

The American Medical Association

Although major cities and states across the U.S. eventually developed their own medical societies, in which physicians gathered to discuss cases and local matters, the country lacked a national organization comparable to the British Medical Association in England until 1847, when the **American Medical Association** (AMA) was formed. It was designed to be a democratic representation of all professional doctors (of the appropriate race and class, however—like European medical societies, the AMA did not treat all doctors equally for many years). The purpose of the organization, as stated by its first president Dr. Nathaniel Chapman, was "the mutual improvement of all members and the advancement of the interests and usefulness of the profession" (Davis, 1877, p. 59). For the mutual improvement of all members, the organization would encourage licensing, higher expectations of education, and a greater respect for the profession. In the advancement of interests and usefulness of medicine, the organization would meet regularly to review cases and professional papers, and most importantly to exchange ideas and experiences to gain a larger perspective on modern medicine.

In the early and mid-1800s, the AMA's goal of advancing the interests of the profession was beset by obstacles from various sources. One popular alternative to contacting a professional physician was the use of one of several common do-it-yourself medical books, available to laypeople everywhere. Texts such as *Gunn's Domestic Medicine or Poor Man's Friend in the Hour of Affliction, Pain, and Sickness*, by John C. Gunn, claimed to reduce the practice of medicine to "principles of common sense" (Gunn, 1860, p. 1). Gunn went on to advocate positive emotions, treatments passed on by word of mouth, and the summoning of physicians as a last resort, if at all.

The AMA began publishing the *Journal of the American Medical Association* (**JAMA**) in 1883, a peer-reviewed periodical that is still a reliable source of medical developments today. It served to counteract some of the laymen publications flooding the market with unstudied or ineffective treatment for medical disorders, and provided another much-needed line of professional communication for physicians. JAMA is now the most widely circulated medical journal in the world. The advancement of medical technique was seen as essential for doctors and their patients alike, and the journal provided a place to publish research nationally; more research results could be analyzed and utilized as quickly as resources and bureaucratic oversight would allow. To facilitate innovation in the industry despite the continued difficulties of making a living in the profession, the AMA founded a grant-distributing Committee on Scientific Research in 1898.

In 1912, the Federation of State Medical Boards was created by merging the National Confederation of State Medical Examining and Licensing Boards and the American Confederation of Reciprocating Examining and Licensing Boards. It accepted the AMA's rating of medical schools as authoritative and backed up their more stringent requirements for obtaining a medical degree. Although it sounds insignificant, this was an important step. The trend at the time was for the government to force as much regulatory responsibility away from the federal government and down to the state governments, which in turn relied on their own state boards for expert council. The Federation of State Medical Boards created the ability to reach a strong consensus at the state level, which gave more power to physicians across the country.

Currently, the Federation of State Medical Boards is a national not-for-profit organization that represents the 70 state and territorial medical boards in the U.S., including 14 state boards of osteopathic medicine (American Medical Association, 2007). It performs a function similar to what was done when it was first created, which is to bring together state authorities to reach a national consensus and further mutually agreed upon values and efforts.

As representatives of doctors as well as medical science, the AMA needed to organize physicians to advocate for the profession. This was the purpose of the Committee on National Legislation, created to represent doctors' interests in U.S. government. The AMA has had a significant impact on medical legislation due to its massive lobbying force. Historically, the AMA has made efforts to limit the number of physicians and discourage nonphysician competition, which critics claim has caused an increase in health care costs to the consumer and a decrease in overall quality of care.

Most recently, the AMA has advocated for patients' rights, as exemplified in 2000, when the AMA supported the Patients' Bill of Rights and was against publicly funded health care. The **Patients' Bill of Rights** limits verbiage in contractual agreements that make it difficult for doctors to communicate with patients regarding treatment options, alternative procedures, risks, benefits, and consequences. It also emphasizes respect and provision of health care and insurance enrollment regardless of sexual orientation, race, age, sex, or genetics (Shalala, 1999).

ADMINISTRATIVE ROLES IN AMERICAN MEDICINE

For thousands of years, health care was distributed one of three ways: religious leaders providing healing as part of a group, healers working one-on-one with their patients, or families banding together to care for sick or injured members. From the beginning of medical care in America, people in need of medical care relied on their relatives (particularly their female relatives prior to the 20th century) for support, and people without close relatives relied on the church or the government, assuming that their government was equipped to provide medical assistance to those in need.

Health care for those who were without families to care for them or money for treatment was unpleasant, at best. Early charity clinics were generally not staffed by doctors, and they allowed for easy spread of contagious disease through poor ventilation and sanitation. They were a last resort of the desperately ill who had no other hope of help.

Another state-run alternative for the sick and destitute were dispensaries, which were low-budget sources of free medicine for those who needed it most. These were staffed by physicians, generally on a part-time basis, but were not well thought of by patients or the medical community. Aside from the unpleasant conditions in early hospitals, the mortality rates were high. Many patients arrived at the hospitals in late stages of illness or after severe trauma, and hospitals became known in the lay population as places for the dying, the plague victims, and orphaned children (Snook, 2003).

Because their services were free, physicians treated both dispensaries and charity hospitals as unwelcome, government-sanctioned competition for patients and the distribution of medical care. Physicians probably overestimated the number of patients lost to these free sources of medical care; however, the standard of care they received for free was noticeably lower quality than that received from a motivated, well-educated physician trying to maintain an active practice (Starr, 1982).

Psychiatric Hospitals

Psychiatric hospitals are institutions that offer short- and long-term care for the mentally ill. Long-term care is often required, as most diagnosable mental illness is chronic. In the past, psychiatric hospitals were more or less storehouses for the mentally ill, as significantly effective treatment of mental disorders is a surprisingly recent development (unfortunately, prisons seem

Internet Exercise 2-2	Locate the American Hospital Association Web site at http://www.aha.org.

1. What hospital-related news is happening in the United States today? Are there any new developments in your state?

2. What are some of the major issues facing hospitals today? Which are the most important to you?

3. What is the total number of U.S. registered hospitals?

4. Where is your nearest hospital? What services does it provide?

to serve a similar purpose today) (Lamb & Weinberger, 1998). Psychiatric hospitals are chronically underfunded and understaffed due to the difficulty of the work in caring for the mentally ill, and the fact that most people with mental disorders also have difficulty maintaining a reliable source of income with which to pay for their own treatment.

In the past, the mentally ill faced even greater challenges. American society viewed the mentally ill as subhuman, or as in some way responsible for their conditions. As such, they received very little aid, even from the many religious organizations that were willing to help the poor and physically infirmed. This became a problem as the populations of cities grew, because the population of the mentally ill increased as well, without any increase in treatment options or even humane care.

It is interesting to note that in the United States, at least, mental-health facilities did not start out unpleasantly. The first American mental hospital was the Asylum for Persons Deprived of the Use of Their Reason in Pennsylvania, founded by Quakers in 1813. Their mission statement included both medical care and "tender, sympathetic attention" as well, as they believed the Bible said it was their duty to look after all people, including those with mental illnesses. It has since changed its name to the Friends Hospital, still operational in Philadelphia, Pennsylvania.

Although there were, and still are, many highly therapeutic institutions for the mentally ill, as recently as the 1950s, investigative journalists were perennially shocked and horrified to discover another poorly run asylum (Belknap, 1980, p. 2). It is for this reason that the United States began the deinstitutionalization of mental health care in the early 1960s. Today, rather than sending people with all types of mental illness to large, government-run institutions in the attempt to provide care to people with a variety of conditions, most mental health care takes place in either the psychiatric ward of a hospital or a specialized, smaller, community-based organization focusing on emergency care, long-term care, or a certain type of disorder (Alzheimer's, schizophrenia, or depression for example). Some types of mental health care are paid for by government agencies such as Medicare or through private insurance companies, but a significant amount of the cost of live-in care is paid for by the individuals with mental illness or their families. One unfortunate result of this deinstitutionalization and privatization of mental health care is that those who have the hardest time getting the help they need are often still without support, and can be found in homeless shelters and prisons across the country. Economic resources are not the only factor affecting the successful management of mental illness. Mental health care is consistently better and more widely available for majority racial and socioeconomic groups (Marks & Scott, 1990).

Care for mental health patients is regulated by the U.S. Department of Health and Human Services and state governments, and Medicare and Medicaid pay for selected treatments. The outlook for those with mental illness has also improved substantially with the development of more advanced psychiatric medication and the availability of outpatient mental health care.

Hospital Administrators: Conducting the Orchestra of Health Care

Hospital administrators have always had a daunting task before them—managing safety and performance of all of the doctors, assistants, staff, facilities, public relations, and the many smaller details that keep hospitals operating day and night. They lead the hospital staff as a conductor leads an orchestra, guiding all of the members to provide accurate, high-quality patient care. They are part of a larger profession referred to as **health care administrators**, managers of clinics, hospitals, nursing homes, and other medical facilities.

Hospital administrators were officially recognized in 1939 when the American College of Hospitals, along with the American Hospital Association, produced an official code of ethics for the profession (Snook, 1997). Today, hospital administrators generally need to have a minimum of a master's degree in a related field, such as public health, health care administration, or business. Health service administration degrees often include a year-long internship (also called a residency) at a health care facility to give future administrators supervised experience on the job (Bernstein, 2004). Health care administrators may also need to maintain current licensure as a health care administrator, particularly if they are employed by or own a nursing home.

DEFINING ALLIED HEALTH

The term **allied health** refers to the fields of health care provision separate from nursing and medicine that contribute to the overall pursuit of health. Allied health professionals are generally specialists who work in fields such as pharmacology, administration, or optometry. Depending on the position, they may require a great deal of education and certification to practice (such as pharmacists), or they may be able to begin working in their field after very short intervals of training (such as surgical technicians or medical assistants).

This variety in training requirements is one way to differentiate allied health professionals from physicians, whose profession requires significant educational commitment whatever the chosen specialization, and nurses, most of whom receive at least a year of training before beginning practice. The requirements to practice in various allied health professions depend upon state, federal, and profession-specific laws and standards. On the following pages you will have the opportunity to explore the development of several major allied health professions.

Pharmacy

As Plinio Prioreschi writes in *A History of Medicine*, "Practically all substances have some pharmacological activity," and will respond to biological systems in some way, even if it isn't immediately noticeable or desirable to the owner of the biological system in question. A great danger in considering the history of pharmacology is the assumptions that ancient humans really understood the usage of plants and minerals in early times (Prioreschi, 2001, pp. 70–71). There have been speculations that medicinal herbs were used to treat internal ailments of the Iceman, the naturally mummified, Copper-Age man discovered preserved in the ice of the Alps. His remains contained bits of grain and pollen and date back to around 3300 BC. Although there is little evidence that the Iceman consumed these substances for medicinal purposes, many members of the scientific community have offered unlikely theories to this effect. The most likely explanation is that he was simply hungry, and had the edible plants on hand for that purpose. However, these are major conjectures about the history of pharmacology to make with such a small amount of evidence.

It would be far more advisable to consider the pharmaceutical therapy and the people who administered it from a better-documented era—the early apothecaries of Babylon, in Mesopotamia. The earliest known record of apothecaries, the precursor to the modern pharmacists, was found in Babylon. Healers from around 2600 BC were religious leaders, pharmacists, and physicians of their time, and they recorded their knowledge of the symptomology of common ancient diseases on stone tablets, which were preserved through the ages. The clay tablets of Babylon included descriptions of specific illnesses and recipes for cures involving both prayer and medicine.

This description of the Babylonian apothecaries' procedures and activities illustrates the main difference in the meaning of the term apothecary as opposed to the term pharmacist—**apothecaries** were untrained purveyors of homemade remedies who sold their provisions to physicians, midwives, surgeons, and laypeople (Troy, Remington, & Beringer, 2005). Although focusing most of their efforts on medicines, apothecaries also provided many services with the limited information available to them. **Pharmacists** today specialize only in the preparation and distribution of medication (Figure 2-6), using a great deal more information now available through modern pharmaceutical research.

In China, the emperor Shen Nung (also known as the Yan Emperor and the Emperor of Five Grains) was making similar progress toward cataloging the symptoms and cures of disease. He was widely known for his botanical and medicinal knowledge. He acquired his knowledge of medicinal herbs by testing several hundred of them on himself and observing his reactions. He recorded 365 drugs in his most well known work, *The Divine Farmer's Herb-Root Classic*. His cures were concocted from native plants including ginseng, rhubarb, and ma huang, which is the plant from which Efedra is derived nearly 5,000 years after Shen Nung's time.

Development of transportation technology that allowed for extensive world travel increased the knowledge base for all types of medical care, but few medical fields benefited more than the developing pharmacy profession. Adventurous Europeans brought remedies from five continents back to their homelands, and shared their own medical knowledge abroad as well. Import of medical plants from other countries, such as guaiac from the Caribbean (used to treat syphilis

Figure 2-6
Pharmacists
today specialize
in the preparation
and distribution
of medication.
*(Courtesy of Getty
Images. Used with
permission.)*

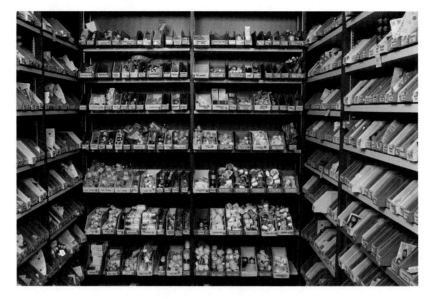

in the early 1500s), cinchona bark (for fevers) from Peru, and sarsaparilla (tried again for syphilis, but also used to treat gonorrhea, herpes, and heart trouble) from the Americas, and most notably opium (a cure for every ailment, if medical literature of the time is to be believed), became viable business for shipping companies (Conrad, 1995).

Early pharmacologists and apothecaries were very concerned with dosage. In fact, **posology**, a branch of medical science entirely devoted to the study of dosage, was a major topic of pharmaceutical conversation in the 1800s. They certainly had a lot to work out. William Hale-White's widely used textbook, *Materia medica, pharmacy, pharmacology, and therapeutics*, advises taking a total of twelve factors into account when considering the dosage for a particular patient, including idiosyncrasy of susceptibility to drugs, "mental emotion" at the time of administration, and the possibility of unpredictable "cumulative action," referencing the sudden onset of unpleasant side effects if the drug in question is taken for too long (1898, pp. 38–41).

Common Medical Ingredients

As with their counterparts in Europe, pharmacists in the United States were generally self employed, many working from home kitchens or small laboratories. Medicine was prepared mainly in the dosage required for individual prescriptions or patients themselves as needed. By the early 1800s, as demand for medicinal treatment grew, chemical manufacturers and pharmaceutical firms began to appear. Then came the Civil War in 1861, and demand for medicine suddenly skyrocketed. By the end of the war, the number of pharmaceutical firms had almost tripled, and mass production of medication became a major industry in the United States (Flannery, 2004, p. 6). Table 2-2 presents common medical ingredients over time.

Modern pharmacists are no longer responsible for the entire process of diagnosis, medicinal research, medicinal preparation, and treatment of patients. Instead, modern pharmacists are

Table 2-2 Common Medical Ingredients Over Time

AD 800–1500	1500–1800	1800–Present
Animal dung	Fish oil	Hormone derivatives
Lavender	Cocaine	Lithium
Extract of human bones	Peruvian bark	Progesterone
Poppy	Opium	Synthetic opioids
Vinegar	Saffron	Custom molecules
Sulfur	Mercury	Sulfa powder
Peony root	Sarsaparilla	Polyenes
Radish	Purple foxglove	Acetylsalicylic acid
Parsley	Antimony	Zinc
Peppermint	Tobacco	Synthesized neurotransmitters

responsible for preparing and dispensing medicine according to the orders of a medical doctor, with the additional requirement of educating patients on the appropriate use of, and safety measures applicable to, the prescribed drugs.

In the early 1800s, apothecaries were banding together and forming local associations to defend their interests against doctors, who were doing the same thing at the time. It is from such associations that schools of pharmacy began to develop. Students learned chemistry, botany, and basic medical concepts before going into business for themselves. Because a degree was not required at the time, nearly all pharmacists practiced without the benefit of formal education anyway, even when college-level programs were available. Some students attended only certain courses, probably at the behest of their employers or mentors, if they were still apprentices at the time (Flannery, 2004).

The most dramatic discovery in pharmacology took place in 1940, and it changed the medical approach to bacterial infections forever. This great event was the discovery of penicillin. This drug has an exciting history, from its unlikely discovery by Alexander Fleming and his associates in Oxford during the height of World War II in England, to its dramatic effectiveness against bacteria without hurting infected patients, to the ground it is losing today against medically resistant strains of deadly bacteria (Lax, 2004).

Most modern pharmacists are employed in the community setting, rather than at a hospital or clinic (Bernstein, 2004). They must pass a state board examination to become licensed to practice. Recently, pharmacy education has become more strenuous for potential American pharmacists. In the past, a baccalaureate degree in pharmacy was the entry-level degree for pharmacy practice. In 1990 the American Association of Colleges of Pharmacy (AACP) increased the requirement to a doctorate-level pharmacy degree to be licensed to practice starting with the class of 2006, also known as the PharmD.

Pharmacists may be assisted by pharmacy technicians, who perform routine pharmacy tasks in the processes of preparing prescribed medicine. Pharmacy technicians may also answer phones, stock shelves, and run the pharmacy cash register. Many pharmacy technicians are trained while working in the pharmacy, but some states require formal training, passage of examinations, and registration before pharmacy technicians may work in the field (Bureau of Labor Statistics, 2008).

Pharmacy Associations

The **International Pharmaceutical Federation** (FIP) is the international organization for both professional and scientifically minded pharmacists, founded in the Netherlands over ninety years ago. Over a million pharmacists and pharmaceutical scientists are members, and enjoy such membership benefits as free access to FIP publications, access to FIP's seven Special Interest Groups, and the opportunity to attend internationally influenced, continuing-education courses. One of the major strengths of the FIP is that it coordinates with the World Health Organization to develop the role of pharmacists and drug therapy in developing countries.

Closer to home, we find the American Pharmacists Association (APhA). Among other activities, the APhA publishes *Pharmacy Today, Journal of the American Pharmacists Association, Journal of Pharmaceutical Sciences*, and *Student Pharmacist*. The APhA was founded in 1852, as the medical doctors were beginning to organize, and currently represents over 60,000 practicing pharmacists and related professionals. The stated mission is "To serve society as the profession responsible for the appropriate use of medications, devices, and services to achieve optimal therapeutic outcomes" (Escovitch & Pathak, 1996, p. 69). A major activity of the AphA today is, as it was when it first began, advocating for professional pharmacists in government and industry.

During the early 1900s, the American Medical Association created the Council on Pharmacy and Chemistry to set standards for drug manufacturing and advertising. As physicians' curative abilities depended greatly on the quality of their medications, standard composition and accurate identification of drugs was necessary to successful treatment. Today, pharmacists are under their own professional organizations and must meet the requirements of the standards that they have developed, but the Council's initial organization efforts were what led to modern pharmacists' organizations today.

Another of the Council's goals was to combat quack patent medicines using various means, including the publication *Useful Drugs*, a regularly updated and comprehensive list of drugs "selected to supply the demand for less extensive materia medica and especially to serve as a basis for examinations on these subjects by state licensing boards, with a discussion of their actions, uses, and dosage" (American Medical Association, 1917, pp. 1–6). Medication was deemed more or less useful based on its effectiveness against the disorders for which it was prescribed and the side effects it inflicted upon the patients. This systematic categorization on a national scale was the first of its kind in American medicine.

The Eye-Care Professionals

Although **optometrists** receive doctoral degrees, the degree is a Doctor of Optometry or OD, which means that optometrists are not medical doctors. However, they are qualified to diagnose eye abnormalities and prescribe and maintain corrective lenses. In some states, optometrists may prescribe medication to treat eye conditions, but this is currently a function generally reserved for ophthalmologists. Optometrists attend two to four years of traditional college and an additional four years of college-level optometric training before they are qualified to practice.

Once an ophthalmologist or optometrist prescribes glasses or contacts, an optician's job begins. **Opticians** are state-licensed professionals who specialize in supplying, fitting, and maintaining glasses and contact lenses. Opticians are not required to be doctors, and are not qualified to examine or treat medical conditions of the eyes.

There are also two major support professions in the field of ophthalmology: ophthalmic medical technicians and ophthalmic assistants. At the moment, the majority of assistants and technicians receive their training on the job or through at-home education provided by nationally accredited educators. Certification is strongly recommended but not required in most states for ophthalmic technicians and assistants.

Podiatry

Podiatry is the medical field associated with the health and care of feet. To practice, one must have a Doctor of Podiatric Medicine (D.P.M.) degree, which requires four years of graduate schoolwork in podiatry. As with other medical professions, a two-year residency is also required, in both medicine and surgery. Once all of the educational and residency requirements have been completed, podiatrists must be licensed by the state in which they wish to practice. They can then diagnose and treat conditions of the feet and ankles. Some podiatrists specialize in certain conditions or treatments, such as conditions related to diabetes or podiatric surgery. Podiatrists also prescribe devices to correct foot deformities and walking problems (American Association of Colleges of Podiatric Medicine, 2007).

Like the ophthalmologic professions, podiatrists have a good deal of autonomy regarding their private practices. However, according to some, podiatrists are not among the most esteemed members of the medical profession (Lucas, McInnes, & Mandy, 2003). Their usual clientele may be one of the causes of this situation. The elderly are a major part of a podiatrist's practice, because foot problems become worse as patients grow older, and conditions like adult-onset diabetes and osteoporosis frequently create new foot problems for older people. Working people who spend a lot of time on their feet on a daily basis are also commonly seen in podiatrist's offices. Because these are not necessarily the wealthiest of patients, and because the work isn't very glamorous, podiatrists are sometimes considered to be on the periphery of the medical community (Lucas, McInnes, & Mandy, 2003).

Chiropractic Medicine

Chiropractic medicine is an osteopathic and holistic medical practice that can be a controversial subject. The object of chiropractic treatment is to improve overall health and cure specific ailments by readjusting the spine and musculoskeletal system to improve the functioning of the nervous system. Daniel David Palmer is recognized as the official founder of chiropractic medicine. In the late 1800s and early 1900s, Palmer claimed to have discovered that most physical problems could be significantly improved or entirely cured by spinal adjustment that would allow what he called Innate Intelligence, meaning the energy of living things, to flow through the body properly (McDonald, 2003).

Research evidence does not support the idea that chiropractic treatments cure medical problems. Some studies, but not all, indicate that chiropractic treatment is useful for relieving lower back pain, some types of tension headaches (which are notoriously difficult to stop using traditional medicine), and other musculoskeletal conditions (McCroy, et al., 2001), but there are not any conclusive, controlled, and replicated research results to conclusively demonstrate that chiropractic care does or does not benefit patients.

Because of this lack of conclusive research into its effectiveness, the American Medical Association did not recognize chiropractic medicine as a legitimate medical practice until 1987. A chiropractor named Chester Wilk sued the AMA under charges of conspiracy and restraint of trade, and the AMA was forced to allow its members to cooperate with and even become chiropractors (Haldeman, 2004).

Today, chiropractors are regulated by state boards, the majority of which require at least two years of undergraduate education, followed by four years of chiropractic training in anatomy, public health, pathology, biochemistry, and chiropractic technique, which leads to a Doctor of Chiropractic degree. In addition to obtaining the doctoral degree, potential chiropractors must also pass a test created and administered by the National Board of Chiropractic Examiners (Bureau of Labor Statistics, 2006).

Midwifery

This profession has gone through many changes through the years. Midwives have been absolutely essential in assuring the successful delivery of children. Women with experience in assisting in childbirth helping new mothers before, during, and after the birth of their children are common in many cultures across the world. Successful midwives need a detailed knowledge of gynecological anatomy and prenatal development, as well as a steady personality to help with the mental challenges involved in childbirth. Although this status quo of experienced midwives helping local mothers was in place for many hundreds of years, the past two centuries have seen major changes in the profession.

As general-practice physicians and surgeons began to develop their skills, they became more involved in the birthing process, slowly reducing (although not wiping out) midwives' career prospects. This happened for several reasons. For one, physicians wanted to curb competition and improve the professional appearance of their profession by preventing, as they saw it, a rival profession from poaching their patients. Once general-practice physicians and surgeons had taken steps to decrease midwives' standing in the medical community, people began to demand more of the physicians' services.

General-practice physicians and surgeons brought other changes than an increase in medical knowledge in training (which, although less generalized than physicians, was not lacking, while midwives were alone in professional childbirth assistance). The relationship between the expectant mother and the physician was somewhat different than with a midwife. Consider this passage from an 1866 guide to midwifery regarding the delivery of twins:

> Dr. Denman states that "it is a constant rule to keep patients who have borne one child, ignorant of there being another, as long as can possibly be done." There is certainly no occasion to frighten the patient, but I do believe that concealments are bad, and that midwifery, as everywhere else, "honesty is the best policy…" It is better neither to inform her abruptly of the nature of the case, nor to make any mystery about it; but certainly to tell her that she will soon give birth to a second; this may be coupled with a congratulation on the fortunate progress of the labor so far; and an assurance that she will have but little more pain to bear, and that the case presents no features calling for anxiety (Churchill, 1866, p. 487).

The mother and child are treated somewhat impersonally as patients in this scenario.

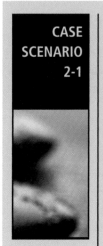

CASE SCENARIO 2-1

Consider the excerpt above regarding the need to inform patients of unexpected news in a stressful situation like childbirth.

CASE ANALYSIS

1. What is wrong with Dr. Denman's approach as described above?

2. What is correct and incorrect about the author's suggestions for handling the situation?

3. How would you react if you weren't expecting to deliver two babies at all?

4. How might you inform the mother of the news? If you were a parent, what do you think you would prefer to hear at the time?

5. What technology is available today that reduces the likelihood of multiple births coming as a surprise on the day of delivery?

The profession of midwifery never died out, and regulation of the profession is as important an issue today as it was hundreds of years ago. Official certification of midwives started in the 1600s in Europe. An Amsterdam bylaw in 1668 insisted that anyone wishing to practice as a midwife needed to pass an examination (likely oral, not written or practical, but that information is not available), and about a decade later another law required prospective midwives to work as an assistant to a currently practicing midwife for four years before she could obtain her own license (Grell & Cunningham, 1997).

In the past two decades, around 22,000 babies per year have been born outside of a hospital in a birthing clinic or home setting without the attendance of a doctor (U.S. Census Bureau, 2006). Many of these new mothers had the benefit of having a midwife or nurse-midwife in attendance instead. Although there are nurse-midwives today who have skill sets that overlap that of a nurse and a midwife, there are also what are called direct-entry midwives, who may practice after completing an applicable education program and becoming licensed by state where required. The modern certification for midwifery is the CPM or Certified Professional Midwife credential, obtained in the U.S. through the North American Registry of Midwives.

Another certification option is the Certified Nurse-Midwife (CNM) certification for nurse-midwives or the Certified Midwife (CM) certification for lay and direct-entry midwives offered by the American Midwifery Certification Board. Individuals interested in either of these certifications must graduate from an accredited midwifery education program and pass a national examination before certification is granted.

According to the American College of Nurse-Midwives, there are over thirty different accredited midwifery education programs the United States, and they can be divided into six major types that can prepare students for certification. There are post-baccalaureate certificates, graduate programs, and pre-certification programs specifically designed for registered nurses and non-nurses to prepare for the appropriate certification for each. These must meet the state standards where they are being offered, which vary widely and are currently in transition as new legislation is pursued in several areas of the country.

In addition to midwives, there are other professionals who assist in the birthing process. These are called **doulas** or birth attendants, and their function is to provide emotional and even physical support to mothers who are giving birth (Rooks, 1999). They serve to offer comfort and instruction in breathing, position, and relaxation, which makes the childbirth process much less stressful, allowing midwives, who often work with doulas due to their complementary philosophy and professional calling, to do their work more peacefully. Doulas are not qualified to diagnose or treat any medical problems related to childbirth.

GENDER

The practice of medicine has historically been a field dominated by men who were supported by competent female nurses and assistants. This has been the case throughout history, although the males involved in the process have been more or less willing to acknowledge women's contribution to the field from century to century. In ancient Rome, for example, women were documented as being involved in treatment of the sick, both by providing hands-on care and by supplying medication (Conrad, 1995), and in pre-Islam Arabic cultures, women were thought to heal sickness through the use of magic (Prioreschi, 2001). However, male names are ascribed to the vast majority of ancient medical treatises, and women's visibility in medical history did not improve for several hundred years.

For much of history, women were primary providers of health care, both for their immediate families and for their neighbors and extended kin. Women used all of the resources at their disposal, from herbs stored for emergency use to the knowledge of older relatives, to heal sick and injured family members (Starr, 1982). The result of this reliance was that women were generally better informed and in possession of more experience in health care delivery than men, with female physicians actually quite common in colonial America (Starr, 1982).

As medical care transformed from a part of household maintenance to a professional system of care and gradually became more lucrative, men began to replace women as the main health care providers. This was not always done in a peaceable or fair manner, but there was a surprising (from our 20th-century perspective) lack of protest from women of the time period.

In *Gunn's Domestic Medicine or Poor Man's Friend in the Hour of Affliction, Pain, and Sickness* mentioned earlier, Gunn included the following rant on midwifery:

> Most midwives of this country, and indeed of most other countries, are those who take up the employment from too great laziness to exert themselves in other walks of life; from utter ignorance of the great responsibilities attached to such a calling, and from a heartless destitution of feeling and humanity, which permits their ignorance and officiousness to entail disease originating from mismanagement on thousands of women for life (pp. 459–460).

In their strenuous effort to remove competition, male doctors were often unmercifully dismissive of their female counterparts, as Gunn's diatribe clearly exemplifies. The difficult task of midwifery, of venturing into all weather and hours of day and night to assist in childbirth with little more than one's hands and a positive attitude, could hardly be construed as work for the lazy. If someone has the nerve to say that nurses work less than other medical professionals, remember that people like Gunn have been saying things like that for years, and they are still mistaken!

Although this negative view of women in medicine was commonplace in the early part of the 1800s, the needs brought about by the onset of the Civil War propelled women into health care once more. Women set up makeshift hospitals and collected medicinal plants near battlegrounds and troop encampments. Some assisted doctors directly in their work, or brought water (and occasionally alcohol) to weary soldiers. Most importantly, women organized the **Sanitary Commission** to promote clean and healthy conditions in army camps, which doubtless saved many lives (Flannery, 2004).

Although women make up almost half of the student population in medical schools, they have a tendency to congregate in some medical specialties more than others. Many allied health professions that require a minimal amount of training (medical assistants, pharmacy technicians, and dental assistants, for example) attract more women than men, and more than half of pediatricians are women as well. On the other hand, surgery is not a popular choice with women—in

2003, over 75% of America's surgical residents were men (Neumayer, et al., 2002). The profession of surgery involves high levels of competitiveness, intensity, and prestige within the community, which seem to be qualities that are valued more highly by men than by women when describing an ideal career. This, in combination with the profession's history of male domination and the slow pace of gender role modernization within the medical community, may account for the number of men in the field of surgery. There is some debate as to whether women are forced into the fields most often described as female dominated, particularly those involving children, or if they choose them willingly.

Medical associations and professional organizations realize that there is room for improvement in terms of the integration of women into the medical field (Figure 2-7). Leadership training is available from many sources, and some programs are geared specifically toward women. They are designed to inspire individuals to become more involved in their field and actively express and meet the needs of women in the medical community. Examples of leadership training opportunities include personal leadership coaching, traveling to meet women leaders, or specific training programs offered by various organizations. The Association of American Medical Colleges publishes a list of national leadership development programs on their Web site so that medical students and new doctors can have easy access to the program information.

One suggested solution for concerns about the professional development of female doctors is a professional mentoring program. Such a system would provide much needed support for female doctors who are at the beginning of their career by pairing beginning professionals with a **mentor**, a more experienced professional who can provide advice, instruction, or moral support as needed. However, aside from personal satisfaction about giving back to the profession, the mentors have little to gain from such an arrangement. For mentoring to be successful in helping new professionals integrate into the medical environment, the mentors involved must be completely supportive of their role and the goals of the program (Delaat, 2007).

Figure 2-7
Women make up nearly half the student population in medical school.

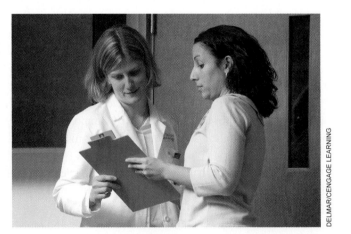

DELMAR/CENGAGE LEARNING

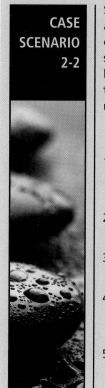

CASE SCENARIO 2-2

Suhaila has just passed her vascular surgery specialty examination with high scores, and has accepted a position at a metropolitan hospital. She enjoys the challenge of her job and is excited about her career opportunities at the hospital since her supervisors have high expectations for her. During her residency experience she had become accustomed to the fact that most of her immediate coworkers are male, but the combination of a new certification, a new job, a new workplace, and all of her new contemporaries are a little intimidating.

CASE ANALYSIS

1. What kind of reaction could she expect from her peers if Suhaila wanted to become a surgeon 100 years ago? Fifty years ago? What would be different than today?

2. If you were one of Suhaila's coworkers, what might you do to make her feel like part of the team?

3. If Suhaila's new surgical team refused to respect her because of her gender, what can she do to remedy the situation? What organizations could offer her support?

4. What incentives are available to encourage Suhaila to take a greater leadership role in her field? Can you think of any new ones that might motivate her to excel?

5. If you were Suhaila's supervisor, how would you go about providing her with a mentor from the hospital staff to help her get started in her new position and keep her excited about vascular surgery?

SUMMARY

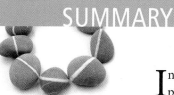

In the beginning, medicine likely developed almost by accident, as humans stumbled across plants and found treatments that cured medical conditions. As culture and technology developed and humans began to think of ways to make their lives better, the war against sickness and injury became a team effort, with families, physicians, apothecaries, and midwives all participating in patient care.

Later, physicians consulted with one another, pooled their information, and worked hard to make medicine an effective and relevant profession. Once the knowledge base became too great for any one person to be an expert in every disorder and treatment, specialists began to appear to supplement the general knowledge of doctors, and assisting personnel became necessary to streamline the process of medical care. These were the beginnings of the allied health professions.

Licensure and education programs were developed to reduce competition from uninformed semiprofessionals and increase patient survivability. Eventually, regulation passed from the professionals exclusively to a partnership between professional organizations and state and federal governments. Standards continue to rise for allied health professionals today, as education requirements increase and more and more successful treatments are perfected. The field of allied health has a long history of constant improvement, and the future ahead is a bright one.

What I do you cannot do; but what you do, I cannot do. The needs are great, and none of us, including me, ever do great things. But we can all do small things, with great love, and together we can do something wonderful.

–Mother Teresa

REFERENCES

AMERICAN ASSOCIATION OF COLLEGES OF PODIATRIC MEDICINE. (2007). *Career zone.* Retrieved September 1, 2007, from http://www.aacpm.org/html/careerzone/index.asp

AMERICAN BOARD OF FAMILY MEDICINE. (2007). *History of the specialty.* Retrieved July 25, 2008, from https://www.theabfm.org/about/history.aspx

AMERICAN MEDICAL ASSOCIATION. (2007). *Physician characteristics and distribution in the US, 2007 edition* (p. 275). Chicago, IL: American Medical Association.

AMERICAN MEDICAL ASSOCIATION. (2007). *State medical licensure requirements and statistics* (p. 1). Chicago, IL: American Medical Association.

AMERICAN MEDICAL ASSOCIATION. (1917). *Useful drugs.* Chicago, IL: Press of the American Medical Association.

AMERICAN SOCIETY OF ANESTHESIOLOGISTS. (2004). *Continuum of depth of sedation definition of general anesthesia and levels of sedation/analgesia.* Retrieved September 2, 2007, from http://www.asahq.org/publicationsAndServices/standards/20.pdf

ANGEL, L. J. (1984). Health as a crucial factor in the changes from hunting to developed farming in the eastern Mediterranean. In Mark N. Cohen & George J. Armelagos (Eds.), (1984), *Paleopathology at the Origins of Agriculture* (proceedings of a conference held in 1982) (pp. 51–73). Orlando, FL: Academic Press.

BELKNAP, I. (1980). *Human problems of a state mental hospital.* Minneapolis, MN: Ayer Publishing.

BERNSTEIN, A. (2004). *Guide to your career.* New York: The Princeton Review.

BUREAU OF LABOR STATISTICS, U.S. DEPARTMENT OF LABOR. (2006). Chiropractors. *Occupational outlook handbook, 2006–07 edition.* Retrieved September 2, 2007, from http://www.bls.gov/oco/ocos071.htm

BUREAU OF LABOR STATISTICS, U.S. DEPARTMENT OF LABOR. (2007). Physicians and surgeons. *Occupational outlook handbook, 2006–07 edition.* Retrieved August 29, 2007, from http://www.bls.gov/oco/ocos074.htm

BUREAU OF LABOR STATISTICS, U.S. DEPARTMENT OF LABOR. (2008). Pharmacy technicians. *Occupational outlook handbook, 2008–09 edition.* Retrieved July 25, 2008, from http://www.bls.gov/oco/ocos252.htm

CARTER, K. C., & Carter, B. J. (2005). *Childbed fever: A scientific biography of Ignaz Semmelweis* (p. 7). Piscataway, NJ: Aldine Transaction.

CHURCHILL, F. (1866). *On the theory and practice of midwifery* (p. 487). London: Renshaw.

COLLINS, C. (2006). Causes of fevers: Miasma versus contagion. *The biomedical scientist.* Retrieved September 12, 2007, from http://ibms.org.cfm?method=science.history_zone&subpage=history_fevers

CONRAD, L. (1995). *The Western medical tradition: 800 B.C.–1800 A.D.* (pp. 49; 61–65; 308). New York: Cambridge University Press.

DAVIS, N. S. (1877). *Contributions to the history of medical education and medical institutions in the United States of America, 1776–1876* (p. 59). Washington, DC: Government Printing Office.

DELAAT, J. (2007). *Gender in the workplace: A case study approach* (pp. 46–55). Thousand Oaks, CA: Sage Publications Inc.

DIGBY, A. (1994). *Making a medical living: doctors and patients in the English market for medicine* (pp. 52–54). New York: Cambridge University Press.

DELAUNE, S., & Ladner, P. (2002). *Fundamentals of nursing: Standards and practices* (p. 232). Clifton Park, NY: Thomson Delmar Learning.

DOWNS, R. B. (2004). *Books that changed the world* (pp. 143–145). New York: Signet Classic.

ESCOVITZ, A., & Pathak, D. S. (1996). *Health outcomes and pharmaceutical care* (p. 69). Philadelphia: Haworth Press.

FLANNERY, M. (2004). *Civil war pharmacy* (pp. 50–64). Binghamton, NY: Haworth Press.

GARRISON, G., Matthew, D., & Jones, R. (May 2007). Future medical school applicants, Part I: Overall Trends. *Analysis in Brief, 7,* 3, (p. 1). Washington, DC: Association of American Medical Colleges.

GEVITZ, N. (2004). *The DOs: Osteopathic medicine in America,* (pp. 1–22). Baltimore, MD: Johns Hopkins University Press.

GUNN, J. C. (1860). *Gunn's domestic medicine or poor man's friend in the hour of affliction, pain, and sickness* (pp. i; 459–460). New York: C. M. Saxton, Barker & Co.

GRELL, P., & Cunningham, A. (1997). *Health care and poor relief in Protestant Europe, 1500–1700* (p. 78). Oxford, UK: Routledge.

HAJAR, R. (2000). Past glories of the Great Library of Alexandria. *Heart Views, 7,* 278–282.

HALE-WHITE, W. (1898). *Materia medica, pharmacy, pharmacology, and therapeutics* (pp. 38–40). Philadelphia: P. Blakiston's Son and Company, Inc.

HALDEMAN, S. (2004). *Principles and practice of chiropractic* (pp. 54–55). New York: McGraw-Hill Professional.

HAWKINS, C. F. (1982). Write the MD thesis. In *How to do it* (pp. 52–61). London, UK: British Medical Association.

KELLY, J. (2005). *The great mortality: An intimate history of the black death, the most devastating plague of all time* (p. 289). New York: HarperCollins Publishers.

KREBS, R. (1999). *Scientific development and misconceptions through the ages: A reference guide* (p. 44). Westport, CT: Greenwood Press.

KUCHARSKI, A., & Todd, E. (2003). Pain: Historical perspectives. In C. Warfield & Z. Bajwa, *Principles and practices of pain medicine* (p. 1). Columbus, OH: McGraw-Hill Professional.

LAMB, H. R., & Weinberger, L. E. (1998). Persons with severe mental illness in jails and prisons: A review. *Psychiatric Services, 49,* 438–492.

LAX, E. (2004). *The mold in Dr. Florey's coat: The story of the penicillin miracle* (p. 2). New York: Henry Holt and Company.

LUCAS, K., McInnes, J., & Mandy, A. (2003). *Psychosocial approaches to podiatry: A companion for practice* (p. 11). St. Louis, MO: Elsevier Health Sciences.

LUNDY, K., & Janes, S. (2005). *Community health nursing: Caring for the public's health* (p. 261). Sudbury, MA: Jones & Bartlett Publishers.

MARKS, I., & Scott, R. (1990). *Mental health care delivery: Innovations, impediments and implementation* (p. 3). New York: Cambridge University Press.

MCCROY, D., Penzien, D., Hasselblad, V., & Gray, R. (2001). *Behavioral and physical treatments for tension-type and cervicogenic headache.* Durham, NC: Duke University Evidence-Based Practice Center.

MCDONALD, W. (2003). *How chiropractors think and practice: The survey of North American chiropractors.* Ada, OH: Institute for Social Research, Ohio Northern University.

Neumayer, L., Cochran, A., Melby, S., Foy, H., & Wallack, M. (2002). The state of general surgery residency in the United States. *Archives of Surgery, 137.11*, 1262–1265.

Nicholson, W. (1999). *Longevity & health in ancient Paleolithic vs. Neolithic peoples: Not what you may have been told.* Retrieved May 18, 2007, from http://www.beyondveg.com/nicholson-w/angel-1984/angel-1984-1a.shtml

Nightingale, F. (1863). *Notes on hospitals.* London, UK: Longmans.

Nutton, V. (2004). *Ancient medicines* (pp. 1; 128). Oxford, UK: Routledge.

Obituary–The late Thomas Barnes, M.D., F.R.S.E. (1872, June). Edinburgh *Medical Journal,* p. 1142.

Prioreschi, P. (2001). *A history of medicine* (pp. 70–71, 201, 214–216, 222–223). Phillipsburg, NJ: Horatius P&R Press.

Risse, G. (1986). Imhotep and medicine: A reevaluation. *Western Journal of Medicine, 144,* 622–624.

Rooks, J. (1999). *Midwifery and childbirth in America* (pp. 10, 79–83). Philadelphia: Temple University Press.

Rotham, D., Kiceluk, S., & Marcus, S. (1995). *Medicine and Western Civilization* (p. 261). Oxford, UK: Rutgers University Press.

Santos-Sacchi, J., & Jahn, A. F. (2001). *Physiology of the ear* (pp. 4–5). Clifton Park, NY: Delmar, Cengage Learning.

Shalala, D. E. (1999). A patient's Bill of Rights: The medical student's role. *Journal of the American Medical Association, 281,* 857.

Shepherd, J. A. (1986). The contribution of Robert Lawson Tait to the development of abdominal surgery. *Surgery Annual, 18,* 339–349.

Snook, D. (1997). *Opportunities in hospital administration careers* (p. 4). Columbus, OH: McGraw-Hill Professional.

Snook, D. (2003). *Hospitals: What they are and how they work* (p. 5). Sudbury, MA: Jones & Bartlett Publishers.

Starr, P. (1982). *The social transformation of American medicine* (pp. 27; 32; 49; 61). Jackson, TN: Basic Books.

Troy, D. B., Remington, J. R., & Beringer, P. (2005). *Remington: The science and practice of pharmacy* (pp. 11–12). Philadelphia: Lippincott Williams & Wilkins.

U.S. Census Bureau. *Statistical abstract of the United States: 2006* (p. 71). Washington, DC: U.S. Census Bureau.

Weil, A. (2004). *The natural mind: A revolutionary approach to the drug problem* (p. 121). New York: Mariner Books.

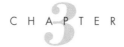

C H A P T E R

PROGRESSION OF THE NURSING FIELD: PAST AND PRESENT

SHEILA COX SULLIVAN

PhD, RN, CNE, Associate Chief Nurse/Research, Central Arkansas Veterans Healthcare System

History is a guide to navigation in perilous times. History is who we are and why we are the way we are.

–David C. McCullough

LEARNING OBJECTIVES

At the completion of this chapter, the learner should be able to do the following:

1. Discuss the importance of understanding nursing history.
2. Trace the history of the nursing profession in the United States.
3. Relate the impact of religion, politics, and socio-economic history on the evolution of nursing practice, education, and research.
4. Identify the contributions of major nursing leaders.
5. Articulate the role of research in nursing practice.

KEY TERMS

American Association of
    Colleges of Nursing
Army Nurse Corps
Associate-Degree Nurse
Brown Report
Cadet Nurse Corps (CNC)
Clara Barton
Diagnostic Related
    Groups (DRGs)
Dorothea Dix
Florence Nightingale
Frontier Nursing Service
Goldmark Report

Harriet Tubman
Health Maintenance
    Organizations
Hill-Burton Act
History
Infection Control
Isabel Hampton Robb
James Derham
Jane Woolsey
Lavinia Dock
Lillian Wald
Managed Care
Mary Adelaide Nutting

Mary Eliza Mahoney
Mary Seacole
National Institute for
    Nursing Research
National League for
    Nursing (NLN)
Nurse Training Act
Nursing Religious Orders
Professional Nursing
Public Health
Sheppard-Towner Act
Sojourner Truth
Susie King Taylor

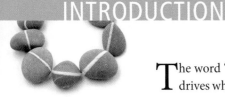

INTRODUCTION

The word "**history**" implies a story; nurses need to know their own story because that story drives who and what we are now. The perspective gained by considering the challenges faced by nursing predecessors assists current and future nurses in understanding our current environment as well as creating a bond between us. D'Antonio (2005, p. 241) asserts that "exploring the past shapes our professional culture," giving us freedom to contemplate why we do what we do the way we do it and with whom. Finally, "history means self-knowledge and as students, that should be one of the most important things to you" (Kreis, 2000).

The purpose of this chapter is to trace the development of **professional nursing**, noting significant religious, political, and socio-economic trends that influenced the current practice of nursing. The chapter will also review the evolution of educational practices that develop learners into practicing nurses. Finally, as nurses have accepted the mandate to base nursing practice in scientific evidence, the chapter will review the development of nursing research. These three branches of nursing (practice, education, and research) enjoy a symbiotic relationship, informing and growing based on advances in the other branches.

HISTORY OF NURSING PRACTICE

The history of nursing in the United States relies on recognizing the contributions made by those in other parts of the world. The practice of nursing is an ancient one, and the identity and role of nurses changed markedly throughout history. The history of nursing in Western Europe and North America may be somewhat familiar to most learners; however, all cultures have a history of health care. This section will provide a brief overview of what is known about these practices.

Ancient Times

Ancient civilizations clearly had some method of providing health care to citizens. Many health care practices coincided with spiritual beliefs and superstitions, the majority rooted in the belief that evil spirits caused illness, or that illness was the consequence of disobedience to the requirements of the spirit world. These beliefs facilitated the connection of those who offered relief from illness and enlightened persons possessing knowledge of spiritual truth. Historians assume family members provided most nursing care inside the home with the guidance of spiritual leaders or medical providers (Joel & Kelly, 2002).

Documentation of nursing appears in the Jewish Pentateuch and Christian Old Testament. The book of Exodus relates the story of Shiphrah and Puah, Hebrew midwives enslaved in Egypt, who defied Pharaoh's edict to slaughter newborn males in the slave camps, thus saving Moses, the Hebrew deliverer. This story of civil disobedience forecast nursing's future as a defender of the underserved. Further, the book of Leviticus functions as a manual for **infection control**, or how to keep infectious diseases from spreading. Far eastern religion also incorporated health care concepts. The Hindu religion recognized hygienic principles, and Buddhists utilized hospitals and disease-prevention strategies (Catalono, 2006). Chinese writings by Confucius teach that health depends on a balance between yin and yang (Ellis & Hartley, 2004), and many alternative treatments, such as acupuncture, used by the ancient Chinese are still practiced today.

Greek society contributed greatly to the development of health care. Hippocrates, known as the Father of Medicine, designed methods for physical assessment and medical record keeping. Importantly, Hippocrates believed natural events caused illness rather than displeased spiritual powers. Approximately 400 BC, Hippocrates began to disseminate his beliefs through oral and written teachings, and he suggested the connection between mind, body, spirit, and environment. Perhaps Hippocrates is best known for the ethical principles he believed should guide the practice of a physician, carefully recorded in the Hippocratic Oath (Catalano, 2006; Beebe, 2007).

Roman culture absorbed many of the practices from conquered peoples, but the empire did not accept Hippocrates' connection between health practices and disease. However, the infrastructure to address **public-health** concerns, specifically clean water and sewage, was a priority (Catalono, 2006). The Roman Empire relied on military might to sustain itself, and providing medical attention to the soldiers stimulated the development of hospital care and pharmacies. Far from being revered, medical personnel were slaves, and both men and women participated in the provision of nursing care (Beebe, 2007; Williams-Evans, Jacob, & Carnegie, 2005).

Middle Ages

The Dark Ages signified a bleak period of little scientific advancement and ubiquitous poverty, illness, and premature death (Catalano, 2006). What survived of the medical beliefs purported by Hippocrates is due to the efforts of Jewish physicians who spread translations of Greek and Arabic documents addressing medical concerns to surrounding physicians. Constantinus Africanus revived Italian medicine with translations of Islamic documents as well as other translated manuscripts from Greek and Arabic sources. In the 12th century, the Italian city of Salerno became a center of healing in Europe under Constantinus' guidance, and women studied midwifery at the school in Salerno (Kalisch & Kalisch, 2004).

Rome adopted Christianity as the official religion of the empire shortly before its demise, and the principles of the Christian faith influenced cultural perceptions toward the value of life and caring for others (Catalano, 2006; Williams-Evans, Jacob, & Carnegie, 2004). During the Dark Ages, the Roman Catholic Church exerted a strong influence over all aspects of life in Europe, and wealthy women would provide food and caring to peasants, traveling from door to door (Catalano, 2006; Williams-Evans, Jacob, & Carnegie, 2004). These activities likely influenced the origin of the word "nurse," from the Latin *nutrire*, translated as to nourish or nurture (Catalano, 2006). Women of lesser means would become nuns and lived together in cloisters.

These convents became places to seek health care, but the members also traveled to rural areas to ensure health care and teaching. These convents became the basis of **religious nursing orders** as early as AD 500 (Catalano, 2006).

The Crusades began as an attempt of Western European Christians to conquer the Holy Land and remove Muslim rule from Jerusalem. This lengthy military effort, lasting for over 200 years, created a need for nursing orders within the military. The Knights Hospitalers of St. John of Jerusalem wore a black robe adorned with a white Maltese cross, so named because their primary responsibility was transportation from the battlefield to the hospital (Joel & Kelly, 2002). These men provided health care not only to the soldiers, but pilgrims and inhabitants of the city (Kalisch & Kalisch, 2004). The Knights Templar, founded in 1118, and the Knights of the Teutonic Order, founded in 1190, also began as nursing orders, but the Teutonic knights became more embroiled in military pursuits. Both orders remained predominately male, although Hospitaler Dames became a female version of the Hospitalers. These women founded numerous hospitals in the Holy Land, providing nursing care for the ill as well as addressing public health concerns (Kalish & Kalish, 2004).

Renaissance

Although a time of great intellectual growth for most other fields, the Renaissance is considered the "Dark Ages" of nursing (Ellis & Hartley, 2004). This dismal title is attributed to the return of the wealthy to tending to their families, and the devaluing of nursing care. Public nursing responsibilities fell to women of lesser repute, specifically prostitutes and prisoners. (Catalano, 2006; Kalisch & Kalisch, 2004; Williams-Evans, Jacob, & Carnegie, 2004.) Male nursing orders began to decrease, and religious orders, comprised of nuns, provided most health care by 1500 (Catalano, 2006). The Sisters of Charity began around 1600, and the Church Order of Deaconesses, who would later train Florence Nightingale, also began to provide formal care as well as training for nurses.

Colonial American Nursing

Nursing in the United States from Jamestown through the revolution fared no better than European nursing at the time. Outbreaks of various diseases limited the expected lifespan to 35 years (Kalisch & Kalisch, 2004), and little infrastructure existed for the provision of health care. Caregivers, if not family members, were those who could find no better employment, and hospitals did not exist until Benjamin Franklin built Pennsylvania Hospital in 1751 (Oermann, 1997). Catholic nursing orders, such as the Daughters of Charity, continued to provide the majority of nursing care outside the home. African-American slaves frequently provided nursing care both to Caucasian masters and other African-American slaves. Of note during this time is **James Derham**, a nurse who worked in New Orleans. Derham used his earnings to buy his freedom as well as pay his way through medical school, becoming the first African-American physician in the United States (http://Nurses.info, 2007).

FLORENCE NIGHTINGALE

Florence Nightingale (Figure 3-1) was born in Florence, Italy, on May 12, 1820, to wealthy English parents. Florence perceived a calling from God to care for the poor and ill from early in life, and Nightingale's father sought to distract her by providing her with an excellent education for a Victorian woman, including math, philosophy, languages, and sciences. Despite her parents' best efforts to secure an advantageous marriage, Florence remained steadfast in pursuit of her goal to become a nurse, and she was allowed to study at Kaiserwerth in Germany, a hospital run by the Church Order of Deaconesses in 1851. It must be remembered that nurses at this time were considered women of poor reputation and circumstance. Charles Dickens personified the state of nursing with his depiction of the drunken Sairy Gamp in *Martin Chuzzlewit*, so one can appreciate the Nightingales' despair. Nevertheless, Florence apprenticed for three months, and she kept copious notes of what she observed and learned about nursing. She left even more resolute to improve conditions for the sick (Kalisch & Kalisch, 2004; Beebe, 2007; Catalano, 2006).

Following her time at Kaiserwerth, Nightingale accepted a position as superintendent of a charity hospital known as the Establishment for Gentlewomen During Illness (Kalisch & Kalisch, 2004). This position was short lived due to Nightingale's conflicts with the board of directors, who refused to envision nursing as Nightingale did. Nightingale began the process of seeking new employment when political forces shaped events that would change health care forever.

Figure 3-1
Florence
Nightingale.
*(Courtesy of
Parke-Davis,
a Division of
Warner-Cambert
Company.)*

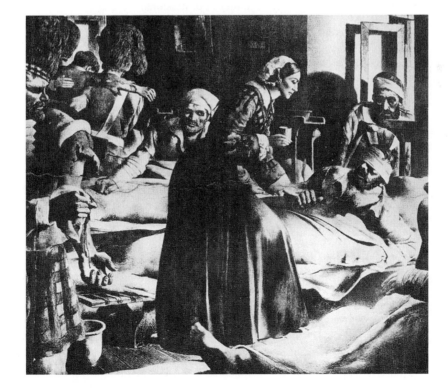

The outbreak of the Crimean War and a cholera epidemic in 1854 stymied Nightingale's pursuit of new employment or opening a school for nurses. Public outcry over reports in *The London Times* regarding the miserable conditions wounded soldiers endured prompted Sir Sidney Herbert, the minister of war, to invite Nightingale to supervise 38 nurses aiding in the provision of care to soldiers. Nightingale carefully chose the nurses from various religious orders through a rigorous interview process; however, the army physicians ignored Nightingale and her nurses upon their arrival at Scutari. Conditions exceeded the reports as the nurses found men lying on cold, bare floors in their own excrement along with inadequate sewage and supplies. However, ten days after their arrival, a massive influx of wounded from the Battle in Inkermann overwhelmed the physicians, and they grudgingly accepted the nurses' help. Nightingale and her nurses operationalized Nightingale's beliefs about cleanliness and good nutrition over the subsequent months and contributed to the decline in the death rate at Scutari from 60% to 1% (Joel & Kelly, 2002). In addition to nursing, Nightingale employed data collection and statistical analysis to provide a basis for political action, such as lobbying politicians in England for supplies and funds to improve conditions for the soldiers. Nightingale often paid for such items from her personal wealth when government officials did not respond in what she considered a timely manner (Cook, 1913).

Nightingale's experience in Crimea left her ill, and she never fully recovered her physical strength. However, she continued to work tirelessly for the advancement of formal nursing education, improved standards of health in India, and writing volumes on military nursing, *Notes on Hospitals*, and *Notes on Nursing*. Her influence set the tone of modern nursing, and Small (1998) honors her as the founder of professional nursing.

Nightingale was not the only nurse leader to serve in Crimea. **Mary Seacole** was born in Jamaica, to a Scottish father and a Jamaican mother. Since her biracial heritage allowed her to be "free," Seacole learned nursing from her mother, who ran a boarding house in Kingston. Seacole attempted to go to Scutari with Nightingale, but she was denied by British government officials. Not deterred despite several failed attempts to join Nightingale's effort, Seacole used her scant personal resources to travel to Crimea, where she opened a boarding house and provided private care to sick soldiers. Although the victim of racial prejudice, Seacole persisted in her desire to care for the ill and wounded, and she was recognized by the English government with a medal of honor (British Broadcasting Corporation, nd; Williams-Evans, Jacob, & Carnegie, 2004; Carnegie, 1995).

NURSING IN AMERICA

The American Civil War

During the Civil War, approximately 2,000 women served as volunteers (Civil War Nurses, 2003), but a total of 10,000 women served as nurses (Kalisch & Kalisch, 2004). Leaders of efforts to recruit a nursing force for the military included **Dorothea Dix** and **Clara Barton**. Dix had already been renowned for her work in mental health, and Barton eventually founded the American Red

Cross. Other nurses who contributed in significant ways include: **Harriet Tubman**, best known for her work on the Underground Railroad; **Sojourner Truth**, better known for her abolitionist activities; and **Susie King Taylor**, who had broken the law prohibiting African Americans from learning to read and write and subsequently taught other African Americans (Williams-Evans, Jacob, & Carnegie, 2004). Sally Tompkins became the superintendent of a Confederate hospital and was given the rank of captain in the army (MacLean, 2006; Bebee, 2007).

The ranks of volunteer nurses during the Civil War included those famous for other reasons. The writings of Walt Whitman, who served as a nurse during the war, captured the experience of military nursing in a riveting way (Kalisch & Kalisch, 2004). Louisa May Alcott, who penned *Little Women*, also volunteered as a nurse briefly (Civil War Nurses, 2003; Williams-Evans, Jacob, & Carnegie, 2004). **Jane Woolsey**, who along with her sister served on the Union side of the war, wrote of her experiences prolifically, highlighting the inconsistencies in care due to lack of standards and training. Following the war, Woolsey and her sisters would be instrumental in developing nursing education.

Post-Civil War

Integration of African Americans into nursing did not occur readily or easily. However, **Mary Eliza Mahoney** graduated from the New England Hospital for Women and Children in 1879, where she had previously worked in a variety of menial roles. Mahoney was one of only four to successfully complete the program, which had admitted forty-two students. Active in the National Association of Colored Graduate Nurses, Mahoney delivered the opening comments at the first convention, and she also served the organization as chaplain. Following graduation, Mahoney worked as a private-duty nurse, finally directing an orphanage on Long Island, NY. The Mary Mahoney award is given by the ANA to nurses contributing to interracial harmony, and Mahoney is a member of the NA Nursing Hall of Fame (Bois, 1997; ANA, 2007).

The next major shift in American nursing occurred in conjunction with the Spanish-American War (see Figures 3-2a and 3-2b). As nursing schools now were producing truly trained nurses, only these graduates were accepted into the military; however, need superseded this requirement, and the military began to accept informally trained applicants (Keeling, 2001). This cadre of nurses provided the beginnings of the **Army Nurse Corps** in 1901, a rich tradition that continues to the present day.

At the turn of the century, **Lillian Wald** established the Henry Street Settlement House in New York City to provide health education, disease prevention, and primary care for infants. However, patients did not have to come to the house; the nurses went to them. This house established the framework for public health nursing throughout the United States (Williams-Evans, Jacob, & Carnegie, 2005). Wald eventually went on to develop public-health courses for nurses at Columbia University (Catalano, 2006). Working with Wald was **Lavinia Dock**, who hypothesized that poverty and squalid environment contributed to health problems (Catalano, 2006). Dock passionately worked to gain suffrage for women and later wrote a text on nursing (Kalisch & Kalisch, 2004).

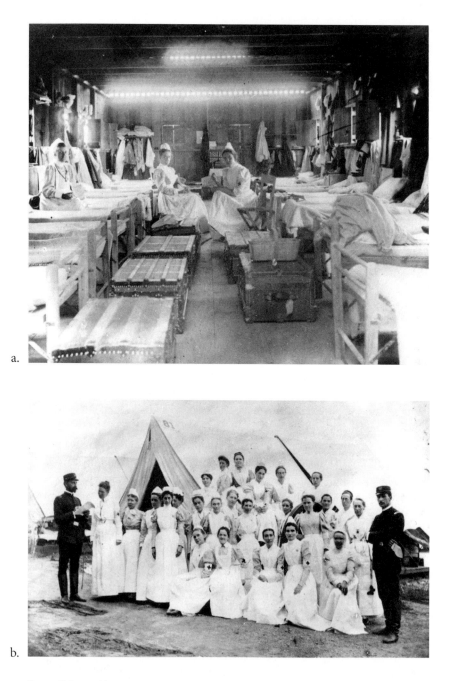

Figure 3-2a and b

These two historical photos of nurses in the Spanish-American War (1898) depict early images of the first truly trained American nurses. 3-2a: U.S. Army. Sternberg General Hospital, Camp Thomas, Chickamauga, GA, "Dormitory C," and 3-2b: The New York Nurses, Sternberg General Hospital, Camp Thomas, Chickamauga, Georgia. *(Photos courtesy of the U.S. Army Center for Military History.)*

Internet Exercise 3-1	Poverty and underserved populations remain a major problem in every community today. 1. Identify the areas and populations of poverty where you are. 2. What is being done to provide health care to the underserved and poor in your area? How is your school involved? How are you involved? 3. Learn more about poverty at http://www.catholiccharitiesusa.org. Click on the "Poverty Campaign" heading. Reflect upon what you have learned and how nursing can help individually and collectively.

World War I and the Great Depression

Nursing again paradoxically benefited from the onset of a war. For the first time, nurse anesthetists participated in front-line surgeries, and over 20,000 nurses ultimately served during the conflict (Oermann, 1997). The need for these nurses resulted in a national recruitment effort organized by the Committee on Nursing under the auspices of the Council of National Defense. In addition, the committee conducted Red Cross training to maintain nursing care on the home front and ultimately established the Army School of Nursing (Keeling, 2001).

In 1921, Congress passed the **Sheppard-Towner Act**, in response to the need to protect women and children. Public health nurses used these funds to promote the health of womenw and infants (Williams-Evans, Jacob, & Carnegie, 2005). Figure 3-3 shows a student nurse and a Junior League volunteer weighing a baby, possibly a result of the effects of the Sheppard-Towner

Figure 3-3

A student nurse and a Junior League volunteer weigh a baby in 1929. *(Photo courtesy of Touro Infirmary Archives, New Orleans, LA.)*

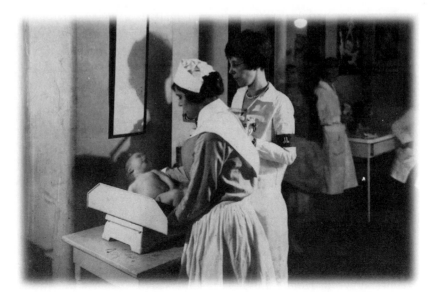

Act. The **Frontier Nursing Service**, founded by Mary Breckenridge, took public-health services to the most rural areas of southeastern Kentucky. The importance of Breckinridge's work exceeds the impact on the lives of the recipients of her care, for she exhaustively documented the impact of her community health project, and proved that even in the most dire conditions, nursing can positively impact the health of a community (Stanhope & Lancaster, 2004).

The stock market crash in 1929 marks the onset of the Great Depression, during which the global economy suffered severely. Millions of American men and women suffered from unemployment and the concomitant inability to provide the fundamental needs of their family members. Roosevelt's social initiatives resulting in the Social Security Act (SSA) of 1935 created numerous employment opportunities for nurses as the government became a significant employer of nurses (Catalano, 2006). The monies from the SSA provided additional care for women and children, and most nursing care transitioned into hospital settings at this time (Williams-Evans, Jacob, & Carnegie, 2005).

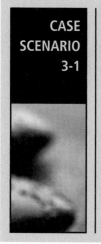

CASE SCENARIO 3-1

For this activity, you are one of the nurses working with a faith-based organization to develop a health care clinic for an underserved population in your area. An individual who opposes this work states that "nurses don't know how to do this kind of work" and continues with the comment "it should be left to physicians and politicians to manage health care problems."

CASE ANALYSIS

1. Prepare a professional letter for the local paper outlining nursing's history with the underserved.

2. Develop a mission statement for the clinic based on ideas found in nursing's history of serving the underserved.

3. Prepare a briefing for your congressional representative regarding nursing activity in the political arena.

World War II

The nature of the attack on Pearl Harbor in December of 1941 galvanized American sentiment toward the war in Europe and Asia, so when President Roosevelt declared war, the citizenry was eager to serve. This included nurses, and while the armed forces had the nurses needed, civilians were left with inadequate or undertrained care. However, due to the heroic efforts of nurses during the war, the military recognized nurses as an essential part of the service, granting them officer status. Colonel Julie O. Filkke was appointed the superintendent of the Army Nurse Corps and was the first woman to attain the rank of colonel (Deloughery, 1998). One source of nurses included those nurses who were no longer in the workforce. The 1942 Labor-Federal Security Agency Appropriation Act funded refresher courses for these nurses to reenter the workforce, in addition to supporting increased enrollment for entry-level programs and facilitating graduate programs in particular fields (Beebe, 2007).

Mid-Century

After WWII, when the men returned home, many women happily returned to homemaking activities. Domestic prosperity abounded, and the baby boom of that era has implications for health care today as those babies age. The Korean conflict reinforced the perception of nurses as valuable members of the military health care team, and strategies developed to treat the wounded soldiers translated into exciting developments in trauma care at home. Further, the advent of widespread antibiotic use meant the prevention of many deaths, but these advantages required additional nursing care.

The advent of defibrillation and advances in cardiology medications necessitated the development of intensive coronary care. These developments created a new specialty branch of nursing practice. Additional education was required for these nurses to use the technology and medications (Keeling, 2001). However, passage of the **Hill-Burton Act** in 1946 exerted one of the largest influences on nursing during the period. This act provided funding to build hospital facilities and for states to plan public health care facilities based on needs assessments (Beebe, 2007). In 1953, Congress passed legislation establishing Medicare and Medicaid, confirming a social commitment to ensuring health care for the elderly and infirm populations (Hood & Leddy, 2003).

Regretfully, nursing was not exempt from the racial intolerance that existed during the times. African-American nurses had been barred from joining the American Nurses Association and had created the National Association of Colored Graduate Nurses (NAGCN). This organization advocated for full membership rights for African Americans. While some northern states had dropped this restriction, southern states persisted in the segregation of African Americans. Indeed, hospitals continued to have separate floors for white and black patients and segregated the nurses as well as the patients. Insensitive comments at the Atlantic City conference in 1946 energized the NAGCN to develop a mechanism to join ANA directly, thus avoiding state membership (Carnegie, 1995).

The war in Vietnam created new opportunities for associate-degree-prepared nurses previously unavailable in the military. Due to medical unit self-contained transportable hospitals (MUST), nurses were near the front lines, resulting in nursing casualties (Catalano, 2006). Further, the women's movement in the 1970s caused nurses to begin to advocate for adequate reimbursement for services. Nurses also began to pursue advanced practice preparation, and nurse practitioners began advanced practice upon successful completion of certification examinations.

Spiraling health care costs resulted in drastic efforts to control costs in the 1980s. One of the first federal efforts focused on the development of **Diagnostic Related Groups**, or DRGs. Whereas services were formally reimbursed based on resources consumed, the DRG allotted a "reasonable" fee for treating a diagnosis. These fees comprised all the compensation a hospital received, regardless of length of stay or resources used (Hood & Leddy, 2003). Hospitals and nurses scrambled to streamline care, and clinical pathways developed guidelines to ensure a cost-efficient, yet thorough, plan of care to facilitate discharge. Home health services became essential as sicker patients received earlier discharges, creating another specialized branch of nursing that required a unique skill set.

During the late '90s and at the beginning of the 21st century, additional efforts at managing health care costs resulted in managed care and **health maintenance organizations** (HMOs). These entities intended to promote wellness, shorten hospital stays, and move care to external settings as much as possible. HMOs achieve these outcomes by paying physicians for caring for patients regardless of the extent of services required. In other words, a physician accepts a patient and an annual fee whether the patient is never seen or requires weekly visits. **Managed care** is a system designed to constrain health care costs and improve quality and access to services (Jecker, 1998). While this idea has obvious merit, as patients were encouraged to assume responsibility for their own health, many services began to be offered on an outpatient basis. Further, patients began to leave hospitals more quickly as home health agencies assumed the role of providing less costly care. For the first time, hospital administrations downsized nursing services. However, facilities such as outpatient surgery centers offered more attractive working hours, and many nurses happily transferred to these environments. Many times, this left nurses working with insufficient staff to meet the demands of a higher acuity population. Park (2003) studied 61 Illinois hospitals in the mid '90s and found a significant relationship between managed care and nurse staffing levels. As the number of managed-care patients increased, nursing positions decreased.

This form of monitoring health care also had a negative impact on relationships between primary health care providers and patients. As the HMOs began to emphasize rapid turnover of patients, many patients felt as thought they did not have sufficient time with physicians during office visits or were not given adequate time to recover in hospitals. One issue became the length of stay after delivering a baby. Women could be discharged less than 24 hours after giving birth. This led to legislation prohibiting "drive through deliveries." As recently as 2007, Congress considered a bill prohibiting discharge less than 48 hours following mastectomies.

Overall, managed care provided a mix of challenges to nursing. New career paths opened in outpatient services, home health, and managed care nurses who help provide oversight to the process. For hospitals, patients remaining in the hospital were far sicker, and fewer nursing staff remained to care for them.

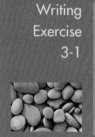

Writing
Exercise
3-1

Reflect over the increasing costs of health care and the nursing shortage.

1. What are some factors driving these forces?

2. How could nurses help control costs?

3. What threats and opportunities affect nursing as cost-control measures are put in place?

THE PRESENT

For a snapshot of the historical events affecting nursing, refer to Figure 3-4. Turning attention to the present, it is clear that nursing continues to face a number of challenges. The babies born during the boom are now entering retirement, and with the advent of the Internet, these consumers are well informed and demand high-quality care at bargain prices. In the context of this rising demand, the current nursing shortage is predicted to worsen, with the Health Resources

Figure 3-4
Events Affecting
Nursing Practice.
*(LoBiondo-Wood &
Haber (2006); Polit &
Hungler (2004); Burns
& Grove (2007);
Williams-Evans, Jacob,
& Carnegie (2005).)*

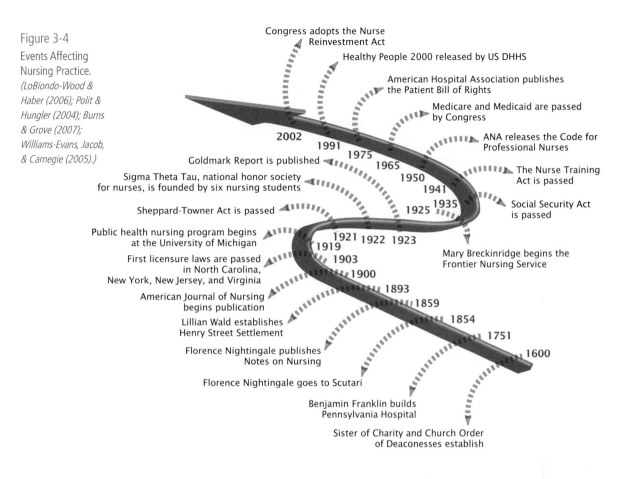

Congress adopts the Nurse Reinvestment Act

Healthy People 2000 released by US DHHS

American Hospital Association publishes the Patient Bill of Rights

Medicare and Medicaid are passed by Congress

ANA releases the Code for Professional Nurses

The Nurse Training Act is passed

Social Security Act is passed

Mary Breckinridge begins the Frontier Nursing Service

Goldmark Report is published

Sigma Theta Tau, national honor society for nurses, is founded by six nursing students

Sheppard-Towner Act is passed

Public health nursing program begins at the University of Michigan

First licensure laws are passed in North Carolina, New York, New Jersey, and Virginia

American Journal of Nursing begins publication

Lillian Wald establishes Henry Street Settlement

Florence Nightingale publishes Notes on Nursing

Florence Nightingale goes to Scutari

Benjamin Franklin builds Pennsylvania Hospital

Sister of Charity and Church Order of Deaconesses establish

2002 1991 1975 1965 1950 1941 1935 1925 1921 1922 1923 1919 1903 1900 1893 1859 1854 1751 1600

and Services Administration (2007) predicting a shortfall of over 1 million nurses by 2020. A number of initiatives to improve diversity among the nursing workforce have met with some success, and Johnson & Johnson developed a very effective advertising campaign to increase nursing school enrollments during the early part of the 21st century.

Despite dire predictions, nursing remains a dynamic and exciting profession. If the profession will speak with a united voice, much will be accomplished to care for the poor, underserved, and infirm.

EDUCATION

Prior to Nightingale, little formal education existed for nurses. Extant education occurred as primarily apprenticeship learning, and these programs were located in the convents of Catholic nuns, such as those developed by the Sisters of Charity in 1600 (Catalano, 2006). The sisters devoted themselves to the betterment of the poor and uneducated, and nursing clearly addresses both of these needs. Due to the teaching style used, education occurred in the illness setting, and learning focused on tasks and observation skills. Early textbooks appeared in these schools.

Following Nightingale's success in the Crimea, she returned to England in 1856, where she founded the Nightingale School and Home for Nurses on the grounds of St. Thomas Hospital. The one-year program, supervised by Mrs. Sarah Wardroper, consisted of apprenticeship learning, although some lectures were given (Florence Nightingale Museum Trust, 2003). The following year, Nightingale established a school for midwifery at King's College Hospital. The mission of these schools was to prepare nurses to educate other nurses by establishing new schools of nursing. Admission standards included moral character as well as physical and emotional attributes (Maggs, 1983). By 1873, Nightingale nurses had arrived in the United States, founding schools of nursing in Massachusetts General Hospital, Bellevue, and New Haven Hospital (Williams-Evans, Jacob, & Carnegie, 2005).

Nursing Education in the United States

The nursing workforce in the United States consisted of apprenticed learners as seen in the Revolutionary and Civil Wars. However, lessons learned from the Civil War and the activism of such women as the Woolsey sisters created an impetus toward formal nursing education, and in 1873, Georgeanna Woolsey participated in the founding of the Connecticut Training School for Nurses (Kalisch & Kalisch, 2004). The Johns Hopkins School of Nursing opened in 1889, led by **Isabel Hampton Robb**. Robb's progressive ideas facilitated improving the status of professional nursing (Taylor, 2007). By 1910, entry into practice required completion of high school, training, and registration (Williams-Evans, Jacob, & Carnegie, 2005).

Isabel Hampton Robb became a vocal advocate of moving nursing education into academic settings in the latter half of the 19th century. Robb believed professional nurses should incorporate theoretical concepts into care provision, and she advocated learning these concepts in an academic setting. Robb operationalized her beliefs at the Illinois Training School for Nurses and later at Johns Hopkins. These schools offered academics in addition to apprenticeships, marking them as unusual for their time.

As discussed earlier in this chapter, the Spanish-American War marked the first time the U.S. Army used an educated nursing workforce, despite the fact that the demand quickly exceeded the supply of these nurses (Beebe, 2007). Annie Goodrich developed a Camp School for Nurses at Vassar to help address this shortage (Catalano, 2006). The program lasted 2 years and was open only to students who had already completed college. The 435 graduates received a commission in the Army Reserves and committed to respond to the needs of the service. Though successful, the school closed when WWI ended (Snodgrass, 1999; Stanhope & Lancaster, 2004).

The concomitant influx of immigrants from Europe around the turn of the century accelerated the development of hospitals in order to meet the health care needs of the expanding population. The paucity of educated nurses spurred these institutions to develop schools of nursing, not only for the development of future employees but a cheap labor force supplied by nursing students. Apprentice learning methodology remained the primary teaching style (Hood & Leddy, 2001). In 1903, four states passed laws establishing standards of education as well as optional licensure for nurses (Shannon, 1975). All the states did not require licensure until the 1940s (Taylor, 2007).

Hampton Robb further aided nursing education by creating the American Society of Superintendents of Training Schools for Nurses, the forerunner of the National League for Nursing (Cristy, 1969). The inception of the **National League for Nursing (NLN)** in 1912 represented a major event in nursing education. The NLN has advocated for standards of excellence among schools of nursing since its inception. The NLN has evolved into a political force on behalf of nurse educators and students. Further, the NLN oversees accreditation of nursing programs at all levels by the National League for Nursing Accrediting Commission (NLNAC), sponsors research from individual studies to multi-site work into educational pedagogy, and disseminates evidence-based nursing practices to faculty via seminars and written publications.

In 1918, the testimony of **Mary Adelaide Nutting** to the Rockefeller Foundation created the impetus for a closer examination of nursing education (Tone, 1999). The 1923 report on nursing and nursing education in the United States, also known as the **Goldmark Report**, discouraged hospital-based nursing education, calling for higher educational standards and relocating professional nursing education into university settings (Goldmark, J., 1923; Nichols, 2001). One impetus for this recommendation was the need for nursing leadership from within the profession, and advocates for university-based education felt that inclusion of more classical elements of education could help develop this leadership. The University of Minnesota began the first baccalaureate nursing programs in 1909, and many others began soon after (Conley, 1973). Although the program lasted 3 years, and the College of Medicine administered the program, the movement of the educational role from the hospital to the academic setting represents a major event in nursing education (Kalisch & Kalisch, 1995). Nursing has still not identified a single educational level of entry into practice, resulting in issues still being debated today. Yale University founded the first independent school of nursing in 1924, led by Dean Annie W. Goodrich.

Learning from the lessons of the Spanish-American War, the Council of National Defense established a Committee on Nursing early in WWI. This committee stressed the importance of educated nurses in army facilities, and the committee's responsibility was to supply these nurses. The Army School of Nursing resulted from these efforts, and intensive national recruiting for the school ensued (Dock & Stewart, 1920). This initiative resulted in an increase in the Army Nurse Corps from 400 at the beginning of the war to over 21,000 nurses by the end (Connelly, 2004; Catalano, 2006).

During the Depression, many schools of nursing foundered. These failures may be attributed to two factors: lack of job opportunities for graduates and inability to afford tuition for potential students. Faculty in these facilities no doubt endured hardships, although literature supporting this supposition is not available. However, as the depression eased, and Congress passed social initiatives including the Social Security Act, a nursing shortage recurred, and the need for production of nurses resumed.

Writing
Exercise
3-2

For this activity, you are a historical researcher. You have a unique opportunity to interview any nurse from the past of American nursing.

1. Whom would you choose to interview? Why this particular nurse? Discuss this person's influence in how you will practice nursing.

2. Prepare a list of questions you would like to ask.

During WWII, the U.S. Congress approved the **Nurse Training Act**, sponsored by Francis Payne Bolton of Ohio. This legislation mandated an expedited education program for nurses (Willever-Farr & Parascandola, 1994). Program length shrank to 24–30 months from 36, and at times even less (Blitzkreig Baby, 2006b). In exchange for agreeing to serve for the entirety of the war, students received an education, financial support, and guaranteed employment upon graduation. The program, known as the **Cadet Nurse Corps** (CNC), was highly successful with 1,125 of 1,300 nursing programs participating by the close of the initiative (Blitzkrieg Baby, 2006a). Figure 3-5 is a historical 1942 photo of representatives of the Army Nurse Corps meeting in Washington to discuss recruiting of army nurses. The Nurse Training Act also prohibited discrimination on the basis of race, creed, or sex. Men began to reconsider nursing, and the corps set aside 56 positions for black nurses (Williams-Evans, Jacob, & Carnegie, 2005). By the end of the war, 3,000 African Americans enrolled, due to action by the National Association of Colored Graduate Nurses (Willever-Farr & Parascandola, 1994).

Schools of nursing that participated in the CNC directive faced few requirements. The major criteria concerned accreditation and affiliation with American College of Surgeon hospitals. However, lack of staff and facilities created a concern for many programs. The CNC supplied funds to participating programs and participation in the CNC helped solve shortcomings in many programs (Willever-Farr & Parascandola, 1994). The CNC exerted a significant influence on the move from nurses' "training" to nurses' "education" and promoted using nurses to lecture on disease processes rather than physicians.

The flux of nurses into the military highlighted inconsistencies among nursing school curricula. As nurses from different locales attempted to perform the same duties, disparity in preparation

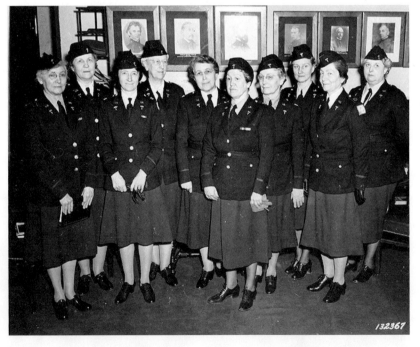

Figure 3-5
Representatives of the Army Nurse Corps from the nine Army Corps Areas meet in Washington to discuss recruiting of army nurses, April 1942. *(Courtesy of the U.S. Army Center of Military History.)*

became evident. In 1948, the **Brown Report** identified nursing education as a pivotal issue in the nursing shortage, and the author called for the examination of every school and for periodic reexaminations to ensure standards remained intact. This controversial report spurred the NLN to begin the accreditation process of schools of nursing. Temporary accreditation status between 1952 and 1957 purposed to help substandard schools rise to the challenge of adequate nursing education. Despite an overall decrease in the number of schools, those remaining offered more consistent curricula while meeting national requirements (Kalisch & Kalisch, 2004).

Following the war, a shortage of nurses persisted; the American Hospital Association documented 22,486 vacant registered nurse positions. Numerous programs to recruit students into nursing appeared around the country, notably in Alabama, Boston, and Chicago (Kalisch & Kalisch, 2004). Causes of the shortage included the return of women to homemaking, an aging population along with the baby boom, and increasing specialization of nursing practice (Catalano, 2006).

To help compensate for this profound shortage of nurses, the **associate-degree nurse** began to appear in 1952 (Nichols, 2001). The Teachers College at Columbia University began the first program directed by Louis McManus. The stated purposes of the program focused on moving nurses into the practice area more expeditiously while facilitating the transition of professional nursing education into an academic environment (Kalisch & Kalisch, 1995). McManus conducted a study using seven community colleges to determine the effectiveness of this new program. After five years, these students had a higher success rate on the board examination than other program types, head nurses confirmed they were adequately prepared, and the students expressed satisfaction with their preparation. Diploma programs began to decrease in number, while there were more ADN graduates than BSN graduates by the 1960s (Catalano, 2006).

The Nurse Training Act of WWII furthered the precedent for governmental assistance in providing a nursing workforce. In 1964, Congress passed H.R. 10042, a bill providing $283 million over five years. An inequitable division of money designated for associate degree versus baccalaureate education created more dissention between the two camps, and in 1965, the American Nurses Association position paper on Nursing Education appeared. This paper clearly states that baccalaureate education is the gateway to professional nursing, a position reinforced by the National League for Nursing position statement of 1982. Nevertheless, associate degree programs continue to provide 60% of entry level graduate nurses annually (Mahaffey, 2002).

In the 1980s, education of registered nurses remained divided at approximately 20.1% diploma programs, 51.8% associate-degree programs, and 28.1% baccalaureate programs (Kalisch & Kalisch, 2004). However, enrollments began to decline, and once again, a shortage of nurses ensued. A proposal for Registered Care Technologists by the AMA in the late 1980s failed largely due to unified nursing opposition to the proposal (Schorr & Kennedy, 1999). The movement of health care to the outpatient setting caused nursing educators to reinforce public health content in the curriculum as well as inclusion of learning activities outside the hospital setting. The onset of AIDS as well as increases in other blood-borne infections accentuated the urgency of educating professional nurses in community settings.

In the early '90s, troubled economic conditions in the U.S. caused many women to reenter the workforce, and enrollment in nursing schools increased, largely due to the job security nurses enjoy. Also, during this decade, the **American Association of Colleges of Nursing** began, positioning itself as the voice of baccalaureate and higher nursing education. Although the organization began in 1969, it became an accrediting agency for BSN and higher programs in 1996. The agency also provides strategies for faculty development and recruitment, and analyzes aggregate data on student and faculty information.

Unfortunately, nursing faculty shortages began to become common, restricting the number of students a program can admit. Faculty shortage continues to plague the profession. In 2004, the American Association of Colleges of Nursing found that nearly 16,000 qualified applicants had been denied admission due to lack of faculty (AACN, 2004). Both NLN and AACN have undertaken initiatives to increase the number and qualifications of available faculty. IN 2005, the NLN published the Core Competencies of Nurse Educators, outlining what expert faculty are doing across the nation. Finally, educators have accepted the challenge to develop a science of nursing education. Many exciting projects are underway to ensure that learners are receiving quality education with evidence-based methodology.

Figure 3-6 recounts the important dates in nursing education discussed in this section.

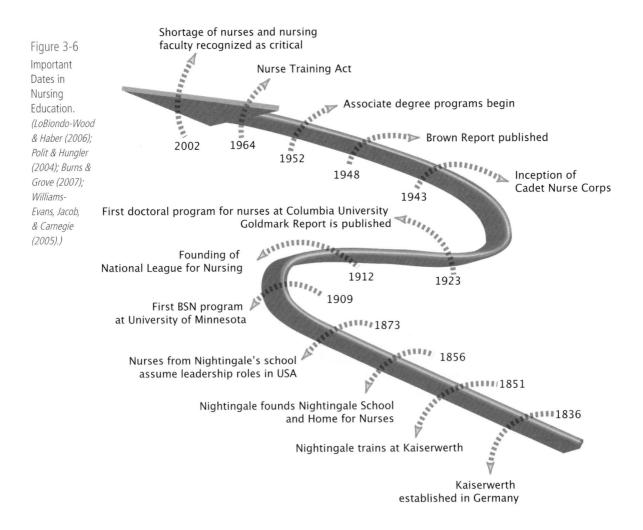

Figure 3-6
Important Dates in Nursing Education. (LoBiondo-Wood & Haber (2006); Polit & Hungler (2004); Burns & Grove (2007); Williams-Evans, Jacob, & Carnegie (2005).)

Shortage of nurses and nursing faculty recognized as critical

Nurse Training Act

Associate degree programs begin

Brown Report published

Inception of Cadet Nurse Corps

2002

1964

1952

1948

1943

First doctoral program for nurses at Columbia University
Goldmark Report is published

Founding of National League for Nursing

First BSN program at University of Minnesota

Nurses from Nightingale's school assume leadership roles in USA

Nightingale founds Nightingale School and Home for Nurses

Nightingale trains at Kaiserwerth

Kaiserwerth established in Germany

1912

1923

1909

1873

1856

1851

1836

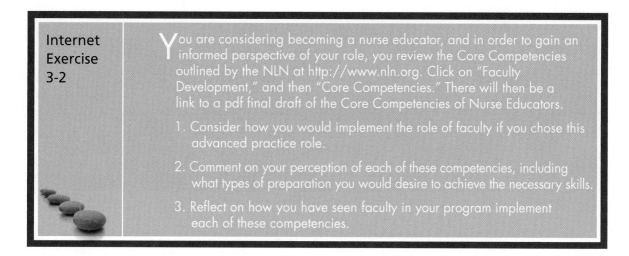

Internet Exercise 3-2

You are considering becoming a nurse educator, and in order to gain an informed perspective of your role, you review the Core Competencies outlined by the NLN at http://www.nln.org. Click on "Faculty Development," and then "Core Competencies." There will then be a link to a pdf final draft of the Core Competencies of Nurse Educators.

1. Consider how you would implement the role of faculty if you chose this advanced practice role.

2. Comment on your perception of each of these competencies, including what types of preparation you would desire to achieve the necessary skills.

3. Reflect on how you have seen faculty in your program implement each of these competencies.

RESEARCH

As with most aspects of nursing, the birth of nursing research can be traced to Florence Nightingale. After exhausting days of organizing care for the soldiers in the Crimea, Florence would document pages of data, later developed into graphic displays to persuade others of the need for controlling disease in the war zone. Her accomplishments in statistics earned her an 1858 election into the Statistical Society, as well as honorary inclusion in the American Statistical Association. Further, Nightingale believed statistics to be a method of uncovering God's laws, and that humans are to discover these laws and then improve society accordingly (Nightingale Museum Trust, 1998). Nightingale's efforts were not restricted to the Crimean War, as she crusaded to improve public water supplies and sanitation using research methods (Palmer, 1977). *Notes on Nursing: What it is and what it is not*, Nightingale's primer on nursing care, was first published in 1859 and largely summarized her conclusions on nursing matters.

Following Nightingale, formal research centered on nursing education with minimal efforts aimed at actual nursing interventions or techniques. The *American Journal of Nursing* began publication in 1900 and began to publish case studies in the 1930s (LoBiondo & Wood, 2006). Studies in the 1940s continued to focus on nursing education due to the profound nursing shortage experienced during World War II. These efforts produced landmark reports such as the Goldmark Report, which criticized basing nursing education in hospital settings. The Brown Report encouraged the move of nursing education from the traditional hospital setting to the academic setting of a university (Polit & Beck, 2004). The Brown Report spawned numerous additional studies on nursing education (LoBiondo & Wood, 2006; Polit & Beck, 2004).

In the 1950s, the number of nurses with collegiate preparation fostered the proliferation of nursing research. Additional factors that spurred on the development of research activities include the establishment of a center for nursing research under the auspices of the army's research

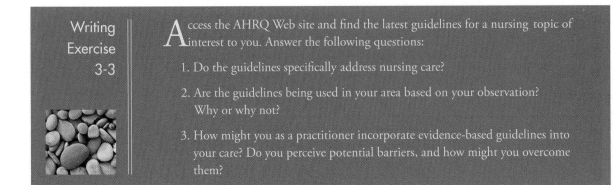

Access the AHRQ Web site and find the latest guidelines for a nursing topic of interest to you. Answer the following questions:

1. Do the guidelines specifically address nursing care?

2. Are the guidelines being used in your area based on your observation? Why or why not?

3. How might you as a practitioner incorporate evidence-based guidelines into your care? Do you perceive potential barriers, and how might you overcome them?

center at Walter Reed, development of governmental and private resources to fund research, and founding of the American Nurses' Foundation in 1955 (Polit & Beck, 2004). Nursing Research began publication in 1952 and remains a prestigious journal today. Also during the '50s, the American Nurses' Association sponsored a study to determine the characteristics and behaviors of nurses, and the results of the project helped determine policy for nurses' standards and qualifications.

In the 1960s, nursing research began to incorporate theoretical models and conceptual frameworks. While theory had existed for some time, nurses began to use theory as a paradigm for viewing problems and then testing those viewpoints with empirical data. This first step toward development of the science of nursing was pivotal, and began to spread beyond the United States (Polit & Beck, 2004). Research into the quality of care also began to develop, and the birth of critical-care units created myriad opportunities for research efforts (Burns & Grove, 2007). Particularly in the 1970s, the focus of research began to shift from education and nurses to how to provide client care. This time frame also witnessed the introduction of qualitative methodology in nursing research (Burns & Grove, 2007).

In the 1980s, the advent of additional doctoral programs created opportunities for enhanced focus on clinical research. Academic institutions founded centers for nursing research and, in 1985, Public Law 99-158 paved the way for the establishment of the National Center for Nursing Research (LoBiondo-Wood & Haber, 2006). Led by the ANA, the passage of this law heralded a major accomplishment for nursing research. The mission of the center was to increase funding for research into patient care topics and facilitate dissemination of these findings. Ably led by Dr. Ada Sue Hinshaw, this center became the **National Institute for Nursing Research** (NINR) in 1993. NINR may be found on the web at http://www.ninr.nih.gov. The reader is encouraged to peruse the site to discover research priorities and note the ways in which nursing research is improving the health and quality of life for the population.

Business initiatives in the 1970s created a public call for documentation of quality in health care as evidenced by outcomes. In 1989, the Agency for Health Care Policy and Research was founded to facilitate outcomes research for all health care practitioners, and in 1999, the agency underwent reorganization and was named the Agency for Health care Research and Quality.

This agency developed patient-care guidelines, which are evidence-based recommendations for patient care. AHRQ maintains a Web site to facilitate finding current guidelines for health care practitioners (http://www.ahrq.gov).

In the 1990s and early 2000s, the demand for evidence-based nursing, and an evidence base for health care in general, continued to grow. This era witnessed a growth from focusing on treatment of illness to prevention of illness and health promotion. (Burns & Grove, 2007). This growth created a need for additional journals focused on evidence-based practice along with increases in funding and calls for faculty involvement in research. Fortunately for learners, the National League for Nursing is also actively involved in developing a science for nursing education. No aspect of nursing is exempt from research, nor should anyone wish to be. The knowledge that one is providing the absolute best based on current knowledge is essential to quality practice and education.

Figure 3-7 provides an overview of some important dates in nursing research.

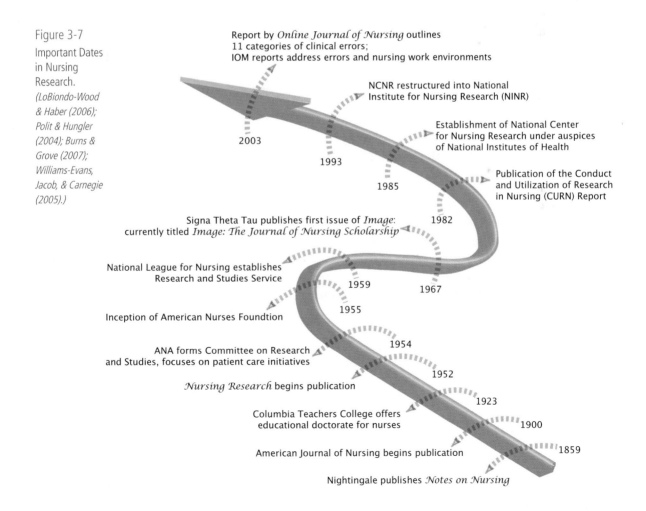

Figure 3-7
Important Dates
in Nursing
Research.
*(LoBiondo-Wood
& Haber (2006);
Polit & Hungler
(2004); Burns &
Grove (2007);
Williams-Evans,
Jacob, & Carnegie
(2005).)*

Report by *Online Journal of Nursing* outlines
11 categories of clinical errors;
IOM reports address errors and nursing work environments

NCNR restructured into National
Institute for Nursing Research (NINR)

Establishment of National Center
for Nursing Research under auspices
of National Institutes of Health

Publication of the Conduct
and Utilization of Research
in Nursing (CURN) Report

Signa Theta Tau publishes first issue of *Image*:
currently titled *Image: The Journal of Nursing Scholarship*

National League for Nursing establishes
Research and Studies Service

Inception of American Nurses Foundtion

ANA forms Committee on Research
and Studies, focuses on patient care initiatives

Nursing Research begins publication

Columbia Teachers College offers
educational doctorate for nurses

American Journal of Nursing begins publication

Nightingale publishes *Notes on Nursing*

2003
1993
1985
1982
1967
1959
1955
1954
1952
1923
1900
1859

SUMMARY

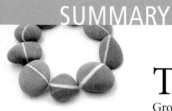

This chapter traced the roots of nursing practice, education, and research. The history of these three branches of nursing are inextricably intertwined, and this is as it should be. Growth in one area stimulates growth in another. Research and education should answer to practice; however, practice must inform researchers and educators whether the current initiatives are producing the results needed by practitioners. No nurse, regardless of practice area, can ever lose sight of the goal of our activities: the promotion of health, restoration of health to clients in a timely fashion, or preservation of choice and dignity in the dying process.

No occupation can be intelligently followed or correctly understood unless it is, at least to some extent, illumined by the light of history interpreted from the human standpoint.

–Lavinia Dock and Isabel M. Stewart

REFERENCES

AACN. (2006). *Nursing faculty shortage fact sheet.* Retrieved July 17, 2007, from http://www.aacn. nche.edu/Media/Backgrounders/facultyshortage. htm

BRITISH BROADCASTING CORPORATION. (n.d.). *Historic figures: Mary Seacole.* Retrieved July 20, 2007, from http://www.bbc.co.uk/history/historic_ figures/seacole_mary.shtml

BEEBE, L. H. (2007). History and evolution of nursing. In Pofliko, K., (Ed.), *Concepts of the nursing profession.* Clifton Park, NY: Delmar Cengage Learning.

BLITZKREIG BABY. (2006a). *Foundation of the Cadet Nurse Corps.* Retrieved July 3, 2007, from http://www.blitzkriegbaby.de.cnc.cnc1.htm

BLITZKREIG BABY. (2006b). *Requirements for joining.* Retrieved July 3, 2007, from http://www. blitzkriegbaby.de.cnc.cnc2.htm

BROWN, E. L. (1948). *Nursing for the future.* New York: Russell Sage Foundation.

BURNS, N., & GROVE, S. K. (2007). *Understanding nursing research: Building an evidence-based practice.* St. Louis: Saunders.

CARNEGIE, M. E. (1995). *The path we tread: Blacks in nursing: 1854–1994.* (3rd ed.). New York: National League for Nursing.

CATALONO, J. T. (2006). Historical perspectives. In Catalano, J., (Ed.), *Nursing now.* Philadelphia: F. A. Davis.

CIVIL WAR NURSES: THE ANGELS OF THE BATTLEFIELD. (2003). Retrieved June 18, 2007, from http://www.civilwarhome.com/civilwarnurses. htm

CONLEY, V. (1973). *Curriculum and instruction in nursing.* Boston: Little, Brown.

CONNELLY, C. A. (2004). Beyond social history: New approaches to understand the state of and the state in nursing history. *Nursing History Review, 12,* 5–24.

COOK, E. (1913). *The life of Florence Nightingale.* London: Macmillan & Co., Limited.

CRISTY, T. (1969). Portrait of a leader: Isabel Hampton Robb. *Nursing Outlook, 17*(1), 26–29.

D'ANTONIO, P. (2005). Nursing and history. *Nursing Inquiry, 12*(4), 241–242.

DELOUGHERY, G. L. (1998). *Issues and trends in nursing.* St. Louis: Mosby.

DOCK, L. L., & Stewart, I. M. (1920). *A short history of nursing.* New York: Putnam.

DOCK, L. L., & Stewart, I. M. (1938). *A short history of nursing* (4th ed). New York: Putnam.

ELLIS, J. R., & Hartley, C. L. (2004). *Nursing in today's world: Challenges, issues and trends* (8th ed). Philadelphia: J. B. Lippincott.

FLORENCE NIGHTINGALE MUSEUM TRUST. (1998). *The passionate statistician.* Retrieved July 3, 2007, from http://www.florence-nightingale. co.uk/stats.htm

FLORENCE NIGHTINGALE MUSEUM TRUST. (2003). *Florence Nightingale.* Retrieved July 5, 2007, from http://www.florence-nightingale.co.uk/flo2.htm

GOLDMARK, J. (1923). Nursing and nursing education in the United States: Report of the committee for the study of nursing education. New York: Macmillan. Reprint in Reverby, S. (Ed.), *The history of American nursing; Vol. 7.* New York: Garland Publishing.

HEALTH RESOURCES AND SERVICES ADMINISTRATION. (2007). *What is behind HRSA's projected supply, demand and shortage of registered nurses?* Retrieved July 20, 2007, from http://bhpr.hrsa.gov/healthworkforce/reports/nursing/rnbehindprojections/4.htm

HOOD, L. J., & Leddy, S. K. (2003). *Conceptual bases of professional nursing* (5th ed.). Philadelphia: Lippincott, Williams, & Wilkins.

JECKER, N. S. (1998). *Managed care: Ethical topic in medicine.* Retrieved March 11, 2008, from http://depts.washington.edu/bioethx/topics/manag.html

JOEL, L. A., & Kelly, L. J. (2002). *The nursing experience: Trends, challenges and transitions* (4th ed.). New York: McGraw-Hill.

KALISCH, P. A., & Kalisch, B. J. (1995). *The advance of American nursing* (3rd ed.). Philadelphia: J. B. Lippincott.

KALISCH, P. A., & Kalisch, B. J. (2004). *American nursing: A history* (4th ed.). Philadelphia: J. B. Lippincott, Williams, & Wilkins.

KEELING, A. W. (2001). Professional nursing comes of age—1859–2000. In K. K. Chitty, *Professional nursing: Concepts and challenges,* 3rd ed. Philadelphia: W. B. Saunders Co., pp. 1–32.

KREIS, S. (2000). Why study history? In *The history guide: A student's guide to the study of history.* Retrieved July 3, 2007, from http://www.historyguide.org/guide/study.html

LOBIONDO-WOOD, G., & Haber, J. (2006). The role of research in nursing. In G. LoBiondo-Wood & J. Haber (Eds.), *Nursing research: Methods and critical appraisal for evidence-based practice* (6th ed), pp. 5–26. St. Louis: Mosby.

MACLEAN, M. (2006). *Captain Sallie Tompkins: Angel of the Confederacy.* Retrieved July 20, 2007, from http://civilwarwomen.blogspot.com/2006/08/captain-sallie-tompkins-angel-of.html

MAGGS, C. (1983). *The origins of general nursing.* Dover, NH: Croom Helm.

MAHAFFEY, E. H. (2002). The relevance of associate degree nursing education: Past, present, future. *Online Journal of Issues in Nursing, 7*(2). Retrieved July 17, 2007, from http://www.nursingworld.org/ojin/topic18/tpc18_2.htm

NATIONAL LEAGUE FOR NURSING. (2005). *Core competencies of nurse educators with task statements.* Retrieved July 25, 2007, from http://www.nln.org/profdev/corecompetencies.pdf

NICHOLS, E. F. (2001). Educational patterns in nursing. In K. K. Chitty, *Professional nursing: Concepts and challenges,* 3rd ed. Philadelphia: W. B. Saunders Co., 33–63.

NIGHTINGALE, F. (1859). *Notes on nursing: What it is and what it is not.* Reprint, Philadelphia: J. B. Lippincott.

NURSES.INFO. (2007). *Men in nursing–historical.* Retrieved June 18, 2007, from http://www.nurses.info/history_men.htm

OERMANN, M. H. (1997). *Professional nursing practice.* Stamford, CT: Appleton and Lange.

PALMER, I. S. (1977). Florence Nightingale: Reformer, reactionary, researcher. *Nursing Research, 26*(2), 84–89.

PARK, C. (2003). *Causal relations among nursing staffing, managed care, and hospital productivity: Case study of Illinois hospitals 1992–1996.* Presented at meeting of AcademyHealth, 2003, abstract no. 920. Retrieved March 11, 2008, from http://gateway.nlm.nih.gob/MeetingAbstracts/ma?f=102275889/html

POLIT, D. F., & Beck, C. T. (2004). *Nursing research: Principles and methods* (7th ed). Philadelphia: Lippincott, Williams, & Wilkins.

SCHORR, T. M., & Kennedy, M. S. (1999). *One hundred years of American nursing.* New York: J. B. Lippincott.

SHANNON, M. L. (1975). Nurses in American history: Our first four licensure laws. *American Journal of Nursing (75),* 40–42.

SMALL, H. (1998). *Florence Nightingale: Avenging angel.* London: Constable.

SNODGRASS, M. E. (1999). *Historical encyclopedia of nursing.* Santa Barbara: ABC-CLIO.

STANHOPE, M., & Lancaster, J. (2004). *Community and public health nursing.* St. Louis: Mosby.

TAYLOR, A. S. (2007). *Educating the profession.* In K. Pofliko (Ed.), *Concepts of the nursing profession.* Clifton Park, NY: Delmar, Cengage Learning.

TONE, B. (1999). *Nursing 101: Nurse education saw many changes in last 100 years.* Retrieved July 17, 2007, from http://www.nurseweek.com/features/99-12/educate.html

WILLEVER-FARR, H., & Parascandola, J. (1994). The Cadet Nurse Corps, 1943–48. *Public Health Reports (109),* 455–457. Retrieved July 11, 2007, from http://lhncbc.nlm.nih.gov/apdb/phsHistory/resources/pdf/cadetnurse.pdf

WILLIAMS-EVANS, S. A., Jacob, S. R., & Carnegie, M. E. (2005). The evolution of professional nursing. In B. Cherry & S. Jacob (Eds.), *Contemporary nursing: Issues, trends, and management* (3rd ed). St. Louis: Elsevier.

CHAPTER 4

NURSING WORKFORCE ISSUES

SHARRON E. GUILLETT

PhD, RN, Associate Professor, Marymount University

None of us can do everything, but all of us can do something.

–Oscar Romero

LEARNING OBJECTIVES

At the completion of the chapter, the learner should be able to do the following:

1. Identify components of a healthy workplace.
2. Identify key recommendations of the Institute of Medicine report related to nursing work environments.
3. Identify current workforce issues facing nurses.
4. Describe organizational factors that affect recruiting and retaining an appropriate workforce.
5. Describe the relationship between nurse satisfaction and patient outcomes.
6. Describe the implications of working in and with a multicultural, multigenerational workforce.
7. Identify behaviors of colleagues and supervisors considered to be "uncivil."
8. Cite research related to the importance of ethical work environments.

KEY TERMS

Baby Boomers	Healthy Work Environment	Maintenance Nap
Bullying	Incivility	Moral Distress
Carefronting	Lateral Violence	Sleep Debt
Dichotomous Thinking	Learning Organizations	Sleep Deprivation
Generation X	Magnet Status	Traditionalists
Generation Y		

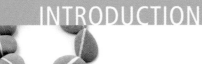

INTRODUCTION

Nurses work in stressful environments. Some stresses are related to the nature of the work itself, assuming responsibility for the well being of others. Some tensions are created by the way we are treated and treat each other as a result of real and perceived inequities in power, value, and respect. These artificial tensions have led to a culture of incivility and conflict that is so commonplace in the nursing workforce it is taken for granted as a way of being. Increasing numbers of nurses are leaving the workforce due to dissatisfaction with the work environment, and another large group of nurses is poised to retire. The workforce that remains will be increasingly multigenerational, multicultural, and of different genders and varied physical abilities. These individuals will be challenged to meet increasing demands with decreasing resources. Many employers, in an effort to put a sufficient workforce in place, are resorting to strategies that will create a number of new tensions for these nurses, such as mandating overtime, placing novice nurses in areas traditionally reserved for seasoned nurses, and increasing the use of agency nurses (Figure 4-1). This chapter will discuss these tensions and other workforce issues facing nurses in the 21st century.

THE NURSING WORKFORCE

Who makes up the nursing workforce? Exact numbers are difficult to ascertain because the number of licensed nurses includes nurses who are not actually working. Additionally, the data often combines nurses in administrative positions, advanced practice positions, and academic positions with nurses in clinical positions, so it is difficult to determine who is actually at the

Figure 4-1

The nursing environment can be stressful, and the anticipated nursing shortage is likely to create new tensions in the future.

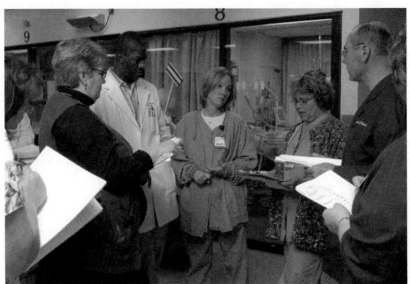

DELMAR/CENGAGE LEARNING

bedside. According to the National Council of State Boards (NCSBN, 2006) the number of licensed RNs in 2005 was about 3.3 million; however, the National Sample Survey of Registered Nurses (NSSRN) reported only 2.9 million nurses licensed in the U.S. in 2004 (Health Resources and Services Administration, 2004). Regardless of the statistics used, the current estimate of the actively working RN population in all settings is about 2.4 million. However, not all of them are working full time. The American Hospital Association (AHA) reported more than 116,000 vacant RN positions in 2007 (AHA, 2007). Not only is the shortage of RNs one of the critical issues facing nurses today, it also creates many of the other issues such as moral distress, incivility, and lateral violence.

Demographics

While males and minorities are increasing in numbers, the nursing workforce has been and continues to be primarily made up of white (88%) females (94%). According to the NSSRN (2004), males make up 5.7% of the nursing workforce, a figure that has not changed substantially over the past decade. One statistic that has changed dramatically is the level of educational preparation. Today the majority of the workforce has either an associate's degree (33%) or a bachelor's degree (34%), and 17% have either a master's degree or a doctorate. Interestingly, more males enter the profession with a bachelor's degree, more females with an associate's. This finding supports the notion that men entering the profession are nontraditional students, many of whom are changing careers (Smith, 2006).

As far as racial/ethnic categories are concerned, according to the NSSRN, 82% of nurses are white non-Hispanic. This statistic is difficult to report reliably, as people increasingly either fail to report a racial or ethnic classification or report belonging to more than one group. Comparisons to data prior to 2000 should be done cautiously, since prior to 2000 survey participants were forced to select one choice from a narrowly defined list of races/ethnicities, and after 2000 they were allowed to select all categories that referred to them. Figure 4-2 shows the racial/ethnic distribution of nurses compared to the general U.S. distribution. These figures illustrate that Black non-Hispanic and Hispanic groups are significantly underrepresented.

The workforce characteristic that is most worrisome is the "graying of the profession." This term refers to the fact that the profession is not attracting as many young applicants as it has in the past. RNs under 30 represent only 8% of the total RN population, compared to 25% just two decades ago (DHHS, 2003). The average age of practicing RNs is 47, which means that as the demand for services increases due to the aging patient population, the actual number of registered nurses able to provide care will decrease due to retirements. Additionally, it is possible that older nurses may simply not be able to perform direct patient-care services any longer. Direct patient care is physically challenging, and one may not have the stamina or the physical strength to perform nursing functions consistently during a twelve-hour shift, such as lifting patients, pulling patients up in their beds, or dealing with simultaneous emergencies.

Macintosh, Palumbo, and Rambur (2006) explored the notion of a "shadow workforce," a group of inactive nurses that could be reengaged through nurse reentry programs. Their research, although limited in scope, suggests that the overwhelming majority of inactive nurses are not interested in returning to practice. Respondents identified free reentry educational

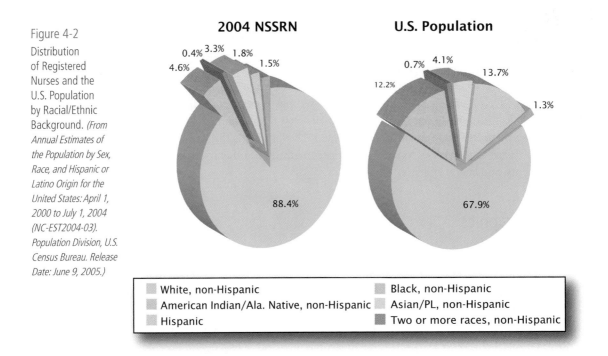

Figure 4-2
Distribution
of Registered
Nurses and the
U.S. Population
by Racial/Ethnic
Background. *(From
Annual Estimates of
the Population by Sex,
Race, and Hispanic or
Latino Origin for the
United States: April 1,
2000 to July 1, 2004
(NC-EST2004-03).
Population Division, U.S.
Census Bureau. Release
Date: June 9, 2005.)*

2004 NSSRN

0.4% 3.3% 1.8%
4.6% 1.5%
88.4%

U.S. Population

0.7% 4.1%
12.2% 13.7%
1.3%
67.9%

- White, non-Hispanic
- American Indian/Ala. Native, non-Hispanic
- Hispanic
- Black, non-Hispanic
- Asian/PL, non-Hispanic
- Two or more races, non-Hispanic

programs and ongoing development programs as key inducements for returning to practice. The expense of such programs coupled with the small numbers of persons willing to reenter led the authors to conclude that such efforts were unlikely to be cost effective. Without a continuous influx of new, younger nurses, the profession certainly will not meet America's future health care needs.

The Bernard Hodes Group and AMN Health Care conducted a study related to the aging nurse workforce titled the *Nursing Management Aging Workforce Survey* (Orlovsky, 2006). Almost 1,000 registered nurses were surveyed as to their projected retirement dates; more than 55% of respondents stated that they intended to retire between the years 2011 and 2020. At this point, it is too far into the future to predict just how long this mass exodus will last. The same concern exists for nursing faculty. According to Berlin & Sechrist (2002), between 200 and 300 nursing faculty retire annually. This is a serious concern in view of the fact that thousands of nursing students are turned away each year due to a shortage of faculty to teach them (Decker, et al., 2003). Delaying retirement will ease the problem in the short term, but long-range strategies are needed to increase the number of young doctorally prepared faculty (Kowalsi, Dalley, & Weigand, 2006).

THE INSTITUTE OF MEDICINE REPORT

In 2004 the Institute of Medicine released the report *Keeping Patients Safe: Transforming the Work Environment of Nurses*. This document presents the findings of the Committee on the Work Environment of Nurses and Patient Safety. It recognizes the "centrality" of nursing care in achieving positive patient outcomes and identifies several threats to the ability of nurses to provide that care: work hours, work spaces, workload, and work processes. The report concludes that **healthy work environments** are essential to quality outcomes and encourages health care organizations to become **learning organizations**, where nurses feel safe and participate in decisions about workflow and design.

HEALTHY WORK ENVIRONMENTS

What is a healthy work environment? According to the American Association of Critical Care Nurses (AACN), it is a place that is "safe, healing, humane and respectful of the rights, responsibilities and needs and contributions of patients, families, nurses and all healthcare professionals." (AACN, 2005, p. 6). The AACN developed six standards for creating healthy work environments that have been adopted as the basis for improving work environments across the world. The six standards address communication, collaboration, decision making, staffing, recognition, and leadership. Each standard has several critical elements attached to it that outline the structures, processes, and behaviors necessary for the standard to be achieved. For example, one of the critical elements associated with skilled communication is that all relevant perspectives will be invited and heard. The standards, along with their defining characteristics and elements, can be found at the AACN Web site (http://www.aacn.org).

Additional attributes of positive work environments identified by the International Council of Nurses (ICN) (Bauman, 2007) include:

- Policy frameworks focused on recruitment and retention.
- Strategies for continuing education and upgrading.
- Adequate employee compensation.
- Sufficient equipment and supplies.

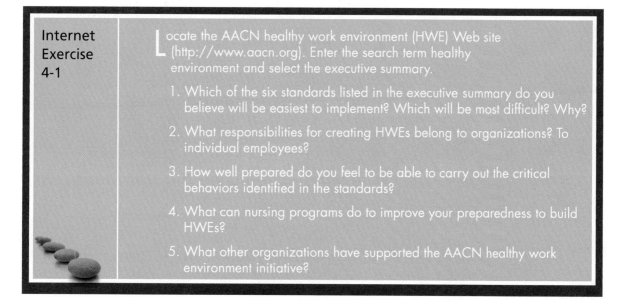

Internet Exercise 4-1

Locate the AACN healthy work environment (HWE) Web site (http://www.aacn.org). Enter the search term healthy environment and select the executive summary.

1. Which of the six standards listed in the executive summary do you believe will be easiest to implement? Which will be most difficult? Why?

2. What responsibilities for creating HWEs belong to organizations? To individual employees?

3. How well prepared do you feel to be able to carry out the critical behaviors identified in the standards?

4. What can nursing programs do to improve your preparedness to build HWEs?

5. What other organizations have supported the AACN healthy work environment initiative?

THE ISSUES

As mentioned earlier in the chapter, there are a number of issues confronting nurses today that have a significant impact on the ability of organizations to provide safe, quality care. Issues related to the shortage of qualified nurses, managing an increasingly diverse workforce, moral distress, and lateral violence must be resolved in order to meet the growing demand for service.

The Shortage

The National Center for Health Workforce Analysis (2003) projected that the need for registered nurses would continue to grow from the need of 2 million in the year 2000 to 2.8 million in the year 2020. Buerhaus, Staiger, and Auerbach (2008) predict that this need will not be met, and that the nursing shortage will triple the current national rate of 8.5%, resulting in an estimated shortage of 500,000 registered nurses by 2025.

The shortage of nurses in acute-care settings is not a new phenomenon. To the contrary, until recently nursing shortages have been viewed as cyclical and amenable to standard organizational remedies such as pay increases and sign-on bonuses. However, the current shortage is unprecedented in scope, character, and duration (Unruh, L., & Fottler, M., 2007). This prolonged, perhaps now chronic, shortage has created organizational cultures, climates, and processes that are not only detrimental to nurses and the clients they serve, but in all likelihood contribute to the declining numbers of nurses recruited and retained. In fact, according to a 2006 survey of American hospitals, nearly 50% of hospital Chief Executive Officers (CEOs) reported that they were experiencing increased difficulty in recruiting RNs to their health care organizations (AHA, 2006). Long-term-care facilities and home health agencies also reported close to 100,000 vacant positions and predict that the shortage of nurses will reach crisis proportions by 2020 (Anonymous, 2005).

| Writing Exercise 4-1 | The predicted shortage of nurses is partly due to the lack of younger nurses in the pipeline to replace nurses that retire. How can we make the profession more appealing to young nurses? To help you think about this, make a list of the factors that influenced your decision to become a nurse. List them in order of importance. Share your list with others in the class. Are the lists similar? Did something on another person's list surprise you? How might this information be used to market nursing more effectively? |

Incivility and Lateral Violence

The concept of workplace **incivility** was first introduced by Anderson & Pearson (1999, p. 457), who defined it as "low intensity deviant behavior with ambiguous intent to harm the target in violation of workplace norms for mutual respect." This differs from workplace aggression where the intent to harm is no longer ambiguous. The fact that there is no clear intent to harm does not mean that incivility is not harmful. To the contrary, lateral violence affects both physical and psychological well-being and may cause trouble sleeping, anxiety, depression, hypertension, apathy, poor concentration, low self-esteem, indecisiveness, and impaired personal relationships.

Incivility in nursing is not a new occurrence. In fact concepts such as rudeness, disrespect, and the notion that nurses "eat their young" have appeared in the literature for decades (Bartholomew, 2006; Farrell, 1999; Krebs, 1976; Smythe, 1984). What places the issue front and center today is the fact that incivility leads to conflict and nurse dissatisfaction, and there is strong evidence that nurse dissatisfaction is correlated to negative patient outcomes. (Hutton, 2006; Lin & Liang, 2007). Furthermore there are economic consequences when nurses work for long periods in hostile environments (Ramos, 2006). These include decreased productivity and quality of care, increased errors, increased absenteeism, higher turnover rates, and increased costs (Johnson & Indvik, 2001).

Many nurses report that they have been victims of verbal abuse from physicians, patients, and families, but sadly, more often than not this abuse comes from fellow nurses (Rowe and Sherlock, 2005). When hostility is expressed between colleagues it is referred to as **lateral violence**. Lateral violence takes many forms, from simple incivility (e.g., rudeness, talking about someone behind their back, refusing to speak to someone, spreading rumors, being uncooperative) to actual physical attacks. When interpersonal psychological violence is motivated by the desire to have power over another person it is referred to as **bullying**. This form of violence can be lateral as well as hierarchical. According to Ramos (2006), one in six workers have experienced lateral violence on the job, and 70% of nurses who feel bullied leave the workplace, 37% of whom claim that they were unfairly evaluated by supervisors who manipulated the appraisal system.

A number of theories have been suggested for why nursing environments are particularly susceptible to the development of lateral violence. Some suggest that nursing is a discipline with a strict hierarchy forcing those at the bottom to feel powerless and strike out at peers to relieve tension rather than expressing dissatisfaction up the chain of command (Leiper, 2005). Others point to a history of oppression dating back to nursing schools when students were treated as second-class citizens forced to work long hours caring for patients and scrubbing floors, receiving little respect from physicians and the public (Farrell, 2001). The theory is that the oppressed students, once out of school and in practice, perpetuate their oppression on new graduates. Another theory is that those individuals who endure the stresses of nursing practice tend to be tough minded with dominant personalities, and that when a number of dominant personalities are in the same work group there is bound to be conflict. Conflict in and of itself is not a negative condition. In fact, without conflict and differing opinions there would be no change. It is the aggressive way that conflict is expressed that creates hostile environments.

Nurses often feel frustrated by the inability to provide the care they would like and powerless to make the changes that would alleviate the frustration (Shaha & Rabenschlag, 2007). These feelings lead to a host of behaviors aimed at regaining control. The pressure created by the time-sensitive, critical nature of the work is another potential reason for the lack of civility. In a high-stress environment with a potential crisis around every corner, treating each other respect-fully seems unimportant, especially when one is struggling just to complete the tasks required to provide safe patient care.

McCallister and colleagues (2007) suggest that the problem goes deeper and involves a cul-tural way of being that is based on **dichotomous thinking**. Dichotomous thinking is having an either/or mind set. It involves culturally derived values that oppose each other and are seen to be mutually exclusive, such as right and wrong, good and bad. For example, one nurse may view the way he or she applies dressings as the "right" (good) way to do it. If another nurse does it differently, it is perceived as wrong (bad) by the first nurse instead of just different. Rather than have a conversation about the merits of each approach, more often than not, these nurses will complain about each other's methods to other nurses and suggest that the nurse acting differently is not "good" at dressing changes. These small acts of incivility breed discontent and interfere with collaboration by keeping nurses locked in competitive relationships. McCallister, et al., suggest that one way to stop either/or thinking is to substitute it with both/and thinking. In the above example, instead of asking which nurse is right (either/or), one would ask if it is possible that both nurses are right (both/and), i.e., you can be both different and right at the same time.

Most organizations have policies related to inappropriate social behavior in the workplace, yet little is done to address disrespectful language and/or actions. Failing to attend to lateral violence early may result in retaliation and create what some have referred to as a "spiral" of incivility, leading to "toxic" environments that end in overt violence costing 4.2 billion dollars and resulting in death for 1,000 U.S. workers in the general population each year (Hutton, 2006; Peck, 2006). Nurse managers are expected to spot incivility, intervene when it occurs, and create environments where civil behavior is expected from all persons. However, the majority of nurses and nurse mangers have not been taught these skills. According to Leiper (2005), gaining control of our own anger is an important first step (Figure 4-3), and Leiper offers these suggestions:

- Step away from the situation and take some time before responding.
- Instead of lashing out, speak to a colleague or friend about your feelings or write them down.
- Act only when you have your anger under control.
- Exercise regularly to relieve tension.

When you are under control, examine the situation from all perspectives, review the policies about harassment or violence to be sure you understand your options, keep records and take the appropriate action outlined in your policies.

Rau-Foster (2007) states that the first step in managing incivility is having a common under-standing of what constitutes incivility and the impact it has on patient care, staff retention, and the bottom line. Arriving at a common understanding, however, is complicated by the nature of today's workforce.

Rudeness and incivility are culturally derived social constructs. For example, some cultures believe it is rude to look directly into another person's eyes, and others believe it is rude not

Figure 4-3

An important first step in combating lateral violence in the workplace is for nurses to gain control of their own anger.

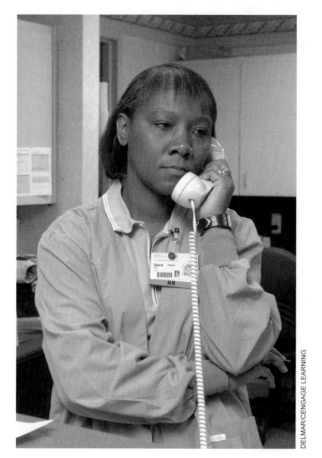

DELMAR/CENGAGE LEARNING

to do so. There are generational differences as well. The work attitudes of the **baby-boomer** generation, which makes up the biggest proportion of working nurses, are markedly different from their **Generation-X** and **Generation-Y** counterparts (Donley, 2005). For example, money, a powerful motivator for the boomers, is less so for the Generation Xers, who value time off and flexible work patterns. Additionally, generational cohorts have preconceived ideas about persons outside their own group (Patterson, 2005). It will be increasingly important for nurse managers to consider the differing values and work ethics of these groups in order to retain current employees and attract younger people to the workforce.

Diversity

Although the first order of nurses was made up of men involved in the Crusades, nursing has traditionally been a profession of women. In the United States these women are primarily Caucasian and middle aged. However, the workforce is gradually becoming more diverse. While this is definitely the desired state, it is not without difficulty. Nurses have been taught how to care for diverse patient populations, but not how to work with or manage people from different age groups or nationalities. Behaviors and speech patterns that are acceptable for one group may be offensive to another. Rapidity of speech, dialects, and direct- vs.-indirect styles sometimes hinder effective communication and create misunderstandings. Idioms are particularly problematic for nurses from other countries. While it is beyond the scope of this chapter to address all of the cultural and ethnic variations one is likely to encounter in practice, one area of diversity receiving increasing attention because of its uniqueness in history is generational diversity.

For the first time in history the nursing workforce is comprised of four distinct generations (Yoder-Wise, 2007): the **traditionalists** born between 1925 and 1945 (also called veterans and the silent generation), the baby boomers born between 1946 and 1964, Generation Xers born between 1963 and 1980, and Generation Yers born between 1980 and 2000 (also referred to as the millennials and netters). The values and attitudes toward work and authority of each generation are shaped by the social and political events of their time. Understanding these historical and sociopolitical forces can foster not only an acceptance of each worldview, but also an appreciation of what each generation has to offer. Table 4-1 compares the generations across a number of personal variables.

Regardless of the generation one belongs to, attitudes and behaviors that demonstrate respect for coworkers as people and professionals must be encouraged, inclusion and community building must be valued, and staff need to be provided with the communication tools and strategies to do so. McCallister, et al., (2007) propose using strategies and gestures found in the practice of modern diplomacy. These strategies were first discussed by Gopin (2002) in a discussion of cultural diplomacy. He asserts "gestures and deeds mean far more in contexts where there is no trust than [do] any words, no matter how convincing … Actions matter." Figure 4-4 lists the strategies and deeds outlined by Gopin and modified by McCallister applied to nursing.

Writing Exercise 4-2

The strategies and gestures outlined in Figure 4-4 were designed to help resolve conflict between countries and religious sects. Go to the original work written by Gopin at http://www.gmu.edu. Look at each strategy and gesture and think about how they might apply to your experiences in clinical situations.

- Make a list of actions, attitudes, or behaviors that you have observed that serve to accomplish each strategy.

- If you have not observed actions or behaviors for a particular strategy or have witnessed actions, attitudes, and behaviors that work against these strategies, indicate that on your list.

- Look at the materials posted in the clinical setting. How do the materials posted support or diminish the strategies listed.

- Identify one concrete activity that would operationalize each strategy.

Table 4-1 The Four Distinct Generations in the Current Nursing Workforce

	Traditionalists	Boomers	Xers	Millennials
STEREOTYPE	Adaptive	Idealists	Reactive	Civic minded
DEFINING EVENTS	World War II The Great Depression Korean War Golden age of radio	Economic boom Suburbia Vietnam War Civil Rights Movement Space Race	High divorce rate Watergate AIDS Corporate layoffs	Multiculturalism High tech Terrorism (Oklahoma City, Columbine) Gulf War
FAMILY CHARACTERISTICS	Traditional nuclear Extended	Nuclear families	Latch-key kids (least kid-friendly generation)	Merged families Very nurtured
HIGHER EDUCATION	A dream	A right	A means to an end	Expensive
PERSPECTIVE	Practical	Optimistic	Skeptical	Confident realism
CORE VALUES	Duty Honor Personal sacrifice	Teamwork Personal growth	Global thinking Self-reliance	Achievement Social responsibility
SOCIAL ATTITUDES	Patriotic	Involved	Balance Informal Fun	Civic duty Morality
COMMUNICATION	Rotary phones Letters Memos	Touch-tone phones	Cell phones	Internet
WORK ATTITUDES	Value authority Support hierarchies Believe seniority matters Loyal to the organization Disciplined	Ambiguous feelings about authority Like to make their own rules Driven, "workaholics"	Not impressed by authority Seek balance between work and personal life	Similar to Gen Xers
MOTIVATORS	Appreciate their experience Recognize with awards Use personal communication	Focus on challenges and their unique abilities to meet them Recognize with status perks	Give opportunities for creativity (break rules) Constructive feedback, fair distribution of perks Invest in technology	Clear goals and the opportunity to work with other bright people Provide mentors

Figure 4-4
Modern Diplomacy
Strategies Applied
to Nursing.

Create a hopeful atmosphere.
Create an environment where people feel safe from physical, emotional, and professional harm.
Treat each other with respect and dignity.
Develop friendships among diverse groups.
Encourage staff members to honestly examine their role in preserving the peace.
Make a peaceful gesture.
Humanize opponents and engage in quiet relationship building.

DELMAR/CENGAGE LEARNING

Moral Distress

Moral distress is the painful experience of knowing what is ethically right to do and not being allowed to do it because of organizational constraints or of being forced to act in a way that is inconsistent with your values (Zuzelo, 2007). Studies have shown that moral distress is common among nurses in all settings (Fudge, 2006), and that there is a direct relationship between the intensity of the distress and the organizational culture (Corley, Minick, Elswick, & Jacobs, 2005).

Nurses continually strive to give patients and their families compassionate, high-quality care based on a common set of values (Figure 4-5) and standards (Table 4-2). However, the demand for services far outstrips the resources available to provide them, and nurses frequently report that they are unable to provide even adequate care and that patient safety is a growing concern (Rodney, et al., 2006; Shaha & Rabenschlag, 2007). The inability to provide the care needed creates inner distress. The distress is increased when nurses are not part of the decision-making process and/or feel that administration does not listen to their concerns. This distress is expressed in a variety of ways, including increased reports of injury, physical illness, emotional exhaustion, absenteeism, and disenchantment with the profession (Kleinman, 2004).

Organizations that fail to respond to this distress send a strong message not only about the importance of the nurses' concerns but ultimately about the value of nursing. For nurses to

Figure 4-5
Nursing
Professional Values.
(Data from Cherry and Jacob, 2005.)

Autonomy	Freedom
Altruism	Human dignitiy
Collaboration	Social Justice
Equality	Truth
Esthetics	

Table 4-2 Elements of ANA Standards of Practice (ANA, 2004)

Patient Care Standards	Professional Practice Standards
Assessment	Quality of practice
Diagnosis	Education
Outcomes planning	Professional practice evaluation
Implementation	Collegiality
Evaluation	Collaboration
	Research
	Ethics
	Leadership

practice safely and effectively, organizations need to create moral environments where the "good" of the patient is central to decision making, and the centrality of nurses in that process is recognized and valued.

A three-year study of Canadian nurses working in two separate sites, one a large emergency department and the other a medical oncology unit, found that nurses also play a part in developing the moral climate of the unit (Rodney, et al., 2006). Nurses in this study admitted that they often treated their patients and each other in ways that were not helpful and at times "demeaning." The researchers suggest that in order to avoid these outcomes and bring about meaningful changes in the workplace, nurses need opportunities to reflect on their practice and their interactions with others, and that it is essential that we move away from thinking that pits nurses against each other based on their roles (i.e., practice vs. administration, clinicians vs. academics, seasoned vs. novice) and engage in collective action.

Health and Safety

According to a health and safety survey conducted by the ANA (2001), 88% of nurses cited health and safety concerns as key factors in their decisions to continue working. This is not too surprising since health and safety are important to everyone. What is distressing is that fewer than 20% of these nurses felt safe in their current environments, with 17% reporting actual physical violence and over 50% reporting verbal abuse. The health issues of greatest concern were related to chronic stress and overwork, with more than two-thirds indicating they worked mandatory overtime every month.

Fatigue related to long hours, mandatory overtime, and rotating shifts with lack of time to recuperate is a significant safety issue for nurses and the patients they serve (Owens, 2007; Surani & Murphy, 2007). While people differ in the amount of sleep they need to function at their best, sleep experts agree that adults typically need between 6 and 10 hours of sleep a day (Lack & Wright, 2007; Rosekind, Gander, & Gregory, 1997). Getting less than the optimal hours of sleep creates a state of **sleep deprivation**. Slower response times have been observed when individuals are sleep deprived for as few as two consecutive days (AHRQ, 2001). Consistent sleep deprivation leads to **sleep debt**. Sleep debt leads to decreased performance as well as altered moods and reduced morale and initiative (Selvi, Gulec, Agargun, & Besiroglu). A meta-analysis of the effect of sleep deprivation on performance by Pilcher and Huffcutt (1996) found that people who are chronically sleep deprived function at the 9th percentile of their non-sleep-deprived counterparts.

The IOM report on safety confirms that long work hours without adequate rest impairs performance and increases human error, and yet over two-thirds of nurses report working overtime every month. In a study by Rogers and colleagues (2004), almost 20% reported working 16 consecutive hours at least once in a 28-day period, suggesting that working double shifts is a common occurrence.

To prevent this practice the IOM recommends that nurses not be allowed to work more than 12 hours in a 24-hour period and no more than 60 hours in a 7-day period. Interestingly, many nurses have protested limiting or regulating the number of hours they can work. The nurses who oppose regulating the number of hours they can work believe that no one should limit their right to work as much and as often as they wish. Nurses expressed the need to work overtime in order to meet family and financial obligations. Many nursing organizations have indicated that the solution for these nurses should not be excessive hours but better pay, stressing that safety for nurse and patient must be the priority. Numerous studies outline the effects of overtime fatigue.

A longitudinal study of the relationship between musculoskeletal injury/disorders and hours worked demonstrated that the risk for injury was increased by working more than 13 consecutive hours, working on scheduled days off, working off shifts, and working overtime on-call (Trinkoff, et al., 2006).

Dawson and Reid (1997) compared the effect of sleep deprivation on psychomotor skills to the effect of alcohol on these skills. Extrapolating the findings of this study would indicate that if a nurse who usually works days and is rotating to nights awakes at 7 am (around the normal waking time) and is unable to nap before reporting to work at 7 pm, that by the end of the shift that nurse will be performing at the same level as a person with a blood alcohol level of .10%. Legal intoxication in most states is a blood alcohol level of .08 to .10%.

Rogers, et al., (2004) found that nurses who worked shifts of twelve-and-a-half hours or more were three times more likely to commit errors than nurses who worked shifts of eight-and-a-half hours or less. Another study conducted in intensive care units found increased overtime was associated with higher rates of urinary tract infections and decubiti (Stone, et al., 2007).

Based on the increasing evidence linking overtime to negative outcomes, eleven states (California, Connecticut, Illinois, Maine, Maryland, Minnesota, New Jersey, Oregon, Texas, Washington, and West Virginia) have enacted laws or prescribed regulations related to workload. In July of 2007, Senator Edward Kennedy introduced the Safe Nursing and Patient Care Act of 2007 (S.1842), which does not pose mandatory limits on nursing hours but would amend title XVIII (Medicare) of the Social Security Act to place limitations on forced overtime for nurses, protect them from retaliation with respect to any aspect of employment, and establish civil money penalties for violations of this act. Chairman of the House Ways and Means Committee, Representative Pete Stark, introduced the bill in the House stating that Congress currently limits the time that truck drivers can drive and the hours that a pilot can fly in order to protect the public, and concluding that "safe nursing is in the public interest as well" (Congressional Quarterly, 2007). The bill also directs the secretary of health and human services to conduct a study to determine the maximum number of hours that a nurse may work without compromising the safety of patients and to report those findings to Congress. To access the bill visit http://thomas.loc.gov.

Another factor related to fatigue is shift work. In fact, a study by Winwood, Winefield, and Lushington (2006) found that the most significant contributing factor to maladaptive fatigue was not age or other family responsibilities as one might suppose, but was indeed shift rotations. This warrants further study, since up to 35% of hospital nurses are required to work "off shifts." A report prepared for the Agency for Health Research and Quality (AHRQ) titled "Making Health Care Safer" (2001) revealed the following about shift work:

- Sleep after night work tends to be shorter than sleep after day work, leading to greater cumulative sleep deprivation.
- Shift workers have poorer quality of sleep and are less likely to feel refreshed after awaking.
- Shift workers tend to perform less well on reasoning and nonstimulating tasks than nonshift workers.

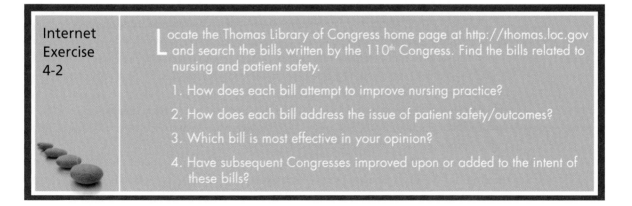

Internet Exercise 4-2

Locate the Thomas Library of Congress home page at http://thomas.loc.gov and search the bills written by the 110th Congress. Find the bills related to nursing and patient safety.

1. How does each bill attempt to improve nursing practice?

2. How does each bill address the issue of patient safety/outcomes?

3. Which bill is most effective in your opinion?

4. Have subsequent Congresses improved upon or added to the intent of these bills?

The AHRQ report cites a study by Gold and colleagues (1992) that found that nurses who rotate shifts, when compared with nurses who predominantly worked day shifts, were more likely to fall asleep at work and nearly twice as likely to report committing a medication error. Sleep deprivation and sleep debt lead to physiologic changes in gastrointestinal function, renal perfusion, hormone release, and immune responses prompting Surani and Murphy (2007) to suggest that there are certain people who should not rotate shifts based on their own health needs, including people with heart disease, diabetes, and GI disorders like Crohn's disease. They also cite studies that show an increase in preterm labor and miscarriage for nurses that work roating shifts.

Given that shift work is a reality unlikely to change in the near future, steps must be taken to decrease the negtive effects of such practices. The AHRQ cites three strategies that may reduce fatigue and improve alertness: forward shift rotation, slow shift rotation, and maintenance napping.

Forward shift rotation refers to the direction of shift work, i.e., rotating from mornings to evenings to nights. The theory behind this is that since circadian rhythms move forward, forward rotaions may be easier to tolerate physiologically. Another consideration in scheduling is the frequency of rotation. Studies suggest that rotaing once every two weeks (slow rotation) allows for better physiologic adjustment than fast-changing shifts every 2–3 days. Slowing shift rotations may result in more sleep at home, less sleepiness on the job, improved performance, and fewer errors (AHRQ, 2001).

Maintenance naps are naps that are taken at work during the shift. The AHRQ report states that while no systematic studies of the impact of maintenance naps exist in shift workers, one investigation did find that short naps during the night improved performance for the remainder of the shift. One potential problem associated with napping is "sleep inertia," a period of time when the person first wakes up from the nap and feels momentary confusion. During this time cognitive abilities and alertness may be impaired, somtimes for as long as 30 minutes (AHRQ, 2001).

ORGANIZATIONAL RESPONSES TO A CHANGING WORKFORCE

According to the IOM report (2004), many hospital restructuring and redesign initiatives emphasizing efficiency over quality and safety, coupled with ineffective communication practices, have damaged trust between nursing staff and management. The IOM report asserts that this loss of trust has serious implications for the ability of organizations to make the changes needed to provide safe patient care. Health care delivery in the United States has become big business. As a result business values related to making and/or saving money have replaced professional values related to the quality of care provided. This shift in organizational values heightens the artificial tensions already in play as well as the stressors of needing to do more with less, creating an environment where many nurses no longer want to work.

Nurse salaries make up the largest percentage of the operating budget of any health care facility. Therefore health care organizations have been reluctant to add RNs to their staff and have chosen instead to replace nurses with unlicensed assistive personnel, increase the nurse-to-patient ratio, require mandatory overtime and extra shifts, and hire agency nurses to fill in the gaps. Studies have shown, however, that hospitals with high numbers of RNs, especially BSN-prepared RNs, have better outcomes (Aiken, et al., 2003). Now that agencies and the public are coming to realize the importance of having an RN at the bedside, there aren't enough of them to meet the demand. As a result health care organizations have stepped up their efforts to recruit new nurses and retain the ones they have.

Recruitment/Retention Strategies

Traditional recruitment strategies have involved sign-on bonuses, trip giveaways, and shift differentials. In other words, more money. Clearly, money is an important consideration, but it is not what attracts people to the field. Lump-sum payments might entice a nurse to choose one organization over another, all other factors being equal, but to choose nursing in the first place requires wage reform. Staff nurses and faculty members are paid much less than other professionals, so in order for money to be an inducement, nursing salaries must be more competitive. Additionally, as discussed earlier, newer generations of nurses have different values and are looking for employment that provides balance in their lives, flexible schedules, personal development, and mentoring programs. A number of organizations are beginning to recognize this and are focusing recruitment efforts on continuing-education needs and tuition reimbursement for advanced degrees and certifications.

While recruitment is important, the need to keep the nurses that are hired is also essential. It costs the organization nearly $40,000 to hire and orient each new nurse. In addition to economic considerations there is a significant impact on the care system and care providers related to the time investment and stress of continually bringing new people on staff, as opposed to solidifying and growing competent teams. New graduates are particularly prone to leave within the first year of employment (Halfer & Graf, 2006), primarily due to dissatisfaction with work schedules, salary, and the inability to bring about change (Casey, Fink, Krugman, & Propst, 2004), as well as patient-care issues (Candela & Bowles, 2005; Greene, 2005).

Organizations must create multiple recruitment and retention strategies to attract differing groups. For example the needs of new nurses may differ from those of experienced nurses, young nurses, older nurses, nurses with disabilities, and nurses from other countries. One size does not fit all. Strategies likely to be successful are those that support nursing practice (resources to provide quality care, shared governance structures), nursing development (tuition reimbursement, opportunity for advancement, mentor programs), and flexibility in scheduling. Those hospitals that report positive outcomes related to recruitment and retention may qualify for recognition as a "magnet hospital."

Magnet Hospitals

In 1981 a task force established by the American Academy of Nursing studied 165 hospitals that seemed to be thriving in an era where most facilities had severe shortages of nurses and high

John is a 28-year-old new grad that has been working in the orthopedic unit of a large inner-city hospital for 6 months and is finally feeling like he has a handle on what is expected of him, although he often feels he is used for his muscle (lifting and moving patients) rather than his mind. He still has a hard time getting his work done on time, but no one seems to complain. The hospital is interested in getting magnet status, and his nurse manager has approached him about joining the magnet task force subcommittee addressing recruitment and retention. She tells him the fact that he is new to the system and part of a minority group will help the committee. Once again John feels he is being used for something unrelated to his abilities, however, he feels that as a new person, he really cannot refuse a direct request from his manager and reluctantly agrees. Meanwhile, the other staff think that it is unfair that John gets to participate and begin to make side comments like "I guess all it takes to get ahead around here is a y chromosome." He notices that since agreeing to be on this committee, his assignments are somewhat heavier than other staff members, and that the oncoming shift members are beginning to complain about him not getting his work done on time. He is confused about what he did wrong and about what to do next.

CASE ANALYSIS

1. What are the diversity issues at play in this scenario?

2. Was the nurse manager right to ask John to be on this important committee?

3. Are the nurses demonstrating uncivil behavior toward John?

4. What should John do, if anything?

turnover rates. Forty-one of 165 hospitals studied were identified as magnet hospitals because of their ability to "attract" and retain adequate numbers of highly qualified nurses (Bauman, 2007). **Magnet status** was based on the presence of fourteen criteria called the "forces of magnetism" (McClure, Poulin, Sovie, & Wandelt, 1983). These forces include management style, quality of nursing leadership, organizational structure, staffing, personnel policies, professional practice models, quality of care, quality improvement, consultation and resources, autonomy, nurses as teachers, image of nursing, community and the hospital, interdisciplinary relationships, and professional development. Figure 4-5 depicts the Magnet Recognition Program Model. It shows the fourteen forces of magnetism supported by the ANA's standards of practice and performance.

In 1990, a national program to recognize magnet hospitals was developed by the American Nurses Credentialing Center. In1998 long-term-care facilities were included, and in 2000 international health care organizations were allowed to participate. Health care facilities that meet eligibility criteria voluntarily apply for magnet status. The criteria and necessary forms can be located on the ANCC Web site: http://www.nursecredentialing.org.

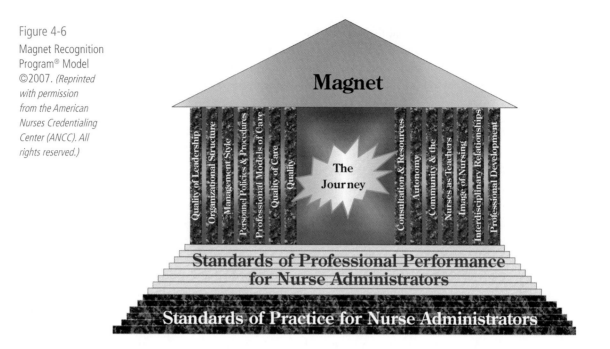

Figure 4-6

Magnet Recognition Program® Model ©2007. *(Reprinted with permission from the American Nurses Credentialing Center (ANCC). All rights reserved.)*

POSSIBLE SOLUTIONS, THE GLASS HALF FULL

Sr. Rosemary Donley (2005) states that nurses and the profession suffer from "negative affectivity." Donley defines affectivity as a "predisposition to perceive and experience events in a negative or positive way" (Donley, 2005, p. 313). She contends that nurses by virtue of their ability to examine all that is wrong within the profession and the health care system have come to view nursing in terms of "deficits" and have developed a world view where "the glass is always half empty." She points out that over time the nursing response to shortages has been the same, "get more nurses!" Getting more nurses in today's world, where there is not only an insufficient number of would-be nurses in the pipeline, but a lack of capacity to increase the pipeline, is unrealistic. She challenges nurses to change their world view and think creatively about to how create systems that support the workforce that we have, instead of lamenting the one we wish we had.

Nurses must begin to see themselves as knowledge workers and create systems that capitalize on their unique knowledge and nursing process skills and leave non-nursing tasks to other workers. Nursing job descriptions that still identify moving furniture as a nursing responsibility and require that they be able to lift 50 pounds in order to be hired must be challenged. The majority of health care no longer takes place in acute-care settings, so the role of nursing in health care must be expanded beyond the acute-care setting. Informatics, technology, and robotics may hold the keys to redesigning work processes. However, most nursing programs are still steeped in traditional content and teaching methods. Educational systems will need significant retooling to meet the needs of future workers. All of these things can be accomplished once we recognize that the workforce we have is made up of highly skilled, intelligent, capable, committed individuals. What are missing are the environments and processes designed to support them. As a profession we need to switch from deficit thinking, i.e., not enough nurses, to thinking about how to best use and support the nurses we have.

Creating Moral Work Environments

Rodney, et al., (2006) describe the moral environment as the implicit and explicit values that shape the climate and context of the work place and drive the care which is given there. Ethical theories address questions of "goodness," e.g., how ought one behave to promote the "good"?, does the good of the many outweigh the good of one?, do the ends justify the means if the end is the common "good"? The ethical principles that guide nursing practice are based on promoting the good of the patient and supporting each other. The American Nurses Association and the International Council of Nurses have developed ethical codes for nurses to follow. Both codes have several common elements: the primacy of the patient, the confidentiality of patient information, respect for human dignity, safety, advocacy for patients and for the profession, and personal responsibility for maintaining competence. Moral environments, then, are those that provide the material, human, and organizational resources required to do quality work, ensure nurse and patient safety, and support ethical decision making (Corley, Minick, Elswick, & Jacobs, 2005).

Promoting Collaboration

One principle of the ICN (1973) code of ethics states that "the nurse sustains a cooperative relationship with co-workers in nursing and other fields." According to a study done by Duddle and Boughton (2007), nurses manage themselves and their client care responsibilities through a number of complex negotiations. Understanding how these negotiations take place, as well as the skills and attitudes that support such negotiation, is essential for creating a self-sustaining work environment. Sherman (2006) discusses how to recognize and use the distinct talents of people from diverse generations and offers a list of questions based on values held by individual cohorts that can be used to engage them in collaborative problem solving (Table 4-3).

Supporting Colleagues that Have Special Needs

Following the passage of the Americans with Disabilities Act in 1990, advocates for disabled persons encouraged the use of person-first language in discussions and in all printed materials. That means that instead of "disabled person," you would say a person with a disability and the "diabetic" becomes a person with diabetes. The intent of person-first language is to focus on the person, not the disability. While it is certainly true that what is of importance is the person, person-first language may not have served this population well, in that it presumes the source

Table 4-3 Questions that Demonstrate Value for Differing Generations

TRADITIONALS	Which tasks require close attention to details?
BABY BOOMERS	Where can we most effectively use teams? Which issues require consensus building?
GENERATION XERS	Where do we need technological skills?
MILLENIALS	How can we be culturally sensitive? How can we use virtual systems?

of the disability is the person, when in fact, the person has an impairment, and the source of the disability (i.e., what is disabling) is the environment (Marks, 2006).

A study of nurses with physical disabilities (Guillett & Neal-Boylan, 2007) found that these nurses were not only capable of providing safe, quality patient care, but many times were recognized as outstanding members of the nursing team. However, the physical environment and the negative attitudes of their colleagues often prevented them from keeping their jobs. In most instances, a simple modification of the environment or the assignment is all that is required to retain these valuable nurses. For example, nurses with mobility issues benefit from reducing the amount of walking required by assigning them to the short hallway, setting up a mini nurse's station in the middle of a long hallway, or assigning a group of patients near the nurse's station or med room. Fatigue has already been discussed as a problem for nurses in general. This is especially true for nurses with physical disabilities. In the above study, a significant portion of respondents indicated that they could do the work, but not for 12 hours. Flexibility in scheduling is a simple solution to this problem.

Of interest is the fact that when the nurses in the study were accommodated with flexible schedules or geographically lighter assignments, they were treated badly by their peers (Guillett & Neal-Boylan, 2007). Nurses must learn to value what each brings to the situation to build a community of professionals. Nurses must develop communication skills that allow them to confront each other in a caring way to solve problems and provide the best care possible. Kupperschmidt (2006) refers to this as **carefronting** (as opposed to simply confronting) and contends that failure to confront negates the importance of relationships and goals. Carefronting uses assertive communication techniques to express what one needs and perceives to be right. The technique assumes that such communications arise from the desire to work together to provide quality care in an environment of mutual respect (Patterson, Grenny, Mcmillan, & Switzler, 2005).

Another group of nurses that require creative policies and work environments are older nurses. Retaining the knowledge, wisdom, and experience of older nurses is imperative. Quality patient care depends on the transfer of "whole knowing" from seasoned nurses to their younger colleagues. According to the Robert Wood Johnson study, *Wisdom at Work* (Hatcher, et al., 2005), older nurses need better ergonomics and lighting at the bedside, more autonomy and recognition for the work they are doing, ongoing education in technology and leadership in order to transition to less physically demanding jobs, and the creation of new roles such as nurse mentor, safety nurse, or research assistant.

Retaining New Graduates

Numerous studies report that 30% of new graduates leave within their first year of employment (Bowles & Candela, 2005). Reasons cited include patient-care issues, workload and scheduling issues, and poor treatment from colleagues and other health care workers. Ferguson and Day (2004) report that new nurses perceive experienced nurses as rude, intimidating, unsupportive, and highly critical of the profession. There are numerous explanations for these behaviors, some of which stem from the enormous pressures created by the shortage. Regardless of the reasons, these behaviors are counterproductive and self-defeating and must not continue. Shirey (2004) discusses the importance of social support to mitigate against stress and burnout. Processes must be put in place to support experienced RNs who are teaching and mentoring novice nurses, so that neither patient care, experienced nurse, nor novice suffer—none are expendable.

New graduates are competent beginners. It takes years to achieve proficiency (Benner, 1984). Most organizations recognize this and provide precepted work experiences to help new grads gain skills and confidence. Less well understood is that new graduates also need help adjusting to the realities of working in a 7-day-a-week, 24-hour-a-day profession, and that this adjustment takes up to 18 months (Greene, 2005). A survey of graduate nurses found that it took a full 12 months for new grads to feel comfortable in the environment (Casey, et al., 2004). Another study reported that dissatisfaction among new nurses was highest at twelve months, but was substantially less at 18 months (Halfin & Graf, 2007). Mentoring programs have been shown to help with both skill acquisition and transition to the profession (Beecroft, et al., 2006; Leners, et al., 2006). Based on the avialable data, it would appear that successful mentoring programs must extend beyond the first year of practice (Hayes & Scott, 2007; Pinkerton, 2003).

Rothrock (2007) also points out that while it is up to the organization to provide incentives and mentoring programs, it is up to each individual nurse to "lead from the middle." As the person in the middle of the situation, each nurse is qualified to lead from that position. That means that each nurse must accept responsibility for creating a work environment that welcomes new nurses, makes them feel valued, listens to their ideas and concerns, supports their educational and adjustment needs, and demonstrates a real desire to keep them as colleagues.

Learning Organizations

In 1990 Peter Senge coined the term "learning organizations" in his book *The Fifth Discipline*, which has been heralded by many as one of the most important books on management in the last 75 years. A learning organization is one where people "continually expand their capacity to create the results they truly desire, where new and expansive patterns of thinking are nurtured, where collective aspiration is set free, and where people are continually learning to see the whole together." Learning organizations are places that encourage employees to create their desired future and give them the tools to do so. The five "disciplines" evident in learning organizations are: systems thinking (taking the long view), personal mastery (continually striving to learn more), mental models (reframing, challenging assumptions), shared vision (shared pictures of the future that foster commitment), and team learning (group think).

Health care facilities that become learning organizations are much more likely not only to survive the coming challenges, but to excel.

CASE SCENARIO 4-2

Stacy is a new grad working on the day shift in a 24-bed surgical unit. She has been on the unit for about 8 months now and is still trying to figure out how to manage a group of patients and leave on time. She feels like she goes from task to task and doesn't really get to know her patients like she did in school, and she thinks maybe she isn't doing a very good job. No one is complaining, in fact no one seems to notice what she is doing as long as she reports off and doesn't leave day-shift duties for the night shift. The nurses she works with have been helpful to a point, but they are all pretty busy, and now that she's out of her preceptorship she is pretty much on her own, which makes her nervous. She is always looking things up which takes a lot of time. At least she isn't close to tears at the end of every shift anymore. She doesn't have any real friends on the unit, and most of the nurses are old enough to be her mother. She doesn't like to go to lunch with them because mostly they just talk about how bad nursing is and complain about the job, the unit, and the nurses on the other shift. They are always good to the patients, but they sometimes talk about them in disrespectful ways. Stacy feels like it is not her place to speak up or question their attitudes, but she is worried that maybe nursing really isn't what she thought it was. She had no idea it was going to be this hard. She thinks maybe she has made a mistake.

CASE ANALYSIS

1. What is Stacy experiencing? Which, if any, aspects of what she is feeling are normal?

2. What workforce-related factors are contributing to Stacy's distress?

3. What organizational policies and programs might have prevented this situation? What can be done to keep Stacy from leaving?

4. How would you characterize the attitudes and behaviors of the experienced nurses? Should Stacy speak up? If so, what approach would you encourage her to take? If you were the nurse manger, what would you do to change the attitudes and behaviors described here?

SUMMARY

This chapter has discussed workforce-related issues that are challenging nurses today. Issues of concern are the nursing shortage, the diversity of the workforce, organizational cultures, moral distress, and incivility. Some recommendations for addressing these problems include expanding recruitment and retention practices, creating mentoring programs, and establishing moral work environments. Organizational responses can add to the problem or lead the way. Positive activities include adopting the principles of learning organizations and embracing the forces of magnetism. Ultimately it is up to the nurses themselves, the people who make up the workforce, to bring about the changes that are desired.

Knowing is not enough; we must apply. Willing is not enough; we must do.

–Johann Wolfgang von Goethe

REFERENCES

AGENCY FOR HEALTH CARE RESEARCH AND QUALITY. (2001). *Making health care safer: A critical analysis of patient safety practices.* Evidence Report/Technology Assessment: Number 43. AHRQ Publication No. 01-E058, Rockville, MD: Agency for Health Care Research and Quality. Retrieved July 23 from http://www.ahrq.gov/clinic/ptsafety/ chap46a.htm4

AIKEN, L., Clarke, S., Cheung, R., Sloane, D., & Silber, J. (2003). Educational levels of hospital nurses and surgical patient mortality. *JAMA, 290*(12), 1617.

AMERICAN ASSOCIATION OF COLLEGES OF NURSES. (2004). *Nursing faculty shortage fact sheet.* Retrieved July 23, 2007, from http://www.aacn.nche.edu/Media/Backgrounders/facultyshortage.htm

AMERICAN ASSOCIATION OF COLLEGES OF NURSES. (2005). *AACN standards for establishing & sustaining healthy work environments: A journey to excellence.* Aliso Viejo, CA: AACN.

AMERICAN FEDERATION OF TEACHERS. (2005). *Recommendations of the AFT nurse faculty shortage task force.* Retrieved March 3, 2009, from http://www.aft.org/pubs-reports/healthcare/NurseFacultyShortage.pdf

AMERICAN HOSPITAL ASSOCIATION. (2007). *The state of America's hospitals—Taking the pulse.* Retrieved June 28, 2007, from http://www.aha.org/aha/content/2007/PowerPoint/StateofHospitalsChartPack2007.ppt

AMERICAN NURSES ASSOCIATION. (2007). *Nursing facts: Nursing shortage.* Retrieved July 20, 2007, from http://www.nursingworld.org/readroom/fsshortage.htm

ANDERSON, L., & Pearson, C. (1999). Tit for tat? The spiraling effect of incivility in the workplace. *Academic Management Review, 24,* 452–471.

ANONYMOUS. (2005). Warning signs for the White House. *Nursing Homes, 54*(10), 26–31.

BARTHOLOMEW, K. (2006). *Ending nurse-to-nurse hostility: Why nurses eat their young and each other.* Marblehead, MA: HCPro, Inc.

BAUMAN, A. (2007). *Positive practice environments; Quality work paces = quality patient care. Information and action tool kit.* Geneva, Switzerland: International Council of Nurses. Retrieved July 21, 2007, from http://www.rcna.org.au/content/ind_kit_final_2007.pdf

BEECROFT, P., Santner, S., Lacy, L., Kunzman, L., & Dorey, F. (2006). Nursing and healthcare management and policy: New graduate nurses' perceptions of mentoring: Six year programme evaluation. *Journal of Advanced Nursing, 55*(6), 736–742.

BENNER, P. (1984). *From novice to expert.* Menlo Park: Addison-Wesley.

BERLIN, L., & Sechrist, K. (2002). The shortage of doctorally prepared nursing faculty: A dire situation. *Nursing Outlook, 50*(2), 50–56.

BOWLES, C., & Candela, L. (2005). First job experiences of recent RN graduates. *Journal of Nursing Administration, 35*(3), 130–137.

BUERHAUS, P.I., Staiger D.O., & Auerbach, D.I. (2008). *The future of the nursing workforce in America: Data, trends, and implications.* Jones and Bartlett Publishers.

CASEY, K., Fink, R., Krugman, M., & Propst, J. (2004). The graduate nurse experience. *Journal of Nursing Administration, 34*(6), 303–311.

CORLEY, M., Minick, P., Elswick, R., & Jacobs, M. (2005). Nurse moral distress and ethical work environment. *Nursing Ethics, 12*(4), 380–390.

DECKER, F., Gruhn, P., Matthews-Martin, L., Dollard, K., Tucker, A., & Bizette, L. (2003). *Results of the 2002 AHCA survey of nursing staff vacancy and turnover in nursing homes.* American Health Care Association.

DONLEY, R. (2005). Challenges for nursing in the 21st century. *Nursing Economics, 23*(6), 312–319.

DUDDLE, M., & Boughton, M. (2007). Intraprofessional relations in nursing. *Journal of Advanced Nursing, 59*(1), 29–37.

FARRELL, G. A. (1999). Aggression in clinical settings: nurses' views—a follow-up study. *Journal of Advanced Nursing, 29*(3), 532–541.

FUDGE, L. (2006). Why, when we are deemed to be carers, are we so mean to our colleagues? *Canadian Operating Room Nursing Journal, 24*(4), 13–17.

GOLD, D., Rogacz, S., & Bock, N., et al. (1992). Rotating shift work, sleep, and accidents related to sleepiness in hospital nurses. *American Journal of Public Health, 82*, 1011–1014.

GOPIN, M. (2002). The practice of cultural diplomacy. Retrieved July 20, 2007, from http://www.gmu.edu/departments/crdc/docs/cultural diplomacy.html

GREENE, J. (2005). What nurses want: Different generations, different expectations. *Hospitals and Health Networks, 79*(3), 34–42.

GUILLETT, S., & Neal-Boylan, L. (2007). Ready, willing and (dis)abled. *American Nurse Today, 2*(8), 30–32.

HALFER, D., & Graf, E. (2006). Graduate nurse perceptions of the work experience. *Nursing Economics, 24*(3), 150–156.

HATCHER, B., et al. (2006). *Wisdom at work: The importance of the older and experienced nurse in the workplace.* Princeton: Robert Wood Johnson Foundation.

HAYES, J., & Scott, A. (2007). Mentoring partnerships as the wave of the future for new graduates. *Nursing Education Perspectives, 28*(1), 27–30.

HEALTH RESOURCES AND SERVICES ADMINISTRATION. (2004). *Preliminary findings: National sample survey of registered nurses.* Retrieved August 1, 2007, from http://bhpr.hrsa.gov/healthworkforce/reports/rnpopulation/preliminaryfindings.htm

HUTTON, S. (2006). Workplace incivility: State of the science. *Journal of Nursing Administration, 36*(1), 22–27.

INSTITUTE OF MEDICINE. (2004). *Keeping patients safe: Transforming the work environment of nurses.* Washington, DC: National Academies Press.

INTERNATIONAL COUNCIL OF NURSES. (1973). *ICN Code for Nurses: Ethical concepts applied to nursing.* Geneva, Switzerland: Inprimeres Populaires.

JOHNSON, P., & Indvik, J. (2001). Rudeness at work: Impulse over restraint. *Public Personnel Management, 30*(4), 457–466.

KLEINMAN, C. (2004). Leadership strategies in reducing staff nurse role conflict. *Journal of Nursing Administration, 34*(7–8), 322–324.

KREBS, R. (1976). Disrespect—a study in hospital relationships. *Hospital & Health Services Administration, 21*, 67–72.

KOWALSKI, S., Dalley, K., & Weigand, T. (2006). When will faculty retire?; Factors influencing retirement decisions of nurse educators. *Journal of Nursing Education, 45*(9), 349–355.

KUPPERSCHMIDT, B. (2006). Addressing multigenerational conflict: Mutual respect and carefronting as a strategy. *Online Journal of Nursing, 11*(2). Retrieved July 21, 2007, from http://www.nursingworld.org/ojin/topic30/tpc30_3.htm

LASCHINGER, S. (2004). Hospital nurses, perceptions of respect and organizational justice. *Journal of Nursing Administration, 34*(7/8), 354–364.

LENNERS, D., Wilson, V., Connor, P., & Fenton, J. (2006). Mentorship: Increasing retention probabilities. *Journal of Nursing Management, 14*, 652–654.

LIN, L., & Lang, B. (2006). Addressing the nursing work environment to promote patient safety. *Nursing Forum, 42*(1), 20–31.

MACINTOSH, B., Palumbo, M., & Rambur, B. (2006). Does a shadow workforce of inactive nurses exist? *Nursing Economics, 24*(5), 231–236.

MCALLISTER, M., Tower, M., & Walker, R. (2007). Gentle interruptions: Transforming approaches to clinical teaching. *Journal of Nursing Education, 46*(7), 304–312.

MCCLURE, M. L., Poulin, M. A., Sovie, M. D., & Wandelt, M. A. (1983). *Magnet hospitals: Attraction and retention of professional nurses.* Kansas City, MO: American Nurses Association.

MARKS, B. (2006). Cultural competence revisited: Nursing students with disabilities. *Journal of Nursing Education, 46*(2), 70–74.

NATIONAL COUNCIL OF THE STATE BOARDS OF NURSING. (2006). *NCSBN research brief 2005 nurse licensee volume and examinee statistics.* Retrieved August 1, 2007, from https://www.ncsbn.org/368.htm

ORLOVSKY, C. (2006). Mass nurse retirement expected in 2011: Survey. *AMN Healthcare.* Retrieved July 30, 2008, from http://www.amnhealthcare.com/News.aspx

OWENS, J. (2007). Sleep loss and fatigue in healthcare professionals. *Journal of Perinatal and Neonatal Nursing, 21*(2), 92–102.

PATTERSON, C. (2005). Generational diversity: Implications for consultation and teamwork. *Monitor on Psychology, 36*(6), 55. Retrieved July 23, 2000, from http://www.apa.org/monitor/jun05/stereotypes.html

PATTERSON, K., Grenny, J., McMillan, R., & Switzler, A. (2005). *Crucial confrontations.* New York: McGraw-Hill.

PECK, M. (2006). Workplace incivility: A nurse executive responds. *Journal of Nursing Administration, 36*(1), 27–28.

PINKERTON, S. (2003). Mentoring new graduates. *Nursing Economics, 21*(4), 202–203.

RAMOS, M. (2006). Eliminate destructive behaviors through example and evidence. *Nursing Management, 37*(9), 34–41.

RAU-FOSTER, M. (2004). Workplace incivility and staff retention. *Nephrology Nursing Journal, 31*(6), 702–703.

RODNEY, P., Doane, G., Storch, J., & Varcoe, C. (2006). Toward a safer moral climate. *Canadian Nurse, 102*(8), 24–28.

ROGERS, A., Hwang, W., Scott, L., Aiken, L., & Dinges, D (2004). The working hours of hospital staff nurses and patient safety. *Health Affairs, 23*(4), 202.

ROTHROCK, J. (2007). Attracting and keeping new graduates. *Association of Operating Room Nurses, 85*(6), 1063.

Rowe, M., & Sherlock, H. (2005). Stress and verbal abuse in nursing. Do burned out nurses really eat their young? *Journal of Nursing Management, 13,* 242–248.

Senge, P. (1990). *The fifth discipline: The art and practice of the learning organization.* London: Random House.

Shaha, M., & Rabenschlag, F. (2007). Burdensome situations in everyday nursing: An explorative qualitative action research on a medical ward. *Nursing Administration Quarterly, 31*(2), 134–146.

Sherman, R. (2006). Leading a multigenerational nursing workforce: Issues, challenges and strategies. *Online Journal of Nursing, 11*(2). Retrieved July 21, 2007, from http://www.nursingworld.org/ojin/topic30/tpc30_2.htm

Shirey, M. (2004). Social support in the workplace: Nurse leader implications. *Nursing Economics, 22*(6), 313–320.

Smith, J. (2006). Exploring the challenges for non-traditional male students transitioning into a nursing program. *Journal of Nursing Education, 45*(7), 263–273.

Smythe, E. (1984). *Surviving nursing.* Menlo Park, CA: Addison-Wesley.

Stone, P., Mooney-Kane, C., Larson, E., Horan, T., Glance, L., Zwanziger, J., & Dick, A. (2007). Nurse working conditions and patient safety outcomes. *Medical Care, 45*(6), 571–578.

Surani, S., & Murphy, J. (2007). Sleepy nurses: Are we willing to accept the challenge today? *Nursing Administration Quarterly, 31*(2), 146–151.

Trinkoff, A., Rong, L., Geiger-Brown, J., Lipscomb, J., & Lang, G. (2006). Longitudinal relationship of work hours, mandatory overtime, and on-call to musculoskeletal problems in nurses. *American Journal of Industrial Medicine, 49*(11), 964–971.

U.S. Department of Health and Human Services, The National Center for Health Workforce Analysis. (2003). *Changing demographics: Implications for physicians, nurses and other health workers.* Washington, DC: Author.

Unruh, L., & Fottler, M. (2005). Projections and trends in RN supply: What do they tell us about the nursing shortage? *Policy, Politics, & Nursing Practice, 6*(3), 171–182.

Winwood, P., Winefield, A., & Lushington, K. (2006). Work-related fatigue and recovery: The contribution of age, domestic responsibilities and shiftwork. *Journal of Advanced Nursing, 56*(4), 438–449.

Yoder-Wise, P. (2007). Key forecasts shaping nurse's perfect storm. *Nursing Administration Quarterly, 31*(2), 115–120.

Zuzelo, P. (2007). Exploring the moral distress of registered nurses. *Nursing Ethics, 14*(3), 344–359.

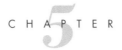

CHAPTER 5

WHERE ARE ALL THE NURSING FACULTY?

BARBARA G. WILLIAMS
PhD, RN, Chairperson, Department of Nursing, University of Central Arkansas

DONNA BRIDGMAN MUSSER
PhD, RN, Assistant Professor of Nursing, University of Central Arkansas

The deficiency of faculty is contributing to the general nursing shortage inasmuch as the inability to recruit and maintain adequate numbers of qualified faculty is restricting the number of students admitted to nursing programs.

–Linda Berlin & Karen Sechrist

LEARNING OBJECTIVES

At the completion of the chapter, the learner should be able to do the following:

1. Identify primary reasons for the nursing faculty shortage.
2. Discuss the impact of the faculty shortage on potential students, the nursing discipline, and society.
3. Discuss the role of the nurse educator.
4. Describe local, state, and national efforts to address the nursing faculty shortage.
5. Identify activities that new graduates can engage in to address the nursing faculty shortage.
6. Identify online resources for future reference.

KEY TERMS

Educational Mobility
Nurse Educator

Nurse Educator Shortage
Nursing Faculty

Nursing Workforce Centers

INTRODUCTION

Graduating more nurses is seen as one of the primary means of addressing the nursing work-force shortage. Nursing education programs need an adequate number of **nurse educators** in order to admit and graduate more students. The problem is much more complex, however, than just hiring more nurse educators, and the implications of not hiring additional faculty affects future nurses, current nurses, and the ability of nurses to provide care to their patients. Consider the following two scenarios of students seeking admission to nursing programs.

Elizabeth graduated from high school two years ago knowing she wanted to be a pediatric nurse. Her high ACT scores earned her an academic scholarship at a regional university, where she took the courses required of students to enter the nursing major. She has no grade less than a B, with a cumulative GPA of 3.43 and a science GPA of 3.2. She was faithful in attending her advising conferences and following her advisor's directions. In the summers she worked as a nurse tech in her community hospital for experience, which reinforced her desire to be a nurse. She scored well on the admission exam, and applied to the nursing major with confidence of being accepted. Elizabeth was devastated to receive a letter from the nursing program telling her that due to the number of qualified applicants, rather than being admitted she was placed on a waiting list. At the beginning of the fall semester, she remained on the waiting list and was not admitted to the nursing major. She later learned that only two of the forty-five students on the waiting list were admitted. Do you know someone like Elizabeth?

Consider Jason—he is 37 years old with a baccalaureate degree in business from a university in another state. He has worked in various management positions in manufacturing and is recognized as being successful and resourceful. However, he has felt unfulfilled for the past five years, wanting to "make a difference" in ways he feels unable to in his current role. After his company suffered major downsizing due to many positions being outsourced overseas, and even though his position remained secure, he decided to return to school to become a registered nurse. Jason took courses online, on the weekends and in the evenings, from various local and national accredited universities to earn the credits that he had not already met with his previous degree. Not wanting to relocate his family, he carefully followed the nursing degree plans and admission requirements posted online for two different universities in his area, even though it meant taking some additional courses not required by both institutions. While Jason admits he played some while earning his first degree, which he completed when he was 22, and his GPA for that degree was 2.99, he earned all As in the additional courses required for the two nursing programs, including several science courses. He confidently applied to both nursing programs. He could not believe it when he received letters from both institutions saying that while he met their eligibility, he was not sufficiently competitive with the other applicants to be admitted to the nursing major.

What is going on here? There is a national nursing shortage, actually an international shortage. Why are students like Elizabeth and Jason, who seem to be capable and qualified, not being admitted to nursing programs? Unfortunately, the cases of these two students are not unique. There are literally thousands of other students, just like them, across the nation, students who fully meet the requirements for nursing programs yet were denied admission (AACN, 2007a). In the majority of these cases, the nursing programs received applications from more qualified students than they had the resources to admit. A primary resource lacking for these nursing programs is a sufficient number of nurse educators (AACN, 2007a; SREB, 2007).

THE SCOPE OF THE PROBLEM

In 1983, a report by the Institute of Medicine (IOM) entitled *Nursing and Nursing Education: Public Policies and Private Actions* recommended that the federal government expand its financial support of graduate nursing education in order to reduce the economic barrier nurses faced in obtaining graduate education (p. 9). In fact, the report stated, "RNs with high quality graduate education are a scarce national resource and... their education merits continued federal support" (IOM, 1983, p. 10). The American Association of Colleges of Nursing (AACN), representing baccalaureate and higher-degree programs nationally, and the Southern Regional Educational Board Council on Collegiate Education for Nursing (SREB CCEN), representing associate, baccalaureate, and higher degree programs in the southern region, collect data annually and have released numerous reports addressing nursing education and the current nursing faculty shortage. The National League for Nursing (NLN) has also examined nursing education, and in 2006 began a major examination of the role of **nursing faculty** in collaboration with the Carnegie Foundation. As with the IOM report, these organizations and individual nursing leaders have consistently pointed out that the only way to address the United States' nursing shortage is to address the capacity of nursing schools and the shortage of adequately-educated nurse educators.

Beginning in February of 2002, Johnson & Johnson and other organizations committed significant resources to bringing national attention to the nursing shortage crisis (Figure 5-1). Donelan, Buerhaus, Ulrich, Norman, and Dittus (2005) found that 81% of all Chief Nursing

Internet Exercise 5-1

Locate the Discover Nursing Web site: http://www.discovernursing.com.

1. Who owns and operates this Web site? Who is the targeted audience?

2. Check under each of the main tabs: Who; What; When; How. Which tab contains a link to "Preparing for Nursing School"? What would you add to their suggestions?

3. Find the page entitled: "Nursing Careers." Click on and read about three different nursing careers. What is the specialty that is related to Nurse Educator?

Figure 5-1

Johnson & Johnson's Discover Nursing campaign brought national attention to the nursing shortage and had a positive impact on the image of nursing. *(Reprinted with permission from Johnson & Johnson.)*

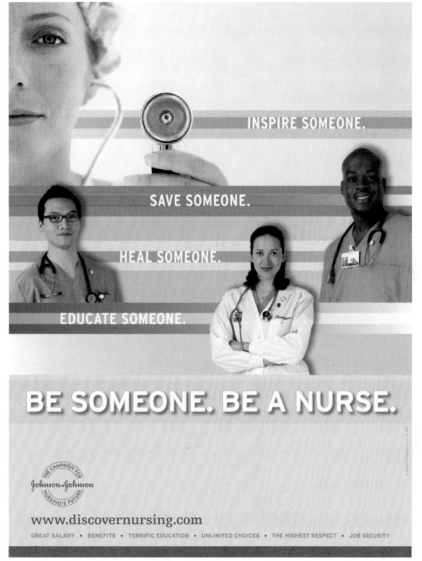

Officers (CNOs), RNs, and nursing students surveyed thought the Johnson & Johnson campaign had a positive impact on the image of nursing. The Johnson & Johnson media blitz and numerous state and local campaigns have been successful in reversing the declining enrollment trend seen from 1995 through 2000. AACN reported an increased enrollment of 10,388, or 13.79%, in entry-level baccalaureate nursing programs from fall 2002 to 2006 (AACN, 2007a, p. 40). SREB reported an increase of 5,083 (23.02%) students in Associate-degree programs in the southern region of the nation during this same period (SREB, 2007; SREB, 2003).

As the interest in and applications to nursing schools increased, another problem became evident, and that was the inadequate capacity of nursing schools to meet the increased demand. AACN's annual survey of baccalaureate and graduate-degree programs started reporting that a growing number of qualified applicants were not admitted, with 49,498 qualified applications not accepted in 2008 (AACN, 2008). The increased number of students pursuing admission to nursing programs and a higher number of qualified applicants denied admission has highlighted a shortage more fundamental than the nursing workforce shortage—the nursing faculty shortage, or the lack of qualified nurses willing to assume the role of nurse educator. Without an adequate number of nurse educators, nursing schools are unable to increase their admission of qualified students.

In 2008 a total of 814 faculty vacancies were reported by 449 baccalaureate and/or graduate nursing programs, nearly two vacancies per program (AACN, 2008). In 2006, SREB found 415 unfilled full-time faculty positions within 249 associate, baccalaureate, and graduate nursing programs, or 1.67 vacancies per program. Schools within the SREB region also reported the expectations that 615 nurse educators would retire within four years (SREB, 2007). The North Carolina Center for Nursing estimates that the state has less than half of the number of nursing faculty needed to educate the number of new nurses that will be required by 2020 (Cleary, Bevill, Laces, & Nooney, 2007).

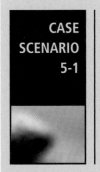

CASE SCENARIO 5-1

You have a good friend who is like Elizabeth and Jason, who were introduced earlier. He met all of the requirements, but was not admitted into nursing school. He wants nursing more than any other profession.

CASE ANALYSIS

1. What would you recommend that your friend do? (Hint: See Discover Nursing Web site.)

2. What resources can you recommend to your friend that will provide him assistance in reaching his goal?

WHO ARE THE NURSING FACULTY?

The nursing faculty consists of individuals who have obtained a graduate nursing degree beyond their basic nursing degree, and who are hired by academic institutions to teach nursing students. (Faculty refers to all of the members of a group, while educator refers to an individual. The nursing faculty is a collective group of nurse educators.)

Most states' board of nursing require nurse educators to have a bachelor's and master's degree in nursing. The National League for Nursing Accrediting Commission (NLNAC) state in their 2006 accreditation guidelines, regarding the qualifications of faculty of diploma, associate-degree, and baccalaureate-degree nursing programs, that "faculty members are credentialed with a minimum of a master's degree in nursing" (NLNAC, 2006, pp. 107, 121, 135). Faculty in an NLNAC-accredited master's program are expected to have a "minimum of a master's degree with a major in nursing, with the majority holding earned doctorates from regionally accredited institutions" (NLNAC, 2006, p. 93). The Commission on Collegiate Nursing Education (CCNE) in their accreditation standards document state that "Faculty members are academically and experientially qualified and sufficient in number to accomplish the mission, goals, and expected outcomes of the program" (CCNE, 2003, Standard II, Key Element II-E). The AACN Board on August 6, 2007, issued a statement, *AACN Guidelines Regarding Faculty Teaching in Baccalaureate and Graduate Nursing Programs,* in which the board states that it is expected that "Consistent with academy expectations that all faculty will hold a terminal degree, faculty with primary responsibility for didactic courses in baccalaureate, master's, and doctoral programs will have doctoral preparation that contributes to their productivity as a teacher, scholar, and clinician" (¶ 3). As evident, it is fairly consistently held that nurse educators will hold the minimum of a master's degree in nursing, and a doctoral degree is preferred, particularly for faculty teaching in graduate programs.

Virginia Partners for Nursing-Nurse Educators (http://www.teachrns.org) describes nurse educators as individuals who serve as role models in implementing evidence-based practice, who combine clinical expertise with teaching, who work in the classrooms as well as clinical settings, and who prepare and mentor future generations of nurses. The Virginia Web site also provides a list of why nurses teach (http://www.teachrns.org/career_profiles.html:)

- Variety of work
- Stimulating work environment
- Their research and scholarship advance the practice of nursing and improve patient care
- Teaching is valued in society, therefore Nurse Educators feel valued
- Flexible work schedules
- Distance learning/teaching opportunities
- To encourage and educate eager minds, and celebrate the achievements of their students
- Nurse Educators express a high degree of satisfaction with their work

Job satisfaction is one of the characteristics assessed in the National Sample Survey of Registered Nurses conducted every four years by the Division of Nursing, Bureau of Health Professions, of the U.S. Department of Health and Human Services (see Tables 5-1 and 5-2). Among the seventeen nursing roles measured, nurse educators are among the top three roles reporting the highest job satisfaction, and nurses with graduate degree(s) have the highest satisfaction relative to other educational preparation levels (Division of Nursing, 2004, Tables 33 & 34).

Table 5-1 Job Satisfaction of RNs Employed in Nursing, by Position Title in Principal Nursing Position: March 2004.

Level of Job Satisfaction	Total Estimated Number	Admin or Assistant	Consultant	Supervisor	Instruction	Head Nurse or Assistant	Staff Nurse	Nurse Practitioner	Nurse Midwife	Clinical Nurse Specialist
Total	2,421,351	125,011	35,617	74,201	62,255	148,210	1,431,053	84,042	7,274	28,623
Extremely Satisfied	651,386	48,057	16,091	19,742	25,405	45,558	316,343	35,588	3,494	11,839
Moderately Satisfied	1,197,997	58,537	13,272	38,121	28,467	77,113	744,673	36,928	2,892	12,685
Neither Satisfied nor Dissatisfied	194,844	5,706	3,940	5,604	2,388	8,580	132,399	3,715	300	1,041
Moderately Dissatisfied	259,147	8,455	1,744	8,072	3,749	12,917	182,774	5,647	294	2,063
Extremely Dissatisfied	68,175	3,046	498	2,465	1,724	3,242	44,276	1,496	135	871
Not Known	49,802	1,209	71	198	521	800	10,588	667	159	124

Position Title

Employment Setting	Nurse Clinician	Certified Nurse Anesthetist	Research	Private Duty	Informatic Nurse	Home Health	Surveyor/ Auditor	Patient Coordinator	Other
Total	32,954	27,287	19,263	11,762	8,570	45,621	12,097	138,404	82,352
Extremely Satisfied	9,678	15,035	6,759	3,722	3,084	14,312	4,411	42,674	23,530
Moderately Satisfied	16,212	9,804	8,772	4,995	3,961	22,044	5,152	66,707	38,849
Neither Satisfied nor Dissatisfied	2,047	732	1,550	2,014	924	3,611	881	11,071	6,969
Moderately Dissatisfied	3,902	1,179	1,583	850	298	4,202	1,122	12,302	6,791
Extremely Dissatisfied	1,017	373	526	182	303	1,293	341	4,675	1,302
Not Known	97	165	73	0	0	159	190	975	4,913

*Includes an estimated 46,753 nurses for whom type of position was not known.

Note: Estimated numbers may not equal totals, and percents may not add to 100, because of rounding.

(Courtesy of Division of Nursing; Bureau of Health Professions, Health Resources and Services Administration, 2004. The Registered Nurse population: Findings from the national sample survey of Registered Nurses.)

Table 5-2 Job Satisfaction of RNs Employed in Nursing, by Highest Nursing or Nursing-Related Educational Preparation, March 2004.

Level of Job Satisfaction	Total Estimated Number	Highest Educational Preparation			
		Diploma	Associate Degree	Baccalaureate	Master's/ Doctorate
TOTAL	2,421,351	369,741	861,949	841,554	310,474
EXTREMELY SATISFIED	651,386	105,340	217,113	207,565	118,717
MODERATELY SATISFIED	1,197,997	180,370	435,068	439,097	139,735
NEITHER SATISFIED NOR DISSATISFIED	194,844	28,868	74,850	72,066	18,032
MODERATELY DISSATISFIED	259,147	39,907	103,040	92,576	22,536
EXTREMELY DISSATISFIED	68,175	10,783	25,117	22,983	8,816
NOT KNOWN	49,802	4,472	6,760	7,266	2,637

* Includes 37,634 nurses for whom highest nursing or nursing-related educational preparation was not known

Note: Estimated numbers may not equal totals because of rounding

(Courtesy of Division of Nursing: Bureau of Health Professions, Health Resources and Services Administration. (2004). The Registered Nurse population: Findings from the national sample survey of Registered Nurses.)

Writing Exercise 5-1

Who are your nursing faculty? What educational preparation do they have? Ask at least three of them when they decided to become a nurse educator, and what were their educational pathways. Select at least one of your faculty members and send him/her a brief note telling how he/she is benefiting your nursing education experience.

REASONS FOR THE NURSING FACULTY SHORTAGE

The AACN, in a March 7, 2007, news release, *Nursing Faculty Shortage Fact Sheet,* addressed the major factors contributing to the faculty shortage, which include: an aging faculty who will retire in the near future, lower salaries in education compared with salaries in noneducation settings, and an inadequate number of graduate students preparing to be nurse educators (Figure 5-2). In 2006 the average age of all full-time nurse educators was 51.9, and the average age of doctoral-prepared faculty was 53.5 (AACN, 2007b, p. 9). Over the next decade nursing education programs are facing a loss of a significant portion of their faculty. Schools within the SREB region reported the expectation in 2007 that 615 nurse educators would retire within 4 years, up from 329 who were predicted to retire 5 years earlier (SREB, 2007; SREB, 2003) (Figure 5-3).

Figure 5-2

There are several factors contributing to a shortage of nursing faculty.

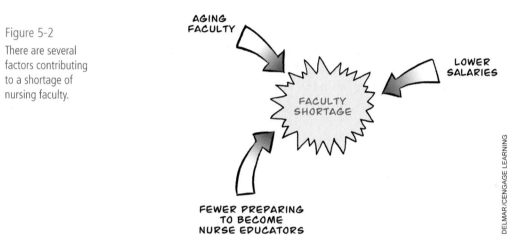

DELMAR/CENGAGE LEARNING

NLN-Carnegie Foundation Study of Nurse Educators

Preliminary findings from the NLN-Carnegie Foundation Study of Nurse Educators (NLN, 2007a) show that nurse educators earn less than faculty in other academic disciplines and less than comparably prepared nurses in noneducation positions, such as nurse administrators, nurse practitioners, and consultants. Higher salaries in noneducation positions result in the educationally qualified nurses seeking employment outside academic institutions. The SREB institutions reported inadequate budgetary and physical resources, as well as a lack of sufficient clinical placement sites for students, as the major barriers to admitting more students. The lower salaries paid nurse educators is viewed, however, as the most important impediment to recruiting adequate numbers of nurse educators (AACN, 2007a, p. 84; Anderson, 2002; Lovell, 2006; NLN, 2007a; SREB, 2007).

Cleary and associates (2007), from the North Carolina Center for Nursing, identified some of the root causes of an inadequate pipeline for nurse educators. After examining

Figure 5-3

Projected
Nursing Faculty
Retirements.
It is expected
that more nurse
faculty will retire
in the near future.
*(Southern Regional
Board Council on
Collegiate Education
for Nursing,
2003–2007.)*

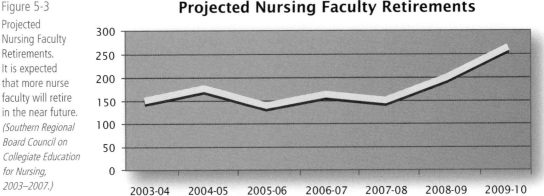

Projected Nursing Faculty Retirements

twenty years of longitudinal data, they found that the "vast majority of nurses never complete additional degrees in nursing beyond the entry and those who do rarely complete more than 1 additional degree" (p. 126). Since the majority of RNs are prepared at the associate-degree level, based on the authors' findings, most will never earn the baccalaureate degree, and very few of those who do earn the baccalaureate will go on to earn the master's, much less the doctorate degree. When the nurse researchers considered the nurses in North Carolina prepared at the master's or doctoral level in 2003, between 76% and 79% (depending on cohort studied) held a BSN as their initial preparation in nursing (p. 128). In addition, they found that only 17.5% earned master's degrees in nursing, and only 0.8% earned doctorates (p. 127). In order to increase the number of graduate-prepared nurses who are qualified to assume nurse educator positions, the entry level to nursing must be considered as leaders and policy makers develop and implement plans to address the nursing faculty shortage.

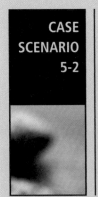

CASE SCENARIO 5-2

You have a friend who is twenty-four years old and does not have a college degree. She tells you she wants to become a nurse practitioner and is thinking about going into a hospital-based diploma program because she can finish in just two-and-a-half years. She then plans to go to a BSN completion program, before entering a graduate nursing program. She asks your advice regarding her plan.

CASE ANALYSIS

1. Review the study by Cleary, et al. (2007), and respond to your friend's plan to enter nursing at the diploma level.

2. If your friend is concerned about the cost of a baccalaureate degree, what resources can you give her for information regarding financial assistance?

IMPLICATIONS OF THE NURSING FACULTY SHORTAGE

The shortage affects not only the number of admissions into, and therefore graduations from, entry-level nursing programs, but has implications for graduate-degree-prepared nurses, the entire discipline, and society (Figure 5-4). Master's and doctoral nursing programs also identify the lack of qualified faculty as the most important reason for not accepting qualified applicants in 2006 (AACN, 2007a, p. 84). The ripple effect of fewer entry-level nurses means fewer advanced-practice nurses providing health care and new nurse educators prepared at the master's and doctoral levels.

The shortage also impacts the preparation, employment, and activities of nurse scientists and nurse leaders (Hinshaw, 2001). Nurse scientists are important to the health and well-being of the population as they conduct and disseminate research, building the body of knowledge used by other scientists and by health care providers and practitioners around the world. Nurse leaders are essential in shaping policy at the local, state, and national levels, impacting education, health, and economics.

Some scientists find that academic career requirements combined with their scientific pursuits are too onerous when their salary potential is compared to the educational debt incurred in obtaining their credentials. As a result, these individuals are finding employment positions in settings other than education, thus limiting the exposure future graduate students have to the nurse-scientist's mentoring and guidance in their professional development.

Figure 5-4

The shortage of nursing faculty has both immediate and delayed effects.

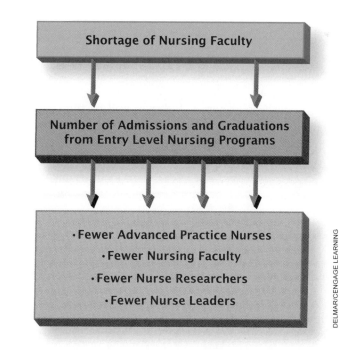

DELMAR/CENGAGE LEARNING

Nurse leaders, shaping policy at the state and national levels, are prepared at the graduate level and are frequently nursing faculty and administrators in nursing education programs. The pressures to address the nursing workforce shortage by educating more students, while struggling with inadequate budgets to employ sufficient faculty and greater teaching loads due to faculty vacancies and faculty turnover, place a strain on these nurse leaders' ability to engage in the time-intensive activities required to influence policy.

HOW IS THE NURSING SHORTAGE BEING ADDRESSED?

The need to increase the number of nurse educators or the need to increase the capacity of nursing schools are phrases used to express the fact that qualified students are denied admission into nursing schools because there are not enough faculty to teach them. To increase the number of new RNs entering the workforce, the nursing faculty shortage must be addressed. These strategies must include multifocal initiatives at the national, state, and local levels. Initiatives addressing the nursing faculty shortage include establishing grassroots media campaigns; lobbying state legislatures to increase faculty salaries and program funding, to provide scholarships, and/or to change state nursing education regulations; and lobbying Congress to fund scholarships and innovative programs and partnerships.

In the remainder of this section, some of the innovative strategies currently in place will be reviewed. The list of strategies is in no way exhaustive, and you are encouraged to check the following Web sites for updated information:

- American Association of College of Nursing (AACN) (http://www.aacn.nche.edu)
- American Nurses Association (ANA) (http://www.nursingworld.org)
- National Council of State Boards of Nursing (NCSBN) (http://www.ncsbn.org)
- National League for Nursing (NLN) (http://www.nln.org)
- Your state board of nursing Web site (available through http://www.ncsbn.org)
- Your state's nursing workforce center Web site (available through http://www.nursingworkforcecenters.org)

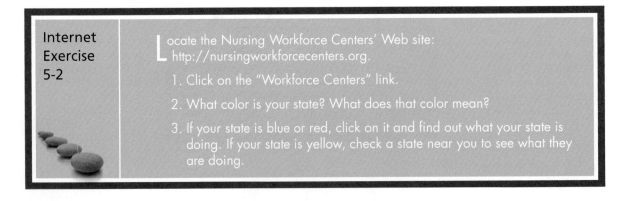

Internet Exercise 5-2

Locate the Nursing Workforce Centers' Web site: http://nursingworkforcecenters.org.

1. Click on the "Workforce Centers" link.

2. What color is your state? What does that color mean?

3. If your state is blue or red, click on it and find out what your state is doing. If your state is yellow, check a state near you to see what they are doing.

The funding of nursing education and workforce development is often the first issue discussed when it comes to identifying the major problem causing the nursing faculty shortage. Funding can come from a variety of sources including the federal government, state government, public and private organizations such as hospitals, or from private foundations. At the federal level, according to AACN (October 2006), the amount of funding for Nursing Workforce Development programs (Title VIII of the Public Health Service Act) doubled from $78.8 million in FY 2001 to $149.7 million in FY 2006 (Figure 5-5).

Nursing Workforce Centers

A number of states have developed **Nursing Workforce Centers** that serve as a clearinghouse for data collection and a means to develop strategies to address the particular needs of their state. By funding these centers, each state can identify the specific needs of their state and develop strategies that will work in their educational and institutional infrastructures. The Forum for State Nursing Workforce Centers Web site (http://www.nursingworkforcecenters.org) provides a link to existing state workforce centers, which enables each state to promote what they are doing to address the nursing shortage. Below is a review of several innovative state programs addressing the nursing faculty shortage. You are encouraged to check and see what your state is doing from the state's nursing workforce center if there is one, from the board of nursing, the state nursing association, and other individuals or organizations.

Arizona's strategic plan (Arizona Governor's Task Force on the Nursing Shortage, 2004) includes addressing the nursing faculty shortage by adjusting salaries to meet market demands, and by encouraging excellent preceptors to pursue faculty position. In May 2005, Governor Janet Napolitano signed into law SB 1294, which increased the funds appropriated by the legislature from fiscal year 2005–2006 through fiscal year 2009–2010, providing $20 million to increase the number of nurse educators at universities and community colleges in Arizona (Arizona Governor's Task Force on the Nursing Shortage, 2006). Updates on

Figure 5-5
Federal funding for Nursing Workforce Development Programs has increased significantly.
(American Association of Colleges of Nursing, 2006.)

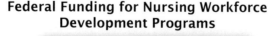
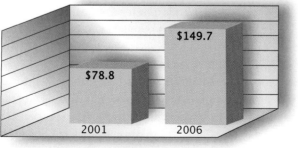

Federal Funding for Nursing Workforce Development Programs

$149.7

$78.8

2001   2006

Millions per Fiscal Year

implemented activities in Arizona can be found at both http://www.azcaringcareers.com and at http://www.azhha.org.

California (http://www.cinhc.org) has developed a unique way of encouraging and enabling baccalaureate- and master's-prepared nurses to become effective clinical faculty by offering a three-hour, graduate-level course to interested nurses in the Bay-City area. The course is offered by the California Institute for Nursing and Health Care (CINHC, 2007) and funded by a grant from the Gordon and Betty Moore Foundation. Individuals who attend this all-tuition-paid program receive a hand-held PDA loaded with clinical databases and a stipend for attending.

Colorado's Center for Nursing Excellence (2007) developed a Work, Education, and Lifelong Learning Simulation (WELLS) Center with grant money from the U.S. Department of Labor. The funds, funneled through the Colorado Department of Labor and Employment, enabled the Center to create a virtual clinic with high-fidelity mannequins at the University of Colorado Hospital-Fitzsimons campus. Using the high-speed backbone of the Rocky Mountain PBS network, the simulation lab provides state-of-the-art clinical simulation experiences to students and educators all over the state. Simulated laboratory equipment is very expensive; by sharing the equipment, both the nursing programs and the hospitals have access to these highly valuable learning and evaluation tools.

Florida's legislature instituted the SUCCEED, Florida! Grant Program in 2005. The nursing component of this program expects to add 765 nurses to the workforce and add 173 new nurse educators over the course of the program's life. In FY 2006–2007, $33.4 million was appropriated to the SUCCEED, Florida! Program, with $10 million of this going to 16 nursing programs (Florida Center for Nursing, 2007). Three of these programs received funding to specifically address the need for more PhD-prepared faculty: Barry University, University of Central Florida, and University of South Florida

In 2002 the Georgia Board of Regents expanded the capacity of the nursing programs and increased the number of graduates by funding year-round education (Georgia Department of Community Health, 2002, p. 22). Working with the Georgia Department of Labor and the Robert W. Woodruff Foundation, the Georgia Department of Community Health also offered a faculty fellowship program to fund 160 RNs for post-master's work; however, they report that few students have taken advantage of this program. As a short-term solution, they are now focusing their efforts on encouraging individuals who are thinking of retiring from clinical practice to consider becoming a faculty member.

Maryland, according to the Robert Woods Johnson Foundation (April 2007), is the only state in the country that has a commission that sets hospital rates. In 2001 Maryland instituted a program called the Nurse Support Program I (NSP I) where, through rate adjustments, hospitals could receive up to 0.1 percent of their gross patient revenues from the previous fiscal year to fund nursing recruitment and retention programs (Maryland's Health Services Cost Review Commission, 2007). By 2005 the commission found existing nursing programs could not accept all of the qualified applicants because of insufficient capacity, so the Nurse Support Program II (NSP II) was implemented to allow hospitals to direct 0.1 percent of regulated patient revenue funds toward expanding the number of nursing faculty. Confusion and duplication between the NSP I and NSP II as well as quantifiable outcomes from the programs will be resolved by the implementation of the Nurse Support Program III in FY 2009, which will combine both programs, streamline the objectives, regulate funding, and create standardized reporting mechanisms.

In Massachusetts, the state is focusing on developing partnerships between health care institutions and schools of nursing. One such grant from the Massachusetts Board of Higher Education funded a dually appointed, full-time, BSN-prepared nurse educator to run a learning skills lab located at the Baystate Franklin Medical Center while maintaining an academic appointment with Greenfield Community College (Massachusetts Board of Higher Education-Nursing Initiative, 2007). This arrangement enabled both institutions to utilize the resource and increased the nursing students' exposure to the clinical setting. Massachusetts has also enacted a waiver program that would allow BSN-prepared faculty without a graduate degree to teach in clinical or skills laboratory settings as long as they are matriculated into a master's program (Massachusetts Center for Nursing, 2007). The waiver could also be sought for BSN-prepared faculty who have graduate degrees in another discipline. BSN-prepared faculty without graduate degrees have five years in which to obtain their graduate education before the waiver expires; the waiver for faculty with non-nursing graduate degrees does not expire.

In Mississippi, nursing faculty salaries were increased by $6,000 each year in 2006 and 2007, when the Mississippi Nurses Association and other nursing groups strongly lobbied the Mississippi legislature to address the nursing faculty shortage, which is double the national average (Mississippi Nurses Association, April 11, 2007).

North Carolina is reportedly the first state to develop an agency dedicated to examining and addressing nursing workforce development. Established in 1991, the center has produced numerous reports and studies that leaders use to develop strategies and policies. In one of the studies, Bevill, Cleary, Lacey, and Nooney (2007) examined the **educational mobility** of three cohorts over a twenty-year span, finding that nurses who began their nursing education with a BSN degree were more likely to pursue master's or doctoral education. They also found that being younger, male, or a member of a racial or ethnic minority increased the likelihood that an individual would pursue graduate education.

Several states have addressed increasing the number of prepared nurse educators by increasing the pipeline through avenues of educational mobility. Increasing distance education programs and the availability of RN-BSN and graduate nursing classes in hospitals and community colleges provides accessibility to graduate education to nurses in communities where otherwise graduate nursing education would not be offered. Virginia and Wisconsin provide examples of promoting educational mobility. Virginia Partners for Nursing-Nurse Educators (http://www.teachrns.org) is a Web site that promotes nursing education by providing links to academic programs and financial resources that can help fund nurses returning to school. Wisconsin has a program called SWIFT, which is an acronym for the State of Wisconsin Initiative to Fast-Track Nurse Educators (2007). It is a partnership program designed and led by the University of Wisconsin-Milwaukee College of Nursing to significantly increase the number of clinical nursing educators available in Wisconsin. The key partners are the U.S. Department of Labor, the Wisconsin Workforce Development

Boards, health care employers throughout the state, the UW System Schools of Nursing, and the Wisconsin Technical College System.

A review of the AllNursingSchools.com Web site reveals online master's-of-nursing programs in almost every state. The Johnson & Johnson's DiscoverNursing.com Web site also lists online programs. According to the DiscoverNursing.com site, there are twenty-six institutions that provide online PhD programs. Almost all of these programs have BSN-PhD entry. Other states are currently developing online programs, so check your board of nursing Web site for a school near you.

A number of states have established scholarships to encourage nurses to pursue graduate education, and some offer added incentives for students to prepare to be nurse educators. Other scholarship and loan programs are available nationally. AACN provides an up-to-date listing of these resources at their Web site http://www.aacn.nche.edu, Click on the Students tab and then select Financial Aid from the list on the left. Check this site or within your individual state to see if scholarships of this nature are offered, such as through your state board, local universities, or nursing workforce center.

Besides federal and state initiatives, the contributions from private organizations, such as Johnson & Johnson and others, are significant. *Nurses for A Healthier Tomorrow* (http://www.nursesource.org) is a coalition of 43 nursing and health care organizations promoting a grassroots media campaign to promote the profession of nursing and the need for nurse educators. This Web site provides downloadable ads promoting nursing education from educators who are passionate about their careers. The latest newsletter on the site is from spring 2004, but the downloadable ads are still timely.

Partners Investing in Nursing's Future (PIN) (http://www.partnersinnursing.org) is a collaborative program funded by the Robert Wood Johnson Foundation (RWJF) and the Northwest Health Foundation (NWHF) that encourages regional foundations to invest in innovative programs that partner public and private entities. One funded project is the Oregon Consortium for Nursing Education (http://www.ocne.org), which partners the Oregon Health and Science University School of Nursing with eight community colleges across Oregon to share resources and curriculum. This program enables students to complete the Bachelor of Science degree through distance education without leaving their local community colleges, therefore addressing the issue of students not having access to bachelor- or graduate-degree nursing programs.

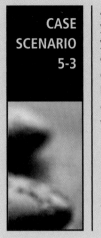

CASE SCENARIO 5-3

As a senior nursing student, you are considering your career goals for the next five years and are drawn to being a nurse educator. Your friends and family suggest that you work, get some experience, pay off your undergraduate student loans, and then consider graduate school. Some even question why you would pursue a graduate degree due to the salary and job opportunities of RNs. At this point in your life you have no real commitments and really want to teach nursing students someday. One of your nurse educators has the Scottish Proverb, "What may be done at any time will be done at no time." hanging on his wall. You have many options.

CASE ANALYSIS

1. What are at least five benefits to being a nurse educator?

2. What is a primary benefit to obtaining your graduate degree in nursing?

3. What do you want from life?

The Robert Woods Johnson Foundation (http://www.rwjf.org) is very committed to researching and funding programs that will improve the health of all Americans. Numerous grant opportunities and research publications can be found on their site, which discusses what needs to be done and what is being done to address the nursing faculty shortage. Their publication, *Charting Nursing's Future (2007)*, provides a synopsis of research and programs from around the United States. A study funded by the RWJF, *The Nursing Faculty Shortage: A Crisis for Health Care* (Yordy, 2006, p. 3), found that less than 7% of all U.S. nursing programs that offer basic RN education also provide research-oriented doctoral training. The costs of relocating and the economic reality of lost income while in school deter capable nurses from pursing graduate degrees. As noted earlier, however, several doctoral nursing programs are now online, allowing nurses to remain in their local community and not relocate.

WHAT YOU CAN DO TO ADDRESS THE NURSING FACULTY SHORTAGE

As a new registered nurse, there are a number of actions that you can take individually to address the **nurse educator shortage** (Figure 5-6). Do not assume that because you do not have a graduate degree or are not a "seasoned" nurse that there is nothing for you to do. Here are a few steps you can take today:

- Be informed about and support proposed state and national legislation to address the nurse educator shortage. Contact your representatives and senator, encouraging them to support the bills. Ask your friends, colleagues, and family to do the same.

- Encourage your place of employment to link with local nursing school(s) to establish partnerships as described earlier.
- Contribute to your alma mater nursing program's scholarship program to assist future students as they obtain their education.
- After you have some practice experience, serve as a preceptor to nursing students in their clinical rotations and to new graduates in orientation.
- Return to school to obtain your master's degree in nursing.
- Obtain your doctoral degree.
- Send a note to your nurse educators thanking them for assisting you in your preparation to be a professional nurse.
- Become a nurse educator! Review the many reasons listed in the earlier *Who Are the Nursing Faculty?* section of this chapter that have been expressed by nurse educators as to why they find satisfaction in the nurse educator role. Also remember that salary and other reasons impeding graduate-prepared nurses from assuming nurse educator positions are being addressed.

Figure 5-6

As a new registered nurse, educate yourself about how you can help address the nurse educator shortage.

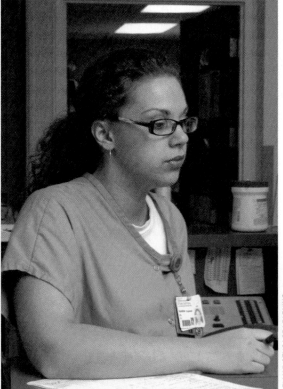

DELMAR/CENGAGE LEARNING

SUMMARY

The nursing faculty shortage must be resolved in order for nursing programs to educate a greater number of students in order to meet the current and future nursing workforce shortage. The lack of qualified nurse educators is the primary reason nursing programs are unable to admit more students. As a result, applicants who meet the admission requirements are being denied admission. A primary reason for the insufficient numbers of nurse educators is the lower salary earned by nurse educators compared with other educators and with other comparably prepared nurses in nonacademic settings. Numerous initiatives to address the shortage are occurring at the national, state, and local levels. New graduates have an important role to play in addressing the nursing faculty shortage, too.

A teacher affects eternity; he can never tell where his influence stops.

–Henry B. Adams

REFERENCES

American Association of Colleges of Nursing. (October, 2006). State legislative initiatives to address the nursing shortage. Washington, DC: Author. Retrieved October 8, 2007, from http://www.aacn.nche.edu/Publications/issues/Oct06.htm

American Association of Colleges of Nursing. (2008). *2008–2009 Enrollment and graduations in baccalaureate and graduate programs in nursing.* Washington, DC: Author.

American Association of Colleges of Nursing. (2007b). *2006–2007 Salaries of instructional and administrative nursing faculty in baccalaureate and graduate programs in nursing.* Washington, DC: Author.

American Association of Colleges of Nursing. (August, 2008). *Nursing faculty shortage fact sheet.* Washington, DC: Author. Retrieved May 7, 2009, from http://www.aacn.nche.edu/Media/FactSheets/FacultyShortage.htm

American Association of Colleges of Nursing. (August 6, 2007). *Draft position statement: AACN guidelines regarding faculty teaching in baccalaureate and graduate nursing programs.* Washington, DC: Author.

Anderson, C. A. (2002). From the editor: Nursing faculty—going, going, gone. *Nursing Outlook, 50*(2), 43–44.

Arizona Governor's Task Force on the Nursing Shortage. (2004). *Statewide strategic plan for nursing in the state of Arizona.* Retrieved October 8, 2007, from http://www.azcaringcareers.com/GovernorNursingShortageTaskForceStrategicPlan.pdf

Arizona Governor's Task Force on the Nursing Shortage. (2006). *Status report: Statewide strategic plan for nursing.* Retrieved October 8, 2007, from http://www.aznurse.org/files/75/documents/NursingShortageFinal.pdf

BERLIN, L. E, & Sechrist, K. R. (2002). The shortage of doctorally prepared nursing faculty: A dire situation. *Nursing Outlook, 50*(2), 50–56.

BEVILL, J. W., Cleary, B. L. Jr., Lacey, L. M., & Nooney, J. G. (2007). Educational mobility of RNs in North Carolina: Who will teach tomorrow's nurses? *AJN: America Journal of Nursing, 107*(5), 60–70.

CALIFORNIA INSTITUTE FOR NURSING AND HEALTH CARE. (2007). *Educational capacity.* Retrieved October 8, 2007, from http://www.cinhc.org/programs/educational.html

CLEARY, B., Bevill, J. W. Jr., Lacey, L. M., & Nooney, J. G. (2007). Evidence and root causes of an inadequate pipeline for nursing faculty. *Nursing Administration Quarterly, 31,* 124–128.

COLORADO'S CENTER FOR NURSING EXCELLENCE. (2007). *Current projects.* Retrieved October 8, 2007, from http://www.coloradonursingcenter.org/CurrentProjects/index.htm

COMMISSION ON COLLEGIATE NURSING EDUCA-TION. (2003). *Standards for accreditation of baccalaureate and graduate nursing programs.* Retrieved July 22, 2008, from http://www.aacn.nche.edu/Accreditation/pdf/standards.pdf

DIVISION OF NURSING: BUREAU OF HEALTH PRO-FESSIONS, HEALTH RESOURCES AND SERVICES ADMINISTRATION. (2004). *The registered nurse population: Findings from the national sample survey of registered nurses.* Retrieved October 19, 2007, from http://bhpr.hrsa.gov/healthworkforce/rnsurvey04

DONELAN, K., Buerhaus, P. I., Ulrich, B. T., Norman, L., & Dittus, R. (2005). Awareness and perceptions of the Johnson & Johnson campaign for Nursing's Future: Views from nursing students, RNs, and CNOs. *Nursing Economic, 23*(4), 150–157.

FLORIDA CENTER FOR NURSING. (2007). *Nurse education: SUCCEED Florida—Nursing education grant program.* Retrieved October 8, 2007, from http://www.flcenterfornursing.org/nurseeducation/grants.cfm

GEORGIA DEPARTMENT OF COMMUNITY HEALTH: HEALTHCARE WORKFORCE POLICY ADVISORY COMMITTEE. (2002). *What's ailing Georgia's health care workforce? Serious symptoms. Complex cures.* Retrieved October 8, 2007, from http://www.georgianurses.org/pac2002fullannualreport.pdf

HINSHAW, A. S. (2001). A continuing challenge: The shortage of educationally prepared nursing faculty. *Online Journal of Issues in Nursing, 6*(1), 3. Retrieved September 23, 2007, from http://www.nursingworld.org/ojin

INSTITUTE OF MEDICINE, DIVISION OF HEALTH CARE SERVICES. (1983). *Nursing and nursing education: Public policies and private actions.* Washington, DC: National Academy Press.

LOVELL, V. (2006). *Solving the nursing shortage through higher wages.* Washington, DC: Institute for Women's Policy Research. Retrieved October 8, 2007, from http://www.iwpr.org/pdf/C363.pdf

MARYLAND'S HEALTH SERVICES COST REVIEW COMMISSION. (2007). *Final recommendations for update to the Nurse Support Program I (NSP I).* Retrieved October 8, 2007, from http://www.hscrc.state.md.us/nurse_support_I/nurse_support_I.html

MASSACHUSETTS BOARD OF HIGHER EDUCATION-NURSING INITIATIVE. (2007). *Inventory of nursing education projects.* Retrieved October 14, 2007, from http://www.mass.edu/p_p/home.asp?id=9&iid=9.17

MASSACHUSETTS CENTER FOR NURSING. (2007). *Board of registration in nursing waiver policy.* Retrieved October 14, 2007, from http://www.nursema.org/become_faculty.html

MISSISSIPPI NURSES ASSOCIATION. (April 11, 2007). *Mississippi nursing faculty secures second phase of two-year salary increase.* Retrieved October 14, 2007, from http://www.msnurses.org/mna/pr/mr04112007.asp

NATIONAL LEAGUE FOR NURSING ACCREDITING COMMISSION. (2006). *Accreditation manual with interpretive guidelines by program type for post-secondary and higher degree programs in nursing.* New York City: Author.

National League for Nursing. (2007a). Headlines from the NLN. Compensation for nurse educators: Findings from the NLN/Carnegie national survey with implications for recruitment and retention. *Nursing Education Perspectives, 28,* 223–225.

Robert Woods Johnson Foundation. (April, 2007). *Charting nursing's future.* Retrieved October 14, 2007, from http://www.rwjf.org/files/publications/other/nursingfuture4.pdf

SREB Council on Collegiate Education for Nursing. (2003). *Annual survey.* Retrieved October 8, 2007, from http://www.sreb.org/programs/nursing/presentations/presentationsindex.asp

SREB Council on Collegiate Education for Nursing. (2007). *Annual survey.* Retrieved October 8, 2007, from http://www.sreb.org/programs/nursing/presentations/presentationsindex.asp

State of Wisconsin Initiative to Fast-Track Nurse Educators. (2007). *State of Wisconsin initiative to fast track (SWIFT) nurse educators.* Retrieved October 8, 2007, from http://www4.uwm.edu/nursing/swift

Virginia Partnership for Nursing. (2007). *Career profile: Why do nurses teach?* Retrieved October 8, 2007, from http://www.teachrns.org/career_profiles.html

Yordy, K. D. (2006). *The nursing faculty shortage: A crisis for health care.* Robert Woods Johnson Foundation. Retrieved October 13, 2007, from http://www.rwjf.org/programareas/resources/product.jsp?id=15889&pid=1135&gsa=1

THE NEWEST NURSING SPECIALTIES

CAROL J. BICKFORD

PhD, RN-BC, Senior Policy Fellow, Department of Nursing Practice & Policy, American Nurses Association

The vision must be followed by the venture. It is not enough to stare up the steps—
we must step up the stairs.

–Vance Havner

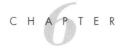

LEARNING OBJECTIVES

At the completion of the chapter, the learner should be able to do the following:

1. Discuss how four components of the definition of nursing relate to specialty nursing practice.
2. Describe the fourteen characteristics of a nursing specialty used by the American Nurses Association for formal recognition of a nursing specialty.
3. Explain how registered nurses can become competent clinicians or nursing role specialists prepared for specialty practice in nursing.
4. Differentiate the characteristics of certification, accreditation, and credentialing related to specialty nursing practice and the associated organizations or agencies overseeing these professional regulatory actions.
5. Identify how ethics and the nursing process are incorporated within one's preferred nursing specialty.

KEY TERMS

Accreditation	Competencies	Role Specialty
Accreditation Bodies	Legal Regulation	Self-regulation
Advanced Practice Registered Nurses (APRNs)	Nursing Domains	Scope and Standards of Practice
Advocacy	Professional Regulation	State Boards of Nursing
Certification	Recognition Criteria	

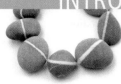

INTRODUCTION

Any discussion about nursing specialties must begin with a firm understanding of the definition of nursing and what constitutes nursing practice. *Nursing is the protection, promotion, and optimization of health and abilities, prevention of illness and injury, alleviation of suffering through the diagnosis and treatment of human response, and advocacy in the care of individuals, families, communities, and populations* (ANA, 2003, p. 6; ANA, 2004, p. 7). This contemporary definition provided by the American Nurses Association (ANA) describes the focus of registered-nurse practice to be far more encompassing than the completion of a series of simple or complex activities that are then enumerated and checked off on a paper or electronic chart form or flow sheet.

The three documents that describe the framework for all nursing practice within the four **nursing domains** of practice—education, administration, and research—also apply to the smaller, more discrete areas of specialty nursing practice. *Nursing's Social Policy Statement, Second Edition* (ANA, 2003) describes how professional nursing is accountable to the public and how the processes of **self-regulation, professional regulation,** and **legal regulation** have been established to maintain that trust. The *Code of Ethics for Nurses With Interpretive Statements* (ANA, 2001) addresses the importance of ethics for all nurses and the necessity of its integration into every setting and every nurse's practice. The third document, *Nursing: Scope and Standards of Practice* (ANA, 2004), presents greater detail to further define the **scope and standards of practice** for all registered nurses by answering the who, what, where, when, how, and why questions necessary for better understanding. This content also introduces the roles held by more experienced registered nurses in clinical specialty nursing practice, by nurses working in a **role specialty,** and by **advanced practice registered nurses (APRNs).**

Schools of nursing have been established to educate undergraduate students in the art and science of nursing and to sufficiently prepare those individuals to demonstrate minimal **competencies** for safe, autonomous practice upon graduation and licensure. Although significant variability exists in the format and presentation of the formal curricula, all schools of nursing must comply with mandates of **accreditation bodies** and **state boards of nursing** for defined content requirements. This translates most often into instruction and clinical experiences related to general categories of nursing care of obstetrical and pediatric patients, public-health or home-health patient populations, and patients with medical, surgical, or psychiatric-mental health diagnoses. Exposure to such diversity provides opportunities for students to begin discovering what areas of specialty practice might be most appealing and interesting. Further validation occurs during the selection of employment settings and actual work experiences.

NURSING SPECIALTY PRACTICE

Nurses moving from novice to experienced levels become proficient in one or more practice areas or roles. Some may focus on patient care in clinical nursing practice specialties, while others function in roles that oversee and influence nursing's infrastructure to support the direct care rendered to patients. The nursing specialty titles may be unique to the profession, or sometimes reflect the historical influence of medical practice specialties. The specialty and name may focus on patient characteristics or an age spectrum, patients within specific health care settings, care of body systems, named diseases or disorders, care delivery processes, or other infrastructure components. Because nursing practice and health care are dynamic and characterized by foundational knowledge bases that are always evolving, the emergence of new nursing specialties creates a constant tension for state boards of nursing in their legal and regulatory oversight responsibilities. Similarly, schools of nursing and other agencies and organizations are challenged to incorporate the appropriate content within undergraduate, graduate, and continuing-education programs to prepare nurses with the necessary competencies for practice in the existing and new specialties.

In an effort to provide some consistency and semblance of nursing's professional regulation of itself, the American Nurses Association's Congress of Nursing Practice and its Committee on Nursing Practice Standards and Guidelines, in collaboration with members of the Nursing Organization Liaison Forum (NOLF), developed and then approved a set of **recognition criteria** for nursing specialties in 1998. The ANA's Congress on Nursing Practice and Economics, which now includes official representatives of organizational affiliate member specialty nursing organizations, regularly reviews the adequacy of the criteria, completed a minor revision in 2004, and continues to use the criteria during the review and decision-making processes to formally recognize an area of practice as a nursing specialty.

The ANA's recognition criteria are listed in Figure 6-1.

Figure 6-1

The American Nurses Association's Criteria for Nursing Specialties. *(Adapted from ANA, 2005.)*

A Nursing Specialty:
1. Defines itself as nursing.
2. Adheres to the overall licensure requirements of the profession.
3. Subscribes to the overall purposes and functions of nursing.
4. Is clearly defined.
5. Is practiced nationally or internationally.
6. Includes a substantial number of nurses who devote most of their practice to the specialty.
7. Can identify a need and demand for itself.
8. Has a well derived knowledge base particular to the practice of the nursing specialty.
9. Is concerned with phenomena of the discipline of nursing.
10. Defines competencies for the area of specialty nursing practice.
11. Has existing mechanisms for supporting, reviewing, and disseminating research to support its knowledge base.
12. Has defined educational criteria for specialty preparation or graduate degree.
13. Has continuing education programs or continuing competence mechanisms for nurses in the specialty.
14. Is organized and represented by a national specialty association or branch of a parent organization (ANA, 2005).

Some specialty areas of nursing practice have not been reviewed through the ANA recognition process for a variety of reasons. The potential specialty may not yet have a sufficiently robust body of knowledge to clearly represent the distinctive characteristics and focus of concern. Without sufficient numbers of registered nurses collectively represented by a national specialty organization, the leadership and resources necessary to formalize a specialty scope-of-practice statement and accompanying standards of practice and professional performance may be lacking. Specialty-specific competencies may not be recognized, firmly entrenched in practice, or included in academic or continuing education programs. A well-established research mechanism is of key importance and often is one of the last criteria to be met. Some specialties may decide application for formal recognition cannot proceed until a specialty **certification** process is present, either offered by the specialty organization itself or by an existing certification body, such as the American Nurses Credentialing Center (ANCC).

PROFESSIONAL REGULATION OF SPECIALTIES AND SPECIALTY PRACTICE

In addition to the demonstrated professional regulation actions offered through formal specialty recognition by the ANA and inclusion of specialty nursing content in educational programs, certification programs are in place to confer recognition of individual nurse expertise in specialty practice, thus serving as another form of professional regulation. Defined criteria must be met and specific application processes completed before certification credentials can be awarded. Most often documentation confirming educational preparation and completion

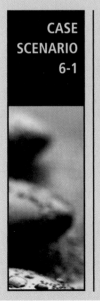

CASE SCENARIO 6-1

Colleagues in your work setting are debating one of the components in the proposal for revision of the nursing career ladder requirements that calls for completion and maintenance of nursing specialty certification. The heated discussions focus on such topics as the actual need for certification, the requirements necessary for initial application and for recertification, duplication of certifications offered by multiple credentialing bodies, the significant diversity in the authorized credentials for those certified, the cost burden, reliability and validity of the certification tests themselves, and "what's in it for me?"

CASE ANALYSIS

1. Discuss the pros and cons of specialty certification.

2. Construct a chart that identifies the economic benefits and costs of certification in a nursing specialty.

3. Identify how a nurse selects one certification over another when multiple options exist.

4. What is in it for me? Should I consider certification in my professional career?

of a set number of continuing education credits constitutes part of the application process. Many certification programs rely on standardized paper-pencil or computer-based tests to be the final proxy for demonstration of specialty-practice competencies. Some specialty certification programs rely on review of professional portfolios rather than completion of certification examinations. Those who have become certified in a nursing specialty can use the designated credentials during the delimited time and must renew that certification after a defined number of years.

Professional regulation also includes an **accreditation** arm that reviews the qualifications, practices, procedures, and outcomes of established certification organizations. Nurses seeking specialty certification should confirm that the selected certification body has met the requirements and passed the rigorous review processes of a recognized accreditation body, such as the American Board of Nursing Specialties (ABNS) and National Commission for Certifying Agencies (NCCA).

Another accreditation arm encompasses the examination of schools of nursing to confirm adequately prepared and sufficient numbers of faculty and educational resources are in place to present the nursing and nursing specialty programs. This accreditation process is provided by two organizations, the National League for Nursing Accrediting Commission (NLNAC) and the Commission on Collegiate Nursing Education (CCNE). Recognition of nursing specialties also becomes part of the purview of state boards of nursing when addressing the oversight and regulation of advanced-practice registered nurses (APRNs).

Writing Exercise 6-1	The staff members in the federal government office preparing the survey instrument for the 2008 National Sample Survey of Registered Nurses have asked for recommendations on how to restructure the questions about nursing specialties. Examine the existing survey instrument available at http://bhpr.hrsa.gov. Click on the link for National Center for Health Workforce Analysis, then on the article "The Registered Nurse Population: Findings from the 2004 National Sample Survey of Registered Nurses." Create at least one new survey question about nursing specialty practice. Remember the results of the survey will be used to quantify the numbers of nurses in specialty practice and will be used to identify what potential educational resources will be needed to prepare nurses who are not enrolled in APRN programs.

OPPORTUNITIES FOR INNOVATION

What nursing specialties exist, and how does one decide which to choose? First begin exploring those areas of instruction in an undergraduate program that may be of particular interest.

Pediatric Nursing

The general category of pediatric nursing involves the care of children from the age of newborn through young adult. Some nurses elect to focus solely on neonatology to care for those newborns who are premature or acutely ill, with special needs within the neonatal intensive care unit (NICU) (see Figure 6-2). Others care for children in pediatric hospitals, pediatric units in general hospitals, ambulatory care clinics, and single-physician or group family practice or pediatrician office settings. Some may choose to work only with adolescents and young adults. The children and their family members are significant partners in the care planning and decision-making processes. Staff nurses may choose to complete graduate-level education in this area to become clinical nurse specialists or nurse practitioners.

School Nursing

School nurses provide care for children in non-health care institutions (Figure 6-3) and must often include public-health approaches to engage families and school administrators as active participants in the health care process. The increased inclusion of children with special needs in mainstream educational programs creates challenges and opportunities for innovative nursing solutions and collaboration. Nurses in college health practice have a significantly divergent spectrum of patients, with ages spanning from adolescent through older adult. Their patients include enrolled students and faculty members.

Figure 6-2
Pediatric nursing is a specialty that involves the care of children from newborn to young adult.

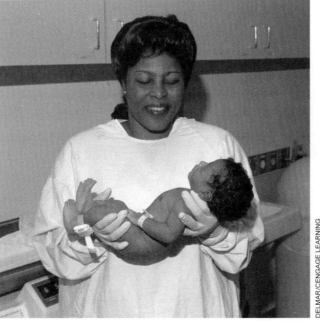

DELMAR/CENGAGE LEARNING

Figure 6-3
School nurses provide care for children in non-health care institutions, as shown in this photo of a nurse administering a vaccine to a 15-year-old female basketball player while her teammates observe. *(Courtesy of the Centers for Disease Control and Prevention/photo by James Gathany.)*

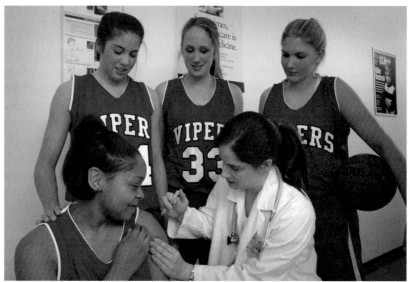

Women's Health Nursing

Nurses engaged in the specialty practice providing women's health services have many options (Figure 6-4). Obstetrical care encompasses services to prepregnant, prenatal, laboring, and postpartum women and their partners and healthy newborn infants. Careful monitoring and extensive health education teaching and coaching are key components in this specialty as women and their families move through significant physiological and developmental phases

Figure 6-4
Women's health nursing provides many options for RNs, including monitoring and health education teaching.

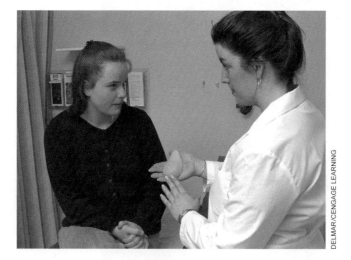

DELMAR/CENGAGE LEARNING

related to childbearing. Women's health services also include the protection, promotion, and optimization of a woman's health and abilities; prevention of illness and injury through regular health screenings, testing, and educational programs; alleviation of suffering through the diagnosis and treatment of human response when illness or disease are present; and advocacy for women's services and rights, including those related to access to reproductive and health services and prevention of abuse and violence. The aging of America's population creates an increased need for women's health specialists well versed in the care of postmenopausal and elderly women. Completion of graduate education and appropriate certification programs prepares certified nurse midwives and women's health clinical nurse specialists and nurse practitioners.

Medical-Surgical Nursing

Medical-surgical nurses most often staff inpatient hospital nursing units. They care for diverse patient populations of varying acuity needing a wide range of different nursing services. Medical-surgical nurses must deal with rapid patient turnover and must be capable of managing very different protocols and clinical pathways with finesse. Excellent people skills are mandatory as patients, families, and clinicians must address tough decisions about difficult care processes and the necessary preparations for care upon discharge (Figure 6-5). When assigned to specialty units, such as shock trauma, cardiovascular, neurology-neurosurgery, transplant, or orthopedic wards, medical-surgical nurses move into other nursing specialties that require new knowledge and skills.

Psychiatric-Mental Health Nursing

Psychiatric-mental health nurses specialize in the area of nursing practice "... committed to promoting mental health through the assessment, diagnosis, and treatment of human responses to mental health problems and psychiatric disorders" (ANA, 2007, p. 1). They rely on the purposeful use of self as the art combined with the science provided by a wide range of nursing, psychosocial, and neuro-biological theories and research evidence. Psychiatric-mental health nurses provide comprehensive, patient-centered mental health and psychiatric care in a wide range of settings and focus on the identification, prevention, and care of mental-health problems and treatment of persons with psychiatric disorders (Figure 6-6). Often these nurses further define their patient population to focus on adult or child-adolescent patients. Psychiatric and mental health care of older adults and elderly patients is gaining increased importance with the recognition of the incidence of undiagnosed depression, dementia, and drug-induced psychoses and other psychiatric disorders.

Figure 6-5
Medical-surgical nurses care for diverse populations in need of a wide range of services, and must rely on excellent people skills to help manage the challenges of this specialty.

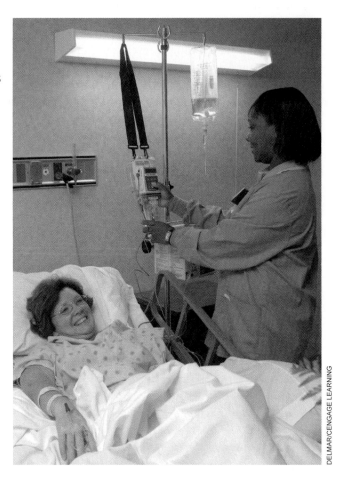

DELMAR/CENGAGE LEARNING

SPECIALTIES ASSOCIATED WITH SPECIFIC HEALTH CARE TREATMENT SETTINGS

A nursing specialty might focus on care of patients within a specific health care treatment setting. These settings are described in the following.

Ambulatory Care Nursing

For example, ambulatory care nurses care for the diverse patient populations that seek services in clinic settings established by government, hospital, health care, or other organizations or agencies. Experienced nurses in this specialty may provide the answers based on defined protocols and algorithms for incoming calls as the staff for health plan, insurance, or health organization telephone call centers, or they may serve in administrative positions managing the

Figure 6-6

Psychiatric-mental health nurses provide patient-centered mental health and psychiatric care in a wide range of settings, and sometimes further specialize by focusing on specific groups such as child-adolescent, adult or, as pictured here, elderly patients.

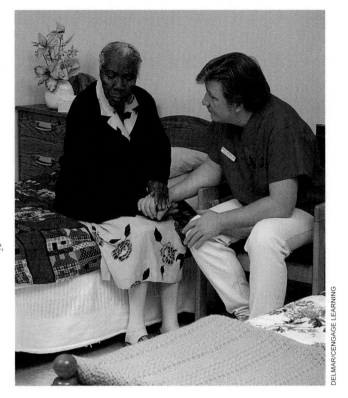

center, clinic, or program services. The centers may service local, state, regional, national, or international patients and may require licensure from more than one state board of nursing.

Home Health Nursing

Home health nurses provide nursing care to acutely ill, chronically ill, and well patients of all ages in their residences. Although not a new nursing specialty, home health nurses are becoming increasingly important health care providers as our aging population encounters the debilitations and challenges associated with chronic illness, disease, and disability. Enlightened communities support efforts to help persons age in place through such things as home modifications, transportation assistance, and provision of social and health services in the home setting. Such initiatives to keep residents out of more expensive long-term-care facilities are gaining momentum. Similarly, decreased use of hospital services because of private insurance and Medicare and Medicaid mandates has increased the need for home care services. Without the luxury of available technologies and resources found in hospital settings, the home health nurse must have creative and innovative problem-solving skills. They are important patient educators, case managers, and patient advocates to help patients identify their preferences and choices related to the use of health care and social services.

Telehealth Nursing

Telehealth nurses participate in the virtual health visit either as the person preparing and presenting the patient for the telehealth visit, or at the other end receiving the transmission and accompanying physiologic monitoring data and information. Telehealth services may include the remote monitoring done by home health nurses or other specialty nurses managing patient populations in nurse-managed clinics, such as congestive heart patient clinics, childhood asthma programs, or diabetes management projects. These technologies permit patient access to services not available in their community or location, enable cost-effective and timely appointment scheduling, and allow for more frequent monitoring, counseling, and education sessions, and actual interventions and therapies. Virtual access to critical-care nurses located in other parts of the country permits the provision of additional patient monitoring capabilities and enhanced professional educational opportunities for just-in-time learning.

Occupational Health Nursing

Occupational health nurses work in clinics or small health care units within manufacturing, industrial, or other environments. Pre-employment health examinations, baseline and recurrent assessments and screenings, health promotion and wellness programs, worker education, injury prevention, workplace monitoring, and emergency services reflect the diversity of the occupational health nurse's responsibilities. These nurses play key roles in helping the employer create a healthy workplace, keep workers healthy, prevent workplace injuries and death, and maintain appropriate clinical and environmental monitoring records.

Corrections Nursing

Corrections nurses provide nursing care to those in prisons, jails, and detention centers. Patients range in age from children to the elderly and include female and male patients. Legislation mandates that health care services comparable to those within the community be available to patients in corrections facilities. Large corrections facilities may provide on-site, acute-care centers that can include critical-care units, dialysis services, and inpatient psychiatric units. Patient education and planning for continued health care services after release are important activities and require public health nursing and case management expertise.

Radiology Nursing

Radiology nurses have a unique patient **advocacy** role as they facilitate a safe interventional and diagnostic radiology experience. Patient and family education before, during, and after the procedures are important nursing activities. Radiology nurses may assist in the preparation of the patient, monitoring during the radiology process and also recovery phases, and often are the staff members who complete follow-up communications and assessments after discharge to home. Radiology nurses in oncology centers provide the continuity of care and psychological support through the many sessions of radiation therapy that may be prescribed as part of the treatment protocol.

Perioperative Nursing

Operating room nurses are now titled perioperative nurses to better describe the role these specialty nurses have in caring for the patient throughout the entire preoperative, operative, and postoperative experience. Circulating nurses have responsibility for the patient and oversight of the operation of the room and all the necessary resources that are not directly under the purview of the anesthesiology team. Some perioperative nurses elect to work only in the preanesthesia staging area and postanesthesia recovery units. With the significant reliance on same-day surgery procedures, the perioperative nurse's work has now expanded to often include next-day telephone communication with the patients and their families to complete a follow-up assessment of their entire operative experience. A select number of perioperative nurses may elect to complete additional preparation to become certified as a registered nurse first assistant, thereby becoming surgical team members directly assisting the surgeons during the operative procedures.

Critical Care Nursing

Critical care registered nurses engage in practice most often in critical-care units within hospitals. Their patients are acutely ill, require very close monitoring and observation, may be attached to many patient-monitoring devices, and usually requite complex and intensive therapies and medication protocols. Critical-care nurses may also work in home settings when critically ill patients have been discharged from hospitals. The registered nurse-to-patient ratio is usually limited to no more than one nurse to two critical care patients. The American Association of Critical Care Nurses has created an intensive educational program to prepare nurses in this specialty practice and ready those individuals for the critical care nursing certification.

Emergency Nursing

Emergency nurses care for those individuals who present to stand-alone or hospital-based emergency departments for emergent care for injury or disease. Sudden, acute injuries or disease include such things as heart attack, stroke, poisoning, hemorrhage, meningitis, severe pain, difficulty breathing, injuries from assault and rape, gunshots and stabbings, and vehicular, home, or industrial accidents. Care focuses on stabilizing the patients' condition and returning them to their home for later follow-up with their private physician or consultant, or getting the person evaluated by a specialist and moved to another health care setting, like an inpatient nursing unit within the facility or transportation to a specialty center. Emergency nurses must be prepared

Figure 6-7

Nurses can become specialized to ground or air transport teams that care for acutely ill or injured patients needing emergency transport.

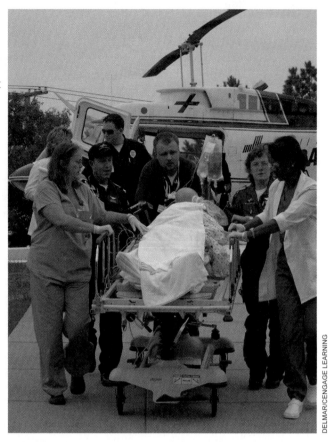

DELMAR/CENGAGE LEARNING

to care for any-age patient with any injury or disease who enters the emergency department. Because some patients use the emergency services department as an ambulatory clinic, triage skills are critical for the emergency nurse to help prioritize which patients need to be treated first and who can wait a bit longer for services. Expert negotiation and communication skills are mandatory because of the tensions and volatile and emotionally laden scenarios present with sudden illness or injury. Some nurses elect to specialize in caring for those acutely ill patients needing emergency transport to other facilities. They may be assigned to ground or air transport teams and may be subject to on-call assignments.

SPECIALTIES ADDRESSING SPECIFIC DISEASES, AILMENTS, OR CONDITIONS

Nursing specialties may bear titles and foci comparable to the medical terminology for the disease, ailment, or condition.

Diabetes Nursing

With the obesity epidemic among adults and children, followed by the greater incidence of diabetes in those patients, the need for diabetes management nurses and diabetes nurse educators is expanding. These nurses have a key responsibility in helping patients learn about their diabetes and its management, and its related health issues (Figure 6-8). Diabetes nurses teach how careful management via diet, exercise, and necessary medication protocols have been shown to reduce the incidence of debilitating complications of end-stage renal disease, blindness, hypertension, and cardiovascular disease. These nurses focus on helping patients appreciate the importance of maintaining compliance of their prescribed therapies to help prevent complications. They also provide consultative services to other staff dealing with unusually complicated diabetic patients.

Genetics/Genomics Nursing

Genetics/genomics nurses are gaining importance as this science evolves. With the increased availability of affordable genomics testing and expanding knowledge bases, more patients are electing to pay for the tests themselves rather than through insurance plans. The genetics/genomics nurses are counselors as families and patients seek to understand and incorporate genomics testing results when making life, therapy, and reproductive choices. They are firm advocates for appropriate confidentiality rules and protections. The International Society of Nurses in Genetics (ISONG) has posted *Essential Nursing Competencies and Curricula Guidelines for Genetics and Genomics* at http://www.isong.org. Click on Resources, then Professional Practice.

Other Examples

Other RNs may elect to provide care for those with specific organ or system health issues such as in the cardiovascular (heart and vessels), pulmonary (lungs and airway), dermatology (skin), nephrology (kidney), and gastroenterology (esophagus, stomach, bowel, liver, pancreas) specialties. Oncology nursing is not a new nursing specialty, but continues to evolve as

Figure 6-8
Diabetes nursing is an expanding specialty area.

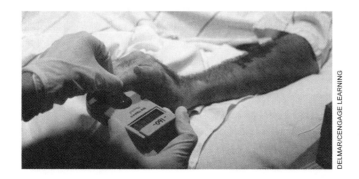

DELMAR/CENGAGE LEARNING

new technologies and research findings change the care of cancer patients. Of key importance are the current and future implications of the genomics revolution. Tailor-made anticancer therapies and new administration methodologies may reduce the complications, improve the odds of survival, and definitely challenge the clinicians to learn the complex technologies and their applications.

HIV/AIDS nurses care for those who range in age from newborns to the elderly and are living with AIDS or have been confirmed to be HIV positive. These patients have ongoing education needs and may have to maintain compliance with complex medication protocols. Plastic surgery nurses, members of a recently recognized nursing specialty, are gaining importance as key patient advocates in a largely unregulated industry. They have an instrumental role in teaching patients about treatment options and postop care and may serve a role quite like that of the perioperative nurse during office-based procedures.

Some nurses specialize in pain management and may elect to further their knowledge through graduate studies culminating in the CNS or NP designation. Others elect to become certified registered nurse anesthetists, master's-prepared registered nurses who provide anesthesia services, including pain management therapies, for patients of all ages and with all types of diseases and conditions. Most often these advanced-practice registered nurses have had a robust work experience history in critical-care and emergency services before becoming a nurse anesthetist. Preparation includes completion of at least a two-year academic program that includes an extensive clinical practicum. These nurses may be the sole anesthesia provider in remote-access and underserved areas.

> **Internet Exercise 6-1**
>
> Specialty nursing organizations have created The Nursing Organizations Alliance (The Alliance). Find the Web site and review the extensive list of specialty nursing organizations. Select two nursing specialties of interest to you and examine the available content at the hyperlinks. Do the organizations have an advocacy committee or staff?

SPECIALTIES CARING FOR A WELL-DEFINED POPULATION

Another way to categorize specialties is by the population served.

Public Health Nursing

Public health nursing has a long and rich history. The first initiatives to address the needs of communities and their disadvantaged members have evolved to today's public health nursing practice focused on promoting and protecting the health of populations through the use of knowledge from nursing, social, and public health sciences. Although local jurisdictions and communities are still important interests, our global economy has forced expansion of the focus of public health nurses to also address international issues and risks. Surveillance, prevention, assessment of risks and threats, identification of strengths and assets of communities and populations, advocacy, and collaboration characterize the practice of public health nurses.

Gerontological Nursing

Gerontology nurses provide nursing care for the elderly who may be at home, attend adult day care, or reside in rehabilitation, assisted living, or long-term care facilities. The increased incorporation of gerontological research findings into practice is changing the long-held myths about aging. Many changes attributed to the aging process are being identified as pathology related to undiagnosed diseases or sequelae of medication and therapies. Care of those with dementias is gaining increased attention, as is the importance of appropriate diet and the use of vitamins and supplements as preventive mechanisms. Gerontology nurses teach the elderly and their families about evaluating Web-based health information resources and serve as patient advocates to help secure appropriate services and therapies.

Faith Community Nursing

Faith community nursing has replaced the title of parish nursing to better reflect the diversity of the population of concern. The faith community may be affiliated with a church, congregation, synagogue, temple, parish, mosque, or other entity. The primary focus of this specialty nursing practice is the whole person and their spiritual and religious concerns. Although these nurses have traditionally been unpaid, their value is becoming better appreciated and they are being reimbursed as salaried members of the faith community. In many locations, faith community nurses have assumed instrumental roles in emergency preparedness planning efforts.

Transplant Nursing

Transplant nurses, because of the associated legal and ethical risks related to transplant services, differentiate their practices into two separate and distinct areas: care for those who are donors and care for those who are recipients. The long duration pre- and posttransplant periods and accompanying emotional and physical challenges and issues require that the transplant nurse demonstrate strong clinical and interpersonal skills. They must care for patients as they struggle with either deterioration of their health and eventual death without receiving the necessary transplant, or alternatively life with the complicated immuno-suppression protocols and the constant threat of potential transplant rejection, infection, or other opportunistic processes that may culminate in death.

Internet Exercise 6-2

Use your information-seeking skills to locate the Web site of the American Nurses Credentialing Center (ANCC).

1. Identify which accreditations ANCC has achieved, and by which accrediting bodies.

2. Then examine the criteria for accreditation from one of the accrediting bodies.

3. Find the nursing specialty of most interest to you and review the posted test content outline that nurses can review in preparation for that specialty certification.

4. Which of those topics have you already studied as part of your current educational program? Which are new?

COMBINATIONS OF SPECIALTIES

RNs may combine specialties and must rely on the synthesis of even more data, information, and knowledge from diverse sources.

Pediatric Oncology Nursing

For example, pediatric oncology nurses care for children and adolescents who have cancer. They must be experts in pediatrics, as well as oncology, to help balance the child's normal developmental needs with the mandates of prescribed therapies and the disease's progression, remission, or cure. Issues associated with maintaining healthy family relationships and cancer survivorship are examples of the concerns addressed by pediatric oncology nurses.

Wound, Ostomy, and Continence Nursing

Wound, ostomy, continence nurses care for patients with wounds and ostomies and also urinary and bowel incontinence. Their expertise proves invaluable in helping ostomy patients learn how to accept their new body image and establish new management activities for bodily functions and social settings. Aggressive wound management protocols lead to healing as the research and science are integrated into practice. That further reinforces the mandate for continuous lifelong learning by all nurses. Strong collaboration with infection-control nurses and physicians is necessary.

Hospice and Palliative Nursing

The specialty of hospice and palliative nursing is gaining increased membership. Although many think this specialty only addresses patient care during the final days immediately before death, hospice and palliative nurses focus on the care for people with life-limiting and terminal illness. That interval may range from days and hours to years. These specialty nurses also assist the families in dealing with the accompanying concerns, thoughts, feelings, and decisions associated with life-limiting or terminal illness. Consider accessing the series of educational materials and professional resources available in the TIPS section of the Hospice and Palliative Nurses Association (HPNA) Web site.

Holistic Nursing

Holistic nursing received nursing specialty recognition by the ANA in 2007. Holistic nursing focuses on healing of the whole person and supporting people to find peace, comfort, harmony, and balance. This person-relationship-centered practice incorporates the nurse as an active and therapeutic partner with the individual, family, community, or population in defining health and the necessary changes and therapies to achieve health. Several undergraduate nursing programs and five graduate programs have been recognized by the American Holistic Nurse Certification Corporation for their programs preparing holistic nurses.

Internet Exercise 6-3

Use your information-seeking skills to locate the Web site of the American Holistic Nurses Association (AHNA).

1. What continuing-education programs are announced on the Web site?

2. Which schools of nursing have been endorsed by AHNA?

3. If you were looking for a new position as a holistic nurse, which one of the job postings would be most enticing and why?

NURSING ROLE SPECIALTIES

Some nurses have little or no direct patient care and focus on assuring effective nursing and health care infrastructures are in place. These positions still require an active RN license.

Case Managers

Case managers help secure and manage resources to ensure that all of the health care needs of patients with severe injuries and severe or chronic illnesses are met. They collaborate closely with insurance plans, community resources, and various health care professionals to create an effective care plan, and then find the necessary services and equipment. Extensive telephone, online, and written communications activities characterize this practice (Figure 6-9).

Forensic Nursing

Forensic nurses address the nursing care of victims and perpetrators of intentional and unintentional injury, including victims of sexual assault, child abuse, or accidental death. They are often instrumental in identifying those who are the victims; establishing educational programs for community and professionals about the issues of abuse, violence and assault; and providing expert testimony in legal cases and investigations.

Infection Control Nursing

The specialty practice of infection control nurses has expanded from the identification, tracking, control, and prevention of infectious and other hazardous outbreaks in health

Figure 6-9
Case managers use their communication and collaboration skills to create an effective care plan and arrange for the resources to meet a patient's needs.

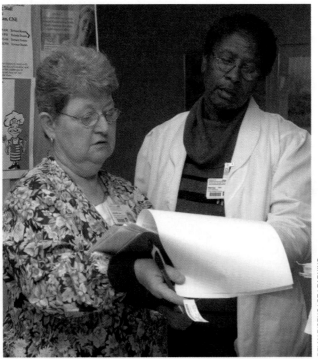

care facilities. These nurses are now key participants in facility, community, state, regional, national, and international emergency preparedness planning and operational activities. They work closely with public health and risk management staff, clinicians, as well as laboratory services providers.

Legal Nurse Consulting

Legal nurse consultants are expert nurse clinicians who assist lawyers in determining the facts associated with medical cases. This involves interviewing patients and witnesses and organizing content found in medical, insurance, and financial records. They help locate evidence and assist in the decision-making process related to determining damages and costs and moving the case forward to litigation. Legal nurse consultants must be expert educators to prepare patients, families, lawyers, and other legal system members about health care, nursing, and medical facts and issues. These nursing specialists may also be case managers and forensic experts.

CASE SCENARIO 6-2

You are a seated member on the ANA's Congress on Nursing Practice and Economics and have been tasked with providing recommendation(s) for action related to three letters received by the congress that call for reversal of the recognition of legal nurse consulting and holistic nursing as nursing specialties. The letter of concern about legal nurse consultants referenced that these nurses do not provide clinical care to patients and work for lawyers, not hospitals or physicians. One letter about holistic nursing focused on the potential for child abuse and neglect related to religious beliefs, cultural traditions, or quackery by this "quasi-voodoo 'nursing' specialty." The second letter about holistic nursing asked if the ANA had confirmed that any state boards of nursing legally allowed holistic nurses to practice.

CASE ANALYSIS

1. Define the stated and potential issues that need examination and action from the Congress on Nursing Practice and Economics.

2. Draft a plan of action to identify the detailed concerns and the resources necessary to inform the response effort.

3. Formulate a collection of questions and criteria that can be used to reaffirm or negate the congress's decisions to recognize legal nurse consulting and holistic nursing as nursing specialties.

4. Identify potential ramifications if a nursing specialty recognition decision was reversed.

5. Develop a summary report to the congress that presents the issues, detailed findings, and your recommendation(s) for action(s).

Nursing Administration

Nurse administrators are most often categorized into two levels: nurse managers and nurse executives. Position titles reflect the diversity of roles and responsibilities of nurse administrators. Nurse managers usually have a prescribed, distinct, limited area of oversight and may supervise nursing staff, establish work schedules and budgets, and maintain medical supply inventories for the specific unit, department, or division. Nurse executives are the most senior-level administrators and may be titled chief nursing officer, chief nurse executive, or vice president for patient services in the clinical setting, dean or assistant dean in academic settings, or be named the chief executive officer, chief operating officer, or chief programs officer in an organization or business setting. Increasing responsibility and accountability characterize the career progression of nurse administrators. Education at the graduate and doctoral levels is now becoming the norm for preparing nurse administrators.

Nursing Education and Professional Development

The professional development specialty includes nurse educators in academic faculty roles who create curricula and teach undergraduate student nurses and graduate-level nurses. Another group of nurse educators are those nurses developing, coordinating, and conducting continuing-education programs for RNs and other health care staff. The nursing shortage is even more evident within this specialty practice, especially as the aging academic faculty elect to leave nursing through retirement or movement into the service sector.

Nursing Informatics

Informatics nurses and informatics nurse specialists are gaining increased attention as greater numbers of facilities, organizations, and agencies integrate the electronic health record into their business and documentation processes. The nursing informatics specialty

Writing
Exercise
6-2

Reflect on your past nursing experiences and identify the type of patient and type of setting you found most interesting and even intriguing. What nursing specialties focus on practice related to your selections? What specialty nursing organizations could you choose to join to help you connect with like-minded nurses? Do they have special membership categories for students and new graduates? Create a table that includes the pros and cons for joining a specialty nursing organization.

integrates nursing science, computer science, and information science to manage and communicate data, information, knowledge, and wisdom in nursing practice. Such efforts support patients, nurses and other providers in their decision making in all roles and settings (ANA, 2008). RNs may also identify themselves as health care consultants, public policy advisors, pharmaceutical and medical supply researchers and salespersons, and medical writers and editors.

PREPARATION FOR SPECIALTY PRACTICE

Most often, preparation for nursing specialty practice begins with at least several years work experience within the specialty area to begin building one's skill set, assessment abilities, and understanding of the patient population and their health-illness experiences. Professional reading in the specialty area must be an integral part of this experience. Membership in an appropriate nursing or other specialty organization is also preferred because this permits exploration of the specialty practice through professional networking opportunities with experts in the field, attendance at conferences, and enrollment in continuing education offerings for preparation for certification in the specialty. Initial or advanced-level certification in the specialty may be available. At some point personal assessment and reflection may prompt investigation of and enrollment in available formal academic programs focused on the specialty practice. Completion of such a graduate program may permit application for APRN recognition, depending on the state board of nursing licensing requirements.

Please note that the sample of nursing specialties presented in this chapter is merely representative of the many, many opportunities available. Some specialty practice areas haven't even been invented. Registered nurses can choose to explore many branches in a career path. Remember, specialty practice is not a life sentence, will involve change over your professional career, and should always reflect your passion for nursing.

SUMMARY

Nursing specialty practice reflects how the registered nurse demonstrates the protection, promotion, and optimization of health and abilities, prevention of illness and injury, alleviation of suffering through the diagnosis and treatment of human response, and advocacy in the care of an identified subset of individuals, families, communities, and populations. The well-derived knowledge base particular to the practice of a nursing specialty serves to guide decision-making in that practice and is reflected in the educational preparation and professional certification programs for that specialty's nurses. Professional organizations and legal entities provide the professional and legal regulatory oversight of specialty practice.

Opportunities for diversity in nursing specialty practice abound for the registered nurse engaged in life-long learning.

Don't be afraid to take a big step if one is indicated; you can't cross a chasm in two small jumps.

–David Lloyd George

REFERENCES

American Nurses Association. (2001). *Code of ethics for nurses with interpretive statements.* Silver Spring, MD: Nursesbooks.org.

American Nurses Association. (2003). *Nursing's social policy statement, second edition.* Silver Spring, MD: Nursesbooks.org.

American Nurses Association. (2004). *Nursing: Scope and standards of practice.* Silver Spring, MD: Nursesbooks.org.

American Nurses Association. (2005). *Recognition of a nursing specialty, approval of a specialty nursing scope of practice statement, and acknowledgment of specialty nursing standards of practice.* Silver Spring, MD: Author.

American Nurses Association. (2007). *Psychiatric-mental health nursing: Scope and standards of practice.* Silver Spring, MD: Nursesbooks.org.

American Nurses Association. (2008). *Nursing informatics: Scope and standards of practice.* Silver Spring, MD: Nursesbooks.org.

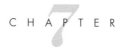

CHAPTER 7

POLICY: ASSESSMENT, DEVELOPMENT, ANALYSIS, AND EVALUATION

LILLIAN WISE

DNS, RN, Professor and Coordinator, RN to BSN/MSN Track, Troy University

AMY SPURLOCK

PhD, RN, Associate Professor, Troy University

Involvement in policy making is not an option for a professional nurse—it is a necessity.

–Dr. Jeri A. Milstead

LEARNING OBJECTIVES

At the completion of the chapter, the learner should be able to do the following

1. Analyze the four steps of the policy process: Assessment, development, analysis, and evaluation.
2. Differentiate between policy and policy process in nursing.
3. Explain why policy is an essential component of nursing practice.
4. Discuss the importance of stakeholders or key players in the policy process.
5. Differentiate between private policy and public policy.
6. Discuss the importance of evidence-based policy process in the nursing policy process.
7. Explain the reasons for a nurse to become involved in the policy process.
8. Discuss the importance of ethics in the policy process.
9. Explain the Step/Stages Model of policy process.
10. Analyze the multiple stream framework and the advocacy-coalition framework.
11. Trace an issue in nursing through the four stages of the policy process.

KEY TERMS

Advocacy-Coalition Framework
Evidence-based Policy Process
Multiple Streams Framework

Policy
Policy Analysis
Policy Assessment
Policy Development

Policy Evaluation
Step/Stages Model

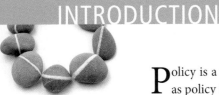

INTRODUCTION

Policy is a topic that many nurses are not fully comfortable discussing. This is unfortunate, as policy is a word that should motivate and inspire nurses. Nurses need to understand and participate in the policy process in order to fully advocate for clients, whether they be individuals, families, or communities. **Policy** refers to "authoritative guidelines that direct human behavior toward specific goals, in either the private or public sector" (Hanley & Falk, 2007, p. 76). In this definition, policy is described as an entity, but policy may also be described in terms of a process (Figure 7-1). When policy is described as a process, it refers to "...taking problems to government agents and obtaining a decision or reply in the form of a program, law, or regulation" (Milstead, 2004, p. 1). These two definitions, when applied to nursing practice, are pertinent and deserve attention (Figure 7-1).

Why is policy an essential component of nursing practice? Nurses are in a unique position to both evaluate policies (Milstead, 2002) and participate in the policy process. Nurses are directly and intimately involved in patient care on an hourly basis, and their knowledge base is such that they are able to educate others about issues that are important to the public's health (Collins, 2006; Steele, Rocchiccioli, & Porche, 2003). Some of these issues include patient safety and satisfaction, access to care, clinical outcomes, health disparities, cost of health care, and quality of care (Abood, 2007; Smith, 2006). Through our direct involvement in client care, we are able to clearly see client needs as well as the impact of policies. According to Abood, nurses should utilize their power, which is "the potential to exert influence" (2007, p. 4). Nurses exert influence through many sources of power, including expert power due to their professional education, legitimate power through their licensure requirements, and referent power through public respect (Abood). And perhaps most importantly, nurses have a natural interest in, and the professional obligation of, advocating on behalf of clients (Abood, 2007; Saikonda-Woitas, & Robinson, 2002; Steele et al., 2003). Engaging in the policy process is an important opportunity for nurses to use their power to provide input and solutions to issues that impact the public's health (Figure 7-2).

Figure 7-1
The term "policy" refers to both an entity and a process.

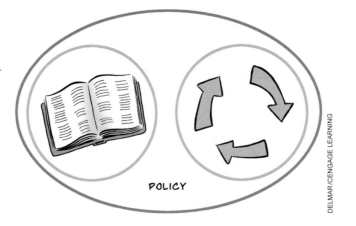

POLICY

DELMAR/CENGAGE LEARNING

Figure 7-2
Nurses must be
involved in policy
in order to fully
advocate for clients.
*(Courtesy of New
York State Nurses
Association.)*

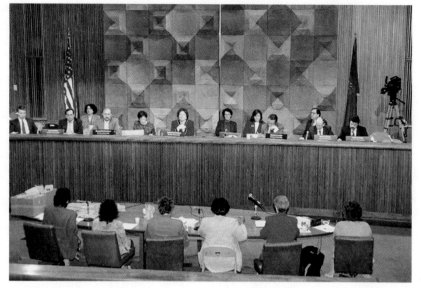

If policy is important, then why are nurses reluctant to become involved? Numerous citations exist in the literature that speak to "the invisibility of nurses in the policy process" (Maslin-Prothero, &Masterson, 1998; Milstead, 2003; Smith, 2006; Toofany, 2005). One reason is that nurses may lack political awareness and knowledge about the policy process itself (Maslin-Prothero et al., 1998; Toofany, 2003). Nurses need to be educated about policy in order to affect positive change, beginning with student nurses in basic educational programs and extending into graduate programs. Another reason is that nurses may feel that policy is not in the role of nursing at the bedside (Maslin-Prothero et al.; Toofany), which implies that nursing practice is somehow removed from policy (Smith, 2006). In fact, nothing could be further from the truth. Each day, the care that nurses provide is influenced by policies and regulations, from resource allocation to evidence-based procedures. Today in the United States, there are over 2.9 million registered nurses, of whom 2.4 million are employed in nursing (United States Department of Health and Human Services, n.d.). If the majority of nurses would become involved in even one policy area, the impact could be enormous. For example, you might be a nurse in a state that does not allow a registered nurse to administer a local anesthetic agent without training beyond basic nurse education for RNs. Yet, you feel that this is a skill that a licensed RN could perform following standardized procedures according to the Board of Nursing in your state. You have heard that the State of Alabama does allow this skill, and have read the Alabama Board of Nursing, Administrative Code, Standards of Practice, which includes the Standardized Procedures and Local Anesthetic Agents (found at http://www.abn.state.al.us). What could you do about this issue? First, you might research the number of potential supporters of this idea by finding out how many RNs currently hold active RN licenses in your state. This will give you an indication of the impact that a policy change might have on the nursing profession in your own state.

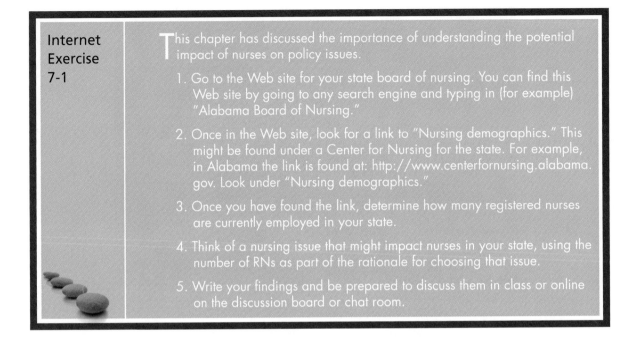

Internet Exercise 7-1

This chapter has discussed the importance of understanding the potential impact of nurses on policy issues.

1. Go to the Web site for your state board of nursing. You can find this Web site by going to any search engine and typing in (for example) "Alabama Board of Nursing."

2. Once in the Web site, look for a link to "Nursing demographics." This might be found under a Center for Nursing for the state. For example, in Alabama the link is found at: http://www.centerfornursing.alabama.gov. Look under "Nursing demographics."

3. Once you have found the link, determine how many registered nurses are currently employed in your state.

4. Think of a nursing issue that might impact nurses in your state, using the number of RNs as part of the rationale for choosing that issue.

5. Write your findings and be prepared to discuss them in class or online on the discussion board or chat room.

Figure 7-3
Diagram of the Four Steps in the Policy Process.

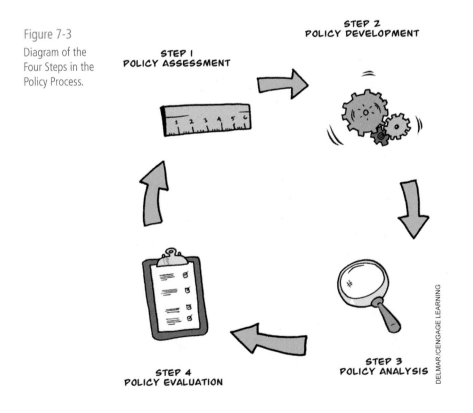

STEP 1
POLICY ASSESSMENT

STEP 2
POLICY DEVELOPMENT

STEP 3
POLICY ANALYSIS

STEP 4
POLICY EVALUATION

DELMAR/CENGAGE LEARNING

POLICY PROCESS

In order to become involved in policy, the first step is to become aware of the policy process. Policy may be divided into four subtopics: (a) assessment, which involves identification and definition of the problem with development of objectives or outcomes; (b) development, which involves supporting data collection and analysis, research review, and recommendation of a plan of action; (c) analysis, which involves a critical appraisal of implications and consequences guided by a model or framework; and (d) evaluation, which involves the evaluation of policy and program implementation and impacts in terms of its goals. The four steps in the policy process in Figure 7-3 reveal an ongoing process.

POLICY ASSESSMENT

Policy may be separated into two broad categories consisting of private policy and public policy (Figure 7-4). Private policy includes health care agencies and institutions that provide more specific guidelines, such as client care or employment; whereas public policy deals at the local, state, and national levels and provides legislation, rules, and laws affecting health care agencies and the public (Hanley & Falk, 2007).

The policy process begins with **policy assessment**, which starts with the first glimpse of a problem, issue, or need that requires action or resolution. Policy assessment is defined as the first step of the policy process in which the problem, issue, or need is identified with initial data.

Figure 7-4
Policy may be categorized as either public or private.

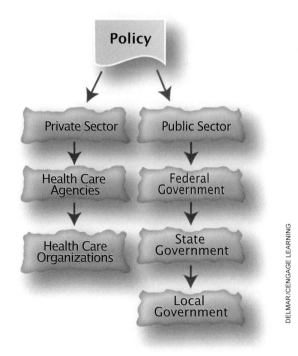

DELMAR/CENGAGE LEARNING

This step is congruent with the first phase of Hanley and Falk's (2007) phases of the policy process or policy agenda setting. In this step the problem is defined, support from stakeholders is gained, and objectives/outcomes are developed (Hanley & Falk).

Once the problem, issue, or need is identified, the nurse will seek support to review the problem and define the policy issue. The support gained from stakeholders who are concerned about the issue will lead to more effective policy assessment. Stakeholders are those individuals or groups who "may be directly affected by the outcome" (Hanley & Falk, p. 76) of the issue. Stakeholders may come from private or public sectors. In the policy assessment step, a nurse might consult stakeholders or key stakeholders such as legislators, board of nursing members, and state nursing association members. Once the stakeholders' support is gained and the problem is defined, then the objectives are developed with measurable outcomes. At this time priorities are discussed and developed and potential implications for governing agencies are included (Hanley & Falk, 2007). Those individuals and groups that support the issue should discuss what is most important and who directly regulates the issue. For example, a group of school nurses is concerned about the policies of delegation of unlicensed personnel. The nurses would identify their state board of nursing as the regulation agency that they will need to work with as one part of their policy development efforts. Other considerations in policy assessment include broader factors such as vision, mission, culture, and values (Randolph, 2006). For example, is the issue in direct conflict with cultural practices? To view policy assessment within the four steps with considerations see Table 7-1, which illustrates the policy process steps.

Policy assessment might begin with a clinical nurse who identifies a need for change. For example, a need might exist in the intravenous procedure (IV) related to the increased rate of IV-site infections; or, a need for change in the cost containment procedures on the clinical unit related to increased unit use of certain items; or, the need for improved safety standards on a clinical unit related to increased needle sticks of nurses. The problem is revealed to the nurse through the initial data, such as increased IV-site infections. Policy assessment could also begin within the public health setting with a nurse who witnessed disparities in health care during a disaster such as Hurricane Katrina, a category-4 hurricane that devastated the Gulf coast between Alabama and Louisiana in 2005. During this major disaster, areas needing improvement became known in the emergency management system, such as the preparedness to manage pediatric emergencies (Huddleston, 2006). Policy assessment could also begin with the nurse who sees the nursing shortage as affecting the workplace, which in turn impacts most health care facilities in his or her individual state. This nurse might join the state and national nurses associations to contribute to efforts to alleviate the nursing shortage at the state and national levels.

Keep in mind that nurses may identify an issue that is either a policy need or a procedural need. Randolph (2006) suggests, "procedures are a chronological series of interrelated steps that are taken to implement a policy" (p. 502). If there is a policy in place, the problem may be with the procedural steps to implement the policy. For example, nurses during a disaster can refer to federal-level policies that give guidance for pediatric emergency management, such as in the 1985 Emergency Medical Services for Children Act (Huddleston, 2006). The problems may occur in the policy or procedure at the federal, regional, and/or institutional level, where preparation may not be adequate for the pediatric needs in the emergency management plan, perhaps due to a lack of funding. The problem may be at the federal level, where emergency management

Table 7-1 Policy Process Steps with Considerations

Policy Process Step	Policy Considerations/ Actions	Evaluation of Actions	Suggested Changes
1. Assessment	Define the problem, issue, or need. Gain stakeholders' support. State objectives or outcomes.	Set criteria to meet objectives or outcomes.	
2. Development	Collect and analyze data. Review research. Consult key stakeholders. State plan of action.	List pros and cons of plan of action. Review outcome of any compromise and/ or negotiation. Review research with proposed options for plan of action. List resource allocation.	
3. Analysis	Describe policy. Review model or framework. Assess impact. Review consequences.	Set model or framework. List impact on different groups.	
4. Evaluation	Evaluate implementation of plan of action. Evaluate performance of plan of action. Evaluate the impact of plan of action. Evaluate ethical considerations. Evaluate impact of research.	List positive and negative aspects of implementation phase. List results related to criteria in plan of action. List ethical impacts. State comparison with outcomes and current research.	

principles and funding have changed since the 2001 terrorist attacks. Currently, many general hospitals spend most of their resources on emergency preparedness for adults, who have very different needs from children (Huddleston). Many general health care agencies may not be adequately prepared with pediatric equipment to meet the needs of children in a major disaster, such as a terrorist attack, flu epidemic, or hurricane. Huddleston, in an analysis of a CDC survey, found that "only 11% of emergency departments answered yes to all of the essential items on their supply list" related to pediatric emergency supplies and equipment (2006, p. 168). These gaps in pediatric emergency care have identified the need for more policy changes and funding at the local, state, and federal levels.

Ethical and Legal Issues

Policy assessment may involve ethical or legal issues that nurses are sometimes faced with in clinical practice, and that may become a highly visible health policy issue for the public. For example right-to-die and end-of-life issues are ethical dilemmas that some nurses have dealt with in their clinical practices. Whether in the home or clinical setting, nurses have had important roles in caring for dying patients and their families. Hospitals have developed policies related to advanced directives that will indicate a patient's wishes related to life-sustaining actions, such as cardiopulmonary resuscitation (Altmann & Collins, 2007). Patients are seeking legal counsel for the development of their own living wills to address their wishes related to end-of-life measures. During the 1990s the issue of euthanasia came into public view through the actions of Dr. Jack Kevorkian, who participated in the physician-assisted suicide (PAS) of up to 130 terminally ill patients (Altmann & Collins). Dr. Kevorkian was eventually convicted and served a prison sentence for a related charge. Altmann and Collins trace the policy process from beginning to end on Oregon's Death with Dignity Act. The PAS issues sparked numerous morality debates, and these issues were passionately debated in many public and political arenas during the 1990s. In 1997 Oregon implemented Oregon's Death with Dignity Act to become law, which legalized PAS, and, since then, 264 individuals have used legal PAS as a method to end their life (Altmann & Collins). Altmann and Collins give recommendations related to PAS for nurses in Oregon. These recommendations begin with "a nurse...understand[ing] their own feelings about PAS" (Altmann & Collins, p. 51). Nurses in Oregon must be knowledgeable and prepared for implications related to PAS and their clinical practice. It is noted that no other state has legalized PAS at this time, but several states are considering some form of PAS. However, the PAS controversy forced states to review their laws related to end-of-life policies. No longer are end-of-life topics taboo for discussion. Nurses should be knowledgeable and prepared for ethical and legal issues in clinical practice that are part of the policy process, including knowing their state laws and institutional practices.

Legal issues in nursing arise sometimes because of failure to follow policy or procedural guidelines. For example the *Legal Eagle Eye* Newsletter for the Nursing Profession reports on the case of Cockerham v. LaSalle Nursing Home, Inc., from 2006, in which a forty-year-old patient with head injuries was left immobile and unable to speak (Anonymous, 2006). The patient was transferred from a nursing home to an emergency department when he pulled out

Figure 7-5
Understanding policy and procedural process leads to safer and more effective nursing care.

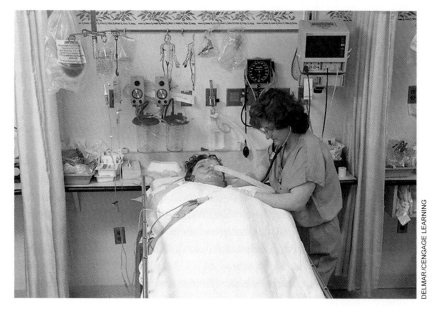

the gastrostomy feeding tube, only to have the tube reinserted (Anonymous). The emergency department nurse replaced the gastrostomy tube, even though she was uncertain of the correct placement of the tube. The patient was returned to the nursing home, however, and the nurse there did not check placement prior to reinstituting gastrostomy-tube feedings. Another nurse at the nursing home discovered problems with the flow and returned the patient to the emergency department. The patient was transferred to a second hospital. The patient developed sepsis after a nutritional formula was infused into the anterior abdominal wall and eventually died (Anonymous). In court the "jury found the nursing home and the first hospital each 50% responsible" (Anonymous, p. 5).

Were the problems in this case with policy or procedures? A critical step the nurse learns in education is to always check placement of a feeding tube before instituting any nutritional type of feeding or medication into a gastrostomy or nasogastric tube. Another critical factor that the nurse learns during education is never to perform a procedure without proper training. Therefore, understanding the policy process will help the nurse understand policy and procedures and the importance of following and participating in the policy process. The nurse who understands the policy or procedural process will be better prepared to deliver safe and effective nursing care that follows specific guidelines and standards of nursing practice (Figure 7-5).

Advanced Nursing Practice Issues

Advanced nursing practice has encountered many issues that have undergone extensive policy assessment and development. Specific regulations on the scope of clinical practice vary from state to state. For example, in 2006 advanced practice registered nurses (APRN) in Georgia gained prescriptive authority, and Georgia became the 50th state to enact this legislation (Phillips,

2007). The Georgia legislation resulted from six years of active work on policy change for APRNs (Phillips). An important development for advanced nursing practice was recommended in 2004 by the American Association of Colleges of Nursing (AACN, 2006). After a long policy process, AACN recommended raising the educational level of advanced nursing practice to the doctoral level by 2015 (AACN, 2006). Skaggs (2006) identifies that positive aspects of the move to the Doctorate in Nursing Practice will be "parity and increased credibility with other professions" (p. 5). These advanced nursing practice policy changes have implications for nursing practice, education, regulations, and research.

Advanced nursing practice policies have global implications. On a global level, Furlong and Smith (2005) report on the national policy for advanced nursing and midwifery practice in Ireland. Several factors led to the development of advanced practice nursing in Ireland, such as financial needs and changes in the health care environment (Furlong & Smith). In 1998 Ireland established guidelines and accreditation standards for advanced practice nursing, which were refined in 2004. Furlong and Smith report that lack of prescriptive authority for the advanced nurse practitioner could be a barrier to effective nursing practice in providing quality care to clients. These are global policy concerns that are dealt with in advanced nursing practice in the United States as well.

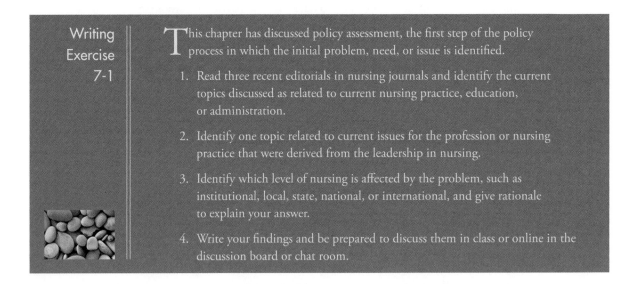

| Writing Exercise 7-1 | This chapter has discussed policy assessment, the first step of the policy process in which the initial problem, need, or issue is identified. |

1. Read three recent editorials in nursing journals and identify the current topics discussed as related to current nursing practice, education, or administration.

2. Identify one topic related to current issues for the profession or nursing practice that were derived from the leadership in nursing.

3. Identify which level of nursing is affected by the problem, such as institutional, local, state, national, or international, and give rationale to explain your answer.

4. Write your findings and be prepared to discuss them in class or online in the discussion board or chat room.

POLICY DEVELOPMENT

Once the policy issue is clearly identified and defined, the policy process moves into the **policy development** phase, in which data are collected and analyzed, research is reviewed, key stakeholders who will advocate for the plan are consulted, and the best plan of action is recommended (Hanley & Falk, 2007). The nurse, such as a nursing manager who has a clinical issue related to his or her clinical unit, may consult with all nursing managers in the hospital who are the key stakeholders or supporters of the problem at hand. As a group they will decide which data should be collected and analyzed, such as data related to the number of nosocomial infections occurring in the patients on each unit or the nurse-patient ratio on each unit. At the same time the supporters could review the latest research on the topic. Through a literature review the nurse will discover what research has been conducted on the problem and what strategies have been developed across the nation and worldwide to resolve the problem. The results from their data collection can be compared with what was found in the literature. How is it being handled in other health care agencies? Networking with nurses in different professional organizations, such as the state nurses associations or national organizations, will bring in ideas related to similar issues being experienced in other agencies.

The best plan of action may require several methods to reach consensus from the group of supporters. Hanley and Falk (2007) recommend that compromise and negotiation should be a part of the decision making process. Compromise and negotiation are important tools to gain support of key stakeholders and are important methods to allow consideration of all options for the plan of action (Figure 7-6). These are important methods as the group considers policy options, such as "What could or should be done about this problem?" (Hanley & Falk, p. 80). This process will allow the pros and cons of the issue to surface and will allow time to consider alternative solutions (Abood, 2007). Other factors should be considered, such as barriers to the actions and resources for the action (DePalma, 2002). Barriers to the actions could be legal issues or political issues. Resources needed for the actions could include budget requirements for implementation or could include the number of individuals needed for implementation (DePalma, 2002).

If the policy process includes a public issue, then the policy development process may move into the legislative arena. At this point the issue may have moved into a professional nursing organization that can lobby for issues in the legislative arena. An important component of policy development is advocacy and coalition building, which broadens the support of the policy issue. The end product of the policy development stage is the policy proposal that clearly states the problem, objectives, and plan for action.

Figure 7-6
Compromise and negotiation are key to effective policy development.

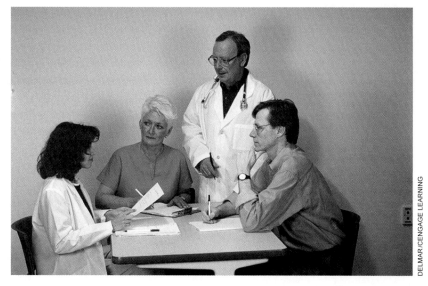

DELMAR/CENGAGE LEARNING

Nurses Who Participate in the Policy Process

Gebbie, Wakefield, and Kerfoot (2000) conducted a qualitative study to describe the effectiveness of nurses related to health policy development in the United States. The participants were nurses in state and national level positions, such as elected officials, national associations, health agencies, and education. Gebbie et al., found that some nurses become involved in the policy development process after "assessment, diagnosis and planning revealed the need for change in the way resources were allocated" (p. 307). One participant reported that the "passion for care" was the factor that moved the nurse from clinical practice into the policy process (Gebbie et al., p. 309). Another nurse was thrust into the policy process when he or she observed an unacceptable hospital policy of "house staff practicing intubations on dead patients" (Gebbie et al., p. 307).

Gebbie et al., (2000) found that some nurses reported important positive attributes nurses bring to the policy process, including: (a) expert nursing knowledge and skills gained from school and practice, (b) understanding the real patient experiences that the data and information are related to, and (c) experience with working and communicating with people. Nurses also reported negative factors for nurses in the policy process, including: (a) some nurses may be viewed as less intellectual than some professionals, (b) nurses do not value political involvement, and (c) nurses may not identify themselves as nurses when they participate in other groups such as a political group (Gebbie et al.). Nurses in the study were most often involved in policy development that related to speaking out for patients who have a limited voice, which speaks to the ethical standard of patient advocacy. Gebbie et al., concluded that "a nurse's knowledge of health issues and unmet needs, coupled with an understanding of what motivates people to get involved, is a potent combination in health policy" (p. 314).

Evidence-Based Policy Process

One change in the policy process is the need for evidence to support the proposed issue. This change has evolved with the development of evidence-based nursing practice. DePalma (2002) proposes that **evidence-based policy process** is "developing changes and improvements with a firm foundation of the best data that exist at the time from the science, the individual performing the service, and the consumer of the service" (p. 55). Evidence-based practice involves the review of the research related to the topic and implementing the best practice principles (DePalma, 2002). Evidence-based policy process should merge the policy process with research that incorporates valid and reliable data (DePalma). As nurses collect evidence to support the policy development, they should consider the credibility level of the evidence. DePalma reported that the most credible evidence was published research with randomized studies at the top. However, in areas of nursing that lack research the nurse could use available data such as quality control data.

DePalma (2002) suggests that policy driven by evidence-based principles should direct the study of policy and the effects on health care practice. Additionally, increased funding should be available for policy process research. A policy proposal that includes an evidence-based policy process will give policy makers, such as legislators, a clearer view of the problem with the latest evidence-based recommendations. The outcomes of nursing research and policy development can lead to policy or procedural changes that improve health care practice at multiple levels.

Evidence-Based Policy Process and Advanced Nursing Practice

One example of evidence-based policy process for advanced nursing practice relates to the education of advanced practice nurses. In 2002, in response to several issues in health care that impacted advanced nursing practice, the American Association of Colleges of Nursing (AACN) began a study of the clinical or practice doctorate. In AACN's 2004 position statement, many health care issues emerged from their evidence-gathering process, including: (a) reports that estimated between 44,000 and 98,000 Americans were dying each year as a result of medical errors, (b) increased health care expenditures as an aging population increased in numbers, and (c) decreased mid-level nurse managers, leaving those remaining with increased responsibilities (as cited in AACN, 2004). At the same time it was noted that many educational programs for advanced practice nurses had extended the degree requirements up to three years to complete requirements for the nurse practitioner track. AACN recommends that "the practice doctorate be the graduate degree for advanced nursing practice preparation, including but not limited to

---

CASE SCENARIO 7-1

In this exercise, you are the BSN-prepared nurse who is working in a hospital that is considering a major health care policy change of seeking magnet status through the Magnet Recognition Program recognized by the American Nurses Credentialing Center (ANCC, 2007). The Magnet Recognition Program is a benchmark that recognizes health care organizations for "quality patient care, nursing excellence, and innovations in professional nursing practice" (p. 1). You have read Shirey's (2005) article that suggested that certification in nursing is "essential to meet multiple standards within the American Nurses Credentialing Center's Magnet Recognition Program for excellence in nursing services" (p. 245). Shirey's article explained the success of one hospital that undertook a commitment to critical care nurse certification. You have been appointed to a committee that is participating in the policy assessment and development phase to develop a plan to establish a professional certification in nursing for your hospital.

CASE ANALYSIS

1. Develop a plan for assessment of the issue. State and define the issue.

2. Craft a policy statement for the issue.

3. Identify potential key supporters of the issue. How will you gain support of nurses who may oppose the issue?

4. Develop the key components for an evidence-based search related to certification in nursing.

5. Formulate a summary of evidence-based research that supports the policy change to present to key supporters.

the four current APN roles: clinical nurse specialist, nurse anesthetist, nurse midwife, and nurse practitioner" (2004, p.13). These recommendations, along with twelve other recommendations, have led to the rapid policy shift for nursing education to develop Doctorate of Nursing Practice (DNP) programs across the United States. The AACN (2004) position statement also included seven essential areas of content. One of the seven essential areas of content included "health policy development, implementation and evaluation" (AACN, p. 14, 2004).

Many changes in nursing created controversy in the 20th century, such as the development of the BSN and ASN prepared nurse. The development and implementation of the DNP has sparked controversy in 21st-century nursing, too. Chase and Pruitt (2006) suggested that caution is needed with the DNP implementation movement until more is understood about the consequences of the policy change for nursing education, health care agencies, and the nursing profession. Hathaway, Jacob, Segbauer, Thompson, and Graff (2006) advocate that DNP programs provide the complex knowledge and skills necessary for advanced nursing practice graduates who will be better prepared to lead the policy process in health care. AACN adopted the goal that the DNP will be the advanced practice nursing preparation by 2015 (AACN, 2006). Nursing has set the path for an evidence-based policy change for advanced nursing practice for education and clinical practice.

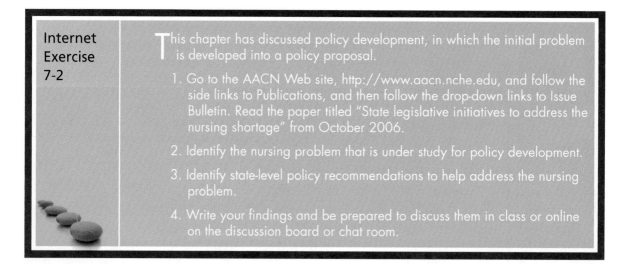

Internet Exercise 7-2

This chapter has discussed policy development, in which the initial problem is developed into a policy proposal.

1. Go to the AACN Web site, http://www.aacn.nche.edu, and follow the side links to Publications, and then follow the drop-down links to Issue Bulletin. Read the paper titled "State legislative initiatives to address the nursing shortage" from October 2006.

2. Identify the nursing problem that is under study for policy development.

3. Identify state-level policy recommendations to help address the nursing problem.

4. Write your findings and be prepared to discuss them in class or online on the discussion board or chat room.

POLICY ANALYSIS

Policy analysis is a critical component of the policy process for nurses to comprehend and participate in. Once the need for a policy has been assessed, and the policy has been developed, there is a need for analysis and evaluation of the policy. **Policy analysis** can be described in terms of both the overall policymaking process, and a specific component within the process, which is how it will be described here (Block, 2004). Policy analysis occurs in many disciplines and may be defined as the description of a particular policy or policy area, assessment of the impact, inquiry into the consequences, and evaluation of the policy's impact (Maslin-Prothero

& Masterson, 1998). Policy analysis can include "informed advice to a client that relates to a public policy decision, includes a recommended course of action/inaction, and is framed by a client's powers and values" (Teitelbaum & Wilensky, 2007, p. 167). A client in this case may be someone who wants advice, such as a policy maker. Informed advice includes research and analysis (including pros and cons); and client values must be considered so that the recommendation is realistic and feasible (Teitelbaum & Wilensky).

Why should nurses become involved with policy analysis? Nursing practice involves policies, regulations, and procedures that are mandated by legislation (federal and state), workplace institutions, higher education, and nursing organizations (Cheek & Gibson, 1997; Hudson, 2006; Milstead, 2002; Milstead, 2003). Nurses may take "policies" for granted, assuming that once a policy is created, it is not to be questioned. This is inherently untrue, as nurses should be the players who analyze policy implications not only for professional issues pertinent to nursing, but also for client welfare issues. As Cheek and Gibson point out, policies can "constrain as well as guide practice" (1997, p. 671), so it is imperative that nurses be able to analyze policies for their applicability.

CASE SCENARIO 7-2

In this exercise, you are the new BSN-prepared manager working in a cardiac intensive care unit that currently has very restrictive visiting hours for the family and immediate friends of the clients. At the present time, visitors are only allowed in to see the client between 10 and 11 am and 7 and 8 pm. You have observed in your practice that the presence of family and friends has a therapeutic effect on your clients, and you are interested in creating new policy with expanded and less restrictive visiting hours. You have read an editorial in *Nursing Management* (May 2004) by Dr. Richard Hader, who concluded that "rules regarding visitation are guidelines, not authoritative or prescriptive in implementation," and that "It's not acceptable for health care institutions to arbitrarily mandate or restrict visitation" (p. 6). As the new nurse manager, you believe that visiting hours are important for your unit and for the health care delivery system where you work.

CASE ANALYSIS

1. Develop a plan for the assessment of the issue. State and define the issue and list two objectives.

2. Craft a policy statement for the issue. Identify the data that should be collected to support the issue.

3. Identify potential key supporters of the issue. Include how you will gain the support of nurses who may oppose the issue.

4. State the plan of action. State the pros and cons of the plan of action.

In order to analyze policy, it is helpful to become knowledgeable about some of the most common models of the policy process. Nursing does not have one model that it relies on; indeed there are many models that have been created, many of which have been heavily influenced by the political and social science disciplines.

There are three policy process models created by other disciplines that are applicable to nursing. The **steps/stages model** (also known as the stages heuristic or rational approach) was created by Jones (1970), Anderson (1975), and Brewer and deLeon (1983) (as cited in Sabatier, 1999). The steps/stages model divides policy into the stages of agenda setting, policy formulation, implementation, and evaluation. Agenda setting occurs when the key players (such as nurses) focus on an issue or problem, which can be brought to attention by a crisis (such as the current care of veterans), a change in a leading indicator (such as smoking prevalence among adolescents), a "hot" topic (such as health care for illegal immigrants), or publicizing by the media (Milstead, 2003). Policy formulation, also known as government response, includes the work of legislators, staff, interest groups, and committees in the crafting of policies and/or legislation. Finally, implementation and evaluation of policies or programs includes oversight by agencies as well as process and outcome measures. A process measure occurs during the evaluation of program or policy implementation, while an outcome measure occurs after implementation and measures program or policy effects (Grembowski, 2001). One criticism of this model is that, traditionally, it is seen as a very linear model, with one stage finishing before the next stage begins. As Milstead points out, though, the policy process is fluid. For example, agenda setting may even occur during evaluation, if a special interest group is petitioning for specific outcomes to be evaluated.

In nursing, Abood (2007) uses a variation of this model to describe a three-stage approach to the policy process: formulation, implementation, and evaluation (Figure 7-7). In the formulation stage, there is an input of information, including research; the issue is framed with a purpose and objectives; strategies are selected; and resources are identified. Implementation involves disseminating information about the policy and the actual execution of the policy, and evaluation involves modifying the policy through both process and outcome evaluation.

Another commonly applied model is the **multiple streams framework**, created by Kingdon (1984; as cited in Sabatier, 1999). This model is based on the Garbage Can Model (GCM) (Cohen, March, & Olsen, 1982), which attempts to understand the ambiguity behind decision-making in large organizations. The multiple streams framework is used to describe how policies are formulated (Figure 7-8). In this model, there are three streams of actors and processes: (a) a problem stream, in which a problem or issue is defined; (b) a policy stream, which offers possible solutions;

Figure 7-7

The modified steps/
stages model of
policy analysis.

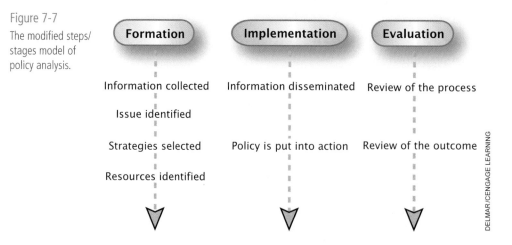

DELMAR/CENGAGE LEARNING

Figure 7-8

According to the multiple streams framework, several forces intersect to create policy.

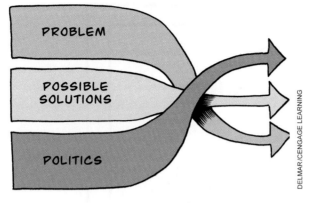

and (c) a politics stream, which includes elected officials and interest groups. These streams are usually independent, but at times the streams may converge and policy change can occur. For example, nurses working in a hospital organization might become concerned with the chronic conditions of children who are being treated for asthma in the emergency room without health insurance. At the same time, hospital administrators might be assessing for ways to decrease "repeat" ER visits for children with acute asthmatic conditions that might be better treated with outpatient clinic services. Finally, if elected officials of the town decided to help fund a low- to no-cost outpatient clinic, after encouragement from nurses, physicians, and administrators, all three "streams" would converge in order to create an alternative to costly ER visits for low-income asthmatic children.

Another model with applicability to nursing is the **advocacy-coalition framework**, created by Sabatier and Jenkins-Smith (1988, 1993, as cited in Sabatier, 1999). This model is based on the interaction of advocacy coalitions within a policy subsystem (Figure 7-9). A policy subsystem is a group of key players from public and private organizations that seek to influence policy. Advocacy coalitions are formed from key players from various organizations who share common policy beliefs within the policy subsystem, and policy change occurs due to "competition within the system and events outside the system" (Sabatier, 1999, p. 9). For example, a town might be concerned with the issue of abused and neglected children who are referred to the local Department of Human Resources (DHR). Suppose many children are referred for investigation, but only a small number of cases are actually brought to trial. Key players in this issue would include: (a) the school system, where many children disclose abuse; (b) DHR, who investigates the claims; (c) the city and county police departments that assist in the investigation and the forensic examiner who assesses the children for abuse; (d) the health care organizations that treat the children, both physically and mentally; and (e) the district attorney's office that prosecutes the perpetrators. All of these key players are composed of advocacy coalitions that operate within the same policy subsystem in order to provide treatment to victims of child abuse and prosecution for the offenders. Once a common mission is created, the advocacy coalitions might realize that victims' interests would be better served through the coordination of all of these services through one entity. Policy change, in the creation of a Child Advocacy Center, would result.

In nursing, one model that has been proposed is the Policy Analysis Model (PAM), created by Steele, Rocchiccioli, & Porche, (2003). The PAM is described as a "cognitive framework for health policy analysis" and developed as a tool for nurse managers (p. 80). The model was

Figure 7-9
Groups of key
players come
together to create
policy according
to the advocacy-
coalition framework.

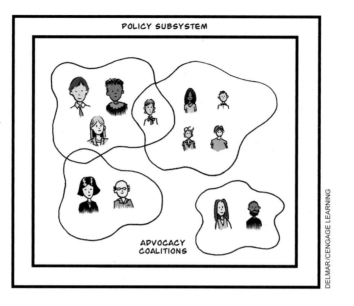

influenced by Hanley's (1998) five-step analysis framework, and consists of problem identification, creation of policy alternatives and objectives, evaluation of findings, and recommendations. Problem identification involves first defining the issue or problem, and then
examining the factors or constraints that may influence the issue, including social factors
(environmental and psychosocial), financial constraints, ethical/legal constraints, and political constraints (Figure 7-10). This step must also include stakeholder involvement, such as
policy makers, nurses, academic institutions, health care organizations, and special-interest
groups. Table 7-2 illustrates Internet links to public and private Web sites for information
related to the policy process.

Figure 7-10
The first phase of
the policy analysis
model involves a
comprehensive
assessment of the
problem and all
related issues.

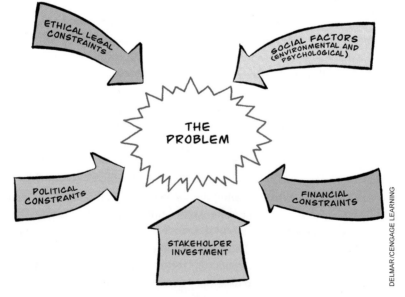

Table 7-2 Internet Links Related to Public and Private Web sites for Policy Process Information

Related Policy Information	Web site
1. Go to federal statistical policy for budget documents, working papers, and federal register notices.	http://www.fedstats.gov
2. Federal statistics: Offering statistics from more than 100 agencies available to citizens everywhere.	http://www.fedstats.gov
3. Thomas: Web site of the Library of Congress that makes federal legislative information freely available to the public. Here, you can learn about congressional activity (federal level).	http://thomas.loc.gov
4. Almanac of Policy Issues: An independent public service that provides background information, archived documents, and links on major U.S. public policy issues.	http://www.policyalmanac.org
5. Go to health policy issues located in the Almanac of Policy Issues: a. Specific issues such as nursing shortage information can be found by entering "nursing shortage" in the search screen.	http://www.policyalmanac.org
6. National Center for Policy Analysis: A nonprofit, nonpartisan public policy research organization to develop and promote private alternatives to government regulation and control.	http://www.ncpa.org
7. National Issues Forum: A nonpartisan, nationwide network of locally sponsored public forums for the consideration of public policy issues.	http://www.nifi.org
8. Policy Agendas Project: Collects and organizes data from various archived sources to trace changes in the national policy agenda and public policy outcomes.	http://www.policyagendas.org

Writing Exercise 7-2

Policy analysis has been described using various models found in the literature.

1. Choose an issue or problem from a clinical area that you feel needs attention.

2. Choose a model or framework from this chapter and use the model to describe how this issue might be analyzed.

3. Write your findings and be prepared to discuss them in class or the discussion board.

POLICY EVALUATION

Policy evaluation is the final phase of the policy process, and one that nurses are well suited to conduct. Policy evaluation shares many commonalities with program evaluation, which is a new discipline that specializes in observing the outcomes of programs. Evaluation impacts nurses everyday, and may occur for a policy, such as a hospital nurse staffing policy, or a program, such as a case management program managed by a nurse. In **policy evaluation**, the policy's "implementation, performance, and impact are evaluated to determine how well [it] has met its goals and objectives" (Hanley & Falk, 2007, p. 82). Nurses are educated to evaluate client outcomes of nursing care on a continual basis, such as response to medication, or oxygenation level. Policy evaluation takes the nurse's natural bent toward evaluation a step further—it examines the response to a program or policy that impacts not one client, but many clients or aggregates. In the practice arena, some hospitals have created a "shared governance" approach to overseeing policies and regulations, in the formation of committees known as Nursing Policy and Procedure Committees (NPPCs) (Hudson, 2006). NPPCs involve the participation of nursing staff members from all clinical areas in decision-making regarding policies and procedures in institutional settings. This type of policy evaluation is especially important for institutions seeking American Nurses Credentialing Center Magnet accreditation.

One issue that must be considered when evaluating policy is ethics. Ethics, including the principles of beneficence (to do good), nonmaleficence (to do no harm), autonomy (the individuals' freedom to choose), and distributive justice (the fair allocation of resources) should be assessed when evaluating programs and policies (Turkel & Ray, 2003; Saikonda-Woitas & Robinson, 2002). Distributive justice, in particular, is an area that nurses should be involved in, as resource allocation is a popular topical discussion in health care. Microallocation, the allocation of resources within an institution, and marcroallocation, the allocation of resources at societal and governmental levels, are both pertinent to nursing practice (Saikonda-Woitas & Robinson, 2002). Nurses have an obligation to evaluate policies and a program on both levels, in order for nursing's input to be heard on behalf of their clients. For example, in an outpatient practice setting, nurses must continually make decisions and evaluate how to allow for same-day client appointments to clinician schedules that are already quite busy. How might the nurse evaluate the appointment policy to make room for those clients with an urgent need to be seen? At the societal level, nurses might provide evaluation input into clinical outcomes, such as the necessity for better prescription coverage for Medicare beneficiaries.

This leads to another issue that must be considered: the importance of research to policy evaluation. According to Sabatier (1991), specific research rarely influences a policy decision. However, shaping a policy agenda through research, as well as evaluating research outcomes, is a most important issue. During the evaluation process, nurses can conduct and publicize outcome findings from studies to legislators, organizations, and key players in the policy arena (Turkel & Ray, 2003). For example, nurses evaluating the impact of a clean air ordinance on the effects of second-hand smoking in public places should disseminate this research to the legislators that passed the ordinance, as well as the public that is impacted by it. According to Turkel & Ray, "research is a powerful tool to address a moral crisis and facilitate change" (2003, p. 24). There is a clear link between research and evidence-based practice, which is becoming increasingly important to health care (Hudson, 2006). Policy and nursing practice are not mutually exclusive; current practice standards are based on research and evidence-based practice standards, which are created through evaluation research. Nurses should conduct both process and outcomes research in order to evaluate policies and programs and show their critical worth as a profession (Milstead, 2003). For example many advanced practice nurses have conducted evaluation research in order to provide rationale for reimbursement. However, barriers can emerge in policy evaluation. Some policies or programs that are approved may not be implemented, or money may not be budgeted for evaluation or may be utilized before evaluation occurs (Milstead, 2003). Methods for evaluating the economic impact of policies and procedures are thus very helpful to the nurse.

If you are a nurse who is charged with evaluating workplace benefits for smoking cessation, performing a cost-effectiveness ratio or a cost-benefit analysis would be very useful. A cost-effectiveness ratio examines an intervention (for example, a tobacco cessation benefit) compared to some other alternative, such as offering no benefit. The net cost of a benefit (the difference in costs between the two, including program costs and averted illness) is divided by the net health outcome (or difference in health outcomes between the two) (Harris, Schauffler, Milstein, Powers, & Hopkins, 2001). Over time, the costs averted by a cost-saving intervention exceed the cost of the intervention and thus it saves money. The cost-benefit analysis examines whether an intervention results in a net benefit (where the benefits exceed the cost) or a net cost (where costs exceed the benefit) for a particular intervention (Harris et al., 2001). For example, a study of the cost effectiveness of a guideline on tobacco cessation found that tobacco cessation treatments were cost neutral, with an estimated Quality-Adjusted Life Year of $1,555 per person (Cromwell, Bartosch, Fiore, Hasselblad, & Baker, 1997). Studies on cost-benefit analyses have found that tobacco cessation treatments have shown a return on investment after four years with evidence of decreased health care utilization (Wagner, Curry, Grothaus, Saunders, & McBride, 1995), and that costs for employers break even after three years (Warner, Smith, Smith, & Fries, 1996).

One last consideration in the evaluation of policy is the role of caring. With our strong link to client advocacy, nursing's motivation for its actions should be the concept of political caring, which relates to "the management of values and the competition of struggle for scarce resources (human and material)" (Turkel & Ray, 2003, p. 17). According to Turkel (2001), there is a dichotomy between nursing expertise in the science and art of caring and the economic environment

---

Writing Exercise 7-3	Policy evaluation, as described in the text, is something that nurses do on a continual basis.
	1. Choose a policy (it can be an institutional policy, found in a health care organization).
	2. Identify specific ways that the policy may be evaluated by a nurse.
	3. Include in your answer the ethical implications, economic impacts, and the roles of research and caring.
	4. Write your findings and be prepared to discuss them in class or on the discussion board.

of today's health care. Evaluating new and existing policies in this context requires that while the economic impacts of policies is of importance, caring (particularly in the nurse-patient relationship) needs to be nurtured through the judicious use of adequate staffing and time management (Turkel, 2001). Any evaluation of a policy or program would benefit from the political caring that nursing could bring to this process. It is imperative for nurses to become involved in policy evaluation to both advance the profession and advocate on behalf of clients.

NURSE INVOLVEMENT IN POLICY

There are examples in the literature of nurses and nursing organizations that have teamed to create policies to better the health of their clients and themselves. Many nursing organizations have recently become involved in environmental health activities and have developed practice resolutions pertaining to drinking water, indoor air quality, and pesticides in schools, among others (Sattler, 2005). The American Nurses Association, the Maryland and Massachusetts State Nursing Associations, and the University of Maryland, among others, have teamed toward improving health care environments with creating policies toward fragrance-free environments (Wolff, 2006).

One policy that is currently impacting nursing practice is the Nurse Licensure Compact (NLC), which allows nurses in member states to practice in other member states without seeking a separate nursing license (Becker, 2006; Wise & Spurlock, 2007). Currently, twenty states are members of the NLC, with implementation pending in two more states (National Council of State Boards of Nursing [NCSBN], 2007). The benefits of the NLC pertain to the advancement of technology that has created telemedicine, nursing call centers, and managed care organizations that allow for the practice of nursing beyond state borders, as well as the mobilization of the nursing workforce, especially in light of natural disasters and bioterrorism (Becker, 2006). The NLC has been endorsed by many nursing organizations, including the American Organization of Nurse Executives (AONE), several state hospital associations, the American Association of Occupational Health Nurses (AAOHN), the U.S. Department of Commerce, the Center for Telemedicine Law, and the Telehealth Leadership Council (NCSBN, 2004). Despite these endorsements, there have been criticisms of the NLC, including the difficulty in coordinating discipline for nursing actions between states, the possible weakening of state-specific standards for nursing (such as continuing education requirements), and the cost of implementing the NLC (Becker, 2006). This is a prime example of a new policy that has been created that requires careful and considerate evaluation to ensure that the compact's mission is met.

So, how can you as a nurse become involved in the policy process (Figure 7-11)? Nurses should first become knowledgeable about the policy process, including determining who the key players are and participating in state legislative days and policy workshops (Abood, 2007; Kitchen, 2004; Smith, 2006; Wolff, 2006). Nurses can educate key players in the policy process on issues important to client health and nursing through the use of e-mail, direct mail, phone calls, and testimony at public meetings or committees (Abood, 2007; Gindel, 2005; Kitchen, 2004; Milstead, 2003; Saikonda-Woitas & Robinson et al., 2002; Smith, 2006). Nurses can also be involved in coalition building for issues that involve many organizations or individuals with a common mission (Abood, 2007; Collins, 2006; Milstead, 2003; Saikonda-Woitas & Robinson,

Figure 7-11
Nurses can become involved in the policy making process in different ways.

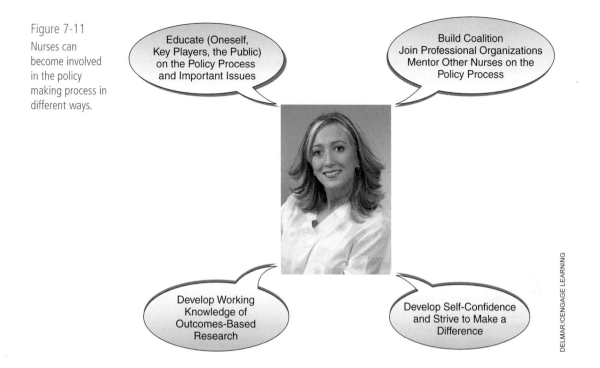

2002; Sattler, 2005; Smith, 2006; Wolff, 2006). Nurses should join professional nursing organizations, and be aware of pending legislation that will impact client welfare as well as nursing practice (Abood, 2007; Grindel, 2005; Smith, 2006). Nurses can also call attention to issues that are important to them through networking with the media to publicize issues, problems, or policies to the public (Abood, 2007; Sattler, 2005). Nurses who are experienced in the policy process should mentor new nurses and be willing to conduct CE programs for novices (Steele et al., 2003). It is imperative for nurses to participate in, be knowledgeable about, and/or direct

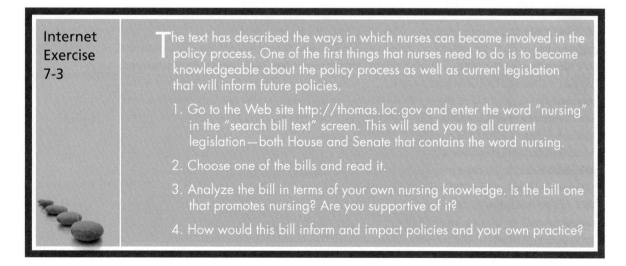

Internet Exercise 7-3

The text has described the ways in which nurses can become involved in the policy process. One of the first things that nurses need to do is to become knowledgeable about the policy process as well as current legislation that will inform future policies.

1. Go to the Web site http://thomas.loc.gov and enter the word "nursing" in the "search bill text" screen. This will send you to all current legislation—both House and Senate that contains the word nursing.

2. Choose one of the bills and read it.

3. Analyze the bill in terms of your own nursing knowledge. Is the bill one that promotes nursing? Are you supportive of it?

4. How would this bill inform and impact policies and your own practice?

evaluative, outcomes-based research (Milstead, 2003; Saikonda-Woitas et al., 2002; Smith, 2006; Wolff, 2006). Finally, nurses must believe that they can contribute to the policy process and make a difference (Smith, 2006). Our clients—whether they are individuals, families, groups, or communities—depend on nurses to ensure that their health care needs are met, and this cannot be done adequately without attention to the policy process.

This chapter has discussed topics that commonly occur in the policy process, including policy assessment, policy development, policy analysis, and policy evaluation. Similar to the policy process, the nursing process is a five-step process well known to all nursing students and nurses, and includes the steps of nursing assessment, nursing diagnosis, nursing plan, nursing implementation, and nursing evaluation. There are many commonalities between the policy process and the nursing process, in both word and meaning. It is time for nurses to participate in the policy process with the same attention that is given to the nursing process.

CASE SCENARIO 7-3

In this exercise, you are a nurse working in an emergency department that currently has a policy stating that no family or significant others may be in the client's room while the client is resuscitated or when the client undergoes invasive procedures. If a client experiences a cardiac or respiratory arrest, the nurse on your unit escorts the family or significant others to a quiet room away from the client. You have observed in your nursing practice experience that the presence of family or significant others has a therapeutic effect on the clients who are having procedures, such as IV insertion. You are interested in creating a new policy that would allow an immediate family member or significant other to be present during invasive procedures or resuscitation. Your interest in the positive effects was stimulated after reading the article by Mian, Warchal, Whiteny, Fitzmaurice, and Tancredi in the February 2007 issue of *Critical Care Nurse*. Mian et al., discuss the current literature related to family presence during resuscitation. Mian et al., implemented family presence during resuscitation, which led to positive results and the implementation as a standard of practice in the emergency department in the study.

CASE ANALYSIS

1. Develop a plan for the assessment of the issue. State and define the issue and list two objectives.

2. Craft a policy statement for the issue. Identify the data that should be collected to support the issue. Identify potential supporters of the issue and include how you will gain the support of those nurses who say "we have always done it this way." State the pros and cons of the plan of action. Identify related research. State the plan of action.

3. Choose a model or framework found in this chapter and describe how the model assists in the analysis of the issue. Who are the key players in the issue? Will it assist or detract from the issue if you involve the media?

4. Develop a plan for the evaluation of the new policy, both in terms of process and outcomes. Consider the implications of ethics and research in the evaluation.

SUMMARY

This chapter provides a general overview of the policy process, including the concepts of policy assessment, policy development, policy analysis, and policy evaluation. Policy may be described as either a process, or an entity, but with either description, policy is an important concept for nurses to both understand and to participate in. Due to nurses' direct involvement in client care, they are able to clearly see client needs as well as the impact of policies. Nurses have influence through professional education, licensure requirements, public respect, and perhaps most importantly, a natural interest in and professional obligation for advocacy on behalf of our clients.

Policy may be divided into the subtopics of assessment, which involves identification and definition of the problem with development of objectives or outcomes; development, which involves supporting data collection and analysis, research review, and recommendation of a plan of action; analysis, which involves a critical appraisal of implications and consequences guided by a model or framework; and evaluation, which involves the evaluation of policy and program implementation and impacts in terms of its goals. There are examples in the literature of nurses and nursing organizations that have teamed to create policies to better the health of their clients and themselves, such as environmental health policies and the Nurse Licensure Compact. Nurses can get involved in policy by becoming knowledgeable about the process, educating key players and the public about important issues, supporting coalition-building, joining professional nursing organizations, mentoring others, and participating in outcomes-based evaluative research. With over 2.9 million registered nurses in the United States, nurses are gaining a significant impact on policies in the health care arena.

The policy of being too cautious is the greatest risk of all.

–Jawaharlal Nehru

REFERENCES

ABOOD, S. (2007). Influencing health care in the legislative arena. *Online Journal of Issues in Nursing, 12*(1).

ALTMANN, T. K., & Collins, S. E. (2007). Oregon's Death with Dignity Act (ORS 127.800–897): A health policy analysis. *Journal of Nursing Law, 11*(1), 43–52.

AMERICAN ASSOCIATION OF COLLEGES OF NURSING. (2004). *AACN position statement on the practice doctorate in nursing: October, 2004.* Retrieved May 24, 2007, from http://www.aacn.nche.edu/DNP/DNPPositionStatements

AMERICAN ASSOCIATION OF COLLEGES OF NURSING. (2006). *DNP roadmap task force report: October 20, 2006.* Retrieved May 26, 2007, from http://www.aacn.nche.edu/DNP

AMERICAN NURSES CREDENTIALING CENTER. (2007). *What is the magnet recognition program?* Retrieved August 5, 2007, from http://www.nursecredentialing.org/magnet/index.html

ANONYMOUS. (2006). Gastrostomy: Sepsis, death tied to nurses' failure to check patency before feeding. *Legal Eagle Eye Newsletter for the Nursing Profession, 14*(6), 5.

BECKER, C. (2006). A license without borders. *AORN Journal, 83*(3), 958–962.

BLOCK, L. E. (2004). Policy: What is it and how it works? In Harrington, C. & C. L. Estes (Eds.),

Health policy: Crisis and reform in the U. S. health care delivery system (pp. 4–17). Sudbury, MA: Jones and Bartlett Publishers.

CHASE, S. K., & Pruitt, R. H. (2006). The practice doctorate: Innovation or disruption? *Journal of Nursing Education, 45*(5), 155–161.

CHEEK, J., & Gibson, T. (1997). Policy matters: Critical policy analysis and nursing. *Journal of Advanced Nursing, 25*, 668–672.

COHEN, M., March, J., & Olsen, J. (1982), A garbage can model of organizational choice. *Administrative Science Quarterly, 17*, 1–25.

COLLINS, S. E. (2006). Nursing and the public policy making process: A primer. *The Florida Nurse, 54*(2), 16.

CROMWELL, J., Bartosch, W. J., Fiore, M. C., Hasselblad, V., & Baker, T. (1997). Cost-effectiveness of the clinical practice recommendations in the AHCPR guideline for smoking cessation. *Journal of the American Medical Association, 278*, 1759–1766.

DEPALMA, J. A. (2002). Proposing an evidence-based policy process. *Nursing Administration Quarterly, 26*(4), 55–61.

FURLONG, E., & Smith, R. (2005). Advanced nursing practice: Policy, education and role development. *Journal of Clinical Nursing, 14*, 1059–1066.

GEBBIE, K. M., Wakefield, M., & Kerfoot, K. (2000). Nursing and health policy. *Journal of Nursing Scholarship, 32*(3), 307–315.

GRINDEL, C. (2005). Influencing health care policy with our children in mind. *MEDSURG Nursing, 14*(5), 277–278.

GREMBOWSKI, D. (2001). The evaluation process as a three-act play. In D. Grembowski (Ed.), *The practice of health program evaluation* (pp. 15–31). Thousand Oaks, CA: Sage Publications.

HADER, R. (2004). Bring hazy visitation policies into focus. *Nursing Management, 35*(5), 6.

HANLEY, B. E. (1998). Policy development and analysis. In D. J. Mason & J. K. Leavitt (Eds.), *Policy and politics in nursing and health care* (pp. 125–138). Philadelphia: W. B. Saunders.

HANLEY, B., & Falk, N. L. (2007). Policy development and analysis: Understanding the process. In Mason, D. J., Leavitt, J. K., & Chaffee, M. W. (Eds.), *Policy and politics in nursing and health care* (pp. 75–93). St. Louis, MO: Saunders.

HARRIS, J. R., Schauffler, H. H., Milstein, A., Powers, P., & Hopkins, D. P. (2001). Expanding health insurance coverage for smoking cessation treatments: Experience of the pacific business group on health. *American Journal of Health Promotion, 15*(5), 350–356.

HATHAWAY, D., Jacob, S., Stegbauer, C., Thompson, C., & Graff, C. (2006). The practice doctorate: Perspectives of early adopters. *Journal of Nursing Education, 45*(12), 487–496.

HUDSON, M. A. (2006). Policy procedure and management: A job that's never done. *Nursing Management, 37*(6), 34–38.

HUDDLESTON, K. C. (2006). Pediatric health policy analysis: The Emergency Medical Services for Children (EMSC) Act and The Wakefield Act, Utilizing social construction of target populations. *Pediatric Nursing, 32*(2), 167–172.

KITCHEN, L. (2004). To impact policy, first prepare. *Nursing Management, 35*(1), 14–15.

MASLIN-PROTHERO, S., & Masterson, A. (1998). Continuing care: Developing a policy analysis for nursing. *Journal of Advanced Nursing, 28*(3), 548–553.

MIAN, P., Warchal, S., Whitney, S., Fitzmaurice, J., & Tancredi, D. (2007). Impact of a multi-faceted intervention on nurses' and physicians' attitudes and behaviors toward family presence during resuscitation. *Critical Care Nurse, 27*(1), 52–61.

MILSTEAD, J. A. (2002). Guest editorial. *Nursing Administration Quarterly, 26*(4), 7.

MILSTEAD, J. A. (2003). Interweaving policy and diversity. *Online Journal of Issues in Nursing, 8*(1).

MILSTEAD, J. A. (2004). Advanced practice nurses and public policy, naturally. In J. A. Milstead (Ed.), *Health policy and politics: A nurse's guide* (pp. 1–36). Sudbury, MA: Jones and Bartlett Publishers, Inc.

NATIONAL COUNCIL OF STATE BOARDS OF NURSING. (2004). Frequently asked questions regarding the NCSBN NLC. *Nurse licensure compact administrators*. Retrieved May 8, 2007, from https://www.ncsbn.org/NurseLicensureCompactFAQ.pdf

NATIONAL COUNCIL OF STATE BOARDS OF NURSING. (2007). Participating states in the NLC. *Nurse licensure compact administrators*. Retrieved May 8, 2007, from https://www.ncsbn.org/158.htm

RANDOLPH, S. A. (2006). Developing policies and procedures. *AAOHN Journal, 54*(11), 501–504.

PHILLIPS, S. J. (2007). The 19th annual legislative update: A comprehensive look at the legislative issues affecting advanced nursing practice. *The Nurse Practitioner, 32*(1), 14–16.

SARIKONDA-WOITAS, C., & Robinson, J. H. (2002). Ethical health care policy: Nursing's voice in allocation. *Nursing Administration Quarterly, 26*(4), 72–80.

SABATIER, P. (1991). Toward better theories of the policy process. *PS: Political Science & Politics, 6,* 147–156.

SABATIER, P. A. (1999). The need for better theories. In P. A. Sabatier (Ed.), *Theories of the policy process* (pp. 3–17). Boulder, CO: Westview Press.

SATTLER, B. (2005). Policy perspectives in environmental health. *American Association of Occupational Health Nurses Journal, 53*(1), 45–51.

SKAGGS, A. (2006). Trends in advanced practice education—Doctorate of Nursing Practice. *Missouri State Board of Nursing Newsletter, 8*(2), 5.

SMITH, K. (2006). Public policy issues and legislative process. In Molzahn, A., & E. Butera (Eds.), *Contemporary issues in nephrology nursing: Principles and practice* (pp. 201–206). Pitman, NJ: American Nephrology Nurses Association.

SHIREY, M. R. (2005). Celebrating certification in nursing: Forces of magnetism in action. *Nursing Administration Quarterly, 29*(3), 245–253.

STEELE, S., Rocchiccioli, J., & Porche, D. (2003). Analyzing and promoting issues in health policy: Nurse managers perspective. *Nursing Economics, 21*(2), 80–83.

TEITELBAUM, J. B., & Wilensky, S. E. (2007). *Essentials of health policy and law.* Sudbury, MA: Jones and Bartlett Publishers.

TOOFANY, S. (2005). Applied leadership: Nurses and health policy. *Nursing Management, 12*(3), 26–30.

TURKEL, M. C. (2001). Struggling to find a balance: The paradox between caring and economics. *Nursing Administration Quarterly, 26*(1), 67–82.

TURKEL, M. C., & Ray, M. A. (2003). A process model for policy analysis within the context of political caring. *International Journal of Human Caring, 7*(3), 17–25.

UNITED STATES DEPARTMENT OF HEALTH AND HUMAN SERVICES. (n.d.). *Preliminary findings: 2004 national sample survey of registered nurses.* Retrieved May 8, 2007, from ftp://ftp.hrsa.gov/bhpr/nursing/rnpopulation/theregisterednurse-population.pdf

WAGNER, E. H., Curry, S. J., Grothaus, M. A., Saunders, K. W., & McBride, C. W. (1995). The impact of smoking and quitting on health care use. *Archives of Internal Medicine, 155,* 1789–1795.

WARNER, K. E., Smith, R. J., Smith, D. G., & Fries, B. E. (1996). Health and economic implications of a work-site smoking-cessation program: A simulation analysis. *Journal of Occupational and Environmental Medicine, 38,* 981–992.

WISE, L., & Spurlock, A. (2007). Professional accountability: Credentialing and accreditation. In K. Polifko (Ed.), *Concepts of the nursing profession* (pp. 137–158). Clifton Park, NY: Delmar, Cengage Learning.

WOLFF, P. (2006). Improving indoor air quality in health care settings by controlling synthetic fragrance: What you as a nurse can do. *The Alabama Nurse, 33*(3), 19–21.

YODER-WISE, P. S. (2006). Professional issues: Creating the challenge of engagement. *Annual Review of Nursing Education, 4,* 67–83.

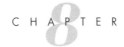

HEALTH POLICY

NANCY L. YORK

PhD, RN, Assistant Professor of Nursing, University of Nevada, Las Vegas School of Nursing

The groundwork of all happiness is health.

–Leigh Hunt

LEARNING OBJECTIVES

At the completion of the chapter, the learner should be able to do the following:

1. Describe how registered nurses can be involved with health policy at the local, state, and national levels.
2. Discuss how various levels of government can work together to promote health policy.
3. Discuss how Healthy People 2010's goals guide and promote health policy.
4. Describe a health policy that protects a vulnerable population.
5. Describe strategies used by special-interest groups to influence health policy development.

KEY TERMS

American Medical
   Association (AMA)
American Nurses
   Association (ANA)
Clean Indoor Air Laws
Health Policy
Healthy People 2010
Insider Strategies
Lobbying

Medicare Prescription
   Drug, Improvement and
   Modernization Act
Nightingales
Nurse Reinvestment Act
Outsider Strategies
Political Action
   Committees (PACs)

Regulation
Special-Interest Groups
Stakeholders
State Children's Health
   Insurance Program
   (SCHIP)
Vaccines for Children
   Program (VFC)

INTRODUCTION

As previously discussed, policy and nursing are intertwined in many ways. Nurses are affected by regulatory policies on a daily basis in their licensure and practice. They are also mandated by hospital policies and those from their national organizations. As important may be the profession's ability to affect policy development. Nurses are in the unique position to influence policies related to health due to their firsthand knowledge and experience of the health care environment.

WHAT IS HEALTH POLICY?

Health policy is a global construct that includes both concrete and abstract concepts and can be viewed as both a process and an entity. Longest (2005) suggested health policy was a collection of authoritative decisions made within any level of government that pertain to health and the pursuit of health. Health policy, in part, relates to a nation's health care system and involves individual patients, caregivers, and health care institutions. It also encompasses such issues as food safety, workplace safety, healthy living environments, and appropriate nurse–patient ratios. There are two chief goals of health policies: to assist citizens in making their choices concerning health easier, and/or to provide an environment that is healthy for everyone. The purpose of this chapter is to assist the reader in recognizing the multiple facets of health policy, as well as to identify ways in which they can become active in the development and enactment of policies that promote health.

Governmental Levels of Health Policy

Health policies are either interwoven between levels of government, such as those policies enacted for childhood vaccinations and tuberculosis (TB) control, or found at a single governmental level, such as a local health department regulation. In many instances the federal government enacts and financially supports health policies, yet requires the individual states, or even local levels of government, to be responsible for carrying out and enforcing these policies (Birkland, 2001). Examples of these include Medicaid, food stamps, and lower-income housing assistance.

Health Policies Throughout Levels of Government

Children's compliance with receiving their required vaccinations has improved significantly as a result of two national initiatives that also require individual state participation, the **Vaccines for Children (VFC)** program through the Centers for Disease Control and Prevention (CDC), and the **State Children's Health Insurance Program (SCHIP)**. The VFC program is coordinated federally through the CDC and National Immunization Program, with the states enrolling physicians to provide vaccinations to VFC-eligible patients. The SCHIP initiative provides federal money to help states expand health care coverage to uninsured children. While the program is jointly financed between the federal government and individual state governments, it is managed solely by the states. These two initiatives cover vaccination costs for children on Medicaid or who are uninsured, as well as American Indian and Alaska Native children. Underinsured children who receive vaccinations at federally qualified health centers also are covered (Figure 8-1). Because vaccinations are low cost or free, these programs help to eliminate cost as a barrier to children receiving their required vaccinations.

Health Policy and Tuberculosis

Controlling the TB epidemic is another example of levels of government working together to promote health. Tuberculosis was the leading cause of deaths in the United States before the development of anti-TB drugs in the late 1940s (Figure 8-2). Drug therapy, along with improvements in both public health and general living standards, resulted in a significant reduction in incidence of TB over the next 30 years. However, between 1985 and 1992, the number of reported TB cases increased by 20%. This increase was attributed to the emergence of the human immunodeficiency virus (HIV) epidemic, deterioration of the nation's health care infrastructure, influxes of immigrants from developing countries, and illegal drug misuse (York, 2008).

At the federal level, the mission of the CDC's Division of Tuberculosis Elimination is to "promote health and quality of life by preventing, controlling, and eventually eliminating tuberculosis from the United States, and by collaborating with other countries and international partners in controlling tuberculosis world-wide" (CDC, 2007, ¶1). The CDC's efforts include disease surveillance, development of prevention and control guidelines, and providing education and training materials to health care personnel and agencies. The federal government is responsible for funding the CDC's work, as well as supporting research related to TB.

While the federal government's role is to manage TB, it is most often at the state and local levels that funding is converted into health policies and programs for TB prevention,

Figure 8-1

The Vaccines for Children program provided by the Centers for Disease Control and Prevention (CDC) is an example of a government-sponsored health policy. *(Photo courtesy of CDC/Photo taken by James Gathany.)*

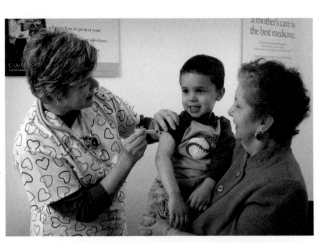

Figure 8-2

This historic photo from 1932 shows a physician conducting a medical examination of a dairy worker at the state tuberculosis sanatorium in Ah-Gwah-Ching, Minnesota. Insuring worker health was an important step in keeping the food supply safe, both for the patients and the staff. *(Photo courtesy of CDC/ Minnesota Department of Health, R.N. Barr Library; Librarians Melissa Rethlefsen and Marie Jones.)*

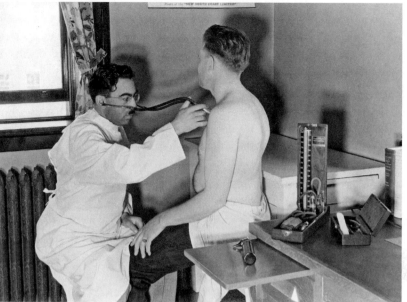

diagnosis, and treatment (Institute of Medicine, 2000). All fifty states and the United States (U.S.) territories have State TB Control offices. The CDC asserts in their Core Curriculum on Tuberculosis that state and local health departments have the responsibility for preventing and controlling TB (CDC, 2001). State and local efforts include working with the CDC to identify and manage individuals diagnosed with, or suspected to have, TB; collecting and analyzing data on incidence and prevalence rates; providing laboratory and diagnostic services; finding the required funding to support TB control activities; educating elected officials on program priorities; and periodically reviewing the laws, regulations, and policies related to TB to ensure that they are consistent with currently recommended medical and public health practices (CDC, 2001).

Health Policy and Secondhand Smoke Exposure

An example of related health policies enacted throughout governmental levels, but independently from each other, are the **clean indoor air laws** enacted to protect citizens from secondhand smoke (SHS) exposure. In 1988 Congress banned all smoking on domestic airline flights. Secondhand smoke laws were strengthened when legislation was passed requiring all federally funded schools, day care centers, libraries, and health facilities for children to be smoke free. In 1998 an executive order was signed that mandated all buildings owned, rented, or leased by the executive branch of the federal government must be smoke free.

While federal policy efforts were being enacted, support for stricter public smoking restrictions were simultaneously occurring at local and state levels. Cities in California were the first to enact smoke-free laws at the local level in 1991. In 1994 both California and Utah enacted statewide laws that restricted smoking to protect citizens from SHS. As of 2008, there

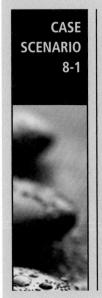

CASE SCENARIO 8-1

In the summer of 2007, a man found to be infected with a drug-resistant form of TB was informed by the CDC to cancel his overseas air-travel plans the following day to Europe. Even though the risk of transmission would be low to other airline passengers and crew members, they would be exposed to TB, as germs are spread by coughing, sneezing, and speaking, and can float in the air for several hours. The man chose to continue his plans and flew to Europe a day after meeting with CDC officials.

CASE ANALYSIS

1. What could the CDC have done to prevent this man from potentially infecting other airline passengers and crew?

2. As a nurse, how would you have educated this man about his disease?

3. Should a health policy be developed that limits the activities of a person with an infectious disease? Provide a rationale for your answer.

4. Are their policies or laws that limit the activities or behaviors of a person diagnosed with HIV/AIDS or infectious Hepatitis?

are over 2,880 municipalities and 28 states that have enacted laws or regulations restricting smoking in workplaces, and/or restaurants, and/or bars, with 13 of these states eliminating smoking in virtually all workplaces (American Nonsmokers' Rights Foundation, 2008). Five additional state legislatures have ratified smoke-free laws; however, they are not yet in effect (see Table 8-1).

Health Policies at One Level of Government

Health policies can also be found at only one level of government, such as a local health department's regulations to protect patrons from poor food handling. A **regulation** is a principle or rule designed to control or govern conduct at the local level. Health departments at the local level have the authority to enter businesses and review their practices that ensure food safety and personal hygiene strategies are maintained. Regulations that ensure proper storage of items, proper hand washing, separation between raw and ready-to-eat food, proper cleaning of fresh fruits and vegetables, and proper washing of cooking utensils are examples of local-level policies developed to protect the public's health.

GOVERNMENT'S ROLE IN HEALTH POLICY

A significant way in which the federal government influences health is through the U.S. Department of Health and Human Services **Healthy People 2010** initiative (USDHHS, 2006). The mission of Healthy People 2010 is to improve the health for all Americans by increasing their quality and years of healthy life and eliminating health disparities. Over 500 national and

Table 8-1 States and Commonwealths that Require 100% Smoke-free Workplaces

States requiring 100% smoke-free workplaces, restaurants, and bars	States requiring 100% smoke-free workplaces, and/or restaurants, and/or bars	States with smoke-free laws not yet in effect
Arizona	California (restaurants and bars)	Montana (added bars to existing law)
Delaware	Colorado (restaurants and bars)	Nebraska (workplaces, restaurants, and bars)
Hawaii	Connecticut (restaurants and bars)	Oregon (workplaces, restaurants, and bars)
Illinois	Florida (workplaces and restaurants)	Pennsylvania (workplaces)
Iowa	Idaho (restaurants)	Utah (added bars to existing law)
Maryland	Louisiana (workplaces and restaurants)	
Massachusetts	Maine (restaurants and bars)	
Minnesota	Montana (workplaces and restaurants)	
New Jersey	Nevada (workplaces and restaurants)	
New York	New Hampshire (restaurants and bars)	
Ohio	New Mexico (restaurants and bars)	
Puerto Rico	North Dakota (workplaces)	
Rhode Island	South Dakota (workplaces)	
Washington	Utah (workplaces and restaurants)	
Washington, DC	Vermont (restaurants and bars)	

(Data from American Nonsmokers' Rights Foundation, 2008.)

Figure 8-3

Examples of Healthy
People 2010
Goals & Objectives.
*(Data from United
States Department
of Health & Human
Services, 2006.)*

Promote health for all through a healthy environment.
- Increase use of alternative modes of transportation to reduce motor vehicle emissions and improve the Nation's air quality.
- Reduce waterborne disease outbreaks arising from water intended for drinking among persons served by community water systems.
- Minimize the risks to human health and the environment posed by hazardous sites.

Prevent disease, disability, and death from infectious diseases, including vaccine-preventable diseases.
- Reduce or eliminate indigenous cases of vaccine-preventable diseases.
- Reduce bacterial meningitis in young children.
- Reduce Lyme disease.

Improve health, fitness, and quality of life through daily physical activity.
- Increase the proportion of adults who engage in vigorous physical activity that promotes the development and maintenance of cardiorespiratory fitness for at least 20 minutes per day 3 or more days per week.
- Increase the proportion of adolescents who engage in moderate physical activity for at least 30 minutes on 5 or more of the previous 7 days per week.
- Increase the proportion of the Nation's public and private schools that require daily physical education for all students.

Reduce injuries, disabilities, and death due to unintentional injuries and violence.
- Reduce firearm related deaths.
- Reduce deaths caused by motor vehicle crashes.
- Increase proportion of motorcyclists using helmets.

DELMAR/CENGAGE LEARNING

state organizations developed 28 health-related goals after the 1979 Surgeon General's Report on Health Promotion and Disease Prevention was published (see Figure 8-3).

Both personal health care and population-based public health prevention efforts are required of citizens to achieve the Healthy People 2010 goals. Specific objectives and sub-objectives have been developed for each major goal and provide strategies for health promotion and disease prevention outcomes. While the CDC's Healthy People 2010 are not laws or regulations, they are the basis and rationale for enactment of many health policies.

Healthy People 2010 is the foundation for coordination of public health action at the national, state, and local levels. The initiative is used by all levels of government, in addition to professional and volunteer organizations, to guide their development of programs to improve health (see Figure 8-4). Nearly all states, the District of Columbia, and Guam have built on the Healthy People 2010 national goals and objectives and adapted them to address their specific needs.

Using the Healthy People 2010 as a general framework, individual states and communities develop their own specific health-related priorities, goals, and outcome measures (see Table 8-2). An example in the commonwealth of Kentucky, which is second only to North

Figure 8-4
Healthy People
in Healthy
Communities:
A Systematic
Approach to Health
Improvement.

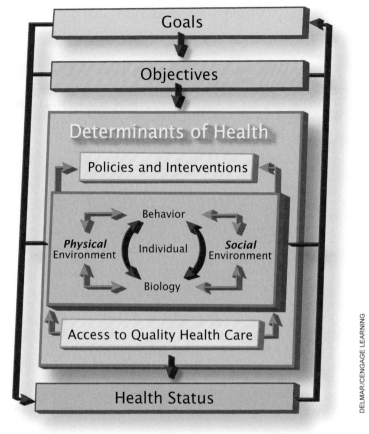

Carolina in burley tobacco production and has smoking prevalence rates consistently above the national average (Kentucky Cabinet for Health & Human Services, 2005b; United States Department of Agriculture, 2005). When Kentucky health care officials wrote their state-specific 2010 goals and objectives to reduce smoking, nearly 33% of the commonwealth's adults smoked cigarettes, compared to 24% of the nation's adults. It was believed that using the Healthy People 2010 goal to reduce adult smoking to 12% would be difficult, if not impossible to attain, since Kentucky's prevalence rates were so much higher than the national average. Therefore, Kentucky developed a more realistic goal to reduce adult smoking prevalence from 32% to 25% by 2010.

Schools, universities, and civic and faith-based organizations have also created activities to improve the health of their communities using the Healthy People 2010 initiative. Schools of nursing, public health, and health care administration have used the Healthy People goals to promote the health of students, faculty, and staff. These groups have initiated mental health programs, diet and nutrition classes, health fairs and dental screenings, and health counseling

Table 8-2 Examples of Healthy People 2010 and State 2010 Goals & Objectives

Healthy People 2010	Healthy States 2010: Selected Objectives
Reduce illness, disability, and death related to tobacco use and exposure to secondhand smoke.	
Objective: Reduce tobacco use (cigarettes) by adults to 12%.	• Maine: Reduce tobacco use (cigarettes) by adults to 19%. • Kentucky: Reduce tobacco use (cigarettes) by adults to 25%. • Delaware: Reduce tobacco use (cigarettes) by adults to 15%.
Prevent disease, disability, and death from infectious diseases, including vaccine-preventable diseases.	
Objective: Reduce or eliminate indigenous cases of vaccine-preventable diseases.	• Maine: Increase the proportion of children who participate in fully operational population-based immunization registries. • Kentucky: Reduce indigenous cases of vaccine-preventable diseases. • Delaware: Increase the proportion of children under 35 months of age who receive all vaccines that have been recommended for universal administration.
Promote health and prevent chronic disease associated with diet and weight.	
Objective: Reduce the proportion of children and adolescents who are overweight or obese to 5%.	• Maine: Reduce the proportion of adolescents who are overweight or obese from 10.3% to 5%. • Kentucky: Increase to at least 20% the proportion of young people in grades K–12 who engage in moderate physical activity for at least 30 minutes on 5 or more of the previous 7 days. • Delaware: Reduce the proportion of adolescents who are overweight or obese from 29% to 11%.

(Data from: Delaware Health and Social Services, 2001; Healthy Maine Partnerships, Bureau of Health, Department of Human Services, 2002; Kentucky Cabinet for Health and Family Services, 2005a; United States Department of Health & Human Services, 2006.)

activities. Professional organizations at the national and state levels, such as the American Cancer Society and American Lung Association, have also used Healthy People objectives to guide their development of immunization reminders, hotlines, fitness programs, and sponsorship of health fairs and health screenings.

Internet Exercise 8-1

Locate the Healthy People 2010 initiative at http://www.healthypeople.gov/data/midcourse.

1. What goals in the Healthy People 2010 initiative affect your life every day?

2. Which of the twenty-eight goals are most important to you personally and why?

3. How should your city, county, or state use these goals to improve citizens' health?

Healthy People 2010 Influencing Policy

While Healthy People 2010 is a federal policy initiative, one of its greatest strengths is that it promotes community-level interventions for what many previously considered as an individual's health issue.

Tobacco and Secondhand Smoke

Reducing tobacco use and exposure to SHS are major Healthy People 2010 goals. Tobacco use, especially cigarette smoking, is the leading cause of preventable death in the United States, accounting for approximately 400,000, or 1 in 5, deaths (USDHHS, 2006). Tobacco use also has consequences that extend beyond the smokers to nonsmokers who are involuntarily exposed to SHS. Exposure to SHS is the third leading cause of preventable death, after only active smoking and alcohol use. With the knowledge that smoking and SHS are deadly, coupled with initiation of the Healthy People 2010 goals, smoke-free policy development (Figure 8-5) has become a major goal of the tobacco control movement (Rabin & Sugarman, 2001).

Efforts to reduce smoking and SHS exposure have shifted from assisting an individual's smoking cessation efforts to more community-wide interventions. Increasing cigarette excise taxes, strengthening youth access to tobacco restrictions, and reducing nonsmokers' exposure to SHS are three tobacco-related Healthy People objectives that have been made into local or state laws throughout the U.S. These policies have been found to decrease smoking incidence and prevalence rates in both adults and teens, as well as reduce nonsmokers' exposure to SHS (Hahn et al., 2006; Heloma & Jaakkola, 2003; Levy & Friend, 2003; Moskowitz, Lin, & Hudes, 2000; Trotter, Wakefield, & Borland, 2002).

Obesity

Healthy People 2010 has also influenced policy development to combat the obesity epidemic in the U.S. Obesity is associated with an increased risk of death from type 2 diabetes, coronary

Figure 8-5
Smoke-free policy
development is part
of the federal policy
initiative Healthy
People 2010.

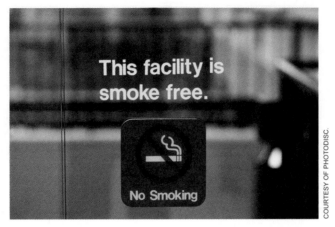

Figure 8-5
Smoke-free policy development is part of the federal policy initiative Healthy People 2010.

COURTESY OF PHOTODISC.

heart disease, cerebralvascular accidents, hypertension, and certain forms of cancers (Kochanek, Murphy, Anderson, & Scott, 2004; USDHHS & United States Department of Agriculture, 2005). However, even with that knowledge, the incidence and prevalence of obesity in children and adults continues to rise. It is estimated that medical costs associated with obesity reached $75 billion in 2003, with approximately half these costs covered through Medicare and Medicaid (Finkelstein, Fiebelkorn, & Wang, 2004, p. 21).

Some people believe enacting policies and laws to regulate the factors associated with obesity are inappropriate. Critics of governmental regulation believe policies such as those that remove vending machines from schools and workplaces, require restaurants to share nutritional content of menu items, regulate advertising and marketing of food to children, or impose taxes on nutrient-poor food should be voluntary. The essence of this reasoning is that individuals who are overweight or obese should be responsible for their own health and welfare. However, others make the case that since taxpayers finance approximately half of all the medical costs associated with obesity and employers are also responsible for a large amount of the costs, the government does have a responsibility to help reduce and treat the obesity epidemic (Gostin, 2007).

Writing
Exercise
8-1

What role should the government have in reducing the obesity epidemic? What are some personal choices that people can make to reduce obesity? Does obesity primarily affect the individual and/or society? What data supports your answer?

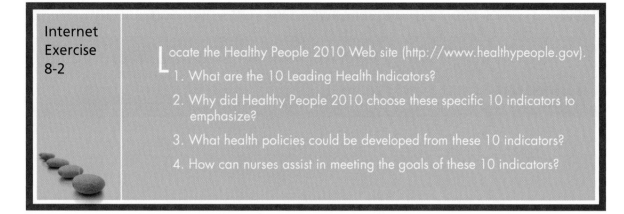

In 2006 state and local governments placed much of their attention on public school districts in an effort to reduce childhood and adolescent obesity. Elected officials, as well as school administrators and teachers, considered a variety of approaches to provide students with healthier diets and more exercise. Seven states enacted new, or strengthened their current, policies to help ensure students had access to healthier food and beverage choices while attending school (see Table 8-3). In addition, ten state legislatures refined or increased physical education requirements, for students during and after the school day (National Conference of State Legislatures, 2007). Other state and local policies enacted to combat obesity in children have included laws and regulations that restrict or remove non-nutritious and/or high-caloric vending machine products from school property, restriction of food sales that compete with healthy school lunch offerings, and closed-campus policies that decrease students' access to unhealthy food choices during lunch periods (Mello, Studdard, & Brennan, 2006).

Government's Role in Health Policy to Protect Vulnerable Populations

The U.S. government also plays a major role in supporting the health of vulnerable populations. These groups include the uninsured, immigrants, infants and children, elderly, mentally ill, homeless, long-term care residents, and populations with chronic illnesses, such as HIV/AIDS. A commonality among these groups is that their health and well-being are either at serious risk or already compromised. There is discussion at the national, state, and local levels about the amount of resources the U.S. government should provide these groups and how much influence it should have over them.

Immigrants

In the 1990s the U.S. was confronted with a massive influx of both legal and illegal immigrants. It is estimated over one million immigrants enter the U.S. yearly (Capps, Passel, Perez-Lopez, & Fix, 2003, p. 4). Unfortunately, immigrants living in the U.S. often do not have health care coverage, making them a high-risk population for maintaining or improving their health. The Kaiser

Table 8-3 States Enacting Tougher Laws to Prevent Childhood Obesity

States with new or strengthened laws to improve children's access to healthy foods and beverages in 2006–2007	States with new or increased physical education requirements for children in 2006–2007
California	California
Colorado	Colorado
Connecticut	Connecticut
Indiana	Delaware
New Jersey	Florida
North Carolina	Indiana
Pennsylvania	Kansas
	Oklahoma
	Pennsylvania
	Tennessee
	West Virginia

(Data from National Conference of State Legislatures, 2007.)

Commission (2004, ¶4) estimates up to 51% of non-U.S. citizens lack health care insurance, compared to the approximately 15% of native citizens. Reasons for the lack of insurance include low-paying jobs or trade occupations without health insurance benefits and legal status in the country.

There is a direct relationship between having health care insurance and using health care services (Carrasquillo & Pati, 2004; Lucas, Barr-Anderson, & Kington, 2003). People without insurance are less likely to seek preventative services and have routine checkups from health care providers. This can lead to higher rates of emergency room visits, medical crises, and chronic disease complications. Medicaid and SCHIP are two programs the U.S. government offers to assist immigrants with health care. In addition, many states have developed programs to provide health care services to immigrants not covered by the Medicaid and SCHIP programs. Even with these programs non-U.S. citizens lack adequate health care access (Kaiser, 2004). In 1996 the U.S. government enacted a law that requires a five-year waiting period until immigrants who legally enter the country may obtain health care benefits. Immigrants in the country illegally are not eligible for any government-sponsored benefits except for emergency services.

Homelessness

Homelessness is increasing steadily throughout the U.S. The most recent estimates from the U.S. Department of Housing and Human Development (2007) find almost 750,000 people are homeless. Whereas men used to be the primary population, woman and children now also occupy many homeless shelters. Those who are homeless have higher-than-average rates of chronic mental illness, acute alcoholism, and physical disabilities (Rossi, 2001).

Various policies have been enacted over the past twenty years in an effort to reduce the homeless population and improve their access to health care. Shelters with family units have been built to accommodate women with their children. Some of these shelters have also implemented emergency services and social services programs to assist those in need. Government agencies have rented motels to house both singles and families. Local and state agencies have collaborated and combined resources and services to assist the homeless and have introduced programs that provide food, transportation, clothing, and health care services. The SCHIP program was specifically developed to provide health care coverage to children who were uninsured.

SPECIAL-INTEREST GROUPS

Special-interest groups that influence health policy have evolved rapidly since the 1960s. These groups have developed into diverse yet powerful **stakeholders** in both federal and state policy development. Political stakeholders are people that have an investment or vested interest in the outcome of a specific policy. Between 1998 and 2006, over 2.2 billion dollars were spent lobbying at the federal level by groups interested in health policies. This amount accounted for over 15% of all lobbying expenditures (Institute for Health & Socio-Economic Policy, 2007, p. 3). Health insurance companies, health care organizations and institutions, and the pharmaceutical industry wield substantial influence on health policy development and enactment through their political and campaign contributions to governmental officials, agencies, and elected officials.

Lobbying

A major purpose of an interest group is to represent the interests of its members by **lobbying** the officials and government agencies that make decisions related to policy development and enactment. Lobbying activities can include informing, educating, persuading and influencing these officials. Some of the more powerful and influential special-interest groups in health policy include the American Hospital Association, the American Medical Association (AMA), the American Dental Association, and various medical insurance and pharmaceutical groups.

Often these groups work collaboratively to combine money, resources, and expertise to influence policy development, while other times these same groups can be vehemently opposed on the same issue. The AMA joined over 60 health care groups in 2007 and encouraged Congress to enact a proposed 61-cent federal tax increase on cigarettes with the funds used to continue the SCHIP initiative (AMA, 2007a). In addition, the AMA is collaborating with special-interest groups to buy print and television advertising, as well as initiating a direct-mail campaign to maintain health insurance access for children.

Political Action Committees

Many interest groups have **political action committees (PACs)** whose responsibility is to fund political campaigns and support elected officials. These committees specifically raise funds to sponsor state and federal congressional, gubernatorial, and presidential campaigns for those who support their interests. Elected officials who receive PAC donations are likely to meet with special-interest groups and listen to their views, but research has shown that PAC money does not translate into officials voting in favor of groups who have made these donations (Malone & Chaffee, 2007). Political action committees have been known to contribute to the campaigns of opposing candidates during the same election. Supporting both candidates provides the special-interest group opportunities to interact with whoever wins the election. Campaign giving through PACs is one of the many strategies special-interest groups use to promote their policies.

Special-Interest Groups' Strategies

Strategies often used by special-interest groups to influence health policy include two approaches: the "insider strategy" of interactions with policy makers, or the "outsider strategy," which focus on mobilization of group members and the public (see Table 8-4) (Kingdon, 2003). Most lobby groups use a combination of strategies, depending upon the amount of resources and time available, as well as the number of elected officials and governmental agencies they need to approach.

Nonoccupational Special-Interest Groups

Other interest groups that influence health policy development, but whose members do not necessarily work within the health care field, include AARP (formerly known as American Association of Retired Persons), Planned Parenthood, and Mothers Against Drunk Driving (MADD). Additional groups not often thought of as powerful within health policy development are the tobacco industry, the American Legion, and the U.S. Chamber of Commerce. All of these groups represent members who lobby government and elected officials because they benefit from the ratification or veto of specific health policies.

Table 8-4 Special-Interest Group Strategies

Insider Strategies	Outsider Strategies
Direct lobbying of elected officials	Initiating grassroots efforts
Educate elected officials and testify at legislative hearings	Mobilizing interest group members
Provide financial contributions to electoral campaigns	Educating the public
Assist elected officials in drafting legislation	Media campaigns
	Coalition building among interest groups
	Obtaining public opinion data

AARP's mission is committed to enhancing quality of life and promoting positive social change to members through information, advocacy, and service (AARP, 2007a). In 2006 AARP's total revenue was approximately $1 billion while it spent approximately $23 million on lobbying both federal and state officials (Birnbaurm, 2007, p. A19). The AARP's lobbying worked against budget reductions in Medicare, Medicaid, and veterans' benefits while supporting prescription drug entitlement.

A recent effort of AARP to influence health policy is their 2007 "Divided We Fail" campaign (AARP, 2007b). One purpose of this initiative is to address the health care needs of people over fifty years of age. AARP is collaborating with the Business Roundtable and Service Employees International Union to encourage elected officials, private businesses, and the general public to develop solutions to ensure everyone has access to quality health care and affordable prescription drugs. AARP's plans to advertise at both the national and state levels, use the Internet, and mobilize members and the public at the grassroots level.

Another special-interest group having a powerful influence on health policy, but with a different priority than AARP, is the tobacco industry. Their lobby typically works against health policies that support clean indoor air while also targeting teenage smoking. The industry uses a variety of tactics, including: claims that removing smoking from public places will cause economic harm to businesses, advocating that smoking is a fundamental right of every citizen, working with the hospitality and gaming industry to promote smokers' rights, and presenting alternative legislation to proposed smoke-free laws. In the 2007 state elections, Ohio, Arizona, and Nevada had smoke-free legislation on their ballots. Alternative legislation, which was less comprehensive and allowed for greater indoor smoking, was placed on each state's ballot thereby giving voters two choices. The intent of this competing legislation was to confuse voters and possibly defeat either both laws or the more comprehensive of the two. The majority of voters from all three states chose the more comprehensive law of the two and enacted strong clean indoor air laws.

Health Care Special-Interest Groups

There are many special-interest groups specific to health care. While some groups promote their business interests, others are there to protect the public's best interests.

Pharmaceutical Industry

While the pharmaceutical industry does not dominate health policy development and implementation, its influence is continuous and substantial. The industry has the largest lobby of any group at the federal level (Angell, 2004). Drug companies and their trade groups spent approximately $155 million in 2006 lobbying government officials and federal agencies such as the Food and Drug Administration and Department of Health and Human Services, as well as donating to political campaigns at both the state and federal levels (Angell, 2004; Ismail, 2005, 4–6).

The industry has received tremendous attention lately. Congressional hearings, investigative stories in the media, and research studies evaluating the industry's practices are widespread. The main reason for this interest is the profits pharmaceutical companies are making. The U.S. House of Representative's Committee on Government Reform estimated the 10 largest drug companies' profits increased by $8 billion during the first 6 months after a new Medicare drug program went into effect in January of 2006 (U.S. House of Representatives, Committee on Government Reform, 2006, p. 1).

The pharmaceutical industry has played a major role in either supporting or blocking passage of several federal laws related to prescription drugs in the U.S. The industry has influenced passage of laws that let drug companies extend their exclusive marketing rights of brand-name prescription medications for an extra thirty months, protect profitable drug patents, and prohibit lower-priced Canadian drugs from being imported to the U.S. (Angell, 2004; Ismail, 2007).

The industry has worked diligently through congress and the FDA to prevent drug importation from Canada. Rationales from the pharmaceutical industry for prohibiting drug importation include safety concerns, such as the improper filling of prescription medications from Canadian pharmacies, and pharmacists in the U.S. losing their jobs to their Canadian counterparts. However, some larger cities and states within the U.S. have attempted to negotiate, or encouraged citizens to purchase their medications through the Canadian pharmaceutical system in an effort to reduce prescription medication costs.

An especially high-profile case that garnered tremendous pharmaceutical industry lobbying was proposed federal legislation to reverse a provision of the **Medicare Prescription Drug, Improvement and Modernization Act**. The act assured citizens who receive Medicare benefits would also be eligible for some prescription drug benefits. However, a portion of legislation added into the act barred the federal government from bargaining for lower medication prices with drug companies. The pharmaceutical industry lobbied Congress intensely to add this piece of legislation, which effectively leaves Medicare unable to negotiate for reducing medication costs like the Department of

Defense and the Veterans Health Administration may do. In 2005 and 2007, legislation was introduced to allow Medicare to negotiate for lower prices, but neither attempt was successful.

The American Medical Association

Physician groups, especially the **American Medical Association (AMA)**, remain influential, though they are not as powerful as they once were. Between 1998 and 2004, the AMA spent over $92 million giving campaign contributions and lobbying federal and state officials. The AMA supported a variety of health care policies, including the Patient Safety and Quality Improvement Act, changes to Medicare and Medicaid, and improvements to SCHIP coverage for children. The 2005 Patient Safety and Quality Improvement Act established a voluntary and confidential reporting structure for physicians, other health care personnel, and health care agencies when medical errors occur (AMA, 2007b).

The American Nurses Association

The **American Nurses Association (ANA)** also has a strong lobby voice at both the state and federal levels of government, though some say nurses have not maximized their potential political impact. The ANA's mission is to advance the "nursing profession by fostering high standards of nursing practice, promoting the economic and general welfare of nurses in the workplace, projecting a positive and realistic view of nursing, and by lobbying the Congress and regulatory agencies on health care issues affecting nurses and the public" (ANA, 2007). There are many other specialty nursing organizations that work either independently, or in collaboration with the ANA, to promote health policy (see Figure 8-6).

The ANA is currently working on several broad initiatives to improve health care in the U.S. Their efforts are focused on delivery of primary health care in community-based settings, expanding registered nurses' and advanced practice nurses' roles in the delivery of health care, obtaining federal funding for nurse education and training, and improving the health care workplace.

One of the ANA's efforts is resolution of the nursing shortage. The ANA suggests reasons for the shortage include inadequate nursing salaries, aging of the nursing workforce, deteriorating working conditions leading to departure of experienced nurses, burnout, and the lack of adequate nursing school enrollment opportunities (ANA, 2006). The **Nurse Reinvestment Act** was one federal policy enacted to combat the nursing shortage and includes strategies such as school scholarships, grants, loan cancellation programs, and advanced training for registered nurses (American Association of Colleges of Nursing, 2005). Many nursing organizations, such as the ANA, National League for Nursing, and the American Association of Colleges of Nursing, collaborated with Congress in 2002 to draft and enact this piece of legislation.

The influence of nursing special-interest groups should not be underestimated. Though not as powerful as the AMA, nursing was successful with its lobbying efforts when over forty nursing organizations joined forces and united to oppose the AMA's proposal to create the role of "registered care technician" in the late 1980s. The AMA supported this newly created role because they believed it would help address the nursing shortage. The nurses successfully argued that this minimally trained, non-nurse health care worker would place patients in jeopardy and

DELMAR/CENGAGE LEARNING

Figure 8-6

Nursing Organizations That Are Politically Active.

American Academy of Nursing—http://www.aannet.org
American Association of Colleges of Nursing—http://www.aacn.nche.edu
American Association of Critical Care Nurses—http://www.aacn.org
American Nurses Association—http://www.nursingworld.org
American Nurses Foundation—http://www.nursingworld.org/anf
Emergency Nurses Association—http://www.ena.org
Hospice and Palliative Nurses Association—http://www.hpna.org
National Association of School Nurses—http://www.nasn.org
National Black Nurses Association—http://www.nbna.org
National League for Nursing—http://www.nln.org/index.cfm
National Student Nurses Association—http://www.nsna.org
Oncology Nursing Society—http://www.ons.org
Tobacco Free Nurses—http://www.tobaccofreenurses.org

increase nurses' workloads. Nursing groups educated elected officials, wrote editorials in local newspapers, generated grassroots support, and participated on radio and television talk shows to share their concerns. It took approximately two years, but the AMA stopped supporting this issue because they were unsuccessful in partnering with health care agencies willing to implement the technician role on a trial basis.

CASE SCENARIO 8-2

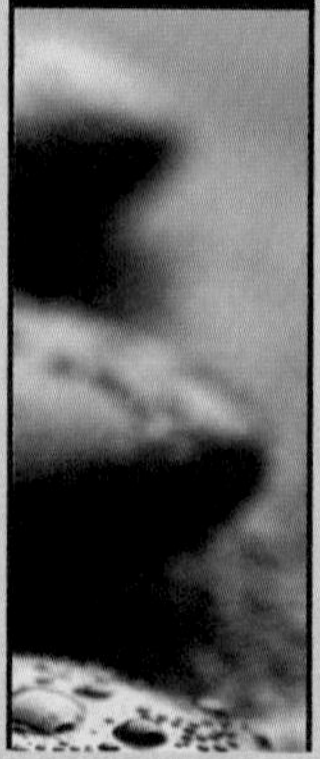

You are joining your state's professional nursing organization and have volunteered to work on their practice committee, which is focusing on the state's current nursing shortage. You are a bedside nurse in a small, rural area that is especially hard hit by the shortage. However, nurses on the committee from the state's larger cities also assert the shortage is affecting their practice.

CASE ANALYSIS

1. What do you believe is the biggest reason for the nursing shortage in your state?

2. How can the state's nursing organization help improve the nursing shortage problem?

3. What policies could be enacted to counteract the shortage in your state?

4. What level of government, or combination of levels, is best suited to address the nursing shortage and why?

Figure 8-7
States Where
Advance Nurse
Practitioners May
Independently
Prescribe
Medications. (*Data
from Phillips, 2007.*)

Arkansas	New Hampshire
Arizona	Oregon
Washington D. C.	Utah
Iowa	West Virginia
Idaho	Wisconsin
Maine	Wyoming
Montana	

A second contentious health policy issue that often divided physician and nurse organization groups was the role of Advance Nurse Practitioners (ANPs). By 2000, NPs throughout the U.S. and the District of Columbia were legally enabled to practice; however, variations in their scope of practice, prescriptive authority, and reimbursement rates remained, with divergent statutory and regulatory limitations. Historically, physician groups in many states were opposed to nurses increasing their scope of practice and lobbied state legislators and governors to be directly involved in the regulation of the ANP role. Physicians argued that their state professional boards should regulate the required legal relationship between physicians and ANPs, and that ANPs should have limited prescriptive authority (Kleinpell, 2006).

By 2007 regulatory authority over ANP practice was predominantly governed by each state's Board of Nursing. Forty-four state Boards of Nursing regulate control of ANP practice, with five states (Alabama, Mississippi, North Carolina, South Dakota, and Virginia), jointly regulated by both the Board of Nursing and the Board of Medicine (Phillips, 2007). All fifty states currently have legislation authorizing prescriptive authority for ANPs. Fourteen states currently allow ANPs to prescribe medications independent of physician authority (see Figure 8-7) (Phillips, 2007).

Writing Exercise 8-2

Determine your state's regulatory authority for ANPs (scope of practice and prescriptive authority). What do you believe are the advantages and disadvantages to your state's regulations? Explain your answer. If you were to become an ANP, would these regulations promote or hinder the way you want to practice?

The Nightingales and Big Tobacco

A true grassroots special-interest group is the **Nightingales**, an assembly of nurses whose purpose is to focus public attention on the behaviors of the tobacco industry and its involvement with tobacco-caused diseases and death (Nightingales, 2007a). The group's goal is to identify

Internet Exercise 8-2

Access the Nightingales' Web site at http://www.nightingalesnurses.net. Review the Web site and answer the following questions:

1. Summarize what the Nightingales say about the tobacco industry.

2. Discuss five activities you could do alone, or in a group, to address the tobacco industry.

3. Locate four anti-tobacco Web sites that the Nightingales suggest as pertinent reference sites.

and challenge the industry's messages that they were "socially responsible" for their products (Malone, 2007). These nurse activists work to educate and advocate for the public's health in many ways throughout the country (see Figure 8-8).

Ruth Malone, RN, PhD, and founder of the Nightingales, started her activism against the tobacco industry by purchasing one share of Altria/Phillip Morris stock and attending their annual shareholder's meeting in 2004. With colleagues and friends joining her at the meeting, Dr. Malone states it was the first time nurses had attended a meeting with tobacco company executives and shareholders. Nightingales nurses addressed the audience by sharing their stories about patients and their own family members who became ill or died due to smoking or

Figure 8-8
Nightingales' Goals to Address the Tobacco Epidemic. (*Adapted from Nightingales, 2007b.*)

1. Real tobacco company social responsibility, demonstrated by voluntary industry commitments to end all active marketing and promotion of products they themselves now admit addict and kill their best customers.

2. 100% smokefree workplaces for employees everywhere, beginning at the local level and including bars and restaurants.

3. Institutional retirement plan divestment from tobacco stock ownership.

4. Full coverage for tobacco cessation treatment programs as part of every health insurance plan, with publicly funded coverage for the uninsured.

5. Divestment of tobacco stock ownership by academic medical centers and their parent institutions.

6. Policies against acceptance of tobacco industry funding for health research and programs.

7. "R" rating for tobacco use in movies.

8. Restoration of full funding levels for comprehensive state tobacco control programs, which have been shown to be effective in reducing tobacco use and changing norms about tobacco.

SHS exposure. They also informed the audience about the negative health effects of smoking on pregnant women and children, as well as the traumatic events that burn victims experience from cigarette-caused fires (Malone, 2007).

Nightingales continue to attend industry shareholder meetings. These nurses, who are bedside caregivers, administrators, and educators, witness first hand the grim consequences that tobacco has on patients and their families, and they are willing to share their experiences. This activism on the part of nurses offers tobacco executives and company shareholders a graphic image of the negative effects these products have on citizens. The Nightingales' willingness to share their experiences and expertise to confront the tobacco industry is a textbook example of nurses advocating for their patients.

EXAMPLE OF FAILED HEALTH POLICY

Physician David Kessler became commissioner of the Food and Drug Administration (FDA) in 1990. Though not initially a main concern, tobacco and the effects it has on health soon became a top priority for Dr. Kessler. What became quickly understood in the early 1990s was that cigarettes were not considered "drugs" and therefore could not be regulated by the FDA. To be a drug, a substance has to affect a function or structure within the body and the manufacturer has to intend that mechanism to occur (Kessler, 2001). It would take Dr. Kessler and his staff years to answer the question of "intent" about nicotine. However, after interviewing tobacco company employees, researching tobacco documents, and conducting laboratory experiments, the FDA determined tobacco manufacturers intended to produce nicotine's addictive effects, making it a drug and therefore possibly regulated by the FDA.

After years of investigating, the FDA stated in 1995 that cigarettes were "drug delivery devices" and proposed they assume jurisdiction over the marketing and sales of tobacco products. Then-President Clinton publicly supported this measure. However, the tobacco industry is one of the most powerful lobby groups in the world. And even though laws and regulations restricting smoking were being passed at the local, state, and national levels, the FDA was not finding the required congressional support it needed to regulate tobacco. The following year the tobacco industry challenged the FDA's proposed jurisdiction of tobacco in federal court. It took nine years of moving through the appeals system for the U.S. Supreme Court to rule 5 to 4 that the FDA did not have authority to regulate tobacco as a drug.

Regulation of tobacco by the FDA became a prominent policy issue again in 2007 when the Institute of Medicine (IOM) called on Congress to allow the FDA jurisdiction over tobacco. The IOM is a private, nongovernmental organization that provides independent, objective, evidence-based advice to policymakers, health professionals, and the public. The IOM recommended the FDA have regulatory control over the manufacturing, distribution, marketing, and use of tobacco products (IOM, 2007). Members of both houses of Congress have introduced new legislation supporting the FDA's control of tobacco.

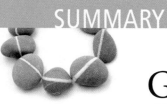

SUMMARY

Governmental agencies such as the CDC and FDA, as well as elected officials and special-interest groups, have a tremendous impact on health policy development and enactment within the U.S. Federal, state, and local agencies and officials often work together to promote the health of U.S. citizens. This does not negate the fact that individuals are also responsible for their health and well being. However, policies, programs, and regulations are in place and supported by the government to promote health.

Nursing has the responsibility to be involved with health policy formation, enactment, and evaluation. Whether at the local level tracking immunization rates, at the state level working to meet state-specific Healthy People goals and objectives, or at the national level educating elected officials or working in federal agencies, nurses understand the health issues the nation is confronting.

There are two things important in politics. The first is money, and I can't remember what the second one is.

–Mark Hanna

REFERENCES

AARP. (2007a). *Overview. AARP mission statement.* Retrieved July, 15, 2007, from http://www.aarp.org/about_aarp/aarp_overview/a2002-12-18-aarpmission.html

AARP. (2007b). *Divided we fail.* Retrieved July 22, 2007, from http://www.aarp.org/issues/dividedwefail

American Association of Colleges of Nursing. (2005). *The nurse reinvestment act at a glance.* Retrieved July 10, 2007, from http://www.aacn.nche.edu/media/nraataglance.htm

American Medical Association. (2007a). *AMA reinforces efforts to cover uninsured kids.* Retrieved July 20, 2007, from http://www.ama-assn.org/ama/pub/category/17767.html

American Medical Association. (2007b). *Patient safety and quality improvement in health care.* Retrieved July 15, 2007, from http://www.ama-assn.org/ama/pub/category/13235.html

American Nurses Association. (2006). *Nursing facts: Nursing shortage.* Retrieved July 10, 2007, from http://www.nursingworld.org/readroom/fsshortage.htm

American Nurses Association. (2007). *About the American nurses association.* Retrieved July 15, 2007, from http://www.nursingworld.org/about/

Americans Nonsmokers' Rights Foundation. (2008). *Overview list—how many smoke-free laws?* Retrieved July 18, 2008, from http://www.no-smoke.org/pdf/mediaordlist.pdf

Angell, M. (2004). Excess in the pharmaceutical industry. *Canadian Medical Association Journal, 171,* 1451–1453.

Birkland, B. A. (2001). *An introduction to the policy process: Theories, concepts, and models of public policy making.* Armonk, NY: M.E. Sharpe.

Birnbaum, J. H. (2007). *On issues from Medicare to medication, AARP's money will be there.* Retrieved

July 15, 2007, from http://www.washingtonpost.com/wp-dyn/content/article/2007/04/23/AR2007042301760.html

Capps, R., Passel, J. S., Perez-Lopez, D., & Fix, M. (2003). *The new neighbors: A user's guide to data on immigrants in U.S. communities.* Retrieved August 8, 2007, from http://www.urban.org/UploadedPDF/310844_the_new_neighbors.pdf

Carrasquillo, O., & Pati, S. (2004). The role of health insurance on PAP smear and mammography utilization by immigrants living in the United States. *Preventive Medicine, 39,* 943–950.

Centers for Disease Control and Prevention. (2001). *Core curriculum on tuberculosis.* National Center for HIV/AIDS, Viral Hepatitis, STD, and TB Prevention. Division of Tuberculosis Elimination. Retrieved July 15, 2007, from http://www.cdc.gov/tb/pubs/corecurr/default.htm

Centers for Disease Control and Prevention. (2007). *Mission statement and activities.* National Center for HIV/AIDS, Viral Hepatitis, STD, and TB Prevention Division of Tuberculosis Elimination. Retrieved July 15, 2007, from http://www.cdc.gov/tb/mission.htm

Delaware Health and Social Services. (2001). *Healthy Delaware 2010.* Retrieved July 12, 2007, from http://www.healthydelaware.com

Finkelstein, E. A., Fiebelkorn, I. C., & Wang, G. (2004). State-level estimates of annual medical expenditures attributable to obesity. *Obesity Research, 12,* 18–24.

Gostin, L. O. (2007). Law as a tool to facilitate healthier lifestyles and prevent obesity. *The Journal of the American Medical Association, 297,* 87–90.

Hahn, E. J., Rayens, M. K., York, N. L., Okoli, C. T. C., Zhang, M., Dignan, M., et al. (2006). Effects of a smoke-free law on hair nicotine and respiratory symptoms on restaurant and workers. *Journal of Occupational and Environmental Medicine, 48,* 906–913.

Healthy Maine Partnerships, Bureau of Health, Department of Human Services. (2002). *Healthy Maine 2010.* Retrieved July 12, 2007, from http://www.maine.gov/dhhs/boh/healthyme2k/hm2010a.htm

Heloma, A., & Jaakkola, M. S. (2003). Four-year follow-up of smoke exposure, attitudes and smoking behavior following enactment of Finland's national smoke-free workplace law. *Addiction, 98,* 1111–1117.

Institute for Health & Socio-Economic Policy. (2007). *Market-based health care: Big money, politics, and the unraveling of U.S. civil democracy.* Retrieved July 22, 2007, from http://www.calnurse.org/research/pdfs/ihsp_marketbasedhealthcare_062607.pdf

Institute of Medicine. (2000). *Ending neglect. The elimination of tuberculosis in the United States.* National Academy of Sciences. Retrieved July 15, 2007, from http://books.nap.edu/html/ending_neglect/reportbrief.pdf

Institute of Medicine. (2007). *Ending the tobacco problem. A blueprint for the nation.* Retrieved July 22, 2007, from http://www.iom.edu/Object.File/Master/43/183/Tobacco%20report%20brief%20general.pdf

Ismail, M. A. (2005). Special report. *Drug lobby second to none: How the pharmaceutical industry gets its way in Washington.* The Center for Public Integrity. Retrieved July 6, 2007, from http://www.publicintegrity.org/rx/report.aspx?aid=723

Ismail, M. A. (2007). *Spending on lobbying thrives: Drug and health products industries invest $182 million to influence legislation.* The Center for Public Integrity. Retrieved July 6, 2007, from http://www.publicintegrity.org/rx/report.aspx?aid=823

Kaiser Commission. (2004). *Immigrants and health coverage: A primer.* Retrieved August 11, 2007, from http://www.kff.org/uninsured/upload/Immigrants-and-Health-Coverage-A-Primer.pdf

Kentucky Cabinet for Health and Family Services. (2005). *Healthy Kentuckians 2010.* Retrieved July 12, 2007, from http://chfs.ky.gov/dph/hk2010.htm

KENTUCKY CABINET FOR HEALTH AND FAMILY SERVICES. (2005). *Tobacco use in Kentucky 2005.* Frankfort, KY: Cabinet for Health and Family Services; Department for Public Health; Division of Adult and Child Health Improvement; Chronic Disease Prevention Control Branch; Tobacco Prevention and Cessation Program.

KESSLER, D. (2001). *A question of intent. A great American battle with a deadly industry.* New York: Public Affairs.

KINGDON, J. W. (2003). *Agendas, alternatives, and public policies* (2nd ed.). New York: Longman Classics.

KLEINPELL, R. M. (2006). Expanding opportunities in ACNP practice. *Nurse Practitioner, S8–9.*

KOCHANEK, K. D., Murphy, S. L., Anderson, R. N., & Scott, C. (2004). *Deaths: Final data for 2002.* Centers for Disease Control and Prevention. Division of Vital Statistics. Retrieved July 21, 2007, from http://www.cdc.gov/nchs/data/nvsr/nvsr53/nvsr53_05.pdf

LEVY, D. T., & Friend, K. B. (2003). The effects of clean indoor air laws: What do we know and what do we need to know? *Health Education Research, 18,* 592–609.

LONGEST, B. B. (2005). *Health policymaking in the United States* (4th ed.). Chicago: Health Administration Press.

LUCAS, J. W., Barr-Anderson, D. J., & Kington, R. S. (2003). Health status, health insurance, and health care utilization patterns of immigrant black men. *American Journal of Public Health, 93,* 1740–1747.

MALONE, P. S., & Chaffee, M. W. (2007). Interest groups: Powerful political catalysts in health care. In J. Mason, J. K. Leavitt, & M. W. Chaffee (Eds.), *Policy & politics in nursing and health care* (pp. 770–771). St. Louis, MO: Saunders Elsevier.

MALONE, R. E. (2007). Taking action. The Nightingales take on big tobacco. In D. J. Mason, J. K. Leavitt, & M. W. Chaffee (Eds.), *Policy & politics in nursing and health care* (pp. 109–119). St. Louis, MO: Saunders Elsevier.

MELLO, M. M., Studdert, D. M., & Brennan, T. A. (2006). Obesity—the new frontier of public health law. *The New England Journal of Medicine, 354,* 2601–2610.

MOSKOWITZ, J. M., Lin, Z., & Hudes, E. S. (2000). The impact of workplace smoking ordinances in California on smoking cessation. *American Journal of Public Health, 90,* 757–761.

NATIONAL CONFERENCE OF STATE LEGISLATURES. (2007). *Childhood obesity—2006 update and overview of policy options.* Retrieved July 5, 2007, from http://www.ncsl.org/programs/health/ChildhoodObesity-2006.htm#phy

NIGHTINGALES. (2007a). *Who we are.* Retrieved July 15, 2007, from http://www.nightingalesnurses.org/who_we_are.html

NIGHTINGALES. (2007b). *Nightingales goals and how you can help.* Retrieved July 24, 2007, from http://www.nightingalesnurses.org/our_goals.html

PHILLIPS, S. J. (2007). A comprehensive look at the legislative issues affecting advance nursing practice. *The Nurse Pracitioner, 32,* 14–16.

RABIN, R. L., & Sugarman, S. D. (2001). *Regulating tobacco.* New York: Oxford University Press.

ROSSI, P. H. (2001). The old homeless and the new homelessness in historical perspective. In E. C. Hein (Ed.), *Nursing issues in the 21st century. Perspectives from the literature* (pp. 311–321). Philadelphia: Lippincott.

TROTTER, L., Wakefield, M., & Borland, R. (2002). Socially cued smoking in bars, nightclubs, and gaming venues: A case for introducing smoke-free policies. *Tobacco Control, 11,* 300–304.

UNITED STATES DEPARTMENT OF HEALTH AND HUMAN SERVICES. (2001). Office of Disease Prevention and Health Promotion. *Healthy People 2010 understanding and improving health.* Retrieved July 14, 2008, from http://www.healthypeople.gov/Document/pdf/uih/2010uih.pdf

UNITED STATES DEPARTMENT OF AGRICULTURE. (2005). *Kentucky tobacco facts.* Louisville, KY: National Agricultural Statistics Service; Kentucky Field Office.

UNITED STATES DEPARTMENT OF HEALTH AND HUMAN SERVICES. (2006). Office of Disease Prevention and Health Promotion. *Healthy People 2010 midcourse review.* Retrieved July 15, 2007, from http://www.healthypeople.gov/data/midcourse

UNITED STATES DEPARTMENT OF HEALTH AND HUMAN SERVICES AND UNITED STATES DEPARTMENT OF AGRICULTURE. (2005). *Dietary guidelines for Americans 2005.* Retrieved July 21, 2007, from http://www.health.gov/dietaryguidelines/dga2005/document

UNITED STATES DEPARTMENT OF HOUSING AND URBAN DEVELOPMENT. (2007). *The annual homeless assessment report to Congress.* Retrieved August 7, 2007, from http://www.huduser.org/Publications/pdf/ahar.pdf

UNITED STATES HOUSE OF REPRESENTATIVES COMMITTEE ON GOVERNMENT REFORM. (2006). *Pharmaceutical industry profits increase by over $8 billion after Medicare drug plan goes into effect.* Retrieved August 8, 2007, from http://oversight.house.gov/documents/20060919115623-70677.pdf

YORK, N. L. (2008). Management of clients with parenchymal and pleural disorders. In J. M. Black & J. Hokanson Hawks (Eds.), *Medical-surgical nursing clinical management for positive outcomes* (8th ed.). Philadelphia: Elsevier.

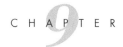

THE POLITICAL INFLUENCE ON THE NURSING PROFESSION

ROSEMARY E. S. MORTIMER

M.S. Ed, MS, RN, Instructor, Johns Hopkins University School of Nursing

Government of the people, by the people, for the people...

–Abraham Lincoln

LEARNING OBJECTIVES

At the completion of the chapter, the learner should be able to do the following:

1. Articulate two reasons why nursing students need to be involved in political activity.
2. Identify and explain at least five key terms in regard to political involvement.
3. Articulate the importance of one person in the establishment of policy.
4. Identify three pieces of legislation that have impacted nursing care.
5. Explain three ways students may have an impact on the political process.
6. Articulate three terms used in parliamentary procedure.
7. Identify and utilize three tips on how to speak at a public meeting.

KEY TERMS		
Collaboration	Negotiation/Compromise	Regulations
Constituent	Networking	Scope of Nursing Practice
Lobbying	Politics	

INTRODUCTION

It may seem strange to nursing students to think about political activity and legislation in terms of the nursing world. While many Americans have studied U.S. government in high school, it is questionable what they remember once they graduate. Nursing students are probably no exception. In the last twenty years there has been an explosion of information, primarily as a result of 24-hour news stations. Yet, a survey by the Pew Research Center (2007) found that the number of citizens who were able to name the current leaders of this country was virtually unchanged in twenty years. Because politics have begun to affect the profession of nursing, and legislation has such an impact on health care, it would appear that nursing students today need to stay abreast of health care issues under discussion in the political arena and to review what they know about the political process and expand their knowledge with new information and awareness.

Nursing students need to learn about the political process so that they can have a direct impact on the care that they are allowed and required to give their patients. Nurses are the best advocates for their clients and need to be sure that laws that are enacted are primarily for the public good. Legislation can be written in such a way that health care is taken out of the hands of providers and given over to others who have no expertise in the field. This is unacceptable to those in the field and those involved in direct patient care. Nurses and nursing students need to be familiar with the legislative process in order to clearly get their ideas across to the powerbrokers and to change how care is delivered. Nurses need to be ever vigilant that their practice is not eroded by others who want to have a say about the way nursing care is administered. Knowledge of and involvement in the process is the only way to have an impact upon the political process.

DEFINING POLITICS

The word **politics** can be defined in any number of ways, but probably the most accurate comment has been attributed to the 19th-century German chancellor of Prussia, Otto von Bismarck, who is believed to have said that politics is the art of the possible (1867). It is unquestionably true that when groups of committed people get together, they will be able to change what is happening in their world.

What legislation has had an impact on the lives of ordinary citizens? When driving an automobile, one must wear a seat belt according to laws in this country. How much a person pays for gas is regulated by laws, because each state collects different amounts for their gasoline tax. Boating is regulated, as are fishing, hunting, and many other aspects of our lives. Where prisons are located and whether the roads and schools are able to keep up with increasing population are all determined by laws. Care of children and mandatory education for our young people are all mandated by legislation.

There has been a variety of federal legislation introduced that would provide additional funds for nursing education. It was thought by policy experts that one way to solve the nursing shortage was to encourage many more people to attend nursing school. State and federal governments have attempted this encouragement in the past by giving money when there have been shortages in teaching and in the military. This money can be used for scholarships and sometimes even for new buildings. Most often this money is given with the caveat that those who are funded will then be required to work for a state or government agency for a specified period of time. It has been recognized that there is a major shortage of nursing educators, and the government has responded by increasing funds for those interested in teaching nursing.

All these pieces of legislation began as ideas and grew into laws. Frequently new legislation is the brain child of a single person or is an attempt by a legislator or an individual to right a real or perceived wrong (Figure 9-1). The aggrieved party discusses the concern with his or her legislator, and the legislator directs staff to write legislation to remedy the problem. These laws then have tremendous impact on daily living.

One nurse practitioner in Maryland was stuck by a needle in the performance of her duties. The patient refused initially to be tested to see if she was HIV positive. Consequently, the nurse practitioner was started on the HIV cocktail to inhibit the disease. She discussed this problem with a state legislator who was a nurse, and they worked on a bill to alleviate this problem. The bill stated that a hospital could test a patient's blood for HIV if the patient's blood was already in the system. Consequently, this law protected hospital health care workers if the patient was already in a hospital and already had blood in the laboratory. The facility did not need the patient's consent for testing (Mooney, 2004). It was no help to those workers who were stuck with a needle when a patient was in another facility, such as a clinic.

A nurse educator in Baltimore discovered that her noninsulin-dependant diabetics were not covered by insurance for monitoring devices. She learned of a law that had been passed in New York mandating that insurance had to cover these devices. She met with the local American Diabetes group and then found her local state senator and convinced him to sponsor legislation to remedy this problem. He agreed to introduce legislation, and then she began lobbying the entire legislature. The bill failed the first year, but after additional education of those legislators who had voted against the bill, it was passed the second year it was introduced. This nurse learned how to advocate for her clients and was resourceful and patient enough to see her idea become a reality (Jossi, 1997). Helping to write legislation is a time consuming and often lengthy process.

Figure 9-1
Ideas for new legislation frequently arise from everyday problems.

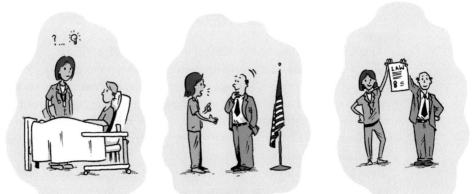

DELMAR/CENGAGE LEARNING

Many times the idea for legislation comes from someone who has suffered a tragedy. Candy Lightner is a woman whose thirteen-year-old daughter was killed by a drunk driver in 1980. She was aghast to realize that the man who killed her daughter had numerous drunken driving arrests on his record but was still allowed to drive. She founded the Mothers' Against Drunk Driving group (MADD), and that group has lobbied legislatures across the country to strengthen drunk driving laws, decrease the blood alcohol level requirements for inebriation, and mandate incarceration and education for repeat drunk driving offenders. This has produced a virtual revolution in the way people feel about driving when they have been drinking. (http://www.madd.org/, 2008). It seems to be common knowledge now that if you have been out drinking alcohol, you need to find someone to drive you home or to get a cab. Many towns even offer free taxi rides on certain nights like New Year's Eve to help eliminate the problem of drinking and driving.

THE NURSE PRACTICE ACT

As has been shown previously, nursing has been and will continue to be impacted by legislation. The most important piece of legislation that the registered nurse and student nurse needs to be aware of is the Nurse Practice Act in the particular state in which they are licensed. The Nurse Practice Act of each state defines what a nurse can and cannot do. It defines the scope of nursing practice. Every state has developed a Nurse Practice Act, which is a law or series of laws whose primary purpose is to protect the public. These state laws regulate who can be a nurse as well as their education and licensing requirements. These laws also define disciplinary measures if a nurse has been found to have violated the law.

Internet Exercise 9-1	Go online to the state board of nursing in your state. Review the disciplinary information provided.
	1. Identify what disciplinary actions might happen if a nurse was discovered to have falsified patient records.
	2. Consider what the implications for one's license would be if a nurse took a controlled substance from the medication cart, signed it out under a patient's name, and put it in his or her pocket to take it home for personal use.

Individual State Boards of Nursing

Historically, a nurse must be registered in the state in which he/she is working and in the state in which he/she resides. Due to the advances in telehealth, the Internet, and people living farther from jobs, this is changing. The National Council of State Boards of Nursing reports that

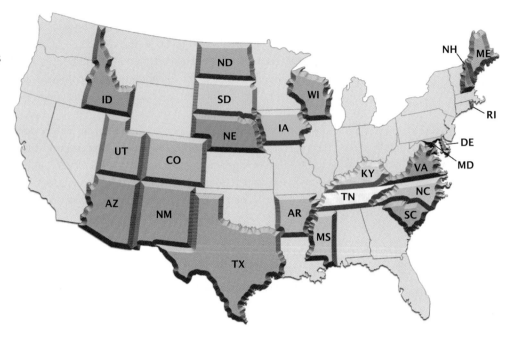

Figure 9-2
A total of twenty-three states participate in the Nurse Licensure Compact. *(Source: National Council of State Boards of Nursing, 2007.)*

as of 2008, twenty-three states had signed legislation to become part of a group known as the "compact states" (Figure 9-2). This is a way to recognize nurses who live in one state and work in another and is extremely helpful for those individuals who commute over state lines for employment. It is also useful for nurses who are involved in telehealth and may be offering advice across state lines. This type of employment is probably only going to expand as technology makes this kind of work more practical, easier, and cost effective. In these states a nurse is licensed in his/her state of residence but must practice according to the Nurse Practice Act of the state in which the care is occurring. This is similar to holding a driver's license in one state but being able to drive in every other state. The person who drives in another state is subject to the laws of the state in which he or she is driving at the time. Student nurses are also impacted by the Nurse Practice Act in the state in which they are practicing.

There are any number of pieces of legislation at the state and national level that affect health care. Legislation that has affected nursing practice includes laws mandating that maternity patients may not be discharged from the hospital within twenty-four hours. Whether your state allows midwives and advanced practice nurses to be paid by third party re-imbursement is decided by law. Do the Advanced Practice Nurses in your state have prescriptive authority? Are any Advanced Practice Nurses prohibited from writing prescriptions? Nursing students need to be familiar with the Good Samaritan Act and be aware if the law has been enacted in their state (Morrison et al., 2004). There are many laws that impact nurses as individual citizens. Do people need to have a car seat for children in the vehicle? What is the age or weight limit and where must this seat be placed? These laws make a difference to nurses who are parents or grandparents. Some of these laws may also have an impact on nurses and their practice. Pediatric nurses need to be aware of such laws before they release a patient to go home from an emergency room. Maternity nurses need to be aware of these laws when they discharge newborns into the care of their families. Laws such as these are plans that the government may put into action and are usually enacted by state legislatures.

Writing Exercise 9-1

Identify one law that has affected your own life. Explain how this law has affected you positively or negatively and how it could be changed. Explain the reason for the change(s) you have suggested. Any suggestions for change need to include a rationale.

WHAT IS LAW AND HOW DOES IT DIFFER FROM POLICY?

Laws are the way we are governed. They are the way we define and institutionalize customs. They are usually enforceable by an authority and may carry with them some measure of punishment if one breaks the law. Policy, on the other hand, is a plan of action that the government may put into action to achieve an end. Policy directs the way in which laws are carried out. One may think of laws as the bricks and foundation of a house. Policy is the paint, furniture, and wallpaper that make it a home. It provides the direction in which the laws will be enforced. If we begin to think of law and politics as issues close to home, it becomes apparent that if nurses do not become involved in the establishment of laws and/or policy, then they will lose a chance to impact their own lives and, potentially, practice.

Participation in the political process can shape policy. Participation in the process can and does determine how bills are written and regulations are adopted. This process affects whatever "house" we are in when we treat our patients. Therefore, as nurses, we need to know how to get our points across to legislators, government officials, and power brokers. This can be accomplished by learning the process and using these skills.

Key Terms in the Political Process

Nurses who want to become more comfortable with the political process need to possess a basic understanding of the language used in the area and will find it helpful to be able to define as well as to understand some basic terms.

Scope of nursing practice is what a nurse can and cannot do and is defined by each individual state. This state law is most commonly known as the Nurse Practice Act. This is a very general civil law. Regulations are more specific and explain how the law is to be interpreted and implemented. The International Council of Nurses (2004) states that, "Scope of Nursing Practice is not limited to specific tasks, functions or responsibilities but includes direct care giving and evaluation of its impact, advocating for patients and for health, supervising and delegating to others, leading, managing, teaching, undertaking research, and developing health policy for health care systems. Furthermore, as the scope of practice is dynamic and responsive to health needs, development of knowledge, and technological advances, periodic review is required to ensure that it continues to be consistent with current health needs and supports improved health outcomes."

Lobbying is the action taken to persuade someone to come to your point of view. Legislators may or may not be familiar with the health care system. A legislator may have never been in a hospital or only occasionally accesses a health care provider. Alternately, the legislator may be a physician and be familiar with the way health care is affecting their own practice. It is up to registered nurses to talk to the legislators and educate them to our point of view. Every one of us lobbies when we want to get our own way. Children lobby for a later bedtime or a higher allowance. Often married folks lobby each other for a new car, or kids lobby parents to help them pay for higher education such as nursing school. Lobbying becomes scary for many people, however, when it is used in the context of dealing with elected officials. Many people seem to feel that legislators are in a class by themselves and are consequently reticent to talk with them or to discuss needs.

Collaboration occurs when two or more parties work together for a common cause. Nurses may find themselves dealing with very different people as issues change. It is important for nurses to keep focused on the goals of nursing and not to align themselves so closely with any one group that sight of the mission or the good idea that the opposition might have is lost. Nurses also want to be sure that they stay independent as registered nurses and nursing students, so it is counterproductive to become very closely aligned with any one group that may not share similar goals.

Negotiation/compromise is similar to collaboration. When one negotiates, he/she discusses and bargains on a variety of issues so that everyone has to give up something for the good of the whole (Webster's, 1997). Usually everyone comes away from a compromise satisfied that they can live with the results, even though they did not get everything that they wanted to be in the final document or law. It is often very difficult and can take a lot of time. No one in the group can be rigid on too many points or the entire project may be lost.

A **constituent** is one who lives in an elected person's district and has the authority to vote to keep them in office (Webster's, 1997). Constituents are the most important people to an elected official because without the individual who will vote for an official, that official will not remain in office. It is, however, also important for nurses to know politicians other than the ones for whom they can vote. Often the nurse can educate them to the nursing point of view, and if the politician respects the nurse and feels that he/she has always given good counsel, the nurse may influence the legislator's vote.

Regulations are rules or laws by which conduct is regulated, and they define the scope of practice in specific terms. Regulations are the ways in which laws are implemented (Webster's, 1997). Standards of care are defined by regulations, as are the standards in the way that students are educated, and in the way that care is practiced. This is how the basics tenets of the profession are upheld. It is often said that the devil is in the details. It is often in writing regulations that a registered nurse or a student nurse may have the most impact. Regulatory agencies like the state board of nursing are often charged with writing regulations; nurses and students may become involved in this process. In some states, however, it is a regulation that assessments may only be done by a registered nurse and this act may never be delegated. These advisory groups allow nurses to participate and have real impact on the lives of their fellow professionals. Many times the people who are asked to write the regulations are drawn from the state nursing organizations. Nurses must be educated and learn to work together so that we can make dramatic changes in the health care arena and in health care policy (Gehrke, 2008).

Because of this important role for nurses, it is important to remember that nurses often are the most informed people to speak for those who have no voice for themselves. Policy makers respond to nurses who can articulate the needs of patients who are less astute in the ways of dealing with powerbrokers. Many times nursing literature has discussed the need for nurses to be taught about and involved in the political process, and yet there has been little research done in this area (Gebbie et al., 2000).

It appears that those nurses who participate in the political process have been exposed to a positive role model who encourages their participation. Gebbie et al. (2000) specifically discusses the major role that nursing faculty have in involving their students in the political process and the impact that involved faculty have on making their students politically aware and adept.

REASONS TO BECOME INVOLVED IN POLITICS

There are three paramount reasons for nursing students and registered nurses to be involved in politics. These are facing issues, the fact that one person can make a difference, and the financial implications of a decision to become or not become involved in the political process.

Facing Issues

Sometimes the only way safe care can be delivered to patients is by having issues resolved through the political process and by making new laws. As has been mentioned, how a nurse may practice, where the nurse may practice, and often the amount he/she will be paid are all issues that are determined by policy. Implementation is often the problem. A case in point is that of Advanced Directives. These are usually written in the statute as a law that allows patients to decide how they want to be treated in their last days of life. Is there such a law in the state in which you are attending nursing school? How is this law implemented in that state? Remember, implementation is defined by policy and by the way the regulations are written. It may be flawed in the particular state in which a nurse finds him or herself.

Are Advanced Directives important in the lives of patients? Health care advocates were distressed during the time when the Terry Schiavo case was in the news. This was the case of a young woman who had suffered severe brain damage in 1990 at age twenty-six when her heart stopped, probably because of a chemical imbalance that was believed to have been brought on by an eating disorder. Court-appointed doctors ruled she was in a persistent vegetative state with no real consciousness or chance of recovery. She had left no written information on how she wanted to be treated, and her husband wanted her to be allowed to die. He was repeatedly thwarted by her parents and brother who demanded that a feeding tube be placed. The case made it through the courts and became a national issue for the Florida legislature. It finally became a national incident when the Congress and President Bush became involved. The Supreme Court refused on several occasions to overrule the local judge in the case, and she was finally allowed to die (MSNBC, 2005). Health providers and politicians realized the importance of health directives on her life and in the lives of any patients, especially the young and seemingly healthy constituents who may not have written instructions.

Internet Exercise 9-2	Go online and download a copy of an advanced directives form in your state of residence. Review the form and then complete the following: 1. Think about yourself and where you are in your life right now. 2. Imagine that without any indicators or notice your family is notified that you are clinging to life in a hospital. 3. Think about yourself. Do you know how you would want treatment to be carried out? 4. Now fill it out for yourself. 5. You might want to write a few notes about what this process feels like before, during, and after.

Patients may not have even considered who should speak on their behalf when they are being admitted to a health care facility. Patients may not have signed advanced directives until they are admitted to a hospital. Yet, coming into the hospital is usually a very stressful time for the average person. It might be preferable that the directive be placed on the driver's license, allowing people to find a more opportune time to discuss what they prefer to happen to them. This seems to be a better topic for people to discuss over the kitchen table with their families as they are re-registering for their drivers' license than in the midst of the emergency room, when time is essential and care decisions may be critical.

One Person Can Make a Difference

It seems very obvious that one person can make a difference in our lives. There are those who might disagree about the importance of one person and believe that it is impossible for one person to make a difference, but history teaches us otherwise. There have been many times in this country when one person has made a difference. A recent example was the 2000 presidential election.

The presidential election of 2000 was not decided for several weeks after the November 7, 2000 election day. The Democratic candidate, Al Gore, had received more popular votes but fewer electoral votes than his Republican challenger, George W. Bush. The election was challenged in the courts, and it was finally decided by the Supreme Court by a vote of 5-4 in favor of Mr. Bush (USNews.com, 2000).

Many historians recount the decision by one senator in the mid-1800s to refuse to vote for the impeachment of President Andrew Johnson. This story was discussed at length during the 1999 impeachment hearings. His action was the determining factor in President Johnson's being allowed to complete his term.

As you read in chapter three, it is important that nurses be aware of the history of their profession. The beginning of nursing history offers a prime example of the difference one person can make. The only reason anyone is in nursing is because of Florence Nightingale, whose writings on sanitation and statistics were so compelling that they revolutionized the care of soldiers in the British Army during the Crimean War. She then organized the first training program for nurses, and that school became the model for other schools. Ms. Nightingale is the reason that nursing is considered a profession today (Donahue, 1996). She faced the issues she saw in her work and found ways to make improvements by advocating for her patients.

Another individual who made a difference to the nursing profession was Isabel Hampton Robb. She was the first superintendent of the Johns Hopkins Hospital Nursing School, and her reforms and standards are still followed today. She instituted grades as a form of showing competency in order to graduate and become qualified as nurses. She became the first head of Johns Hopkins Nursing School in 1889, and later she was one of the founders of the American Nurses Association and the National League for Nursing (Donahue, 1996). Clearly she understood the issues facing students being prepared to enter the profession and did what she could to improve the training and status of nurses.

Nurses who work in Community Health often emulate Lillian Wald. Ms. Wald was a nurse who worked in the tenements in New York City at the turn of the 20th century. She faced the issue of the deplorable conditions in the New York tenements and arranged for health care to be delivered in the home (Donahue, 1996). Another individual, Mary Mahoney, faced massive discrimination when she completed her coursework to become a nurse in 1879. She persevered and was the first African-American graduate nurse in this country (Donahue, 1996). These were individuals who found that something was wrong, faced the issues squarely, and discovered ways to change the environment.

The history of the nursing profession is studded with individuals who have not been afraid to face critical issues and thus have made a difference. Mary Breckinridge discovered how appalling the care of pregnant women and their children was in the hill country of the Appalachian Mountains and was determined to change the care that they were receiving. She founded the Frontier Nursing Service in 1925, based on a model from England. Eventually, there was a school of midwifery established to train nurses for midwifery services in rural areas (Donahue, 1996).

Research by Dr. Linda Aiken from the University of Pennsylvania in 2003 promulgated nursing data that shows how important registered nurses with baccalaureate degrees are in the care of patients. This research states that in hospitals with higher proportions of nurses educated at the baccalaureate level or higher, surgical patients experienced lower mortality and failure-to-rescue rates (Aiken et al., 2003). She also, along with Dr. Peter Buerhaus, has validated for the world the impact of the nursing shortage on our facilities and, most importantly, on patient care. Dr. Buerhaus and his colleagues documented that when registered nurses provided more hours of patient care, the care of hospitalized patients was improved (Needleman et al., 2002). Dr. Aiken and her colleagues found that nurses in hospitals that have high patient-to-nurse ratios experience more dissatisfaction with their jobs and burnout (Aiken et al., 2002). Insufficient numbers of nurses can only be stretched so far, and any stretching at all lessens the optimum ratio of nurses to patients. As has been shown in Chapter 3, nursing has come a long way, but still there are issues of crucial importance facing both nurses and patients today. If these issues are not faced, then all will pay enormous prices.

Finally, it should be mentioned that some nurses, especially those who serve in or with the military, are perhaps involved in the most political ways of all. Edith Cavell was a nurse who established the first school for nurses in Brussels, Belgium. She was executed in Belgium by the Germans as a spy because she was caring for soldiers from both sides of the war during World War I (Donahue, 1996).

Having moved back now to the present tense and reasons for us to become involved in politics, think of a time when we are at our most vulnerable. Concern about personal security easily transfers to concerns about safety when being treated for illness or injury. People who are hospitalized often feel a loss of control of their lives very quickly when illness or accident strikes. They become dependent on the health care system that is fraught with the potential for errors. Many nurses will anecdotally say that they will only go into a hospital with a nursing colleague with them to act as a patient advocate. These concerns can become the basis for new laws when legislators find themselves or their constituents in situations that they object to and decide to write a law to change an area in health care that they find difficult to understand or to navigate. Nurses need to be in the forefront of explaining health care to these legislators and determining whether a new law is warranted or would be unduly cumbersome for health care as a whole.

Financial Concerns

The third reason one needs to be involved politically is financial. Whether one is a student or has been practicing nursing for many years, all nurses are obligated, as are all other members of society, to pay taxes. It is unquestionable that money runs the government, yet few of us know how it is spent. It might surprise the average nurse to realize that in many local jurisdictions, over half of each tax dollar goes to fund the local department of education and the schools. If asked, many would probably say that their taxes go to public safety and to the debt left at the local community hospital by those who cannot pay but receive health care. In actuality the funds that do reach hospitals and health care may be no more than twenty cents out of every dollar. It is interesting to note that many people who do not have children in public schools often express the feeling that they have no need to vote in the school board elections because members of the local school boards have little or no impact on their lives. Yet, it is these folks who are spending well over half of the local tax dollars (Howard County, Maryland Tax Bill, 2008). This is

Writing Exercise 9-2

Consider your own involvement in the political process. Reflect on the following questions and then describe your involvement as accurately and as honestly as you can. If answering the questions first helps your reflection, then go ahead, but your written reflection is the key work here.

1. Are you a registered voter? When and where did you first register? Was there a specific reason that you registered when you did, or someone who influenced you to register to vote?

2. Did you vote in the last general election? What criteria did you use to decide for whom to vote? (These elections are held in November every other year.)

3. Did you vote in the last primary election? How did you review the individual candidate's positions on the issues? (These are usually held in September of every other year, except for the presidential primary years.)

4. During an election year, what publications or Internet sites do you read or access to find out information about political candidates?

5. What are the names of the two U.S. Senators from your state? To which political party do they each belong? How do they and their parties feel about universal health care insurance for everyone?
   What are the names of your state senators or delegates, and representatives or assemblypersons? To which political parties do they belong? What is that group's stance on emergency contraception being allowed to be dispensed over the counter? Do you agree with their stance?

6. Name one local or state issue that you have worked on or are interested in working on? Why does this particular topic interest you?

7. On what topic have you sent a postcard, letter, or e-mail to an elected representative? What was it that made this topic important enough for you to contact them? If you have never done this, what topic could you address with your elected representative and why does it matter to you?

8. Have you worked on a candidate's campaign? What attracted you to that candidate? If you have never worked on a campaign, what characteristics about a candidate would encourage you to do so?

9. What organization do you belong to that studies issues and takes positions on them? Why did you join this group?

10. Have you visited a legislator's office? If so, what was the visit like, and what did you discuss?

something for those in nursing to consider, and to ask local powerbrokers what more could be done to help the health community.

INVOLVEMENT IN POLITICS

How does a nurse or a nursing student become involved in politics? It is easier than one might think. Initial involvement is fairly straightforward: registering to vote and then voting. Beyond that, becoming involved in professional organizations allows awareness of and involvement in issues of current concern, which may be handled within or through the organization. Other steps include working within the legislative process and networking to strengthen your case among others.

Voter Registration

Anyone interested in becoming involved in the political process must first be registered to vote (Gehrke, 2008). It is a matter of public record as to who is registered, and legislators will pay much more attention to those who are able to vote for them than to those who complain but have not even bothered to register to vote. Voter registration is easy and can even be accomplished online for many states. Many public agencies, including the department of motor vehicles and the local public library, have applications. Many times state residents can register to vote by mail. Every state has different criteria for residency and dates by which you have had to register in order to vote in the next election. Many candidates are voter registrars and will have the necessary paperwork. Often local and state fairs will have a registration booth.

Voting

The importance of nurses voting in every election must not be minimized. Voting is the primary way for all members of society to make their opinions heard. Those who do not vote when they are able allow everyone else to make decisions for them. It is imperative that nurses vote in every election no matter how many seats are in contention. Nurses have an obligation to themselves and to their patients to educate themselves in order to make a well reasoned vote. Nurses will discover by networking and educating themselves how other nurses feel about issues that directly affect their practice. Nurses and student nurses who are active in their professional organizations will get written and e-mail information to help them make more informed choices. Nurses need to prioritize what issues are most important for them when they are voting and vote accordingly. It is helpful to know the national platform for the various parties in order to help guide decision making. Over the last twenty years there has been a virtual revolution in the delivery of health care, and it has affected every aspect of nursing. One example is the dramatic change in length of stay in in-patient facilities, and how insurance companies have directly impacted patient care. In the early 1990s hospitals were told by insurance companies that patients who had had vaginal deliveries were to be allowed only twenty-four hours post-delivery care in in-patient facilities. This led to many concerns among providers and patients that mothers and babies were unsafe when they were discharged this quickly. Some mothers had significant problems with post-partum hemorrhage, and there were a number of babies who were not tested for Phenylketonuria, which can be easily diagnosed by a simple blood test. Laws were passed in some states to allow patients to stay in a hospital for forty-eight hours and to even extend hospital stays when the patient and their providers felt that being discharged would be hazardous to the patient's health.

Nurses need to decide for themselves if they vote as health care advocates. If they decide to vote this way, then they need to be aware of how a candidate feels about health care and vote for the one that is most closely aligned with their philosophy. Nurses need to educate themselves on the various stands of candidates. A nurse may want to attend a candidates' forum and ask very specific questions of each candidate and vote for the candidate who seems to have the interests of patients as his or her paramount idea.

Professional Organizations

Nurses and nursing students need to be members of a professional nursing organization. Why is it necessary to join a professional organization? It is a way of finding people who have a common interest. It is a great way to network. It is a way to find out about jobs, conferences, new equipment, and ways of practicing. Since many nursing leaders are members of professional organizations, it is a wonderful way to initiate and to maintain professional contacts. It becomes a place for nurses to meet old friends and for nursing educators to see where their students have gone.

The American Nurses Association (ANA) is the professional organization that represents professional nurses. The ANA represents almost 2.2 million nurses. Every state has a group that is a sub-group of the American Nurses Association. "One in 44" is the ANA slogan to show that 1 out of every 44 female voters is a nurse (Figure 9-3). If nurses would take the ball and run with it, there are incredible changes that could be made in health care. The American Nurses Association works with congressional leaders and all federal representatives to write laws that will help patient care. They lobby the powerbrokers most responsible for issues concerning the

Figure 9-3
One out of every
44 female voters
is a nurse.

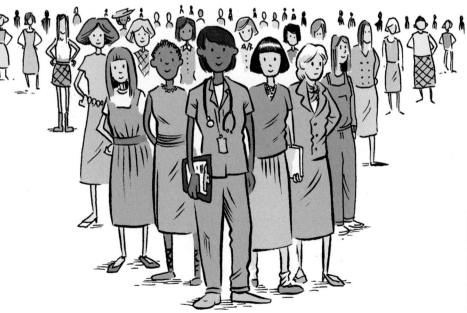

profession and their patients. Laws are often very general and lack the specific language that details how the legislation will be implemented. Federal agencies are then charged with writing the rules and regulations that make the general law specific. It is at this point that groups like the ANA have tremendous impact.

There is power in the number of registered nurses in this country. When nurses become involved with a professional nursing association, they set the agenda for the activities and are able to advocate for the things in which nurses believe. By being involved in professional nursing groups, these nurses learn skills to advocate for their group when they meet the power brokers. It is by this involvement that nurses help make the decisions that will affect practice for years to come.

The American Nurses Association represents all nurses. Almost every group of nurses has a professional group organized around an area of practice or interest, that advocate especially for practice issues. Nurses can be involved in writing bills about these issues. Health legislation is a big priority in the state capitols and the Congress every year. Nurses need to find a topic that is important to them and make their voices heard on it if they want to protect their care and the public at large.

While qualified nurses may belong to the ANA, many students join the National Student Nurses Association (NSNA), which has a membership of over 45,000. Students from across the country can become involved in the National Student Nurses' Association. Some schools and universities have a stronger presence than others in this organization. The NSNA provides leadership opportunities and career guidance through mentoring the professional development of future nurses and facilitating their entrance into the profession by providing educational resources (NSNA, 2007). The NSNA meets as a national organization twice a year; the student leaders meet in the fall for leadership training and hold a convention in the spring.

This student-run organization holds an annual convention at which resolutions are passed. Resolutions are documents that are written to further enhance the goals of the organization and to bring ideas for action to its members. Many of these resolutions deal with practice and professional issues. These resolutions are shared with other national groups and have an impact on legislators as they grapple with health concerns (Mason, Leavitt, & Chafee, 2007).

Over the past several years the NSNA has joined with other health care organizations to discuss ways in which they can impact the nursing shortage and clinical practice issues. Some student leaders represented the organization in 2007 at the International Congress of Nurses in Japan. Student leaders come to these national meetings and have the opportunity to interact with leaders in nursing about whom they may have read. The meetings showcase nursing leaders, and these leaders give speeches regarding many ideas and changes in the field. The students often have an opportunity to interact with the leaders after meetings and in small focus sessions. Students often find that their involvement with the NSNA makes them much more aware of how to use parliamentary procedure. They begin to understand that correct utilization of these rules is a way of organizing meetings and keeping a meeting on schedule. They see that it is a way of functioning so that everyone may have his or her opinions heard. These students have an opportunity to practice these skills in meetings with students from all over the country. Students may find themselves speaking and giving their opinion to over a thousand other students at one time.

Students begin talking with other students from around the country and realize that the problems that they are seeing in the facilities in which they work are just a microcosm of concerns in health care. These students often return to their home schools with an appreciation of the broader world of nursing. Many students consider the high point of their involvement with NSNA to be the chance to get to know their faculty on a more individual basis. They often look up to these faculty as mentors, who in turn follow the students' careers with interest and are often called upon for advice as the newer nurses rise in the profession.

Many students who become involved with the NSNA continue utilizing the skills they have learned when they become registered nurses. Students who join NSNA often go on to become members of the American Nurses Association and specialty nursing practice groups. Many of these groups are called upon by the regulatory agencies in the states to provide expert witnesses for practice issues. Other nursing leaders from these organizations may serve on regulatory bodies and decide issues that directly impact the nursing profession.

Internet Exercise 9-3	Go to the National Student Nurses Association Web site at http://www.nsna.org.

Review information regarding resolutions.

1. Identify one resolution that deals with a clinical practice area that you are working in or have recently worked in.

2. Explain how this resolution could assist in dealing with a concern for patients.

Those nurses who are active in their professional organizations are often the ones who are asked to testify when a bill is being heard at the state legislature. Many times these groups have difficulties finding nurses who are able to testify due to time and other constraints. Having a large organization from which to identify a nurse with expertise in a certain field makes for stronger legislation that is more clearly focused on high-quality patient care. Nurses from these state organizations are often the ones asked to testify regarding bills and to sit on boards that deal with new regulations that impact practice.

Nursing organizations often have the financial resources to hire a paid lobbyist whose job it is to track legislation that is important to nursing. Membership in nursing organizations usually entails a financial commitment. Part of the dues goes to this endeavor. Consequently, if a nurse or a student nurse cannot find the time to be active, they are able to participate by paying their membership dues, which will in turn fund the activities of a lobbyist. Therefore, just by being dues-paying members of a nursing organization, nurses may impact policy with their membership dues.

It is imperative for nurses and nursing students to remember that the way nurses are allowed to practice is often decided by those who have no idea about nursing and know very little about health care. Participation in the process can and does change that. Those at the table decide the practice. If nurses want to be the ones who determine their own practice, then they must make the effort and learn the skills to be at the table.

LEARNING THE LEGISLATIVE PROCESS

Many groups hold classes to explain to people how to become involved in politics. The League of Women Voters is one such nonpartisan group. The League's Web site explains that it "is a nonpartisan political organization, which has fought since 1920 to improve our systems of government and impact public policies through citizen education and advocacy…The League of Women Voters is strictly nonpartisan; it neither supports nor opposes candidates for office at any level of government. At the same time, the League is wholeheartedly political and works to influence policy through advocacy" (LWV, 2007). Many other nonpartisan groups, including the National Parent-Teacher Association, explain to their members in detail how to lobby their legislators.

Some colleges and universities will also hold classes to explain the legislative process to their students. Individual faculty may be committed to teaching about health care policy and students can learn from their advice and involvement (Gebbie, 2000). Many of these faculty will also model techniques on how to work with legislators. Some will encourage students to join them while they lobby legislators in their home offices or in their district offices and in the state and national capitols (Waldron, 2003).

Nurses need to learn who the appropriate official is for the problem they are seeking to remedy (Figure 9-4). It is counter productive when the wrong person or agency is contacted to resolve an issue. U.S. Senators deal with federal legislation that, for example, makes money available to help deal with the nursing shortage. They would not be the correct officials from whom to request a stop sign near a community clinic or a cross walk for that area. This is a situation that would be covered by a council member or city manager. Accessing the correct office or individual saves everyone's time and lends credibility to the person asking for assistance.

Nurses also need to know the correct period in which to ask for help. The time to ask about sidewalks in front of the hospital is early in the budget hearing process. It is not correct to ask for

Figure 9-4

Learning whom to contact and when to contact them is an important part of understanding the legislative process.

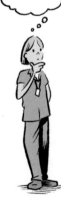

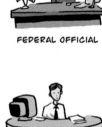
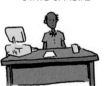
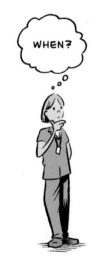

WHO?

FEDERAL OFFICIAL

STATE OFFICIAL

LOCAL OFFICIAL

WHEN?

DELMAR/CENGAGE LEARNING

sidewalks when the budget is being voted upon. Asking at the wrong time also is counter productive as it wastes everyone's time and may make officials annoyed that their time and efforts are being wasted. Often questions on timing and appropriateness can be answered by making a simple phone call to a public official's office.

Many state nursing organizations hold an annual day or night in their state capitols at which time they interface with lawmakers. Frequently, nursing students join these groups and are involved with the registered nurses meeting their legislators and explaining to them how their actions affect the management of health care and patient care. Nursing students are usually very welcome in these groups as they are looked upon as the future of the profession.

Networking to Influence Legislation

Once one has an understanding of the legislative process, one may want to know how to connect with as many people as possible to help spread the word or to help persuade legislators to consider and act upon a particular concern. By reaching out to those who share the same concerns but who may not act on them or know the legislative process themselves, nurses can create their own network of people who, working together, have a stronger voice. Nurses who utilize networking often have a better chance of having legislation passed than those who do not, simply because many more people are involved through networking. It is also helpful for nurses to know their legislators personally. A familiar name will be recognized as a known entity, while an unknown name may register nothing and be ignored. Legislators will listen most to their own constituents because they vote for them (Cardoni, 2004). Imagine the power of a network of such constituents!

Networking is accomplished by introducing oneself to a legislator and talking with him/her about a variety of topics. One way to do this is by offering to assist a legislator with health issues. Legislators often rely on others for information about a specialty area such as business or health care. Nurses can engage legislators when they are present at their work sites or at church or social events. Networking is a way for people to expand their own knowledge base. Nurses can become invaluable to legislators when they are open, genuine, and willing to share their knowledge. They can offer to work on a committee for a legislator and exchange ideas (Mason, Leavitt, & Chafee, 2007).

When a legislator personally knows someone who comes forward with opinions regarding pending legislation, he or she is more likely to seriously consider voting for the legislation that the person thinks is important when it deals with practice issues. This is an example of networking (Mason, Leavitt, & Chafee, 2007). It is also a reason to step forward and become involved politically.

Nurses need to remember very practical suggestions when they are networking. First, they need to introduce themselves as nurses. They also need to carry business cards with them and give them to the legislators or staff members. It would help if nurses got into the habit of calling their legislators and leaving their names and phone numbers. As a courtesy, but also as a networking strategy, nurses need to be sure that they call a government official back promptly when they receive a phone call. If a nurse has agreed to do research or find a legislator an expert in a specific field, the nurse needs to be sure to follow up on the assignment and get back to

CASE SCENARIO 9-1

There was a piece of legislation pending that the nursing community was interested in getting passed. Nursing leaders put out action alerts to motivate fellow nurses to advocate for the legislation. One registered nurse knew that her own delegate and state senator were in favor of the bill because they were co-sponsors of the legislation. She first called her own legislators and left her name with their staff members, thanking them for their support in co-sponsoring the bill, and said that she was so pleased that they would be voting for the bill. She then called the rest of the members of her county delegation and talked with their staff members. She left her name and asked that they let the senator or delegate know that she had called and was very interested in this legislation and would like the legislator to vote for it. She explained to each of the legislator's assistants that though she didn't live in that member's district but was very active in the community and would be very appreciative of the vote of the legislator. She had been president of both the county PTA council and the League of Women Voters in the county, so knew all the members of the county-wide district, and they knew her. The legislation eventually did pass.

Several weeks later she happened to run into one of the legislators who mentioned to her that he had received her phone call. He commented that he had not voted for the legislation when it was before him in his committee. However, when he received her call, he said that he looked at the legislation again and could find nothing objectionable in it. He said that he reasoned that the nurse who called knew about nursing and had taken the time to call him to say it was a good bill. Because he knew and respected her and her nursing knowledge, he decided to change his vote and vote for the legislation after all.

CASE ANALYSIS

1. Identify how the nurse networked in this example.

2. What made the difference to the legislator and affected his vote?

3. How would you have improved on this interaction?

the legislator with a phone call or e-mail with the information or a reason why the information is delayed. Good communication is of paramount importance and will enhance a nurse's credibility. It is imperative here as elsewhere that the credibility of nursing is always upheld.

Applying the Nursing Process to Influence Legislation

Most nursing students learn the tenets of the nursing process from their early days in nursing school. This is a good model for use when dealing with the legislative process. The steps in the nursing process as defined by the American Nurses Association Standards of Clinical Practice (1998) rely on the application of the nursing process, which are assessment, diagnosis, planning, implementation, and evaluation. Nursing students learn to assess when they discover a problem with the health care system. They collect data about the situation in an organized way. They begin to ask questions and to establish if there is really a problem or if they perceive something that is not necessarily true (Hood & Leddy, 2003). These skills can continue to be utilized when the students become registered nurses and are a good basis for working on many situations in the legislative arena. Nurses need to utilize their resources as professionals as well as the organizational and listening skills they have learned and continue to refine as professionals. Nursing students and professional nurses can learn to utilize data they collect and can organize the data objectively and in a focused way that will address a health concern. This identification of a problem is often called a diagnosis (Hood & Leddy, 2003).

Once there is a diagnosis, nurses and nursing students need to decide the best way to remedy the situation. They may be able to make a phone call and discuss the information that they have with a public official. The problem may have already been identified and a solution may be in place or in process. Informal discussions will often lead the way to quick resolution of a problem. If it is discovered that the problem has not been identified previously or has not had any attention paid to it, then a student or nurse may want to develop a plan to remedy the situation. It is at this point that the student or registered nurse needs to involve others in the profession in their consultations. It is often good to brainstorm a problem with others and for a variety of interventions to be selected that may resolve the problem. Goal setting at this point is important (Hood & Leddy, 2003).

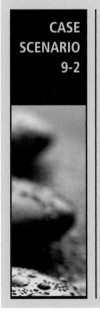

CASE SCENARIO 9-2

Every semester the maternity nursing students at this particular university are assigned one day in an out-patient facility as an enrichment activity. One student came back to the clinical area after her experience and reported on her day to her instructor. She felt that the care that the patients had received in the county health department was exceptional. However, she expressed concern that the clients who attended the clinic by bus had to get to the agency by taking a long walk once the county bus let them off. The clinic was about a half-mile walk from a major bus terminal. This was proving problematic for mothers-to-be who were in the later stages of pregnancy and for those who may have had another child in tow. The instructor knew the county well and expressed surprise that there was not a bus stop closer to the clinic.

CASE ANALYSIS

1. How would the instructor and the student work on this problem and help the patients to access bus service that would be more advantageous for the patients as they went to the clinic?

2. Who is impacted by the lack of a bus stop?

3. What public officials could be identified and contacted to remedy the problem?

Implementation occurs in the action phase. A decision for a plan is made. The plan is set in motion. The plan itemizes in priority those actions that will most likely bring results. The plan with the most probability of success will be the first action that is undertaken. The plan may include making phone calls, setting up an appointment with a legislator or a staff member, and may include testifying before a committee.

Once the plan has been implemented the nurses need to collect more data. Data collection is imperative because that is the only way one can know what happened when the plan was implemented. Once the data is collected, it is helpful for those nurses who have been involved in the situation to get together and to discuss what they have learned. The nurses need to share the collected information and to discuss the results. At this point the nurses can decide what part of the plan worked and what did not. This is known as evaluation. It is at this point that a new plan may be developed (Figure 9-5).

Other Methods of Using the Nursing Process to Affect Change

There are many other ways in which a nurse can work with public officials and impact legislation and regulation (Figure 9-6). It is helpful to keep in mind the nursing process and the steps of assessment, diagnosis, planning, implementation, and evaluation. Utilizing good communication skills during this process is vital to success.

Figure 9-5

Nurses can apply the nursing process to political issues.

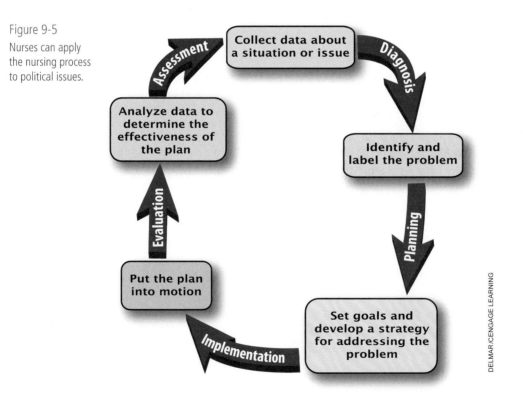

DELMAR/CENGAGE LEARNING

Figure 9-6
There are multiple
ways to work with
public officials.

	Pros	Cons
Telephone Calls	Efficient	Any messages left may not be received
Personal Visits	Helps establish a relationship with the legislator	Can be rushed if held during the busy legislative session
Letter Writing	More effective than phone calls or emails	Form letters are usually disregarded
Attending Meetings	Can see first-hand how the legislative process works	May involve scheduling conflicts
Testifying at Meetings	Nurses are highly-regarded speakers	The process can be intimidating
Using the Internet	Efficient	Older nurses may not be proficient with computers
Electioneering	Helps establish a relationship with the legislator	Time consuming
Running for Office	Potential to influence health care significantly for years to come	Requires substantial time and resources

DELMAR/CENGAGE LEARNING

Telephone Calls

Phone calls regarding bills are counted for the purpose of informing legislators how their constituents feel about an issue. Callers may just need to state their name and their support or nonsupport for a bill. The problem with phone calls is that the message may not be delivered correctly, and the caller has no actual record of the call. It is often good to keep a phone log of the date and time of the call that can be referenced for additional calls. It is important for the nurse to know who they have spoken to every time an office is called. That way they will be able to speak to that person again or refer to the information that was gleaned from them (Mason, Leavitt, & Chafee, 2007).

Personal Visits

It is extremely helpful if a nurse has developed a personal relationship with a legislator prior to there being an issue important to nursing. When nurses have an ongoing relationship with politicians, they can speak to them about issues often without going through staff people. The credibility of the nurse is already established and they have access.

Nurses and nursing students can make appointments with their legislators to discuss issues. These visits are usually more helpful if they are held at the legislator's home office prior to the start of a busy legislative session. Always dress and act in a professional manner. Be sure that the agenda is well known and that a specific time limit is adhered to. It is very helpful to have written material to leave with the legislator or their staff members. A follow-up with a thank-you note always leaves a positive impression, even if the legislator was not convinced of the correctness of the nursing position (Mason, Leavitt, & Chafee, 2007).

Many states' nursing organizations sponsor a lobby time for nurses at their state capitol during the legislative sessions. This is often the first experience in which many nurses are exposed to the legislative process. Students and practicing registered nurses are briefed by nursing leaders on the current issues before the legislature. Legislators meet with the attendees in both formal meetings and during receptions for an exchange of views. This is often the first step in continuous involvement by nurses in the political process (Cardoni, 2004).

Internet Exercise 9-4

Go to the Web site for your local government.

1. Find out who your local delegate, representative, or assembly person is.
2. Discover on which committees they serve.
3. Find one piece of legislation they have sponsored that pertains to health care or policy.
4. Explain to the class how this legislation will help or harm nursing.

Letter Writing

Legislators are very impressed by hand-written letters that are from their constituents. Letters need to be legible and need to be addressed to the legislator with the correct title. They may be typed as long as the information is unique and not a form letter that can be mass-produced. Arguments for or against a bill should be well-reasoned. Letters tend to have more impact on legislators than phone calls or e-mails. Form letters are not useful. E-mails are becoming more widely used to set up meetings or to make a quick point. E-mails that are sent out en-mass are usually disregarded.

Again, be sure that contact information is included in all letters (Mason, Leavitt, & Chafee, 2007). Be sure to give facts as well as anecdotes. Explain why this is an important issue to the legislator's constituents. When referring to an exact bill, it is helpful to use the bill number. Explain exactly what action the legislator is requested to take (Hood & Leddy, 2003). Utilizing all academic credentials has an impact on the legislators and shows that the writer has academic qualifications and an area of expertise. Letters should be limited to no more than two pages and bulleting is helpful. Be precise and succinct in your writing and mindful of using correct grammar.

> **Writing Exercise 9-2**
>
> Write a one-page letter to your legislator discussing the bill that you identified on the Internet and give your opinion on this legislation. Follow suggestions given above.

Attending Meetings

Nurses need to attend meetings to see in person how the legislative process works. One can read about meetings and watch meetings on television, but in person one is able to grasp a more complete idea of what is really happening. Most states and county agencies hold open meetings, and the public is invited to attend and to see their government in action. It is by attending a series of meetings on a topic that nurses will begin to understand who the players are on both sides of an issue and what the opinions of each side are. Often a nurse will be able to speak to the principals on both sides after the meetings. This is when it is essential for a nurse to have business cards in order to obtain the cards of the other interested attendees. Dressing professionally helps as well.

Nurses will learn the ground rules of testifying by attending multiple meetings. Those people testifying may be allowed to read the written testimony or they may be told that they can only give a piece of the material. It is a good idea to have notes when testifying in order to make points, keep organized, and stay within a time frame. Many find it helpful to practice their testimony before a colleague or a family member, or at least a mirror. It is always important for someone who is testifying to submit information in writing. That way the legislators will be able to refer to the material and to glean more information about a topic. There may be a time limit for each person to speak, and this may or may not be enforced with great rigidity. Each agency is different, and it is by sitting in the audience that an astute nurse can pick up this information. These guidelines are a matter of public record, and they may be found online or by a phone call to the agency.

Testifying at Meetings

Testifying before a government agency or a legislative body may seem daunting at first. Government officials usually encourage citizen participation and will most likely be quite kind to someone who they can tell is testifying for only the first or second time. As with any activity, testifying becomes easier with continued practice.

The Gallup Poll, as recently as December 2006, again discovered that nurses are the most highly respected of all the professions. Eighty-four percent of those polled rated nurses highest in the values of honesty and ethical standards among all professionals, including pharmacists, veterinarians, and physicians. Consequently, when nurses testify, they are often listened to by the powerbrokers. Nurses need to be heard. Legislators and others like nurses!! Nurses and nursing students have statistics and anecdotal information. It is imperative to use both in testimony. Research-driven data is an absolute necessity in testimony. What nurses then need to do is to put a face on the statistics by using anecdotes. Anecdotes are like war stories. These are the actual stories about the patients that nurses have cared for and about what has happened that has changed their lives. Statistics are facts; anecdotes change minds.

One legislator felt that having family leave was an unnecessary mandate for a business. However, when his wife became ill after the birth of their first child, he understood the necessity of such an act. His employer was upset that he needed to take time off to care for his wife and child, and he realized that if he had had the option of family leave, he would not have been concerned about his job. He was aware of the facts and had made one determination, but when the situation became real to him, he was able to come to a different conclusion. Statistics tell part of the story. Anecdotes, especially personal anecdotes, touch the heart.

Nurses can give compelling testimony that is both fact driven and a clear example of how circumstances affect patient care. These can change the minds of legislators. Try and find a hook or a sound bite that people will remember. Often nurses and other health providers testify wearing scrubs or with a stethoscope around their necks. Otherwise, dress in a business suit or other professional attire. Wearing a white lab coat over clothes is often eye-catching. Use whatever makes an impression. Nurses just need to take the opportunity to deliver the testimony. Be sure to have copies of your testimony in writing for each member of the committee and hand it to the clerk or chairperson. Having copies for the press is often helpful for everyone concerned.

Electioneering

Electioneering means helping someone run for office. This may not be everyone's choice, but legislators remember those who gave them help in a campaign and will be in their debt. It will give you access and a friendly ear when you have a problem. A nurse may contribute time and/or money as both are needed by candidates (Mason, Leavitt, & Chafee, 2007).

Running for Office

There are many more nurses and other health professionals running and being elected to political office today than in the past. Running for office is an exciting, exhausting, and exhilarating experience. Nurses are well liked, usually organized, and know a lot of people in a community. Nurses are considered very honest and believed to be in a political race for the greater good. They make good candidates. Nurses, however, need to be able to find the time, the staff, and the financial resources to run for office. It takes a tremendous amount of time and commitment, as well as shoe leather, as one may want to walk to voters' homes and discuss the issues directly with them. Not everyone can be elected, but nurses who choose to run for office will learn a lot about themselves, their families, their communities, and the strengths and weaknesses that they possess. They will also learn who their friends are. They will learn that the sun will come up the next day, even if they are not elected, and that they can be role models for other nurses to follow. Being elected to political office is well worth the time and energy and is the way nurses can make the most dramatic and long-term decisions that will affect health care for years to come.

COMMUNICATIONS

One of the most important skills learned as nursing students is the ability to communicate. Nurses need to be able to ask important questions, listen keenly to answers given, and assess whether or not the material given is pertinent or complete. Then they must understand their audience, be very clear about the information they need to impart, explain it clearly enough to be understood, and be ready to answer any questions asked of them. These skills are excellent tools to help nurses when they speak publicly about issues that concern them.

Dealing with the Media

Dealing with the press is similar to working with patients, their families, or elected officials. Nurses can utilize the same skills of organization, networking, and research when talking with the press as they sometimes do with patients or politicians. It is imperative that facts are correct and checked before they are given to the press. It is helpful to have enough copies of testimony for each public official when testifying at a meeting, and additional copies for the press with correct contact information included. Nurses who are the president of an organization or the designated spokesperson for the group should be the only ones delegated to speak with the press. Other nurses and students should refer any and all questions from the media to them.

Nurses may decide when they want to speak to the press, and they may want to do this when they are not stressed and can think about their words. Words said in haste can be detrimental to a cause when printed in a newspaper. Few people read a correction made a couple of days after the quote. The print press may call for a quote when they are on deadline. This means that what the reporter is working on is going to press almost immediately. It is up to the nurse whether he/she wants to respond, and sometimes it is better not to do so if the timing does not feel right. It is usually better not to speak to a member of the press "off the record," as there is no guarantee that the words will not be quoted. When a nurse establishes a long-term relationship with a reporter, the nurse may be willing to give background if there is a level of trust that has been built between the two. This needs to be done cautiously and very judiciously and is not a technique that is useful for the neophyte.

Radio shows are a good way of getting one's point across, but it is imperative to be prepared for this media as much as for any other. Questions on the telephone or from the host may come as a surprise, and it is a good idea to know both sides of the argument and who else will be on the show. It is also wise to ask for a list of questions in advance in order to be prepared. This is a good time to interact with the experts so that all the information will be current and accurate.

Television is the fastest way to expose a point about an issue and may be widely viewed. Again, it is imperative to be well prepared, to choose one's words extremely carefully, and to say enough to get the point across without becoming flustered. It is helpful to come up with a few sound bites that capture the essential elements of any argument. This is another situation when looking professional or wearing scrubs is eye-catching and makes a point. It is often a good idea to practice presentation style and wording with trusted colleagues prior to speaking with the press.

Public Speaking

Many people seem to be afraid to speak in public. Like any skill, from inserting catheters to starting an intravenous line, public speaking is an art that takes practice. When speaking in public for the first few times, it is important to have some notes to refer to in case of trouble remembering what to say. Index cards with bullet notes are a good way of keeping one's place and making sure that all points are covered. It is not wise to tell a group that one is nervous. Nurses tend to be very warm and need to show that to their audience. Establish yourself as a human being and as a person by explaining who you are and why you are testifying. Often a committee chairperson will ask those testifying to give their name and their address. This is a good time to mention that you are a nurse and that you are testifying as a nurse expert or a student nurse concerned about an issue. Be yourself. Don't put on airs or pretend that you have more credentials than you possess.

Nurses are on the front lines of health care. They need to talk about their patients while being careful to observe HIPPA regulations. One must never identify a patient by name and must couch comments about patients with care so as not to identify a particular patient. Nurses may choose to verbally draw the legislators a picture of the sites in which they are working or may have actual pictures of the area. Make the legislators understand what it is like to go to work every day. Use examples of good care or problems in the settings. Everyone enjoys a quick story, and it is a way of explaining a point.

Be sure information is current. Health care changes quickly, so it is imperative that the research and the information be up-to-date. Use anecdotes throughout the speech. Use visual aides as long as they do not take away from the message. Using emotion is fine as long as it is controllable. It is fine to show passion for a topic as long as the nurse is rational. Showing emotion validates for the listener that the speaker is human. Be organized and never apologize. If a person is organized, it will help make the points clear and concise. Nurses need to be sure that they are conversing with their audience and not talking at them, as most people react negatively to being talked at or down to. Begin with confidence and end strong. The audience will remember what you said at the end of your speech. As with any skill, public speaking takes practice, practice, practice. It is often good to give a speech to a small group of trusted colleagues or a significant other (Mason, Leavitt, & Chafee, 2007). Teenage children may not be the best judge of the skill, but they may be quite creative when thinking of a special way to make a speech memorable.

RUDIMENTARY PARLIAMENTARY PROCEDURE

Nurses interested in political activity need to have a working knowledge of parliamentary procedure. Some of the terms with which a nurse will first become familiar when dealing with parliamentary procedure are *agenda, motion, quorum*, and *debate*. As with any activity, parliamentary procedure is a skill that can be learned. It is helpful to have the latest copy of Robert's Rules of Parliamentary Procedure (2000) and to read and study this book. Many questions about these rules are also answered online. While using parliamentary procedure initially may seem a bit confusing, it is a good way of keeping an organization running smoothly and of making sure that the rights of all will be preserved.

Well-run meetings will have an agenda and a time period. Meetings should be started and ended at the designated times. A meeting can be continued for a certain time period if there is a motion made to extend the meeting and if the approval of the group is given to continue. An agenda has the items to be covered in bullet form and may often have a time period for each item. There will be discussion and motions made, which will move the business of the organization along.

Nurses need to use the appropriate language of making a motion, which is "I move …" and then add whatever the suggestion is. This should be done with a few words so as to identify the problem. When a motion is made, the maker of the motion then stops and waits for the chairperson to repeat the motion and ask for a second to the motion. It is often a good idea for the maker of the motion to line up someone who thinks the same way to second the motion. After that the maker of the motion asks permission to speak to the motion. It is at this time that the rationale for the motion can be given. Debate may continue for a while, and the chairperson has the right to restrict people speaking on an issue to a certain number of times. It is usually up to the chairperson to decide when the debate has run its course. The motion is then repeated by the chairperson or the secretary and the vote is taken. In order for a vote to be taken, there must be a quorum. Quorum is the term given to the number of people required to be present in order to vote on a motion. Usually a quorum is considered to be one more than half of those who are eligible to vote. Majority rules in this situation. An astute nurse or nursing student will not debate an issue unless there are enough supporters for the proposal in the room.

The chairperson or presiding officer may state that there is a quorum by just looking out over the group. If challenged, it is possible for a quorum count to be taken to be sure that the people who are present are members of the body and allowed to vote. Asking for a quorum count is a procedural issue called a point of order. If there is no quorum, then no vote can be taken. Also, if a significant number of those who are allowed to vote choose not to, then the vote can also fail due to lack of a quorum. This can only be used when an actual count of those present and voting is taken.

When a motion is controversial, it is a good idea to have discussed the idea outside of the meeting with supporters. It is helpful to have an idea how a vote will go before it is taken. Using correct parliamentary procedure can move along the agenda of an astute nurse (Mason, Leavitt, & Chafee, 2007).

CONCLUDING THOUGHTS

Determined people can make changes for good or ill. Nurses must become aware that the power to improve their working conditions is in their hands. They can directly impact the care of patients by being involved in legislation and politics. Those in the seats of power around the table are those who make the change. If those in nursing are not in the role of policymakers and in the seats of power, then they will always be forced to stand behind the chairs. If nurses refuse to become involved, then behind the chairs is exactly where they deserve to be.

SUMMARY

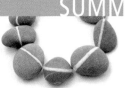

This chapter delineates reasons why nursing students and nurses need to be involved in political activity. Terms utilized in the political process are explained. The importance of one person, such as a nurse or nursing student willing to face issues he or she sees in the field, and willing to become involved in the establishment of policy and law, is explained. Several pieces of legislation that have impacted nursing care and the lives of nurses as providers and individual citizens have been discussed. Some of the ways that students and registered nurses can impact the political process are explained, along with several terms utilized in parliamentary procedure. Tips are given on how nurses might speak at public meetings and how to deal with a variety of media. All of this information is provided to focus attention on the pivotal role nurses and nursing students can have politically on the work they do and the care they provide as members of a proud and important profession.

Man is by nature a political animal.

–Aristotle

REFERENCES

Aiken, L. H., Clarke, S. P., Sloane, D. M., Sochalski, J., & Silber, J. H. (2002). Hospital nurse staffing and patient mortality, nurse burnout, and job dissatisfaction. *The Journal of the American Medical Association, 288*(16), 1987–1993.

Aiken, L. H., Clarke, S. P., Cheung, R. B., Sloane, D. M., & Silber, J. H. (2003). Educational levels of hospital nurses and surgical patient mortality. *The Journal of the American Medical Association, 290*(12), 1617–1623.

The American Nurses Association, Inc. (1998). American Nurses Association — Home. Retrieved March 14, 2008, from http://nursingworld.org

Brannan, R. (2000). Unfair trade practices: prohibit discrimination against victims of family violence in insurance coverage, rates, and claims. *Georgia State University Law Review, 17*(1). Retrieved July 29, 2008, from http://law.gsu.edu/lawreview/index/archives/show/?art=17-1/17-1_Insurance_Brannan.htm

CARDONI, K. (2004). MD nurses being heard. *Advance for Nurses, 6*(6), 15.

CROFTON, J. (1977). John Crofton (1912–). The James Lind Library. Retrieved July 29, 2008, from http://www.jameslindlibrary.org

DONAHUE, M. P. (1996). *Nursing the finest art: An illustrated history* (2nd ed.). St. Louis, MO: Mosby.

GALLUP POLL. 2006. *Nurses top list of most honest and ethical professions.* Retrieved April 13, 2009, from http://www.gallup.com/poll/25888/Nurses-Top-Most-Honest-Ethical-Professions.aspx

GEBBIE, K., Wakefield, M., & Kerfoot, K. (2000). Nursing and health policy. *Journal of Nursing Scholarship, 32*(3), 307–315.

GEHRKE, P. (2008). Civic engagement and nursing education. *Advances in Nursing Science, 31*(1), 52–66.

GETTYSBURG ADDRESS. (2009). In *Encyclopaedia Britannica.* Retrieved April 13, 2009, from http://www.britannica.com/EBcheeked/topic/232225/Gettysburg-Address

HOOD, L. J., & Leddy, S. J. (2003). *Conceptual bases of professional nursing* (5th ed.). Philadelphia: Lippincott Williams & Wilkins.

INTERNATIONAL COUNCIL OF NURSES. (2004). *Position statements (revised 2004) [scope of nursing practice].* Retrieved March 14, 2008, from http://www.icn.ch/psscope.htm

HOWARD COUNTY GOVERNMENT. (2008). *Information for Howard County Taxpayers,* Howard County, MD.

JOSSI, K. (1997). Diabetes educator influences lawmakers. *Nursing Spectrum, 7*(15).

LEAGUE OF WOMEN VOTERS. (2007). *About us.* Retrieved March 14, 2008, from http://www.lwv.org/AM/Template.cfm?Section=About_Us

MASON, D., Leavitt, J., & Chafee, M. W. (2007). *Policy and politics in nursing and health care* (5th ed.). Philadelphia: Elsevier.

MOONEY, B. (2004). Needlestick protection. *Advance for Nurses, 6*(2), 35–36.

MORRISON, H., Bagalio, S. (2004). Being a good Samaritan. *Advance for Nurses, 6*(21), 19–20.

NATIONAL COUNCIL OF STATE BOARDS OF NURSING, INC. (2007). *Nurse Practice Act.* Retrieved March 14, 2008, from http://www.nursing.about.com/od/glossary/g/nursepracticeac.htm

"MEETINGS." National Student Nurses' Association. (2008). Retrieved March 14, 2008, from http://www.nsna.org/meetings

NEEDLEMAN, J., Buerhaus, P., Mattke, S., Stewart, M., & Zelevinsky, K. (2002). Nurse-staffing levels and the quality of care in hospitals. *The New England Journal of Medicine, 346,* 1715–1722.

PEW RESEARCH CENTER FOR THE PEOPLE AND THE PRESS. (2007). Public knowledge of current affairs little changes by news and information revolutions. *What Americans Know: 1989–2007.* Washington, D.C.

ROBERT, H. M. (2000). *Robert's Rules of Order Newly Revised.* Reading, MA: Addison-Wesley.

SKIRBLE, ROSANNE. (2006). *Madd founder Candice Lightner: Grassroots activist turns personal tragedy into national movement.* Retrieved April 13, 2009, from http://dui.com/dui-library/victims/personal-tragedy

"TERRY SCHIAVO DIES, BUT BATTLE CONTINUES." (2005, March 31). *MSNBC,* Retrieved April 13, 2009, from http://www.msnbc.msn.com/id/7293186

"ELECTION 2000." USNews.Com. 2000. Retrieved March 14, 2008, from http://www.usnews.com/usnews/news/election/home.htm

VON BISMARCK, O. (1867). Remark on August 11. Retrieved March 14, 2008, from http://www.quotationspage.com/quote/24903.html

WALDRON, T. (2003). Nurses vote! *Johns Hopkins Nursing,* 1(2).

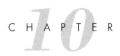

C H A P T E R

10

THE FINANCIAL HEALTH CARE ENVIRONMENT

AILEEN WEHREN

Ed.D., Vice President Systems Administration, Porter-Starke Services, Inc.

MARY JO REGAN-KUBINSKI

PhD, RN, Dean Division of Nursing and Health Professions, Indiana University South Bend

…the majority of care averts death, pain, and erosion of functional health status. However we must be careful not to discount quality or access in the name of economic efficiency. There is a delicate balance to maintain between health care as a social good and health care as a consumer good.

–Steven R. Eastaugh

LEARNING OBJECTIVES

At the completion of the chapter, the learner should be able to do the following:

1. Identify the financial sources of support for health care.
2. Discuss the context of health care in the economy as a whole.
3. Have working knowledge of key terms regarding health care financing.
4. Discuss public policy implications of health care financing.
5. Articulate current trends in health care and their potential impact on the nursing profession.

KEY TERMS

Bundled Charges
Capitation
Care Management
Centers for Medicare and
   Medicaid Services (CMS)
Charity Care
Clayton Act
Consumer Directed Health
   Plan (CDHP)
Coinsurance
Co-pay

Diagnostic Related
   Group (DRG)
Disease Management
Dsproportionate Share
Emergency Medical
   Treatment and
   Active Labor Act
Employer Sponsored
   Insurance (ESI)
False Claims Act
Fee for Service
Fiscal Intermediary

Gross National
   Product (GNP)
Health Insurance Portability
   and Accountability
   Act (HIPAA)
Health Literacy
Health Reimbursement
   Accounts (HRAs)
Health Savings
   Accounts (HSAs)
Joint Ventures
Managed Care

Pay for Performance
Price Transparency
Prospective Payment
    System (PPS)
Regional Health Information
    Organization (RHIO)

Resource-Based Relative
    Value Scale (RBRVS)
Self-Insured Plans
Sherman Anti-Trust Act
Specialty Hospital
Stark

Third Party Administrator
    (TPA)
Tiered Health Plans
Usual and Customary

INTRODUCTION

Health care finance is often thought of as the business of paying for health care and of the earning of income from the delivery of that care. That is much too restrictive a definition. To consider health care finance thoroughly it is necessary to examine not just the methods of paying for care. It is critical to examine factors that influence the cost of health care, including factors that may be considered more "social" in nature. An example is disease management, the process of proactively engaging patients in their own care in such a manner as to decrease the long-term cost of the care of that individual while also improving the outcome of that care. In this chapter some factors that are clearly more financial in tone will be reviewed. Trends that appear more social, but because of their impact on the health of the individual have longer-term cost implications, are also examined. It is more difficult for nurses to have an immediate influence on the more financial factors. There are more opportunities to participate in activities that improve community or individual health, thus influencing cost. Improved patient education so there is greater adherence to medication regimens is a good example of how nursing can influence long-term cost in the health care environment. Your challenge is to determine those opportunities, opportunities that may occur at the management and/or at the delivery level.

DEFINITIONS AND TERMS RELATED TO HEALTH CARE FINANCING

Health care is an industry that is full of specialized terminology and acronyms. Such language facilitates communication within the field but limits it with others that are not knowledgeable about the "shorthand" that such language use implies. To understand the business of health care and to read within the literature of the field requires an understanding of that terminology. Some key terms related to health care financing and the insurance industry follow.

Bundled Charges: Charges for health care services are discrete. For instance in a hospital environment, each service delivered, whether it is an x-ray or a pill, will result in a charge. Payment to the health care provider, however, is often bundled. Instead of paying for these discrete charges, insurance (particularly managed care) negotiates to pay for service on a "bundled" basis. They may pay a specific "per diem" amount that effectively ignores those individual charges. The incentive to the provider is to deliver only that amount of care absolutely necessary to treat the patient, keeping the cost of that health care down.

Capitation: Capitation is a payment system whereby a provider is paid a specified (contractual) amount of money to meet the health care needs as defined in a written contract for members of the health care plan. The payments are typically paid on a monthly basis for the number of "covered lives" in the plan. The calculations are complex as each party to this agreement is working to manage a combination of capital outlay and risk. The insurance company is trying to pay the least amount per member and the provider is trying to determine risk and ensure that the level of care provided will not exceed the amount of money paid. Ideally, from the perspective of a provider, they will make a profit. This system of payment shifts substantial risk to the provider of care, particularly if the patient population is sicker than anticipated and the level of care exceeds that paid for by the plan.

Diagnosis Related Groups (DRG): Diagnosis Related Groups (DRG) is the system used by Medicare to pay for most inpatient care. Under the DRG system hospital procedures are rated in terms of intensity and cost, and providers are paid a specific amount to care for a patient treated in that DRG, regardless of the cost to the hospital.

Fee for Service: Fee for service was the prevailing system for payment of health care services until the not-too-distant past. Providers of health care services set rates for each service, and billed the patient and/or their insurance for the charge. The expectation was that in most cases the provider would be paid for the service as charged, and payment would be received at the time of service. The system potentially encourages overuse of service and therefore increased cost. This system for payment of care is relatively rare now, although there are medical supplies that continue to be paid for in this manner.

Fiscal Intermediary: A fiscal intermediary is a company that is contracted by payers (or providers) to, at minimum, process claims for services. They also frequently are contracted to deliver education to providers, to interpret regulatory or rules changes that affect providers, and to perform other administrative functions such as an audit of records of providers. The Medicare program uses regional fiscal intermediaries to manage the Medicare business.

Managed Care: The term managed care refers to those insurance and payment systems that typically have provider networks, have utilization management systems that may require preauthorization of care (which demands evidence of medical necessity), and that attempt to control cost through systematic application of care protocols and price negotiation with providers. They may or may not involve capitation, but always work to share risk between the insurance carrier and the provider of care. The design of the coverage will vary but there are a couple of predominant designs. Health Maintenance Organizations (HMO) are organizations that offer or arrange for coverage for certain health care service for enrolled plan members for fixed premiums. Preferred Provider Organizations (PPO) contract with specific providers (preferred providers), have negotiated rates with those providers that are less than the full charge, and encourage their covered members to use the preferred providers through use of financial incentives. If patients use providers outside the network of preferred providers, there are additional costs that they incur "out-of-pocket."

Resource-Based Relative Value Scale (RBRVS): This is the physician payment scale that Medicare uses to determine the reimbursement to doctors for the services they render, with the calculation based upon the amount of time and resources used, adjusting for overhead and geographic variation.

Self-Insured Plans: Companies may elect to self insure through their own resources combined with the contributions from their employees, rather than purchasing commercial insurance. When companies self insure they often hire companies to manage those benefits while retaining the financial risk for the health coverage. Since they are assuming financial risk, they buy stop-loss insurance or re-insurance to protect them against unforeseen financial liability that results when their pool of covered lives exceeds a certain defined cost in health care claims.

Third Party Administrator: Third Party Administrators (TPA) manage benefits, claims, and administration of health insurance for self-insured companies and entities. TPAs do not assume financial risk. Companies that self insure usually do not have the infrastructure or expertise to manage the benefits and hire TPAs to do the day-to-day management of the benefit.

FINANCING THE HEALTH CARE INDUSTRY

There is a general misunderstanding that health care is largely paid for by private insurance. In fact that is not the case. There are three primary sources of reimbursement for health care: the patient, private insurance, and government (Figure 10-1). The largest percentage of reimbursement comes from a different sector depending upon the type of service received. For instance, a higher percentage of the cost of pharmaceuticals and dental care comes from the patient, not from insurance (California Healthcare Foundation, 2004). So what does it mean to say that reimbursement for health care in the United States comes from these three sources?

The Patient

Patients contribute to health care through a couple of primary mechanisms: they pay out of pocket for some or all of health care costs, and/or they pay some or all of the cost of health care premiums (Figure 10-2). In terms of out-of-pocket expenses, if individuals are uninsured, then the entire cost of the health care service is often borne by the patient themselves, unless they are fortunate enough to have access to and qualify for low-cost clinic services or charity care from a health care provider. If insured, they pay deductibles and **coinsurance** or **co-pays** for specific services received. Even for individuals employed and fortunate enough to have health insurance provided by their employer, as health care costs have increased and premium costs have increased, employers have shifted more of the cost of health care to the employee. These cost shifts come in the form of higher deductibles,

Figure 10-1

Primary Sources
of Reimbursement
for Health Care.

Primary Sources
of Reimbursement
for Health Care

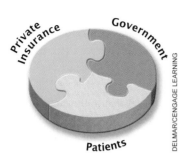

lessened or more restrictive coverage, and higher percentages of the charge shifted to the patient in the form of higher coinsurance and co-pays. Goldman and McGlynn (2005, p. 25) note the co-pay required by most Health Maintenance Organizations was $10 in 1996 (87% of employees), while in 2003 only one-third of employees had a co-pay that low. Likewise deductibles have been increasing over time. They indicate that the average deductible was $175 in 2000, but was $275 in 2003. This is illustrative of an ongoing trend of shifting the costs to patients.

Often employers will offer different plans with different levels of risk to the employee. Generally, the lower the financial risk the higher the cost to the patient. The assumption is that if you are healthy, you will select a plan that may result in higher out-of-pocket expenses because you are not anticipating actually using the insurance. Alternatively, if you have higher demand for health care services because of illness or because you have a family and therefore more exposure to risk,

Figure 10-2

Patients are
responsible for
paying for health
care in several ways,
including paying
out of pocket for
some or all of the
expense and/or
paying some or all
of the health care
insurance premiums.

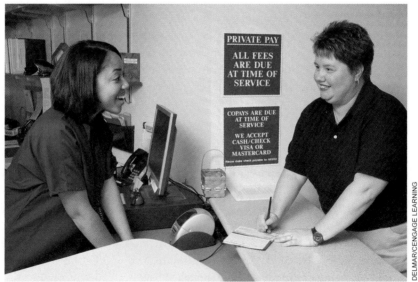

you are more likely to select a plan that costs you more but that also pays a larger percentage of your health care expenses. Whether or not these assumptions are correct is a matter of some debate, particularly as the cost of health care increases. The cost of the patient portion of premiums is increasing at such a rate that there is increased risk of individuals selecting lower-cost or no coverage because they cannot afford the insurance plans that pay more of the cost of care. This effectively continues the cost shifting from insurance to patient. Data cited by Goldman and McGlynn (2005) indicate that the uninsured population is increasing. The percentage increase was from 13% in 1987 to 18% in 2003, a number equal to 45 million individuals. While they also indicate that younger adults (who are on average more likely to be healthy) are the groups most likely to be uninsured (30% aged 18 to 24, about 25% aged 25 to 34, and 16% aged 35 to 54 were uninsured in 2004), it is true that many of these individuals are working (Goldman & McGlynn, 2005, p. 22). In 2003 only 20% of the uninsured had no one working in the family (Goldman & McGlynn, 2005, p. 21). Obviously personal choices about how to use disposable income influences whether or not health insurance is purchased. Other factors may be equally influential. Cost of insurance to the individual or family relative to total income is also a significant factor. Families or individuals may simply not be able to afford the cost of the premium. Factor in the high cost of coverage for the immediate family and the out-of-pocket expense may be prohibitive, causing people to "take their chances" that they will continue to be relatively healthy.

The Government

Government pays for health care in a number of ways. There are the two insurance plans that are government sponsored: Medicaid and Medicare. Government also supports health care through the purchase of private health insurance for government employees. The third method of support is the Veterans Administration health services, a very large and comprehensive health care delivery system. Finally, government supports health care delivery in a number of direct and indirect ways: support of medical teaching institutions, through Federally Qualified Health Centers, through various subsidy systems for medical education, and systems designed to deliver needed medical services to areas of the country where those services are in short supply. As the definition of health care changes, services historically not considered or paid for as health care by government (e.g., residential mental health treatment for children) become part of the government cost of health care.

The share of health care expense borne by government is not likely to decrease. Medicaid and Medicare are the largest source of dollars for nursing home placement. As the population ages and the actual number of elderly in real numbers goes up, nursing home or other health care later in life will increase even if the delivery systems for that care change. The elderly (those 65 and over) also spend more on health care than most other individuals—about four times more according to Goldman and McGlynn (2005), and are more likely to be insured through Medicare. Also, the number of very old continues to increase and, as a rule, health care costs increase with age. Thus, the percentage of costs attributable to government insurers is likely to increase.

This increase in stress to government sources is also being felt in the Medicaid system. States have seen an annual increase in their Medicaid expenditures. Since Medicaid is a federal/state cost-sharing program, there have been annual increases in Medicaid expenditures at the federal level as well. Some of the increases have been a function of other changes in health care delivery systems. For instance, states during the 1980s and 1990s began to apply to the federal government for waiver programs that allowed them to offer more community-based programs to specific populations, for instance the mentally retarded and mentally ill. This allowed the movement of individuals out of state-supported institutional settings and into the community. Medicaid often paid for the community support services necessary for this transition to occur. The result was cost shifting from state resources to a federal/state mix. Now there is increased pressure from the federal level to slow the growth in the Medicaid program, forcing states to look at how they will rein in those cost increases. They are turning more and more to the institution of managed-care programs for Medicaid-paid services. Such efforts are complex and require examining the role of Medicaid as a safety net provider and the impact of managed care on the financial viability of the insurers and provider (Ku et al., 2000).

At the same time there is a trend toward managed Medicaid to limit the percentage growth in expenditures from this payer source, and there is also increased attention on the uninsured. Consequently states are looking at ways to use existing funds to extend coverage to populations that are presently uninsured (Brodt et al., 2007). This usually takes the form of a government-sponsored plan with some premium cost to the individual and provision of basic insurance coverage. More focus on illness prevention is also pursued in an effort to decrease health care costs in the future (Bella, Goldsmith, & Somers, 2007).

Private Insurance

Private insurance is the third significant source of dollars to support health care delivery in the United States. In 2004 private health insurance paid 35.1% of the total cost (California HealthCare Foundation, 2006). Sources cited by Goldman & McGlynn (Olin & Maclin, 2003) indicate that there is variation (as expected) by age of the patient. For those individuals under 65 years, private health insurance makes up 54% of the total paid, while for those over 65 private insurance covers only 14%. This variation is expected because most people over the age of 65 years are now covered by Medicare, and in most cases Medicare is the primary insurer.

Clemans-Cope and Garrett (2006) have done extensive research on changes in **employer sponsored insurance (ESI)**. ESI are insurance plans that patients access through their employer, with the employer paying part of the premium and the employee paying part. They conclude that between 2000 and 2004, there has been a decline in the percentage of nonelderly individuals insured through their employer (from 66% to 61% respectively). They cite a number of reasons for the change, including a decrease in the number of employers offering ESI, increases in the number of individuals unable to afford to purchase insurance through their employer, and increases in the number of part-time workers and others not eligible to purchase the ESI. Over this same time period there were increases in the number of uninsured adults and, if the Medicaid and State Children's Health Insurance Program (SCHIP) programs were not available for children, there likely would have been the same increases in number of uninsured children. The individuals most likely to be uninsured are those that are working in smaller companies, those with lower incomes, those not working full time, and younger people. Significantly, they note "the share of all businesses offering health benefits declined from 69 percent in 2000 to 60 percent by 2005, driven largely by decreases among small to mid-size firms (3 to 199 employees)." (Clemans-Cope & Garrett, 2006, p. 13).

Internet Exercise 10-1	1. Go to the Kaiser Family Foundation Web site at http://www.kff.org.
	2. Search for "Health Care Cost: A Primer."
	3. Read the publication and suggest three ways in which nurses could participate in the management of health care costs.

ISSUES IN HEALTH CARE FINANCING

The health care market includes many parties: the individual consumer of health care services or patient, the provider of care, insurance companies, secondary suppliers such as providers of durable medical equipment, manufacturers of medical devices (such as the orthopedics industry), pharmaceutical companies, pharmacies, and the government. There are also significant numbers of other professions and businesses that specialize in the area of health care finance. A nonexhaustive list includes accounting firms that provide audits of the health care providers, legal firms that specialize in health care, software companies that support the health care industry, as well as disease management firms and other secondary businesses that are an outgrowth of the health care industry. So, when one speaks of the health care market, it is conceivable to be including or excluding any one of a number of these businesses and members.

Supply and Demand

The health care market responds to the same principles as do other markets. If the demand is there, then the market expands to fill that void. This applies directly to the providers of health care as well as the secondary businesses that depend upon the health care industry. Currently there is growth in **care management** or **disease management** companies (Mechanic, 2004) that are responding to specific market conditions. The market is looking for methods of preventive care as a mechanism to reduce cost and improve outcomes rather than simply trying to reduce cost through management of services to patients who are already ill.

The health care industry not only responds to demands, it also creates demand in a number of ways. One example is the relatively new phenomenon of direct marketing to the patient.

Marketing is in part an effort to create demand for the products and services provided. Particularly where there is some level of competition for services or a need to continue to create "door demand" in order to maintain the supply of new consumers of the health care product, there is often advertising of health care products. Presently there is advertising for pharmaceuticals, hospitals, doctors, and medical procedures. There is also a continuing offer for various screening services designed to detect health care concerns and then provide easy access to providers of service who can manage the health care concern just detected. In all of these instances the desired outcome is self referral and increased sales.

Marketing directly to physicians is conducted by the pharmaceutical industry, the biomedical engineering industry, and others. The American Medical Association has raised ethical concerns about this trend, fearing that physicians, who are seen by the public as objective individuals whose role is to simply provide the best care possible without outside influence, may in fact make or be perceived as making medical decisions based upon factors other than purely medical considerations. The Kaiser Foundation (Kaiser Foundation, 2004) has published data that illustrate the increase in what they term "promotional spending." Furnishing of samples to physicians was the largest category of expense and the category that showed the greatest increase, from $4.9 billion dollars in 1996 to $15.9 billion in 2004 (Figure 10-3). Direct marketing to pharmacies and doctors was the next largest category, growing from $3 billion to $7.3 billion in 2004. Direct-to-consumer marketing increased from $0.8 billion in 1996 to $4 billion in 2004, while

Figure 10-3
Growth in
Promotional
Spending. *(Data
from Kaiser
Foundation, 2004.)*

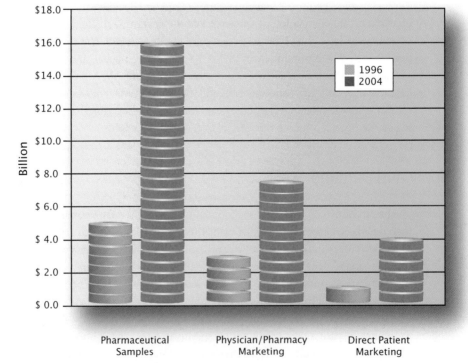

Growth in Promotional Spending *

advertising in professional journals remained about steady at $0.5 billion. Woo et al., (2007) notes that spending for prescription drugs grew more than 12% each year from 1990 to 2000, and while those expenditures have slowed some, there was still a 6% increase from 2004 to 2005. They also note that marketing of drugs tends to focus on newer, more expensive drugs. According to data published by the National Association of Chain Drug Stores, total retail prescription sales increased by 7.7% (from $232 billion to $249.8 billion) from 2005 to 2006. Clearly, research on the impact of marketing on prescribing patterns is needed.

Hospitals and medical practices advertise directly to the public through television, radio, print, and mail. They now use results of satisfaction surveys, outcome data, and other third-party reports to encourage use of their facility for various medical procedures and to structure the services and the environment of care to achieve higher customer satisfaction (Figure 10-4). High customer satisfaction may have the side benefit of assisting in negotiation with physicians, managed care companies, etc. Hospitals and doctors are competing for business. As the use of hospital-based services declines and outpatient surgeries increase, as the number of hospital days for procedures decreases, and as other factors impact their inpatient business, both the doctors and the hospitals need to compete more and more for what might amount to a scarce resource: inpatient business. As a result, they are developing other medical offerings to maintain their fiscal viability and their competitive advantage.

If there is an assumption that there is a finite need for specific services such as outpatient surgery, then providers of health care must try to secure a part of that market, or market share, in order to remain financially viable. There is also advertising for market share among ancillary industries, such as pharmacies and other medical suppliers. Changes in demographic makeup may shift competition to different services. Hospitals and other health care providers must constantly determine where there is market growth, and therefore the potential for additional business. They then work to secure a part of that new or expanding business.

Figure 10-4 Hospitals use surveys, outcome data, and other third-party reports in advertising to generate business in an increasingly competitive environment.

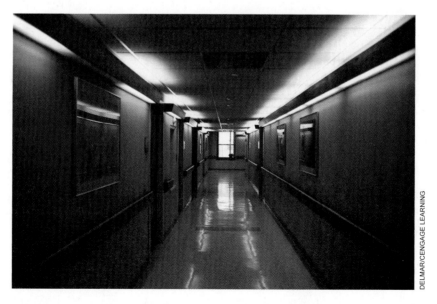

DELMAR/CENGAGE LEARNING

Marketing in health care is often perceived in negative terms. Eastaugh (1998) argues that health care should be engaging in what he terms "social marketing," with social marketing defined as a shift from selling simply the product to selling products that promote and establish better health to the consumer. The marketing is social in that it promotes a social good rather than simply a product. His perspective is that this shift will offer opportunities for diversification in the health care industry that will also have the impact of developing feeder systems into the core product.

> **Writing Exercise 10-1**
>
>
>
> Marketing and advertising health care service is prevalent in today's health care environment. Does this have an impact on the care provided? Does marketing serve the need of informing the public and making them better consumers of care, or does it "sell" services that may be unnecessary and therefore drive up all health care costs? Is the answer somewhere "in between"? Do you have a professional role in resolving this conundrum?

Competition and Regulated Competition

Health care is heavily regulated. Even though there is a lot of competition among health care providers for business, it remains one of the most closely regulated industries. Some of the federal regulations (laws and rules as published at the federal level) regarding health care are listed in Table 10-1. In addition there are a multitude of state regulations that vary from state to state.

Health care includes both private and public good, perhaps one of the basic reasons for this level of regulation. Private good is the benefit afforded to the individual through improved health, while public good refers to the positive benefit that accrues to the community when the citizens are healthier. Government also pays a **disproportionate share** of the cost, another reason for the regulatory environment of health care. As governments become more concerned about the status of the uninsured portion of the population and look for ways to meet the health care needs of this segment, the level of regulation may increase because costs may shift to the government even more.

Some individuals advocate a free market in health care, assuming that free competition will result in lower cost and higher quality. A free market in health care may have the unintended consequence of increasing health care delivery, though not always for improved patient care. An unregulated market risks delivery of care for financial gain rather than for health improvement reasons.

In addition to the risk described above, Cimasi (2005) has listed a number of barriers to free-market competition in his discussion of specialty and niche hospitals. In part, his list is as follows (p. 77):

1. Patients don't purchase services directly from providers. Instead their health care plans may direct them to specific providers, and their health care insurance may pay the bulk of the expense.

Table 10-1 Select Federal Health Care Regulations

Health Care Regulation	Description
SHERMAN ANTI-TRUST ACT	Prohibits collective restraint of trade and monopolies
CLAYTON ACT	Prohibits price discrimination and mergers, acquisitions, and joint ventures that decrease competition
FALSE CLAIMS ACT	Establishes civil liability for knowingly presenting false or fraudulent claims to government payers, and for reckless disregard of the accuracy of the claims
ANTI-KICKBACK	Establishes as a felony knowingly or willfully soliciting or receiving payment in return for referral of a patient for services paid for by a government health plan
STARK	Prohibits physicians from referring patients to entities with which they have a financial interest
MEDICARE MODERNIZATION ACT	Among other things, establishes payments for ambulatory surgery centers from Medicare
EMERGENCY MEDICAL TREATMENT AND ACTIVE LABOR ACT	Established the legal responsibility of a hospital to screen patients and stabilize emergency medical conditions if they have the capacity
HEALTH INSURANCE PORTABILITY AND ACCOUNTABILITY ACT (HIPAA)	Established privacy and security requirements for health care providers and set time frames for implementation of those requirements

2. Patients don't compare prices between providers. Unlike a retail environment that allows easy comparison between products, health care does not offer this simplicity or transparency, making price comparisons very difficult.

3. The government is the largest purchaser of health care. Because Medicare and Medicaid are two of the largest insurers of health care, there is less pressure for a free market.

4. Private purchasers often lack market power. Health insurers wield considerable power over the pricing for services. Individual consumers, on the other hand, are more isolated and are less able to use their collective power for decreased prices.

5. Patients, purchasers, and providers lack information. On what basis should an individual consumer of health care base demands for lower prices or improved outcomes? Information on either is limited and difficult for most people to understand.

6. Many providers have monopoly or near-monopoly power. How many hospitals are in your community? Is there real competition for hospital or physician services?

7. Providers are rewarded for increasing costs. The only method of increased reimbursement for service is to increase the charge for the care..

8. Certificate of need, regulation, and licensing laws are an entry barrier to competing and substitute providers and services. It is very expensive and difficult to enter the health care market due to the plethora of regulations and complexity of the reimbursement environment, discouraging competition.

Pricing

Pricing is a complex interplay among a number of factors.

- The government sets many prices through implementation of the Medicare program. Medicare pays for most services that are provided in a hospital setting using a **Prospective Payment System (PPS)** that relies on **Diagnostic Related Groups (DRG)**, resulting in payments that are based upon the "norm" for treatment of medical conditions. Theoretically, since payment is the same regardless of the level of care, lower cost and more efficient care are rewarded.
- Medicaid pricing (and what they will and will not pay for) is a major influence.
- Managed-care companies use their considerable market strength to negotiate the lowest prices possible.
- The medical community "pushes back" against these pressures to lower prices and, through membership in various advocacy organizations, works to maintain prices that allow continued growth and investment in health care delivery.
- The need to provide charity care to uninsured or underinsured individuals places pressure on prices. Since some patients must receive discounted or free services, the cost to deliver those services gets "shifted" to other payers such as insurers.
- **Usual and customary** is a term often heard. This refers to the practice of setting allowable prices based upon prevailing charges in a region. Usual and customary prices are often used by insurance companies in their negotiations with providers.

A focus on cost containment in health care has been apparent over the past couple of decades. Part of the rise in health care costs reflected increased expenses unrelated to the direct cost of health care delivery. Costs also included the increased expense of managing managed care, advertising to attract new customers as a function of a more competitive environment, and increasing ancillary costs to make sure that the health care provider did not run afoul of regulations. While the emphasis on cost containment was likely a positive influence in many respects, Cimasi (2005) makes a good argument that cost containment is not a reasonable long-term solution for rising health care costs because health care cannot be evaluated in the same manner as other industries. He provides three reasons for this: First, health care is more "people dependent" and not as amenable to automation for cost efficiencies; second, health care is local and cannot be moved out of the community or country to decrease costs; third, quality bears some relationship to the amount of time spent in delivery of service. Also, improved health care has a benefit elsewhere in the economy (e.g., lowered absenteeism) that is difficult to measure.

However, price for health care exists in the general market, and therefore does respond to some market considerations. Eastaugh (1998) identifies three primary considerations in pricing: competition in the market area, the possibility of new providers entering the market, and the strength of the bargaining power of the buyers of health care, primarily the insurance industry and their capacity to negotiate discounts. He believes that the traditional pricing strategies of health care providers may not be effective in the current health care environment. Instead in a competitive environment, he suggests that there be increased emphasis on marketing and pricing that is consumer focused, particularly "customer satisfaction, marketing, discovering what the patients wanted, cutting excess costs and offering the service at a favorable price" (p. 97).

Still, price will continue to be examined critically. As the patient portion of health care charges increases, there is increasing pressure to hold down costs. As long as someone else is paying the bill, people tend not to pay as much attention as when they are paying the bill themselves. It is probably true though that price only plays a role when people have the time and the luxury of price comparison. In emergency situations this is not realistic, nor is it realistic when risk increases.

Rising Costs and Cost Containment

It is well known that health care expenditures are rising. In 1980, $255 billion was spent on health care. In 1990 the amount was $717 billion, and in 2000 it was $1.359 trillion. By 2004 the amount was $1.878 trillion (California HealthCare Foundation, 2005, p. 2) (Figure 10-5). These increases

Figure 10-5
Rising Health Care Expenditures (in Billions). *(Data from the California HealthCare Foundation, 2005.)*

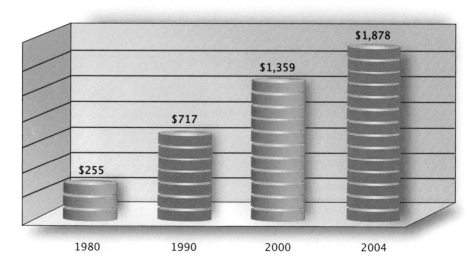

Rising Health Care Expenditures (in Billions)

$1,878

$1,359

$717

$255

1980   1990   2000   2004

occurred despite efforts of the health insurance industry to rein in those costs. There are many reasons for these increases.First, there have been significant technological advances in health care, advances that improve the outcomes of care but also increase costs. As cited by Goldman and McGlynn (2005, p. 23), according to the American Hospital Association, the cost of one day in the hospital in 1965 was $128, while in 2002 (adjusted for inflation) it was $1,289, with technological advances accounting for most of this increase.

Second, inflation plays a role in health care cost increases, although it is the case that health care costs have been increasing at a rate that exceeds that of inflation. Third, the administrative costs of health care have increased in part in response to increased pressure to control payments from the insurance industry. Hospitals and doctors' offices have had to hire staff and spend more resources on management of service delivery; for instance, prior authorization management. Fourth, shortages in critical fields, most notably nursing, have at times driven up salaries faster than they might otherwise have increased. Fifth, medical care requires people, most of whom cannot be replaced by machines. Consequently, efficiencies that other businesses can achieve because of mechanization are not possible in the same way or to the same extent in health care (Figure 10-6).

Demographic changes also have an impact on overall health care costs. The growing number of older Americans is increasing the overall cost of health care because this group tends to have a higher level of chronic illnesses and requires more medical care. According to a Rand report (2006), by 2030, 22% of the population will be over age 65, and 2.5% will be over 85. This change to a higher percentage of older persons has already begun and will change the nature of health care substantially, because the needs of this group of individuals are different from that of a younger group.

There have been a variety of efforts made to contain the rising cost of health care. Managed care came about in direct response to rising costs. As costs increased, employers found that insurance premiums were rising and becoming unaffordable. The insurance industry responded by developing products to help employers manage their costs. One expectation was that by managing the care delivered, there would be a reduction in the total volume of service. Additionally, managed-care companies began to establish provider networks with whom they had negotiated

Figure 10-6

Despite advances in medical technology, medical care depends on people to deliver care and services, which contributes to the increasing cost of health care.

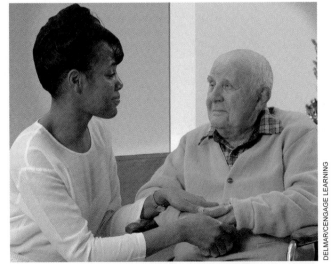

DELMAR/CENGAGE LEARNING

pricing structures that allowed them to pay less than full charge for the services rendered. In order to gain market share, health care providers found it necessary to participate in managed-care contracts. Otherwise they would find that they were "out-of-network" and were not able to treat a sizable number of patients without additional expense to the patient and, at times, with no reimbursement from the patient's insurer.

Managed care was somewhat effective in helping to slow the rate of cost increase. However, patients often were frustrated by the administrative requirements in order to receive medical care and by the restrictions on what care they could receive. This dissatisfaction resulted in some softening of managed care, in particular expansion of networks and somewhat easier authorization of service. Additionally, tight management of service is expensive for insurers. Therefore, insurers determined the circumstances under which authorizations made a cost difference. They then determined which services did not require authorization, thus decreasing costs to the insurer.

Other cost-containment measures included negotiation of lower rates for services and exclusion of certain services from reimbursement at all. These efforts had the unintended consequence of shifting cost from payers that paid less for service to those that would pay more. Recently there has been a great deal of concern that the uninsured are the patients who have assumed more than their fair share of the health care cost, primarily through cost shifting. Since the uninsured do not have collective clout, they are unable as a group to negotiate favorable terms for payment of health care expenses. They are therefore more likely to be charged the full price. Individuals that are insured, on the other hand, benefit from the fact that they have an insurer who is working to ensure the lowest possible price for care. Cost shifting for them comes from their employer, who is trying to minimize premium costs by shifting ever-larger shares of the health care charges to their employees, either through deductibles or other measures.

The **Centers for Medicare and Medicaid Services (CMS)** is often the leader in changes in health care systems. Diagnosis-related groups (DRGs) were part of an attempt on the part of CMS to reduce or slow expenses to the Medicare program. DRGs, as described earlier, are an attempt to determine payment for specific procedures in such a manner that efficiency of care is rewarded. APCs establish a similar payment system for physician services.

Prospective payment systems (PPS) also are used to contain costs. With PPS certain characteristics of the patient (for instance diagnosis, age, or other complicating factors) combined with the care received are used to determine payment. If care is provided efficiently and in fewer than a specified number of days, then the hospital makes a profit on the care, while if care exceeds a certain level, either in terms of services or days in the hospital, then the hospital either breaks even or loses money depending upon their costs. The risk is therefore shifted to the health care provider.

Percentage of Gross National Product

The cost of health care in the United States has been growing faster than the gross national product. In 1960 it represented about 5% of the total, while by 2002 it was about 15% of the **gross national product (GNP)** (Goldman and McGlynn, 2005). GNP is the value of all goods and services produced in the nation. According to a Kaiser Foundation report (2007, p. 1), health care expense as a share of GNP leveled off in 2004 at about 16%. Per capita health care expenditures also rose during this time period, more than doubling from 1990 to 2004 (up 123%), with an average annual increase of 9.9% from 1970 to 2004 (Kaiser, 2006), or about 2.5% faster than GNP. However, the spending is without the requisite improvement in health status of the population (Kaiser 2007). Some questions surface as a result. Is it possible to continue to afford this increase, and is it reasonable for these increases to continue? Are we getting the quality of health care that the price tag would presume? Cimasi (2004) argues that because health care has fewer opportunities to decrease the cost of a service, the price of health care will naturally go up. While there is concern about the percentage of the GNP accounted for by health care, other industries are able to benefit significantly from technological advancement and other factors that decrease the cost of production. Therefore, while costs increase for health care, costs decrease for other segments of the economy, effectively increasing the share of GNP that is attributable to health care. Problematic, however, is that although the United States spends more per capita on health care than many other countries, overall health is not better than many other countries that spend less. (Goldman & McGlynn, 2004, p. 4).

Quality Access Debates

In 2006 the Rand Corporation summarized the findings from a variety of research reports concerning health care quality in the United States. Those studies indicated that only about half of adults received the recommended care.

Despite the huge investment of financial resources in the health care system in the United States, there is ample evidence that, compared to other countries, the United States is not buying quality. Infant mortality is higher than in other industrialized countries, and our life expectancy is less (Eastaugh, 1998). Goldman and McGlynn (2005, p. 36) reported data from *The Dartmouth Atlas of Health Care* (2004) that indicated that variation of rates of different surgical and diagnostic procedures is unrelated to the health care needs of the patients. They also report that failure to provide needed medical procedures is more of a problem (46% of the time) than provision of unnecessary service (11% of the time). There are many statistics that indicate that there is much room for improvement in the quality of care delivered in the United States. Schoen et al., (2005, p. 1) compared health care across six nations, including the Untied States, and conclude "…one-third of U.S. patients with health problems reported experiencing medical mistakes, medication errors, or inaccurate or delayed lab results—the highest rate of any of the six nations surveyed. While sicker patients in all countries reported safety risks, poor care coordination, and inadequate chronic-care treatment, with no country deemed best or worst overall, the United States stood out for high error rates, inefficient coordination of care, and high out-of-pocket costs resulting in forgone care." Discerning how to change the health care system to effect improvement is the challenge.

The Role of Insurance in Access/Use of Health Care

Hadley (2007) conducted a study that demonstrates what intuitively was suspected. Individuals who are uninsured are much less likely than those that are insured to receive medical care after an unintentional injury or at the start of a chronic illness. In addition, although the two groups received the same level of referral for follow-up care, persons with insurance were considerably more likely to receive that care than were the uninsured. The uninsured that had chronic-care conditions were more likely to use emergency room services (a very expensive form of health care) than were the patients with insurance. He also found that patients who were uninsured were more likely to not have adequate recovery from either chronic conditions or unintentional injuries. These data point to the greater health risks incurred by people without insurance and, from a public-policy perspective, indicate that lack of insurance can have a significant impact on the health of a community. As the numbers of uninsured rise (from 44.8 million in 2005 to 47 million in 2006, a 15.8% increase), the possible impact also increases (DeNavas et al., 2007). Compounding the problem is the evidence that there is an increasing level of uninsured children. Between 2005 and 2006, the increase was from 8 million to 8.7 million, an 11.7% increase (DeNavas et al., 2007).

Access to and/or effective use of health care can also be affected by demographic variables. Rural poor will have a more difficult time accessing providers and may have fewer options. Status as a legal or illegal resident of the country can have an impact on access to Medicaid or other insurance. According to Goldman, Smith, and Scod (2007, p. 1), illegal immigrants actually consume very little health care—they represent about 3.2% of the population, but only consume 1.5% of medical costs. If you are illegally in the country, it is more likely that the job you hold will not offer health insurance. Language and cultural differences can also make a difference in access to and use of health care; if patients cannot communicate effectively with a health care provider, they are less likely to use that provider or receive/use health care information.

> **Writing Exercise 10-2**
>
> Some medical technologies decrease costs of care by cutting the number of inpatient days required to treat a condition, while other technologies may have the opposite impact. Identify one in each category and formulate an argument as to what the access to that medical technology should be for a person who is insured versus one that is uninsured.

Changes in Medicaid Management by States and the Push to Expand Coverage for the Uninsured

States are faced with increased pressure to decrease costs or slow the increased costs of the Medicaid program. They are also under pressure to improve the heath status of the population and ensure some standard of health insurance coverage for the presently uninsured. Therefore, they are looking for new methods of managing the systems, and the costs of providing publicly-funded health care. Emphasis appears to be shifting to the promotion of health rather than simple access control through prior-authorization programs. Health promotion involves lifestyle changes, however—changes that are difficult to achieve and difficult to maintain, despite the fact that lifestyle changes are the key ingredient to decreasing overall long-term health care cost. For instance, decreasing levels of obesity among children will result in long-term decreases in health care costs for the treatment of a myriad of diseases that are associated with obesity, such as hypertension and diabetes. In other words, drop the number of individuals with chronic illness in the future. Greene (2007) has examined the efforts of two states to provide incentives such as cash or gift certificates for healthy behavior and finds that while promising, the approach requires much more research to determine if it is effective on a long-term basis. She also indicates the need for states to be aware of the existing barriers to healthy behavior. Specifically listed are factors such as difficulty accessing specific health care providers, such as dental care, because of Medicaid program restrictions and difficulty of locating participating dentists, problems with access to preventive care because of transportation problems, and program costs that are prohibitive, such as the charges for sports programs for children.

Bella, Goldsmith, and Somers (2007, p. 1) have listed particular endeavors that offer the potential for significant savings in state Medicaid programs, while still recognizing that Medicaid is a safety-net program that serves a proportionately large group of frail and elderly, who consume a very high percentage of Medicaid dollars (20% consume 80% of the cost). They suggest the following actions by the states; efforts that focus on improved care management of specific consumer groups. First, improve prenatal outreach in order to increase the likelihood of a healthy birth. Second, enroll children with asthma in care management programs so as to reduce emergency room admissions of these patients and increase the likelihood of uninterrupted schooling. Third, implement care management for those who are aged, blind, and disabled, who collectively consume about 70% of the total Medicaid expenditures. Fourth, better manage the health care needs of individuals who require long-term care, so as to better coordinate Medicare and Medicaid and to drop emergency room and other costs. Finally, focus on the provision of intensive care management for those people with multiple chronic-health needs, reducing the need for both hospital and nursing-home care. The argument is that since these groups use a disproportionate number of Medicaid dollars, focusing on the management of care to these groups will have the most significant and rapid cost benefit. According to data presented by Crippen (2007) regarding acute care, the top 1% of Medicare and Medicaid recipients account for 33% of the cost ($52,500 per member versus $1,500 annually). "The bottom 50% of members (188,000 members) account for only 1.5% of total costs and have an average cost of $50/member" (Crippen, 2007, p. 9). He defines hospitalizations for asthma as preventable and hospitalizations for diabetes and chronic heart failure as avoidable, emphasizing the need to focus on prevention and illness management.

Both approaches rely on the involvement of Medicaid recipients in their own care through care management, or cash, or other incentives. They reflect the trend in the commercial insurance market toward health savings accounts and other mechanisms to make individuals knowledgeable consumers of health care and not just purchasers of health care. In the case of Medicaid recipients the task may be more difficult since there is a lower level of literacy overall, difficulty in reaching the population in a meaningful manner so that they understand and participate in new programs, and a history of lack of opportunity for involvement in program design by Medicaid recipients. However, states are pursuing these partnerships with consumers in order to have improved community health and budget predictability (Barth, 2007). States are also using performance profiling to motivate doctors to meet quality targets that are often focused on improved preventive care. Literature (Hibbard, Stockhard, & Tusler, 2005) supports the perspective that motivation to improve the quality of care can be affected by a desire to protect one's reputation. Financial risk (discussed in the next section on "Pay for Performance") may provide an effective motivator.

Additionally, some states are looking at implementation of what are called Defined-Contribution and Limited-Benefit Arrangements. Rosenbaum (2006, p. 2) defines these: "... 'defined-contribution' means the payment of a flat, per-capita amount toward the cost of health plan enrollment, regardless of benefit design or actual health care utilization and cost. The term 'limited-benefit' plan means a health plan whose benefit and coverage design is narrower and more restricted than that utilized under 'traditional' Medicaid benefit design." The idea is to use commercial insurance strategies to manage the growth in Medicaid expenditures. While laudable on one level, she also makes the case that Medicaid, as a safety-net program, is fundamentally different from the commercial insurance market and provides health coverage for a high percentage of individuals whose health care needs are serious and chronic. She states, "In reality, Medicaid operates in accordance with unique rules that have been designed for a low income population in relatively poor health, who enroll in the program at the highest point of need, and whose enrollment is often tied to the receipt of specific medical and health treatments.... In essence, Medicaid is built to serve people whose living and health conditions place them outside of population norms" (p. 8). While this should not discourage states from looking for ways to better manage costs and to improve health care outcomes, it does urge caution and care in design and implementation of different coverage plans.

The savings from these efforts to improve the health status of the Medicaid population can theoretically be used to expand coverage to those who are currently uninsured. This then fulfills the public responsibility to ensure health care for those that have limited access.

Internet Exercise 10-2	Locate the Web site http://www.kff.org. 1. Locate the publication: "The Faces of Medicaid II: Recognizing the Care Needs of People with Multiple Chronic Conditions." 2. What data have the authors presented that argue against a fee for service payment system? What payment systems do they advocate? What is the support for those alternative payment systems, and would the quality of care be improved, stay the same, or decline?

EMERGING MARKETS AND TRENDS IN HEALTH CARE

The U.S. health care market is dynamic and ever changing. Changes come about through technology, through pressure from patients, from the need to maintain profits in the insurance industry, and in response to societal determinations about value and what the government should pay for and for whom, among other considerations. Whatever the source of change it is important to recognize that health care is not static, either in terms of what defines health care or in terms of what is paid for and by whom. Following is a discussion of a number of changes and trends that are presently underway. Their significance long term in the health care industry is unclear, but at least some of them will likely have a significant impact on health care and the cost of that care in the future.

Pay for Performance

People like to get their money's worth. Historically this adage was not applied to health care. Instead you received care, got the bill, and managed to pay the bill. While there may have been a question as to why a pill that was inexpensive in the drug store could cost so much more when provided in the hospital, there were relatively few challenges to costs. That perspective has changed over the past three or four decades.

Providers of health care are being asked not just to deliver care with the assumption that the quality and outcomes of care will be good; they are instead being asked to assume some level of financial risk regarding the outcomes of the care provided (Thrall, 2004). **Pay for Performance** refers to the concept of paying for quality and efficiency in health care rather than paying for simple delivery of a service. It shifts financial risk to the provider and, by paying differentially, strives to focus on the results of care, frequently in a comparative manner. The comparison is often against other providers of the same service and against evidence-based standards of care. This continued shift in risk from payer to provider is occurring not just in the commercial/managed care market, but also in the public payer system. Both Medicare and Medicaid are becoming involved in Pay for Performance, and there is a growth in literature and guides to states to implement Pay for Performance as part of a strategy to manage quality and cost. For example, the Center for Healthcare Strategies published a Pay for Performance guide for states (Llanos et al., 2007) that wanted to establish these programs for physician services. Pay for Performance systems have at their heart the same goal that has been driving change in the U.S. health care system for an extended period of time. Goals include improvement in health care outcomes, improved disease management and disease prevention, and lowered costs or slowing of the rate of cost increase.

With Pay for Performance, the payer, unilaterally or through negotiation, establishes performance goals and then links payment of care to whether or not goals are met. At this time there are relatively few medical conditions that are subject to payment of this variety, but as evidence-based practice gains ground it is likely that there will be an increase in the number of medical conditions subject to Pay for Performance.

Pay for Performance can be configured in two primary ways: bonuses paid from a pool of extra money for meeting defined performance targets, or the withholding of a percentage of contract dollars with payment of those withheld monies only if performance meets or exceeds established benchmarks. Use of the bonus payment system is intended to create incentives to meet performance benchmarks because additional income can be realized. This methodology carries lower financial risk for the provider of care (versus the alternative payment system) and may be successful in reducing use of some higher-cost medical procedures that are not medically compelling. Thus, two goals may be met, improved care and lowered cost.

When Pay for Performance is managed by withholding a portion of contracted dollars as an incentive for achieving specific outcomes, the provider carries greater financial risk. This is because some of the money the provider would ordinarily earn is now tied to performance. If those performance targets are not met, then the provider does not receive all of the income that would otherwise have been earned. Hospitals, typically having low profit margins (1 to 4%), may not be in a position to assume this type of risk.

There may be some unintended consequences of Pay for Performance systems. When providers are paid for specific health care outcomes they may work to select those patients that are healthier, more responsive to educational efforts, more able to make healthy lifestyle changes and in other ways "assist" the provider in achieving the intended outcomes. While that select group of patients will, as a group, benefit from this payment model, many other patients will not.

Another difficulty in implementing Pay for Performance concerns the fact that there are a multitude of different payers, each conceivably with a different perspective on what the outcome measures should be and each with different, and sometimes onerous, reporting requirements. It is no secret that the U.S. health care industry does not collaborate in ways to assist providers in meeting universally agreed upon goals.

| Writing Exercise 10-3 | What is Pay for Performance? What is a measurable goal that nurses could participate in that would help evaluate the success of care and be a reasonable evaluative tool (and therefore a determinant of reimbursement) in a Pay for Performance environment? |

Care Management or Disease Management

Disease Management can be related to Pay for Performance. The concept of disease management involves targeting specific chronic conditions and improving overall care by following evidence-based practices, engaging patients in their own care, and creating incentives for patients to improve their self care, for instance, increased attention and adherence to medication regimes resulting in lowered risk of complicating medical conditions. Shactman (2004, p. 2) notes that "In the year 2000, 125 million Americans, or 45 percent of the U.S. populations, had at least one chronic condition and accounted for 75 percent of U.S. health spending. It is estimated that by 2020 over half of the population will have a chronic condition and account for 80 percent of spending." If that estimate at 2020 is accurate, then implementing some method of disease management that improves health care outcomes and reduces health care expenses for chronic diseases could have a significant health and financial impact. Interestingly, the major impact may be in cost avoidance, an outcome that is difficult to measure and quantify.

Good disease management provides evidence-based care combined with empowerment of patients to self manage their own health care, particularly for chronic conditions such as diabetes. An obstacle to this trend is that U.S. health care is fragmented, with little communication and coordination of care across different providers (Mechanic, 2004). In addition, as noted by Schactman (2004), health care in the United States is reactive and focused on the treatment of acute conditions, while disease management programs seek to coordinate care across medical providers and to enable the patient to improve their health in such a way that chronic episodes are diminished in number or intensity. A fee-for-service payment system that requires that there be an acute medical condition that is diagnosable to enable payment of a service does little to assist in movement toward a disease management approach to chronic care. In fact the payment system is based upon illness. Without illness the health care industry earns no income. Insurance companies have a financial incentive to support disease management systems if they can see the financial results of those systems in a relatively short period of time; Mechanic (2004) indicates six to twelve months. This is due to the fact that annually most patients who are insured have an opportunity to change or alter their coverage.

Disease management also requires that there be technological support in the form of information management systems, including but not limited to electronic records. Further there needs to be computerized systems to track patients and outcomes and, in the end, to provide that information to payers. These systems are very expensive, however, and often do not communicate effectively across providers due to software differences, again limiting the possible impact of disease management. Still it is likely that disease management will become more prevalent in the future.

Regional Health Information Organization (RHIO) and Advances in Medical Technology

Regional Health Information Organizations, or **RHIOs**, are comprised of health care providers whose patient information is electronic, with providers connected to one another for the rapid exchange of health information about shared patients (Figure 10-7). The objective of RHIOs is to improve the rapid transmission of health care information in order to improve patient care. Improved patient care leads to improved outcomes that then decrease cost, possibly immediately and into the future. For instance, having a physician's office connected electronically to other health care providers allows the physician to communicate health information about a patient to another provider for rapid consultation. It allows communication of medication information from different prescribing doctors to one another, decreasing the risk of inadvertent drug interactions. It allows transmission of x-ray information electronically to a radiologist many miles away for that radiologist to read the x-ray and inform the treating facility, potentially assisting facilities that are unable to have the necessary specialty on-site. There are many other ways in which the electronic exchange of health information will likely transform the health care environment in the future and improve the care of patients.

Several ingredients are required to develop RHIOs. Health care providers must determine that there is a business value in establishing electronic prescription management systems and/or

Figure 10-7
Example of a
Regional Health
Information
Organization.

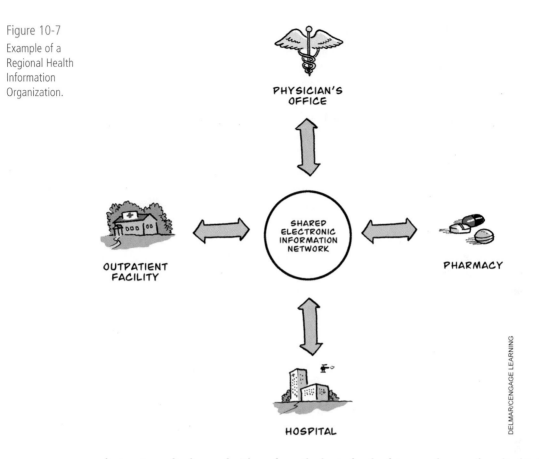

electronic medical records. These form the basis for the future exchange of medical information about patients and for electronic consultation among doctors about particular cases. It is very expensive to invest in the technology to allow exchange of information electronically, an investment that many smaller medical practices find difficult to afford. Further, the investment is not a one-time expense, but rather continues into the future with additional purchase of equipment and software upgrades or changes. This limits their ability to participate and is one of the most significant deterrents to the development of RHIOs. The federal government has periodically indicated that they have interest in the expansion of electronic medical records but thus far has done little to support that development financially, either through grant programs or tax or other incentives.

Another factor in the development of RHIOs is a reflection of the behavior among health care providers themselves. They must recognize that there is inherent value in this method of information exchange and recognize that patient care can be improved and cost lowered. There is increasing emphasis on coordination of care from within the medical community and from insurers. In some instances, as part of the quality improvement program, insurers require that there be exchange of information. To be able to do so "automatically" through electronic means is more efficient and more likely to come closer to "guaranteeing" that exchange.

The community must in some way invest in the infrastructure necessary to make this information exchange relatively simple and cost effective. The most common (though expensive) solution is the investment in fiber loops in the community. Establishing these loops provides business, including the health care business, with less expensive access to linkage with each other and to the Internet. The linkage is also reliable and fast, so data can include images, a necessary component of medical information.

So far RHIOs are largely conceptual in nature. There are many roadblocks to their implementation. Cost is a factor mentioned earlier. Many medical practices do not have the funds needed to make the necessary investment. Even when they have invested in technology, smaller offices do not have the technical knowledge base in their practice to develop the means to exchange information securely with other health care providers. There are also many different software packages, resulting in issues of compatibility. Overcoming incompatibility between different software packages requires technical knowledge and expertise, again often lacking in smaller medical offices. Even when there is the money, knowledge, and desire to affect this exchange, there are issues of data security and patient privacy to consider. There are federal and state laws and regulations designed to ensure that private health information remains just that, private. Any exchange of health information must occur in conformance with those laws and regulations.

A Kaiser Family Foundation Snapshot (2007) provides a good discussion of the impact of medical technology on health care costs. While defining health care technology broadly (including new procedures, drugs, medical devices, and support systems), noted is both the ability of technology to decrease cost (e.g., a drug that reduces invasive surgical procedures), as well as to increase cost (e.g., a new test that requires expensive equipment and expertise). The conclusion, however, is that technology has generally increased cost, but that the increased cost has usually been worth the expense. Two Rand reports (both 2005) appear to support those conclusions and urge the federal government to assist in development of policies that will help with the adoption of health information technology. Into the future, cost-benefit analysis of advances in medical technology will have an impact on the health care financing policies and covered benefits by health insurance plans.

Consumer Directed Health Plans

Consumer Directed Health Plans (CDHPs) attempt to decrease health care expenditures by making consumers share more of the financial risk and burden (Figure 10-8). The logic is that as cost to the patient increases, so do the incentives to choose health care carefully, considering both the cost and the quality in making these decisions. The end result is more efficient (less costly, less unnecessary care) and more effective health care (because considerations of quality are considered in the decision-making process).

The most common methods of designing CDHPs are through the use of high-deductible plans and tiered benefit designs. These are often combined with either **Health Reimbursement Accounts (HRAs)** or **Health Savings Accounts (HSAs)** as a mechanism to offset the financial liability of the patient with the higher out-of-pocket cost incurred with the high deductible or tiered plan. As defined by Buntin et al., (2004, p. 10) "HRAs are employer-funded and employer owned accounts...," they continue: "Unused funds carry over from year to year for employees to use, but unused funds revert to employers when the employee retires or leaves the firm." (p. 10).

Figure 10-8
Consumer Directed
Health Plans shift
more financial
risk to patients.

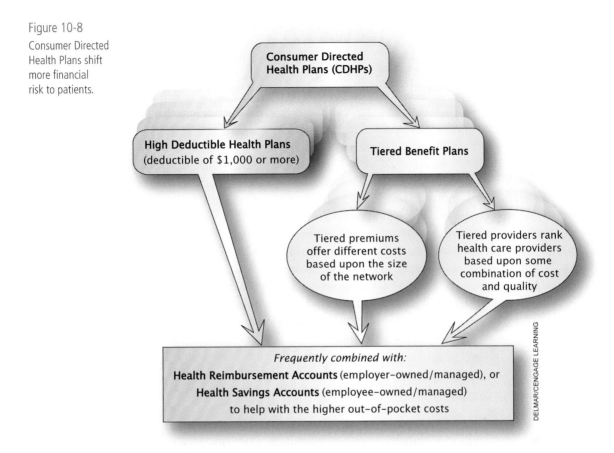

HSAs are designed differently and offer more flexibility. They must be combined with higher-deductible insurance plans and have federally defined maximums on how much money can be deposited into the account. They are "owned by" the employee regardless of who makes the contribution to the account and can be used for purposes other than heath care, with some penalties if the person who owns the account is under 65 years of age.

High-deductible plans are defined as those with deductibles of $1,000 or more. High-deductible plans are becoming more common as health insurance premiums increase and employers look for ways to manage benefit costs for their employees. Their use, though, remains limited as a percentage of the total market (about 3% of the commercial insurance market according to Buntin, et al., 2006). When combined with an HRA or an HSA, a mechanism for saving to meet the deductible and other out-of-pocket health care expenses is created. So, what it the impact on health care of these high-deductible plans?

The goal is for patients to become more knowledgeable about their own health care **(health literacy)**, "shop" for the best quality at the best price (price transparency, to be discussed later), and to therefore make good decisions about both preventive and sick care. The goal for the employer is to satisfy the need to provide health insurance at reasonable cost to the business and with sufficient value to the employee.

What is the real impact of high-deductible plans? There is some evidence that high-deductible plans, when not combined with a HRA or HSA, do in fact decrease health care expenditures, at least until the deductible is met. The next logical question is whether or not people diminish just their use of unnecessary care or their use of necessary care as well. Buntin et al. (2006) reviewed the literature, including discussion of the Rand Health Insurance Experiment (HIE), and determined that although the evidence is limited, there are indications that higher-deductible plans do result in decreased expenditures on health care, particularly in comparison to more traditional plans. Unfortunately, there is also some evidence that there may be a negative impact on use of both necessary and unnecessary care, particularly for poorer individuals with chronic medical conditions. It is critical that research to determine the impact on more vulnerable populations take place for many reasons, including the fact that if there is a negative impact on this group, there will be a shift in cost from private insurance and the patient to government, possibly in the form of Medicaid and Medicare.

Is it true these plans help make patients better "shoppers" and "consumers" of health care? Since these plans regularly place greater emphasis on preventive care, often by not requiring payment of a deductible for these services, and greater emphasis on education of patients to improve their own self management of their health, particularly for prevention of and management of chronic illnesses such as diabetes and hypertension, logically it would seem that this may be the case. Research indicates, where the information is relatively clear and accessible, these designs may be creating better "shoppers." Goldman et al. (2004) determined that increased patient cost for prescription drugs reduced use of prescriptions.

Another option in CDHP is **tiered health plans**. There are two types of tiered plans: those that offer tiered premiums, and those that offer tiered providers. Tiered premiums offer different cost to the individual based upon the openness of the network, with lower costs for premiums in more restrictive provider networks. Alternatively, individuals could choose to select a broader network at a higher price. They then would not need to change doctors if their treating physician is not part of the more restrictive network.

Tiered providers rank health care providers into tiers based upon some combination of cost and quality, such as desired outcomes and patient satisfaction. The expectation is that patients will select lower cost combined with high quality since there are financial incentives to do so. Tiered provider plans are difficult to manage when considerations other than cost are included. There are limited data concerning quality, particularly comparable data across providers. How does use of tiers accommodate differences in the patient base for different hospitals or different medical practices? Do "poorer" outcomes reflect a difference in the level of complexity of the medical conditions or real differences in the quality of the care delivered? Even when the information is available, comparable, and accurate, patients need to be capable of understanding and evaluating the information provided. Thus, there is a need for health literacy in order for this approach to be effective from a cost and a care perspective.

The chronically ill population is at greatest risk in a CDHP environment because of the degree of cost shifting to the patient. In order not to have negative consequences on this group, Yegian (2006) has made several suggestions to the health insurance industry. She suggests altering contributions to HRAs (this variation is not permissible with HSAs) based upon health status and income. Also, definitions of preventive care (and consequently services covered in full) could be broadened so that some required products for treatment of chronic conditions are included as preventive. Prevention of more serious illness or complications becomes the goal rather than occurrence or early detection of the illness itself. Finally, increase use of co-insurance is suggested instead of deductibles. Out-of-pocket expense is leveled over time, resulting in reduction of out-of-pocket costs for care that is necessary while increasing cost for care that is not. Regardless, close monitoring and more complete research on the real outcomes of these new approaches is needed.

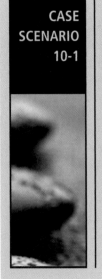

CASE SCENARIO 10-1

A long-term patient enters the for-profit health care clinic where you are working and is determined to have a significant health care condition that will require extensive medical intervention, although there are different treatment options that vary in cost. This patient, having been healthy in the past and in a relatively low-earning job, selected insurance coverage by a high-deductible HSA, and so will bear much of the cost of any medical procedures before his insurance begins to pay.

CASE ANALYSIS

1. Do you inform the treating physician of the economic and insurance position of the patient? If yes, how would you do so?

2. The higher-cost treatment option is more aggressive and, on average, has better outcomes. In combination with the insurance position of the patient, how does this information effect how options are presented to the patient? Should his insurance have any impact on this?

3. Is there an opportunity for the patient to receive some form of charity care, or should there be, even though the clinic is for profit?

Price Transparency

Price transparency at its simplest refers to providing patients with actual or, at least, estimated charges at or before the time of service. It is akin to getting an estimate on repairs to your car. After a brief diagnostic evaluation, a possible repair cost is provided with the understanding the actual cost may vary from the estimate if they find additional problems. It seems simple enough and in some instances is: a dentist can often provide an estimate of cost for a filling, a charge to clean your teeth is relatively fixed, and an eye exam may be a standard price. In fact in medical care estimating cost can be much less easy to accomplish, particularly when the question is often not "what will it cost" but rather "what will it cost me."

Ginsburg (2007) has provided an excellent analysis of price transparency in health care. He points out that many consumers are already participants in price shopping, albeit generally on a secondary level. They have already had prices negotiated for them by their insurer and then make decisions on care primarily based upon whether or not a provider is in network or out of network, with cost to the patient being higher if they select an out-of-network provider. So, price transparency in this context reflects not the actual charges for procedures, which are meaningless to the patient, but rather how much their out-of-pocket expense is paid as coinsurance or co-pays. Of course, if an individual is uninsured then price can become of much more significant concern.

Ginsburg also differentiates between choice of provider (often a function of factors other than price, such as practice style) and the medical service required, where shopping can become more of an option if the care is not an emergency, or a variety of other factors apply. He points out that there are circumstances under which price shopping is more likely to be effective: when the procedure is of defined and lower complexity and so there is less variability in treatment, when the medical intervention is planned rather than urgent, when the medical care is after the diagnosis has been made so care options can be more clearly defined, when bundled services are provided and patients do not need to evaluate individual medical procedures or costs, and when the patient's insurance provides some incentives for lower-cost care. These considerations restrict the value of price transparency and also redefine it for the insured population. In any case it is critical that the information must be usable to the consumer of health care in order for it to be used and to be of value in the decision-making process.

Providing public disclosure of prices may drive up prices rather than depress them. This is because when providers become aware of prices paid to their competition, lower-priced providers will have a basis to request payment increases. Despite this there continues to be momentum toward price disclosure. The Health Finance Management Association, through their Patient Friendly Billing Project, has taken the position that health care providers have a responsibility to assist patients in knowing their potential out-of-pocket costs. This despite the fact that there are many barriers, including federal anti-trust considerations—there is a risk of price collusion when engaging in price disclosure. Also it is very difficult to know exactly how much a specific patient may owe given the variation in possible charges, the variations in specific insurance plan coverage, and the patient's deductible status, among other things.

Charity Care and Benefit to the Community

While health care is a business, it is a business that carries a great deal of emotional baggage for the consumer and for the community in which the care occurs. This is most true for hospitals and less so for individual medical providers. There is an expectation given the nonprofit status of most hospitals that they return benefit to the community. Generally this is defined in terms of the level of **charity care** provided to individuals. Charity care refers to pricing discounts to a patient that are typically determined by income, family size and, at times, debt level. The level of charity care provided by a hospital as a percentage of their total income has been the object of recent scrutiny, with some indications that hospitals may risk losing their nonprofit status if they do not provide "adequate" levels of charity care (Pryor, 2005; Austin et al., 2005).

Focus on charity care has led to increased focus on some pricing practices of hospitals and other health care providers. Hospitals set gross charges for all goods and services. Insurers either set the price that they will pay (e.g., Medicare) or negotiate the amount that they will pay (managed care). It is rare that an insurer will pay all or a percentage of the charge. Uninsured patients, in contrast, have no such leverage in price setting. Therefore they will receive a bill for the actual charge, an amount always higher than that paid by an insurance company. The insurance company has also negotiated the charges that will be paid by individuals insured through them, resulting in lower charges for the insured patient as well. When combined with difficult-to-decipher charity care procedures and/or aggressive collection policies on the part of hospitals, pressure to reevaluate community benefit and tax-exempt status may occur.

Specialty Hospitals and Outpatient Surgery Centers

Specialty hospitals capitalize on a small but influential market, luring patients that have the means to make a selection in health care provider and who want less of a "big hospital" environment. The emphasis is on customer service, satisfaction, and outcomes. Since the scope of the service is more defined than a full-service hospital, specialty hospitals are smaller, more focused in their care, develop expertise in a particular area, have fewer beds, are less likely to have emergency departments and the overhead associated with them, and are more likely to be for-profit rather than not-for-profit.

The National Health Policy Forum (2005) identified three types of specialty clinics: national chains, joint ventures between hospitals and physicians, and physician-owned hospitals. Care tends to be in the areas of orthopedics, cardiology, and surgery. While the number of specialty hospitals remains small in comparison to the total number of general hospitals, they represent a significant influence on health care. Concerns have been raised about the growth in specialty hospitals and the potential impact of those hospitals on the ability of the general hospitals to remain financially competitive and to continue to offer high-quality health care. If, as is posited, specialty hospitals tend to draw the healthier and more affluent patient, then the general hospitals would be left with those patients that are more difficult to treat. Under the Medicare DRG system of payment, the general hospital would therefore be financially penalized for treating the more ill patient. This appears to be the case. Specialty hospitals also treat a smaller percentage of Medicaid and uninsured patients. So, it is possible that the growth of specialty hospitals will have a deleterious impact on the ability of general hospitals to provide the broad range of medical services that communities depend upon. To quote Dummit (2005, p. 10), "Specialty hospitals are the most recent provider group to create a niche by delivering services that had been provided in the general hospital. This situation has played out before with respect to outpatient surgeries, ancillary services, and even post-acute care. In the case of specialty hospitals, competitors to the traditional hospital may have improved service delivery through innovations and efficiencies. However, they may also have reduced the ability of general hospitals to profit from providing certain services. As the delivery of discrete services becomes more efficient, the cross subsidies that often finance unprofitable services or care to unprofitable patients may become more difficult to sustain."

A secondary concern has to do with physician referral to facilities in which they have a financial interest. The risk is that physicians will refer selectively to those hospitals or outpatient surgery centers since they stand to gain financially from the transaction. Finally, there have been questions about comparative quality, although the research at this point indicates that quality is comparable, while patient satisfaction is higher in specialty facilities. Again further research is needed to determine the overall impact of this change in the health care landscape. Do these hospitals have an overall positive, negative, or neutral impact on health care in the community? How does their growth affect the general hospitals, not limited to the areas in which the specialty hospitals operate, but more broadly in terms of services, patient mix, and ability to continue to provide uncompensated care?

Joint Ventures

Since the health care industry is very competitive and hospitals are constrained by both revenue decreases and cost increases, hospitals are continuing to initiate **joint ventures** with other providers to the health care industry, including physicians. As the percentage of surgeries performed in a hospital setting (versus an ambulatory surgery center) has declined to about 22% in the early 2000s, hospitals need to develop business lines that reflect the new realities of the health care market. Oftentimes, the propinquity of the organizations forming the joint venture can result in additional cost savings from resulting efficiencies. Joint ventures with physicians have the added advantage of creating a strategic alliance between the two entities, potentially strengthening the economic position of both. It is possible to strengthen the existing business while growing the business in new ways by expanding a particular service, improving access, or moving into new market areas. Joint ventures between hospitals and physicians must be developed carefully so as to meet federal regulatory requirements (Stark law and the Anti-Kickback Statute), and also to not jeopardize a hospital's tax-exempt status. While all such arrangements require legal review to ensure compliance with the various state and federal regulations, a basic principal of any joint venture is that it should involve new expense, new service, and a contribution by the physicians of money, expertise, or business risk. Otherwise the endeavor will be suspect and potentially perceived by regulatory agencies, particularly the Office of the Inspector General (OIG), as for the primary benefit of referrals. The Healthcare Financial Management Association provides a report that analyzes the risk-benefits of joint ventures while reviewing the legal framework and making suggestions for structuring such relationships in a mutually beneficial manner (Healthcare Financial Management Association, 2006).

Changing Population Demographics and Long-Term Care

Meeting the health care needs of the growing number of elderly is a national concern (Figure 10-9). People are living longer. Older people also have a higher likelihood of having chronic illness or of developing a health need. They also are more likely to need higher levels of support in meeting those health care needs. Coupled with changes in payment for hospital-based care that has resulted in discharge of Medicare recipients earlier and with more immediate medical care needs, there is increased demand for home health care, assisted living, and nursing home care. Long-term care, broadly defined as including nursing homes, assisted living, home health care, rehabilitation, hospice and care provided by friends and family, is a growth industry (Spillman, Liu, & McGilliard, 2002; Brodt, 2007; Eastaugh, 1998).

Figure 10-9
The expanding elderly population makes long-term care a growth industry. *(Image copyright Orange Line Media, 2009. Used under license from Shutterstock.com.)*

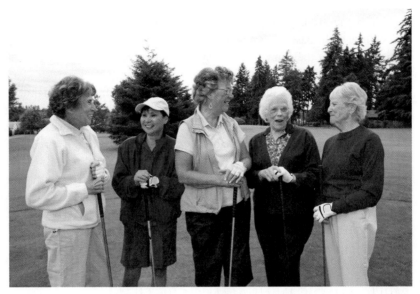

Long-term care, especially nursing home care, is very expensive. Tucker, Kassner, Mullen, and Coleman (2000) estimated the annual cost of care at that point in time at $56,000. Even those with reasonable financial resources would have them drained quickly. Thus, most nursing home care is paid for by Medicaid and Medicare (Eastaugh, 1998; Tucker et al., 2000). Designing options for care that combine some cost efficiencies (and less of an institutional environment than a nursing home affords) with higher levels of consumer satisfaction and autonomy have led to the development of assisted living facilities and communities that offer a range of housing and supports that enable an individual to continue to live in the same basic community, but to "graduate" to higher levels of care as the need occurs. Eastaugh terms these continuing health care communities (CHCCs). There has also been some growth in home health care, including such care paid for through public means. The risk in the expansion of public payment for home health care is that there will be an increase in demand for those services, an increase that actually represents cost shifting. Instead of the care being provided through friends and family, existence of a publicly supported payment system will shift that care to home health care agencies and therefore shift payment to public resources.

Growth of the Long Term Care (LTC) insurance industry is another option. So far this has been a slow-growth industry, perhaps because it is unclear if the insurance as defined thus far will be worth the investment, and because there are other demands on the income that would be used to pay these premiums. Eastaugh (1998) suggests that combining acute with chronic care coverage may be a more reasonable approach. It spreads risk for the insurance company and may be more marketable.

Lynn (2004) and Lynn and Adamson (2003) have examined the needs of the growing aged population and concluded that there needs to be change in the health care delivery system for the growing number of elderly. To put this in context, in Across the States (Gibson et al., 2004, p. vi), the estimate is that in 2005 only 3 states had 15% of their population over age 65, but by 2020, 42 states will have 15% or more of their population over age 65. In addition, the number of individuals over age 85, people who are most likely to have more and more significant health care needs, is growing as well. Continuing to provide medical care to these individuals as we have in the past will not necessarily be a good strategy for the future. It is also important to recognize that the growth of this segment of the population will require an expansion of the personnel needed to provide the care.

Lynn (2004) indicates that the number of older adults that have extended periods of diminishing capacity and who live for extended periods of time while needing a high level of support and care (e.g., dementia patients) is growing. Unfortunately, the health care community is ill prepared to respond. Both the health care system and the health care reimbursement system are designed to provide acute care and care in clearly defined periods of time. Hospice care is not reimbursed for longer or intermittent periods of time when death might occur, limiting the ability of that care provider to intervene. Payment systems that reward episodic care will not be most effective in treating the elderly. Needed are coordinated systems of care that are able to both anticipate what care is needed, and to extend that care in a coordinated fashion that includes integration of care and flexible funding (Stone, 2000).

NURSING IMPLICATIONS IN HEALTH CARE FINANCE

There is no question that existing and anticipated growth and changes in health care will continue to increase the demand for nurses. Population trends alone, such as growth of the elderly, will mean that more nurses with geriatric specialty will be needed. Those services will be delivered in a variety of settings and will be of differing levels of complexity. Technology may allow the elderly that presently need to go into a care environment to remain in their home or in a less institutional setting. Nurses will be needed to provide some of that care. Continued growth of less invasive surgical procedures, procedures that have allowed patients to leave a hospital setting earlier, will likely continue to be developed. This may result in an increased need to have nurses provide some post-hospital care and to educate patients more thoroughly in self care.

Additionally, increased emphasis on care management and preventive health care will require nurses to manage those programs and to deliver the required services. Effective preventative care and disease management, an area that is expected to receive increased emphasis in the future, will require that nurses be available to support these efforts. So, there may be a market for nurses that are providing less direct care and more management and monitoring of care.

Emphasis on cost and shortages of physicians will increase the demand for more Nurse Practitioners and Advanced Practice Nurses, particularly as the focus shifts to preventive care. More and more Nurse Practitioners and Advanced Practice Nurses are substituting for doctors in their areas of expertise and are furnishing the front line of medical care in geographic areas where there are shortages of doctors. This trend is apt to continue, again as the need for medical personnel increases while the supply of physicians does not grow to meet the demand.

Nurses will need to work more independently in more community-based settings and will be less reliant upon physicians. Again, this is a function of a shift from reactive to proactive health care.

As technology develops, nurses will need to become more and more fluent in that technology, requiring additional training and skill development. More educated and informed consumers will result in the development of new jobs in marketing and educational environments. Technological growth and the growth of technology to exchange health care information among different providers will provide nurses with an opportunity to work in software development that meets the needs of the provider and consumer communities as well as in RHIOs.

Nurses already are in high demand in accounting and the legal field, especially if they also seek the additional degrees (CPA, JD) to work fully in those fields. Health care is unlikely to become less regulated, so these opportunities will continue to expand.

Nurses will need to be able to be flexible in their pursuit of career goals. What they train for today may not be the work that they perform in the future. They need to be able to respond to shifts in demand, gain education throughout their career, and to continue to work as a patient advocate. This advocacy role will become more important as the complexity of the health care system and the decisions that individual patients need to make continue to multiply.

SUMMARY

It is important to understand health care financing in order to respond to changes in health care delivery that may be driven by cost considerations. Health care is paid for from three sources: the patient, the government, and the insurance industry. Pricing and cost considerations respond to market conditions that include a host of factors. Included are pressures to limit expense as a percentage of the GNP and to make health care affordable to individuals, employers, and insurers, including the government. The public good makes the push to decrease the number of uninsured individuals a goal. It also makes the pressure for price transparency and accountability to the patient likely to continue. Additional current drivers of change in the market include various methods of tying quality of care to payment for that care. At the same time providers of care need to be able to cover their actual costs in order to continue to exist and continue to deliver care, making joint ventures and marketing of their service more likely. Demographic changes in the country will cause providers and insurers alike to examine the methods of service delivery and payment. It is an exciting time in the field and one that offers many opportunities within the nursing profession.

Policy makers face significant challenges, short and longer term, as they think about how the nation will pay for the growing cost of health care... Developing the philosophical, ethical, and political framework necessary to balance the benefits of future advances with our ability to pay for them is one of the next great challenges for health policy.

–Kaiser Family Foundation

REFERENCES

AUSTIN, B., Burton, A., DeFrancesco, L., Frieden-zohn, I., Patel, S., Patterson, M., & Trinity, M. (2005). State of the states: Finding alternate routes. *AcademyHealth*, January 2005. Retrieved April 14, 2009, from http://govinfo.library.unt.edu/chc/resources/papers/stateofstates2005.pdf

BARTH, J., & Greene, J. (2007). Encouraging healthy behaviors in medicaid: Early lessons from Florida and Idaho. *Center for Health Care Strategies, Inc.* July 2007. Retrieved April 14, 2009, from http://www.chcs.org/publications3960/publications_show.htm?doc_id=507380

BELLA, M., Goldsmith, S., & Somers, S. (2006). Medicaid "best buys" for 2007: Promising reform strategies for governors. *Center for Health Care Strategies, Inc.* December 2006. Retrieved April 14, 2009, from http://www.chcs.org/usr_doc/Medicaid_Best_Buys_2007.pdf

BRODT, A., Burton, A., Cohn, D., Cox, B., Folsom, A., Friednzohn, I., Martinez-Vidal, E., & Trinity, M. (2007). State of the states: Building hope, raising expectations. *AcademyHealth*, December 2007. Retrieved April 14, 2009, from http://www.rwjf.org/pr/product.jsp?id=15929

BUNTIN, M., Damberg C., Haviland, A., Kapur, K., Lurie, N., McDevitt, R., & Marquis, M. S. (2006). Consumer-directed health care: Early evidence about effects on cost and quality. *Health Affairs*, October 2006. Retrieved April 14, 2009, from http://content.healthaffairs.org/cgi/content/abstract/25/6/w516

BUNTIN, M., Damberg, C., Haviland, A., Lurie, N., Kapur, K., & Marquis, M. S. (2005). "Consumer-directed" health plans: Implications for health care quality and cost. *California HealthCare Foundation*, June 2005. Retrieved April 14, 2009, from http://www.chcf.org/documents/insurance/ConsumerDirHealthPlansQualityCost.pdf

CALIFORNIA HEALTHCARE FOUNDATION. (2005). *U.S. health care spending: Quick reference guide.* Retrieved April 14, 2009, from https://broker.beerepurves.com/News/Newsletter/pdf/Apr2005/NHEQuickReference.pdf

CIMASI, R. J. (2005, November). *The attack on specialty and niche providers.* Paper presented at Physician Agreements and Ventures, Chicago, IL.

CLEMONS-COPE, L., & Garrett, B. (2006). Changes in employer-sponsored health insurance sponsorship, eligibility, and participation: 2001 to 2005. *The Henry J. Kaiser Family Foundation*, December 2006. Retrieved April 14, 2009, from http://www.kff.org/uninsured/upload/7599.pdf

CRIPPEN, D. (2007). Identifying Medicaid's best buys. *CHCS/Harvard Government Innovators Network "Best Buys" Call*, February 2007. Retrieved April 14, 2009, from http://www.chcs.org/usr_doc/DCrippen.pdf

DAMBERG, C. (2005). Statement of Cheryl L. Damberg, Ph.D. Senior Policy Researcher, The RAND Corporation Before the Department of Insurance State of California. *The RAND Corporation*, September 20, 2005. Retrieved April 14, 2009, from http://www.rand.org/pubs/testimonies/2005/RAND_CT249.pdf

DeNAVAS-WALT, C., Proctor, B., & Smith, J. (2007). Income, poverty, and health insurance coverage in the United States: 2006. *U.S. Census Bureau, Current Population Reports*, 60–233.

DUMMITT, L. A. (2005). Specialty hospitals: Can general hospitals compete? *National Health Policy Forum*, 84, July 2005. Retrieved April 14, 2009, from http://www.nhpf.org/library/issue-briefs/IB804_SpHospitals_07-13-05.pdf

EASTAUGH, S. (1998). *Health care finance: Cost, productivity, and strategic design.* Gaithersberg, MD: Aspen Publishers.

GIBSON, M. J., Gregory, S., Houser, A. N., & Fox-Grage, W. (2004). Across the states: Profiles of long-term care 2004. *AARP Public Policy Institute*, December 2004. Retrieved April 14, 2009, from http://www.aarp.org/research/reference/statistics/across_the_states_profiles_of_long-term_care_2004.html

GINSBERG, P. B. (2007). Shopping for price in medical care. *Health Affairs, 26*(2), w208–w216.

GOLDMAN, D., & McGlynn, E. (2005). U.S. health care: Facts about cost, access, and quality. *RAND Health*, January 2005. Retrieved April 14, 2009, fromhttp://www.rand.org/pubs/corporate_pubs/2005/RAND_CP484.1.pdf

GOLDMAN, D., Smith, J. P., & Sood, N. (2006). The public spends little to provide health care on undocumented immigrants. *RAND Labor and Population Fact Sheet,* November/December 2006. Retrieved April 14, 2009, from http://www.rand.org/pubs/research_briefs/2006/RAND_RB9230.pdf

GOODMAN, J. C. (2006). What is consumer-directed health care? *Health Affairs, 25*(6), w540–w543.

GREENE, J. (2007). Medicaid efforts to incentivize healthy behavoirs. *Center for Health Care Strategies, Inc.*, July 2007. Retrieved April 14, 2009, from http://www.chcs.org/usr_doc/Medicaid_Efforts_to_Incentivize_Healthy_Behaviors.pdf

HADLEY, J. (2007). Insurance coverage, medical care use, and short-term health changes following an unintentional injury or the onset of chronic condition. *The Journal of the American Medical Association, 297*(10), 1073–1084.

HEALTHCARE FINANCIAL MANAGEMENT ASSOCIATION. (2006). *Consumerism in health care: Achieve a consumer-oriented revenue cycle.* Retrieved April 14, 2009, from http://www.mckesson.com/static_files/McKesson.com/MPT/Documents/PFB%20Brochure_FullRevise.pdf

HIBBARD, J., Stockard, J., & Tusler, M. (2005). Hospital performance reports: Impact on quality market share and reputation. *Health Affairs*, July/August, 1150–1160.

THE JOINT COMMISSION. (2007). *"What did the doctor say?:" Improving health literacy to protect patient safety.* Retrieved April 14, 2009, from http://www.jointcommission.org/NR/rdonlyres/D5248B2E-E7E6-4121-8874-99C7B4888301/0/improving_health_literacy.pdf

KAHN, J., Kronick, R., Kreger, M., & Gans, D. (2005). The cost of health insurance administration in California: Estimates for insurers, physicians, and hospitals. *Health Affairs*, 24(6), 1629–1636.

KAISER FAMILY FOUNDATION. (2007). *Heath care costs: A primer.* Retrieved April 14, 2009, from http://www.kff.org/insurance/7670.cfm

KAISER FAMILY FOUNDATION. (2007). *Health care spending in the United States and OECD countries.* Retrieved April 14, 2009, from http://www.kff.org/insurance/snapshot/chcm010307oth.cfm

KAISER FAMILY FOUNDATION. (2007). *Health coverage for low-income Americans: An evidence-based approach to public policy.* Retrieved April 14, 2009, from http://www.kff.org/uninsured/upload/7476.pdf

KAISER FAMILY FOUNDATION. (2007). *How changes in medical technology affect health care costs.* Retrieved April 14, 2009, from http://www.kff.org/insurance/snapshot/chcm030807oth.cfm

KAISER FAMILY FOUNDATION. (2006). *Comparing projected growth in health care expenditures and the economy.* Retrieved April 14, 2009, from http://www.kff.org/insurance/snapshot/chcm050206oth2.cfm

KAISER FAMILY FOUNDATION. (2005). *Trends and indicators in the changing health care marketplace.* Retrieved April 14, 2009, from http://www.kff.org/insurance/7031/index.cfm

KRONICK, R., Bella, M., Gilmer, T., & Somers, S. (2007). The faces of Medicaid II: Recognizing the care needs of people with multiple chronic conditions. *Center for Health Care Strategies, Inc.,* October 2007. Retrieved April 14, 2009, from http://www.chcs.org/publications3960/publications_show.htm?doc_id=540806

KU, L., Ellwood, M., Hoag, S., Ormond, B., & Woodridge, J. (2000). Evolution of Medicaid managed care systems and eligibility expansions. *Health Care Financing Review,* Winter 2000, *22*(2), 7–27.

LLANOS, K., Rothstein, J., Dyer, M. B., & Ballit, M. (2007). Physician pay-for-performance in Medicaid: A guide for states. *Center for Health Care*

Strategies, Inc., March 2007. Retrieved April 14, 2009, from http://www.chcs.org/publications3960/publications_show.htm?doc_id=471272

LYNN, J. (2004). *Sick to death and not going to take it anymore: Reforming health care for the last years of life.* Berkeley, CA: University of California Press.

LYNN, J., & Adamson, D. (2003). Adapting health care to serious chronic illness in old age. *RAND Health White Paper,* WP-137, 2003. Retrieved April 14, 2009, from http://www.medicaring.org/whitepaper

MECHANIC, R. (2004). *Will care management improve the value of U.S. health care?* Paper presented at the Eleventh Annual Princeton Conference, Princeton, NJ.

McGLYNN, E., Asch, S., Adams, J., Keesey, J., Hicks, J., DeCristofaro, A., & Kerr, E. (2003). The quality of health care delivered to adults in the United States. *New England Journal of Medicine, 348*(26), 2635–2645.

NATIONAL ASSOCIATION OF CHAIN DRUG STORES. (2007). *Industry facts-at-a-glance.* Retrieved April 14, 2009, from http://www.nacds.org/wmspage.cfm?parm1=507

PRYOR, C. (2005). The hospital billing and collections flap: It's not over yet. *Journal of Health Care Compliance,* May/June 2005, 25–30.

THE RAND CORPORATION. (2006). *Cutting drug co-payments for sicker patients on cholesterol-lowering drugs could save a billion dollars every year.* Retrieved April 14, 2009, from http://www.rand.org/pubs/research_briefs/RB9169/index1.html

THE RAND CORPORATION. (2006). *The first national report card on quality of health care in America.* Retrieved April 14, 2009, from http://www.rand.org/pubs/research_briefs/2006/RAND_RB9053-2.pdf

THE RAND CORPORATION. (2005). *Electronic prescribing systems: Making it safer to take your medicine?* Retrieved April 14, 2009, from http://www.rand.org/pubs/research_briefs/2005/RAND_RB9052.pdf

THE RAND CORPORATION. (2005). *Health information technology: Can HIT lower costs and improve quality?* Retrieved April 14, 2009, from http://www.rand.org/pubs/research_briefs/2005/RAND_RB9136.pdf

ROSENBAUM, S. (2006). Defined-contribution plans and limited-benefit arrangements: Implications for Medicaid beneficiaries. *The George Washington University Medical Center,* September 2006. Retrieved April 14, 2009, from http://www.gwumc.edu/sphhs/departments/healthpolicy/chsrp/downloads/Rosenbaum_AHIP_FNL_091306.pdf

ROSS, M. N. (2006). Consumer-directed health care: It's not whether the glass is half-empty, but why. *Health Affairs, 25*(6), w552–w554.

SCHOEN, C., Osborn, R., Huynh, P. T., Doty, M., Zapert, K., Peugh, J., & Davis, K. (2005). Take the pulse of health care systems: Experiences of patients with health problems in six countries. *Health Affairs,* November 2005.

SCHACTMAN, D. (2004). *Managing cost and quality through the health care delivery system.* Policy Brief at the Eleventh Annual Princeton Conference, Princeton, NJ.

SPILLMAN, B. C., Liu, K., & McGilliard, C. (2002). Trends in residential long-term care: Use of nursing homes and assisted living and characteristics of facilities and residents. *U.S. Department of Health and Human Services,* November 2002. Retrieved April 14, 2009, from http://aspe.hhs.gov/daltcp/reports/rltct.pdf

STONE, R. I. (2000). Long-term care for the elderly with disabilities: Current policy, emerging trends, and implications for the twenty-first century. *Millbank Memorial Fund,* August 2000. Retrieved April 14, 2009, from http://www.milbank.org/reports/0008stone/LongTermCare_Mech5.pdf

THRALL, J. (2004). The emerging role of pay-for-performance contracting for health care services. *Radiology, 233,* 637–640.

THOMPKINS, C., Altman, S., & Eilat, E. (2006). The precarious pricing system for hospital services. *Health Affairs, 25*(1), 45–46.

TUCKER, N., Kassner, E., Mullen, F., & Coleman, B. (2000). Long-term care. *AARP Fact Sheet,* May 2000. Retrieved April 14, 2009, from http://www.aarp.org/research/longtermcare/trends/aresearch-import-672-FS27R.html

UNITED STATES GENERAL ACCOUNTING OFFICE. (2003). Specialty hospitals: Geographic location, services provided, and financial performance. *United States General Accounting Office Report to Congressional Requestors*, October 2003. Retrieved April 14, 2009, from http://www.gao.gov/new.items/d04167.pdf

WOO, A., Ranji, U., Lundy, J., & Chen, F. (2006). Prescription drug costs: Background brief. *The Henry J. Kaiser Family Foundation*, 2006. Retrieved April 14, 2009, from http://www.kaiseredu.org/topics_im.asp?id=352&parentID=68&imID=1

YEGIAN, J. M. (2006) Coordinated care in a "consumer-driven" health system. *Health Affairs*, October 2006. Retrieved April 14, 2009, from http://content.healthaffairs.org/cgi/content/short/hlthaff.25.w531v1

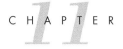

INSURANCE AND ITS EFFECTS ON HEALTH CARE IN THE U.S.

MARY JO REGAN-KUBINSKI

PhD, RN, Dean, Nursing and Health Professions, Indiana University South Bend

AILEEN WEHREN

EdD, Vice President Systems Administration, Porter-Starke Services, Inc.

I have an almost complete disregard of precedent and a faith in the possibility of something better. It irritates me to be told how things always have been done... I defy the tyranny of precedent. I cannot afford the luxury of a closed mind. I go for anything new that might improve the past.

–Clara Barton

LEARNING OBJECTIVES

At the completion of the chapter, the learner should be able to do the following:

1. Relate the history and evolution of health care insurance in the United States.
2. Explain how patient insurance coverage may influence treatment decisions.
3. Discuss the implications of employee-provided health insurance as a major means of financing health care.
4. Describe the various types of public funding for health care insurance.
5. Discuss the implications of a mixed public/private model for provision of health care insurance in the United States.
6. Outline implications for health policy and political action; participate as an informed citizen.

KEY TERMS

Beneficiary
Capitation
Co-Payment
Fee-For-Service
Group-Model HMO
Health Maintenance
   Organization (HMO)

Indemnity Plans
Insurance
Managed Care
   Organization (MCO)
Medicaid
Medicare
Medigap

Parity
Premiums/Group Premiums
Risk
Service Plans
Staff-Model HMO
State Childrens' Health
   Insurance Program (SCHIP)

INTRODUCTION

The complexity of the health care system in the United States is illustrated by financing structure for health care in this country. In this chapter, you will examine the various insurance models that pay for health care in the United States, and the historical and social contexts in which they developed. You will explore the systems of insurance coverage that have evolved to meet the expense of health care services for different groups of people in the United States. Hopefully, you will find yourself thinking about this structure, and its effects and consequences on your patients and your career.

The United States remains the only large, industrial nation that does not provide national health insurance for its citizens. The mix of the private, employer-based insurance and various forms of governmental insurance programs is uniquely American. The current structures to pay for health care rely on employers, who provide health care as a part of benefits packages, and governmental programs, which provide coverage for groups that are considered in need of such coverage. There are no mechanisms in place to assure that coverage is available or equitable for all citizens, and the cost of providing medical care in the United States continues to be a social and political issue.

The employer-based system for providing health insurance coverage places a financial burden on those employers who choose to or who are required by law to provide medical coverage. Meanwhile, as costs continue to rise, health insurance is becoming increasingly unaffordable for employers. Small companies require higher out-of-pocket costs of their workers than do large employers. Employers pass on the increase in cost of coverage to workers in the form of higher premiums, or they offer less coverage for the same price. The cost of providing insurance is also passed on to consumers in the often hidden means of higher prices. Employers who provide retiree health benefits also face the challenge of increases in premiums, with some reducing or eliminating retiree coverage.

At the same time, the profits of health insurance companies are increasing; the industry average was from 3 to 5%, and rose to 6% in 2007 (*The Washington Post*, "Rise in Cost of Employer-Paid Health Insurance Slows," 9/12/07). At the same time, executive compensation of many of the large health insurance providers has skyrocketed. As examples, in 2006, the CEO of Humana earned $3.3 million and the CEO of Aetna earned $2.2 million (*Forbes*, "Executive Pay: What the Boss Makes," 2006).

Since 2001, premiums for health insurance have gone up 78%; wages have increased 19% (Figure 11-1). The average annual premium for family coverage in 2007 was $12,106, roughly equivalent to the salary of a full-time worker making minimum wage (*Washington Post*, "Cost of Employer Provided Insurance," September 12, 2007).

Federal and state programs that provide health care coverage have been developed to address gaps in the employer-based model. For groups of people who are not employed or who cannot be employed due to age, disease, or disability, governmental programs provide a safety-net so that paying for health care becomes more feasible. However, offering more health care benefits to more people increases the burden on tax payers, and raises questions about who should be

Figure 11-1
Since 2001, increases in health insurance premiums have outpaced wage increases. *(Source: Washington Post, "Cost of Employer Provided Insurance," September 12, 2007.)*

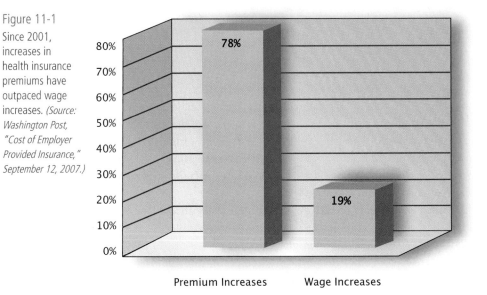

provided coverage, and what that coverage should include. The same cost increases that affect the ability of employers to provide coverage also affect governmental programs, and similar cost-containment measures are taken by both the private and the public sectors.

Since businesses are trying to compete in a global economy, and as risk-pools shift with the aging of the population, the context and conditions that had existed when health insurance plans were first introduced have all changed dramatically. Change is a constant. Perhaps the health care insurance and health care delivery system are so intertwined that they can no longer be considered as separate issues. It may be that a quality, effective health care delivery system is dependent upon—or may be the same as—an effective means of providing health care insurance for the American people. Solutions for the complex systems that have evolved cannot be simple. Solutions must be both practical and political, and when costs are high, strategies must be bold.

The current health care insurance debate in the United States illustrates the importance and the complexity of the matter of paying for health care in this country. It is important for nurses to be knowledgeable about health insurance for many reasons (Figure 11-2). First, it is important for nurses as individuals to comprehend the coverage that they have, and to be able to make informed decisions when choices are available. Second, nurses increasingly need to explain coverage to patients. Third, nurses need to recognize how and why treatment decisions may be made on the basis of the kind of coverage a person has. Fourth, nurses need to understand the history of the insurance evolution in the United States, compare and contrast that evolution with other models, and participate as informed citizens in political and policy discussions about health insurance. Finally, nurses may be in the position of one day exerting influence on future models for payment for health care and the provision of insurance coverage. Knowledge is power in these discussions.

Figure 11-2

Nurses must be knowledgeable about health insurance not only for their own benefit, but so they can explain a patient's coverage and can participate in shaping political and policy discussions in the future.

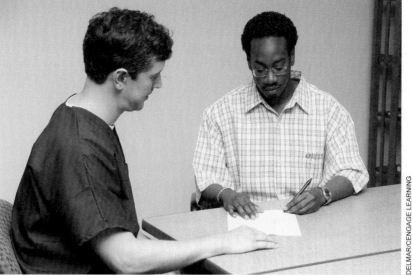

DELMAR/CENGAGE LEARNING

INSURANCE: FUNCTION AND DEFINITION

Discussions about health insurance usually take place without much thought or consideration given to the actual function and the true definition of insurance. Perhaps it is assumed that everyone "knows" what insurance is, and what it is designed to do. However, the history of health care in the United States has been accompanied by variations in the conceptualization of medical insurance, as well as unique in the many permutations in available or typical insurance coverage for medical conditions and health care. Continuing and current political discussions about health care, health insurance, and paying for health care have kept insurance in the public view, and on nurses' minds.

Insurance is, at its most basic, a protection from **risk**. Insurance presupposes that conditions will occur at random. Using a common example, when tornadoes strike, they hit objects at random. No one can know for certain what will be hit, even if the tornado itself has been forecast. Some events can be predicted, or their rate of occurrence can be estimated within a certain, defined group. We know that the Midwestern section of the country is more susceptible to tornadoes than the coasts. The Gulf Coasts, on the other hand, are more susceptible to hurricanes. We are all familiar with car insurance. Insurance companies predict the rate of accidents, estimate their costs for repairing damages and paying for injuries, and then base the premium they charge on the number of people who will be insured. A **premium** is the amount paid to the insurance company to provide selected coverage. We know that certain groups of drivers, such as teen boys, are more likely to be involved in accidents. While any one boy may be accident free, the cost of insuring the entire group increases because teen boys are members of the group. The cost of covering all is shared by the group, but some group members may be charged higher premiums for the same coverage.

In health care, the consumers or the holders of health insurance seek to protect themselves from the financial risk resulting from a major medical problem. Health insurance plans were developed in the United States as a means of ensuring that individuals and families were not economically devastated by a catastrophic illness. They became popular only after the 1930s, when the Great Depression brought financial ruin to many. Most policies covered catastrophic care, or provided coverage for illnesses and injuries that required hospital care. But, governmental policies in the 1940s created incentives that lead to the development of a rather unique arrangement for medical care coverage, and expanded that coverage beyond catastrophic care (Starr, 1982).

Governmental policies set limits on consumer prices and on wages. In 1952, legislation was enacted that made fringe benefits tax free. Together, these policies supported an employer-based model for the provision of medical coverage. Employers could increase the amount of coverage they provided for their employees instead of giving them pay raises. Employees liked the benefit instead of a pay increase because those benefits were not taxed. As a direct result, medical coverage became—and remains—a powerful tool for recruitment and retention of workers. And, also as a direct result of these governmental policies, workers came to expect more and better insurance coverage, coverage that is probably more comprehensive than if individuals purchased coverage on their own (Barr, 2007).

Risk Management

Insurance plans attempt to spread the risk of the cost of providing health care across the group that is covered. A basic premise of the insurance industry is to shift the heavy burden from those who need the most care to the group as a whole (Figure 11-3). The healthy subsidize the care of the unhealthy. Larger pools spread the risk across more people, and pools that represent or contain more healthy individuals have lower initial risk. Health status is a key factor in assigning risk to any group, but the goal is always the same: to reduce and to share risk.

The price of any individual insurance plan is determined by the risk assumed to be present among those who will be insured under that plan. Ratings seek to predict the needs of the group as a whole, with premiums based on the projected expense for the group. The insurer can use the actual experiences of a group to set the rates, or can project the rates based on past experiences with similar groups. Premiums are the cost to the insured; premiums may be the entire responsibility of one party, such as the employer or employee, or a shared responsibility. For employer-provided insurance, the most common model today is a shared model, with employers covering the larger portion of the premium and the employee responsible for the remainder (Barr, 2007).

Types of Insurance

Health insurance can be purchased privately, by individuals, for their own financial security. Private insurance is voluntary coverage. It also can be purchased by groups or by individuals. In the United States, the major purchasers of health insurance are employers. The group concept

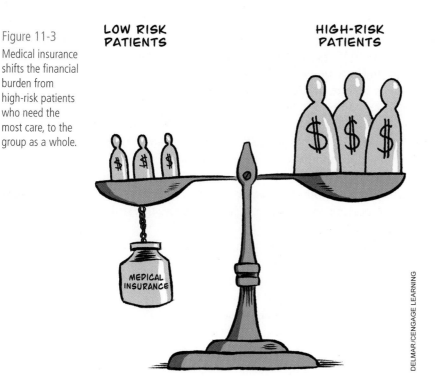

Figure 11-3

Medical insurance shifts the financial burden from high-risk patients who need the most care, to the group as a whole.

LOW RISK PATIENTS

HIGH-RISK PATIENTS

MEDICAL INSURANCE

DELMAR/CENGAGE LEARNING

evolved to a high degree in the United States because of tax incentives and pressure from workers' unions for coverage for workers. Plans vary in their cost to the purchaser, the coverage provided, and the amount of the cost that is born by employer or employee (Barr, 2007).

Health insurance plans also vary in regard to how health care providers are reimbursed for giving care to the insured. Regardless of plan type, each attempts to maximize profits for the parties involved, and the rate of success in actually doing so depends on a number of complex factors, including the health services that are actually used by the beneficiaries.

With **indemnity plans**, the insured, or **beneficiary**, would seek medical care, pay for it, and be reimbursed by the insurance company. The physician or service provider would be paid for each procedure on a **fee-for-service** basis (Barr, 2007), that is, payment is received for each service rendered by the provider. Incentives to provide more care are built into indemnity plan models. The more services provided by the individual physician provider, the greater the profit realized by that individual.

In contrast, **service plans** pay for a set of agreed-upon services that are provided to the insured, as needed. A hospital or physician is paid and is responsible to provide all of the specified care for the beneficiary at the negotiated price. The money received to pay for provided services is pooled and spread out among all of the beneficiaries. In service plans, physicians typically work for a salary, rather than being paid per service. Any cost savings are profit for the provider, while cost overages are their responsibility. It is a simple deduction that providing care to healthier beneficiaries or limiting the services provided under the plan increase profits for the provider.

Although indemnity plans continued as the dominant form of health insurance, some service plans did emerge as early as 1929 (Kongstvedt, 1995). These plans provided medical coverage for well-defined groups, and paid for that care directly to the care provider, as compared to providers billing beneficiaries for care after it was delivered. Service plans arose to cover medical costs for groups such as farm cooperatives, or large factories, or even towns.

In the United States, service plans were actively discouraged by the American Medical Association (AMA) since as far back as the 1930s (Barr, 2007; Starr, 1982). The AMA stated that it was unethical for physicians to be paid a salary instead of being paid on a fee-for-service basis. Physicians who violated the AMA ethical standards lost hospital privileges, and could no longer practice medicine. Together with the governmental policies that favored employer-provided insurance, these AMA pronouncements created powerful forces that shaped how medical care is paid for in the United States.

The extent to which service or **capitation** plans might have grown without the interference of the political and medical systems is, of course, not known. Although service plans in general did not proliferate in the early 20th century, on a large part because of AMA opposition, such plans did in fact survive and eventually became the model for managed care in the United States in later years. The most well-known of these plans is the Kaiser-Permanente system in California, founded in 1942. Also established at about the same time, in 1947, was the Group Health Cooperative of Puget Sound in Seattle, Washington (Kongstvedt, 1995). These service plans were designed to spread out the risk of providing health care for a defined population, those enrolled in the plan, and to shift responsibility of care from the solo provider to the corporation that formed the plan. Service plans were intended to address issues such as quality, cost, and professional performance by adding a structure that could monitor and spread costs among multiple providers, monitor outcomes, and hold providers accountable for those outcomes (Barr, 2007; Kongstvedt, 1995).

Fee-for-Service

Initially, medical insurance followed the existing standards and practices used for other types of insurance by the insurance industry. In this model, either an individual, or more often, a group (such as an employer) purchased a policy. Insurance companies had nothing to do with the provision of medical care. The beneficiary sought care wherever they chose, and was reimbursed after care was provided. Insurance companies made a profit when the costs of care used by beneficiaries were lower than the premiums paid by the purchaser of the policy.

In this model, physicians were paid on a fee-for-service basis; the more services they provided, the higher their pay. Insurance providers paid physicians at negotiated rates and their incentives to keep costs down were minimal. Fee-for-service stands in contrast to salary as a form of payment. With a salary, the provider is paid for time at the same rate regardless of the number or type of services provided during that time frame.

Premiums charged by insurance companies were negotiated; not every individual or company purchasing insurance paid the same price for that coverage. When large companies sought to provide coverage for their employees, the corporation was often able to negotiate lower purchase prices based on volume. A larger volume of beneficiaries allows costs to be spread out among many people. There are presumably more healthy individuals to share the burden of cost of those in the group than those who require medical services, and this cost sharing allows for lower premiums for all (Barr, 2007).

Group premiums are based primarily on past use of medical services by the group itself, with overhead costs for managing the processing of claims factored in. As long as group membership and health status of members remain fairly stable, premiums could be set with a good deal of accuracy. However, another factor also influences the cost to insurers: the actual cost of delivery of health care. With technological advances, the cost of care provision can dramatically increase the cost of doing business for insurance companies. In turn, the insurance companies pass along the cost increases in the form of higher premiums to provide coverage.

Historically, in the traditional model, insurance provided coverage for high-cost medical events. After payment of a deductible by the beneficiary, insurance paid for the rest of the covered care. In the early years of health care insurance there was no coverage for visits to doctors' offices, preventive services, or medications. Ancillary treatments such as radiology services and laboratory services were covered for hospitalized patients, but only while they were hospitalized and in emergencies. But routine diagnostic testing for any outpatient services was not covered by insurance plans. As a result, patients were hospitalized for diagnostic testing because insurance coverage paid for hospital-based testing. Additionally, this particular arrangement created a financial incentive for the physician, whose income was based on a fee-for-service model. Hospital care is more costly than outpatient care, and so hospitalizing a patient was in the physician's best financial interest.

Nurses did not directly benefit from a fee-for-service model, but nursing jobs were created in response to the need to provide more inpatient care for those whose insurance covered all hospital-based services. The practice of nursing evolved in tandem with the fee-for-service model for payment of health care, but the profession of nursing was not a significant factor in determining how health care was paid for in the United States.

MANAGED CARE

In the 1980s, the costs to provide medical care rose dramatically. In the early 1990s, employers, the primary providers of private insurance coverage in the United States, were financially challenged to cover the increased cost of premiums. Some large corporate employers began to provide health care insurance for their own employees rather than purchase insurance from traditional insurance companies, essentially forming their own insurance company. These employers funded health care coverage by using the dollars that they would have spent on insurance to pay for the health care of their employees. The insurance company was no longer used as an intermediary, and the corporations were able to reduce their overhead costs. However, the fee-for-service or indemnity model of payment was still in effect. Physicians and hospitals continued to charge for each service provided, and there were few constraints placed on spending. Self-insurance did not provide the financial relief that corporations sought when they initiated it.

Unlike indemnity plans, service plans paid for all medical care for those covered under them. The beneficiary had no out-of-pocket costs for the negotiated coverage. The money collected from premiums was pooled and used to pay for care. Service plans were funded on a yearly basis.

The money collected in any given year was the amount available to pay for care provided during that year. There was no carry over of losses to the next year. These plans are also called capitation plans. There is a cap, or limit, on the money available in a given timeframe for care. Physicians were salaried and contracted to provide all of the care for the group members.

However, despite local success, such service plans and the system of managed care that they provided only slowly evolved in the United States. Not until the 1970s did managed care emerge as a social and political issue. Due to rising costs and a confluence of events that included the introduction of Medicare and Medicaid in 1965, a number of organizations sought health care reform and endorsed prepaid insurance plans. Efforts failed to bring forth any true health care reform, but the United States Congress did enact the Health Maintenance Organization Act in 1973 (Barr, 2007; Kongstvedt, 1995). Prepaid group plans became known as **Health Maintenance Organizations (HMOs)**. Although no system-wide reform was enacted, for the first time, providers had financial incentives to reduce the use of their services (Starr, 1982). In the HMO model, all care for a certain group of beneficiaries would need to be paid from the premiums paid to the plan. As a result, it was in the best financial interest of a provider to limit or decrease use of services. Now, providers would not be paid more because they provided more services but rather, providers had a fixed amount of money to use to provide that care.

The HMO Act removed barriers to the provision of managed health care, including all state laws prohibiting HMOs. It provided funding for new HMOs, which were required to be non-profit organizations for certification as a federally qualified HMO. Restrictions were lifted so that if HMO coverage was available in a geographic area, employers who offered health insurance were required to offer the HMO option to employees. And, in a compromise with the AMA, physician payment could include a fee-for-service payment component. This fee-for-service feature is called an Independent Practice Association, or IPA (Barr, 2007).

Managed care continued to develop in the United States, supported by the federal government and large businesses. There was little political support for any national health care plan, and no large-scale call for reform to the health care delivery system until 1993. The proposed national managed care system failed to receive political support and although, once again, no large-scale health care reform occurred, what did result was a wide-spread shift to cost containment using the managed care model (Barr, 2007).

Managed Care Models

All managed care plans offer health care services to beneficiaries from a selected group of providers who work under a capitated system. This means that all negotiated services are provided from a fixed budget, and beneficiaries are not themselves billed for the services that they use that are covered under their plan. The capitation rate is the key feature distinguishing HMOs from traditional insurance plans. HMOs must provide all contracted care for the negotiated rate (Barr, 2007).

Managed care organizations (MCOs) are not a singular entity. Just as traditional insurance plans implement different payment structures, there also is variation in managed care payment and organizational structures. Table 11-1 summarizes the major models of Health Maintenance Organizations that currently function in the United States.

Table 11-1 Models of Health Maintenance Organizations

HMO, HEALTH MAINTENANCE ORGANIZATION	Organization that provides or arranges for negotiated health coverage for its members.
PPO, PREFERRED PROVIDER ORGANIZATION	A managed care organization that contracts with select providers to give care to its members. The providers are "preferred."
MCO, MANAGED CARE ORGANIZATION	A collective term referring to a number of different health plans, including HMO, PPO, and IPA, as well as others.
IPA, INDEPENDENT PRACTICE ASSOCIATION	A group of providers that contract services to managed care plans, typically for a negotiated fee.

Provider-Agency Relationships

Typically, the financial structure of HMOs is based upon the physician relationship to the total organization: as staff, part of a group, or as an independent provider.

In a **staff-model HMO**, physicians are employees of the HMO. The staff-model HMO may own its own hospital. All premiums go to the HMO. The HMO sets a fixed budget and resources from premiums collected must cover all costs for an entire year. Employers or individuals contract directly with the HMO to provide services.

Group-model HMOs directly hire physicians to provide care for their beneficiaries. The HMO contracts with hospitals and physician practices. There is wide variation in those contracts, but in each, contracted services are supplied for a negotiated rate. Some examples of the kinds of negotiated arrangements include paying physicians a set amount for each patient cared for (regardless of medical status), fee-for-service, or a salary. The group is also responsible to negotiate with hospitals to provide inpatient services for a set price.

The Independent Practice Association (IPA) models of HMO are financial arrangements made by physicians to provide contracted care for fixed capitation payments. Physicians stay in their typical practice environment and contract with the managed care agency to provide care for enrolled beneficiaries for either a fixed cost per person, or on a discounted fee-for-service basis.

Keep in mind that managed care organizations rarely exist in a "pure" form (Hicks, Stallmeyer, & Coleman, 1993). There is a great deal of blurring of the distinctions that have been presented here and in your readings, and they may be described differently elsewhere. In addition, another potentially confusing factor is that managed care organizations may be either profit-making ventures or have not-for-profit status. Profit status can have a huge impact on the demographics of beneficiaries (who joins or is able to join), the negotiations with providers (the payment providers receive), and comprehensiveness of the benefits provided by a plan.

Features and Advantages of Managed Care Structures

All managed-care models function on the basis of prepayment, or the assurance of such payment, from beneficiaries for a defined set of benefits. HMOs build in incentives for providers to keep medical costs down. Savings are realized by limiting hospitalizations, and by providing only needed services. HMOs have structured review procedures that analyze and compare the number and kinds of services prescribed, financial implications of prescribing practices, and their outcomes. In contrast to independent models for health care delivery, there are formal checks on the practice patterns of individual practitioners.

HMOs promote the use of primary care and other outpatient treatments, in comparison to hospitalization. HMOs attempt to reduce the use of costly medical treatment by paying for preventive care, including regular screenings and immunizations. Health promotion is another common feature of HMOs. Coupled with preventive care, health promotion measures seek to keep plan beneficiaries healthy and, thus, less likely to need more expensive care.

Nursing was directly impacted by the shift to managed care. Many nursing jobs in hospitals were either eliminated or shifted to outpatient settings. But, new opportunities arose. The emphasis of nursing services broadened to include health promotion and prevention in a new and vigorous way. And, the shift to primary care and cost containment paved the way for the rise of advanced practice nurses, particularly nurse practitioners.

> ### Writing Exercise 11-1
>
> 1. Examine your own insurance coverage. Write down the out-of-pocket costs to cover you, as an individual, for that insurance policy. If you are a part of a family plan, determine the cost for yourself, and for the family coverage. Find out exactly what your policy covers. If you do not have coverage, find out how much a policy would cost and what it would cover.
>
> 2. Figure out what your insurance coverage and your out-of-pocket costs would be if you broke your wrist. Be concrete and detailed in identifying costs, including any lab tests, office visits, x-rays, and medications, including over-the-counter medications.

PUBLIC FINANCING FOR HEALTH CARE

Public Financing supports what are called categorical programs; each program is specifically developed to benefit a certain category or group of people. The federal government adds coverage for new categories as it determines that the group is vulnerable and/or its medical needs are not being met. Keep in mind that there may be overlap in group membership, which complicates the application of rules governing program eligibility and its benefits.

Medicare

Medicare was designed to provide medical care coverage for all persons over the age of 65. Medicare is run by the Centers for Medicare and Medicaid Services (CMS), a federal agency that is part of the Department of Health and Human Services (www.medicare.gov). It was instituted by Congress in 1956 and is a part of the Social Security network that was designed to protect people as they moved out from the work force (and having an income) and into retirement. Medicare was initiated because just over half of people over the age of 65 had no medical insurance. The political feeling at the time that Medicare was introduced was that the elderly should not be faced with financial ruin due to medical problems. Since instituted, Medicare has expanded to cover persons with certain disabilities and all persons with end-stage renal disease, in addition to those persons age 65 or older (www.medicare.gov).

Medicare is universal health care coverage (Barr, 2007) for persons in this age group; that is, all persons over age 65, regardless of income or any other status, are eligible for the program. Medicare is funded by withholding wages from each employee in the United States. Beneficiaries of Medicare pay a premium, based on established income and tax-filing status. The cost for Medicare coverage for the beneficiary is based on income and marital status; premium costs for those with lower incomes are a larger percentage of their income than for those who are financially better off. Table 11-2 lists the fees by income and tax-status criteria.

Table 11-2 2006 Medicare Fees by Income and Tax-Filing Status

Beneficiaries who file individual tax returns with income	Beneficiaries who file joint tax returns with income	Income-related monthly adjustment amount	Total monthly premium amount
Less than or equal to $80,000	Less than or equal to $160,000	0	$93.50
Greater than $80,000 and less than or equal to $100,000	Greater than $160,000 and less than or equal to $200,000	$12.30	$105.80
Greater than $100,000 and less than or equal to $150,000	Greater than $200,000 and less than or equal to $300,000	$30.90	$124.40
Greater than $150,000 and less than or equal to $200,000	Greater than $200,000 and less than or equal to $400,000	$49.40	$142.90
Greater than $200,000	Greater than $400,000	$67.90	$161.40

Source: CMS Medicare Program Rates and Statistics.

The initial plans for Medicare were consistent with a traditional model for medical insurance, that is, it would provide hospital coverage. Political and social forces, including AMA insistence that the plan cover physician services, created a hybrid model. As a result of these pressures, Medicare became both a service and an indemnity plan (Barr, 2007). There are now four parts to the Medicare system, each part providing coverage for different services (Figure 11-4).

Medicare Part A

Medicare Part A provides coverage for hospitalization. It is the service part of the Medicare model. The patient pays only a deductible, and then Medicare provides full coverage for all hospital-related expenses beyond that cost for 60 days. But, if a hospital stay extends beyond 60 days, the patient once again becomes responsible for a fixed daily cost. And, if hospitalization continues beyond 90 days, that fixed daily cost increases. When 150 days of hospitalization is reached, there is no longer any Medicare coverage for hospital expenses.

Medicare Part A also provides coverage for up to 20 days in a skilled nursing facility if, and only if, the patient is admitted for rehabilitation or skilled care after an illness. Medicare does not pay for people who live in nursing facilities because they cannot care for themselves. After 20 days, the above-mentioned payment model is implemented; patients pay a fixed rate per day. Coverage lasts for 100 days, beyond which time there is no longer any Medicare payment for care.

The final feature of Medicare Part A is hospice care, care given during the last 6 months of life of terminally ill patients. Physicians must certify that hospice services are required, and the affected patients must give up any extraordinary measures to prolong their lives.

Medicare Part B

Medicare Part B, Supplementary Medical Insurance, is the indemnity portion of the Medicare Model. Part B pays for outpatient bills and physician visits. It covers the ancillary services such

Figure 11-4
There are four
parts to the
Medicare system.

Medicare	
A • Coverage for hospitalization • Patient pays deductibles	**B** • Coverage for outpatient bills and physician visits • Patient pays premiums and/or deductibles
C • Includes the benefits of Parts A, B, and possibly D • HMOs or PPOs that require the use of certain physicians and/or hospitals • Provided by private insurers • Patient pays premiums and/or deductibles	**D** • Outpatient prescription plan • Voluntary • Patient pays premiums and deductibles • Complex system with gaps in coverage

as x-ray and laboratory fees. There is no coverage for vision care, physical exams, preventive services, or dental care. The funding mechanism for Part B is structured so the beneficiary pays approximately 25% of costs through premiums and/or deductibles, and the government pays for the remaining 75%. An important difference between Part A and Part B is that Part B is voluntary. However, most Medicare recipients opt for both Part A and Part B.

For both Part A and Part B, insurance companies act as fiscal intermediaries in the payment process. This means that the government does not actually pay hospitals or physicians directly. Rather, the government contracts with insurance companies in just the same way employers do, and the insurance company handles billing and payment services.

Medicare Part C

A third option that Medicare enrollees can select, Part C of the Medicare plan, is the Medicare Advantage Plus plan. It is sometimes called Medicare + Choice. Medicare Advantage is solely provided by private insurance companies, who in turn must be approved by Medicare to offer this coverage. Medicare Advantage plans are either HMO or PPO, requiring the use of specific physicians and/or hospitals. These plans must provide all of the benefits of Medicare Parts A and B; they may or may not provide Part D, prescription coverage, which is explained below. The cost and the services provided vary by plan. Advantage Plus plans can offer convenience and cost-saving advantages for services received, but often these plans carry a higher price tag. Eligible participants may choose a Medicare Advantage Plus plan because it consolidates their medical coverage into one plan for all of their hospitalization and medical needs. Another reason for selecting an Advantage Plus plan is satisfaction with the quality and services offered by a particular HMO or PPO.

Medicare Part D

Beginning in January 2006, all Medicare recipients became eligible for a voluntary program, Medicare Part D, an outpatient prescription plan. For some Medicare recipients, Part D offered coverage for medications for the first time. For those who were enrolled in Medicare HMOs, Medigap, or had Medicaid prescription coverage, Part D replaced those benefits (Kaiser Family Foundation, Medicare Fact Sheet. The Medicare Prescription Plan Benefit, June 2006). For Medicaid recipients, coverage automatically changed to Part D as of December 31, 2005. If an individual on Medicaid did not choose a Part D plan, they were assigned to one. All Medicare recipients with prescription coverage from a retirement plan or another source that was at least as good as the Part D coverage could keep that coverage and not sign up for Part D. Some Medicare recipients chose to forego prescription coverage. If at some later point in time they decide they would like coverage, they will have to pay a late enrollment fee, an extra one percent of the national base premium for each month until they joined the plan. This late fee was intended to act as a financial incentive for timely enrollment.

Medicare Part D is not simple. As with other forms of coverage under Medicare, Part D is contracted to providers, and the beneficiary pays a monthly premium. Premiums are not standardized, which means that the cost to the individual varies depending upon the plans available to them in their state or region. The plans may be stand-alone prescription plans, or be a part of a Medicare Advantage plan (an HMO model). Persons with incomes below 150% of poverty are eligible for a subsidy to help them pay for Part D coverage. Low income subsidy forms are available from the Social Security Administration (http://www.socialsecurity.gov) or by calling a local Social Security office.

These Part D plans also vary in terms of which drugs or classes of drugs that they cover, as well as at what level they are covered (tier). Plans are free to choose not to cover certain drugs. Other drugs—cough suppressants, barbiturates, benzodiazepines—are not eligible for coverage by Medicare. So, if a plan provides coverage for its beneficiaries that are not deemed eligible by Medicare (providing above standard benefits), those costs cannot be passed along to Medicare.

Medicare pays the plan providers (e.g., insurance companies, HMOs) to provide what is considered to be the standard benefit. Plans can also offer services that exceed the standard in order to attract additional enrollees, increasing their income from premiums and increasing their risk pools.

In 2007, the standard benefit is a $265 deductible and 25% coinsurance up to a limit of $2,400. Persons who have over $2,400 in drug costs then pay 100% of their further drug costs out of their own pockets until they spend $3,850 out of pocket (excluding premiums). Once the $3,850 is spent, the person pays 5% of the drug cost, or a **co-payment** ($2.15 for generic or $5.35 for brand name) for each prescription for the rest of the year (Kaiser Family Foundation, Medicare: A Primer, 2007). A gap in coverage occurs when the individual reaches the $2,400 limit. Spending on drugs must then reach a total of $5,451 ($3,850 of which is out of pocket) before Part D coverage resumes. This gap is infamously known as the "doughnut hole," an issue that raises both individual consternation and political deliberation. The following year, the schedule resumes; the deductibles, out-of-pocket costs, and limits on spending begin to accrue all over again. Keep in mind that the terms of Part D may change yearly, and that there is great variability among available plans. For up-to-date information about Medicare, see the primer on Medicare on the Web site of the Kaiser Family Foundation (http://www.kff.org) or the U.S. Centers for Medicare and Medicaid Services (http://www.cms.hhs.gov).

As you read this, you are probably somewhat confused. Think about the position of an elderly person who is trying to understand their Part D coverage. Also, think about explaining Part D coverage to an eligible recipient, or of helping someone select a plan. Your knowledge of the workings of this complex health care delivery system is truly necessary for you to assist your patients as they maneuver through this system.

Writing
Exercise
11-2

It is predicted that in the future, the number of current American workers cannot sustain the Medicare system. Keeping in mind that the Medicare trust fund does not put aside enough to pay for the care of current workers, are you willing to continue to pay a portion of your wages for coverage for those who are currently the beneficiaries of Medicare? Why or why not? State the facts that lead you to your conclusion.

Medigap

Perhaps you noticed that Medicare does not cover all of the costs of medical care for its beneficiaries. In fact, it is estimated that about 90% of beneficiaries have some form of supplement to their Medicare coverage (Barr, 2007). That supplemental coverage is collectively referred to as **Medigap**, that is, to cover the gap between Medicare coverage and out-of-pocket cost to beneficiaries (Figure 11-5). There is not yet any Medicare-approved plan that covers the "doughnut hole" gap in Plan D coverage, but many plans are offered to supplement standard Medicare coverage.

Medigap coverage is typically purchased on an individual basis by beneficiaries who can afford it. One source of such insurance is the American Association of Retired Persons (AARP). Some individuals have Medigap coverage as a part of their retirement benefits. For beneficiaries whose income is below federal poverty limits, Medicaid provides coverage that can be conceptualized as Medigap coverage; these individuals receive both Medicare and Medicaid. Or, individuals can enroll in a Medicare managed care program that provides greater coverage than the traditional Medicare plan. These beneficiaries did not need Medigap insurance because of this expanded coverage, which was less costly than purchasing insurance. There are some trade-offs for the beneficiary enrolled in a managed care Medicare plan, most notably limitations in physician selection. In many plans, beneficiaries must obtain consent from their primary physician if specialist care is needed.

Social and Political Issues

In 1997, Congress passed the Balanced Budget Act, legislation that altered the course of the original Medicare plans. The policy changes were intended to stop a dramatic increase in Medicare spending, and the cost of providing coverage to beneficiaries. Hospitals and physicians were reimbursed at lower rates than previously, and payments to HMOs were likewise decreased. The effect of this policy change was to drive HMOs out of the Medicare market. The HMOs were no longer so eager to enroll Medicare beneficiaries because they stood to lose profits. Beneficiaries saw their choice of plans diminish, hospitals were faced with decreasing payment rates and many closed, and the cost of remaining plans increased in the form of increased premiums.

Congress acted to reverse these negative effects of the Balanced Budget Act, but the quandary of how to hold down medical costs for the elderly remained. Further confounding the Medicare issues is the fact that a small proportion of Medicare recipients are responsible for

Figure 11-5
Medigap coverage helps Medicare patients with out-of-pocket costs.

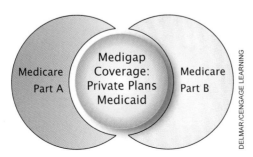

DELMAR/CENGAGE LEARNING

a high percentage of the costs incurred. The increased life span of Americans, in addition to advances in life-prolonging medical technology, resulted in demands on the Medicare system that are far greater than the system was designed to manage. The longer-lived Americans are using more resources than they paid into the Medicare system through their payroll contributions, shifting further the cost of the care of present-day recipients onto current workers. The shift means that fewer resources will be available for present-day workers when they become eligible for Medicare. Predicted results include higher premiums, less coverage, and perhaps the collapse of the system (Figure 11-6).

Another strain on the Medicare system is Graduate Medical Education. In 1983, the federal government accepted an increase in responsibility for paying for graduate medical education (GME), training for physicians after they graduate from medical school. The funding for this program was money diverted from the reserves accumulated for Medicare Part A. Hospitals embraced the program because it provided them with a much less expensive means of staffing. They could hire medical residents who were supervised by staff physicians at a much lower cost than hiring the same number of physicians—and have the cost of those residents paid by the federal government. Funding for GME has also increased the number of specialists trained in U.S. hospitals (in comparison to primary care), and increased the number of foreign-trained physicians in the U.S., who are eligible for GME positions upon their graduation from medical school. There are no comparable programs to fund nursing education at any level.

Figure 11-6
Multiple forces
are stressing the
Medicare system.

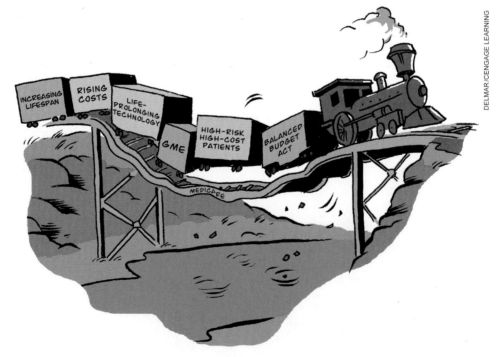

DELMAR/CENGAGE LEARNING

Medicaid

Medicaid was instituted in the same year as was Medicare, 1965. Medicaid was designed to provide health care coverage for persons living in conditions of poverty. Even though both programs were created at the same time, they were not created equally. Indeed, the model for Medicaid is quite different from that of Medicare (Figure 11-7). The complexity challenge continues!

Unlike Medicare, Medicaid was originally designed as an indemnity program, with no service component. Medicaid is not a universal coverage program; persons must meet eligibility requirements to receive Medicaid coverage (Barr, 2007). Medicaid is not entirely a federal program. It is administered by the states, with variable amounts funded at the federal level, and states are free to decline participation. However, the federal government offers incentives to states to participate in the Medicaid program by reimbursing states for those services that the state does provide. The federal contribution rate is based on the rates of poverty in a given state. States with more citizens living in poverty receive reimbursement for a greater percentage of the Medicaid spending than do states with fewer poor citizens. There is also state-by-state variation in the provided coverage, and in eligibility requirements. Each state determines which of its citizens are eligible for Medicaid coverage, and each state determines the coverage it will provide for eligible beneficiaries (Barr, 2007).

However, the federal government does set guidelines for services that must be covered in order for the state to qualify for federal Medicaid funding. These services include hospitalization, nursing home care, physician services, laboratory and x-ray services, family planning services, immunizations and preventive care for children, and services at federally-approved community health centers (Barr, 2007). A notable feature is the inclusion of reimbursement for services provided by nurse practitioners and nurse midwives.

There are also federal guidelines for Medicaid eligibility. The main groups that are covered by the Medicaid program are low-income families with children, the elderly who meet income requirements, and the disabled. States can choose to provide coverage to individuals who do not fall into the federally designated categories, but who have incomes below a designated level or meet other criteria. For example, single people who fall below a certain income level can be covered in a certain state. But, keep in mind that eligibility in one state does not guarantee eligibility in another, and that most states do not cover all poor people (Barr, 2007).

Figure 11-7
Medicaid's structure differs from Medicare in several ways.

Medicaid	Medicare
• Provides coverage for low-income persons	• Provides coverage for persons over 65, certain disabilities, and end-stage renal disease
• Enrollees must meet eligibility requirements	• Provides universal coverage for targeted populations
• Combination federal/state program	• Federal program
• Funded by federal and state governments	• Funded from employee wages

There are multiple features of the Medicaid plan that create problematic and complex issues for the health care delivery system. Payments to physicians for providing care to Medicaid recipients are very restricted compared to the prevailing market; as a direct result, many physicians do not accept Medicaid as a form of payment.

Lack of access to a physician often means that beneficiaries delay or forego care. It also means that providing care shifts to emergency rooms when medical needs become severe—and cost of providing that care is higher. And, although intended as a program primarily for families (and children in particular), most Medicaid recipients are elderly poor, a group that is more expensive to cover than children.

Parallel to the movement to managed care by the federal government with the Medicare program, state governments introduced managed care plans for Medicaid recipients in the 1990s. States contracted with HMOs to provide coverage for Medicaid beneficiaries and paid a negotiated amount for the HMO to deliver that care. In effect, states were able to shift cost increases to the HMO while fixing the cost to the state. Yet, Medicaid continues to burden state budgets and efforts continue to find ways to reduce that burden.

For up-to-date information on Medicaid, see the Web site of the Kaiser Family Foundation (http://www.kff.org), as well as that of the U.S. Centers for Medicare and Medicaid Services (http://www.medicare.gov). Keep in mind that you must supplement this information with state-specific information. In addition to resources you might find on your state governmental Web site, the Kaiser Family Foundation also publishes some state health facts.

Internet Exercise 11-1

Go to your home state Web site and locate the information about Medicaid coverage in your state.

1. Prepare to explain your state's coverage to a client who seeks health care.

2. Where can you refer a patient who is not eligible to receive treatment at a facility that does not accept Medicaid?

3. In you local community, is there any discussion about provision of care for persons living in poverty?

STATE CHILDREN'S HEALTH INSURANCE PROGRAM

In 1997, Congress enacted the **State Children's Health Insurance Program (SCHIP)**. Earlier health care reform efforts in 1993–1994 brought to the light that millions of children lacked health insurance and, as a result, did not access medical care or preventive services. As a group, children are less expensive to insure and stand to gain the most from preventive services (Figure 11-8). Children need immunizations, and regular examinations could reveal potential problems before those problems escalated. It was also deemed socially/politically unacceptable

Figure 11-8

The State Children's Health Insurance Plan (SCHIP) is aimed at reducing the number of uninsured U.S. children by half, a population that is less expensive to insure but has the most to gain from preventative services.

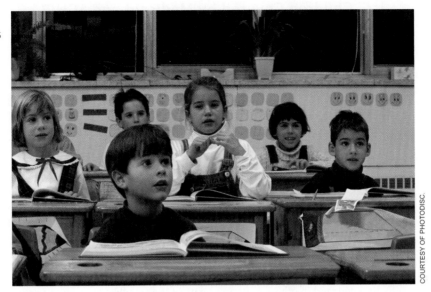

COURTESY OF PHOTODISC.

for so many children to be without basic medical care. The SCHIP program was launched with a specific goal: to reduce the number of uninsured American children by one half by providing access to coverage for children in families whose incomes were too high to qualify for Medicaid but who could not afford private health insurance (Barr, 2007).

SCHIP is a joint federal and state program, akin to Medicaid. As when Medicaid was initiated, states were given financial incentives to create programs that would reach out and provide more coverage for children. States were also given options in designing their own SCHIP programs. There were three basic options for states: expand Medicare, establish a separate program for SCHIP-eligible children, or a combination of the two. All three variations were enacted. States then applied to the federal government for funding of their programs. The federal government stipulated that funds had to be spent within three years or be returned.

The initial response to SCHIP by the states was positive. Programs were developed and children enrolled. But things did not continue so smoothly. Reports arose that the application process for the program in some states was too cumbersome, that outreach efforts were ineffective in locating eligible children, and that some states were not funding the programs properly. An unanticipated problem occurred as the result of the fact that states had to pay higher amounts of the medical costs for children enrolled in Medicaid than they paid for those enrolled in the SCHIP program. States then enrolled Medicaid-eligible children in SCHIP to shift the higher cost burden to the federal government. Figure 11-9 illustrates the percentage of children covered under Medicaid and under the SCHIP program. Observers noted that some of the children enrolled in SCHIP had previously been covered under their parents' policies. This shifting of financial burden from private to public funded insurance coverage put additional pressures on the public system. Some parents lost private coverage because they lost their jobs. Others decided to enroll their children in SCHIP because of the increased cost of purchasing employer-based coverage.

All in all, after the first three years of the program, over half of the state-allocated funding for SCHIP was returned to the federal government. The 4 million children covered are many less

U.S. Children Covered by Medicaid and SCHIP

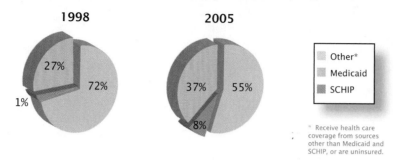

Figure 11-9

U.S. Children Covered by Medicaid and SCHIP. *(U.S. Department of Health and Human Services. Centers for Medicare and Medicaid Services, "The State Children's Health Insurance Program," PowerPoint Presentation, March 5, 2007, pp. 19–20.)*

than the target goal of 10 million. Problems continue with funding shortages; state budgets cannot easily absorb the mandate to provide this coverage. In some states, state-imposed enrollment gaps emerged, and in others, the complexity of the enrollment process discouraged applications. Despite a decade of advertising by both private foundations and the federal government, nearly 30% of eligible children are not enrolled in the program (*New York Times*, "Many Eligible for Child Health Plan Have No Idea," August 22, 2007).

When the SCHIP program was up for renewal in 2007, it became the centerpiece of the larger political discussion of who should be responsible for paying for health insurance—the government or the private sector. The argument revolved around the possibility that families would enroll their children in the SCHIP program due to the rising cost of premiums for private health insurance policies. In effect, this shift to SCHIP is a shift from private to public insurance. SCHIP remains a political issue, one that highlights the unresolved debate over whether health care is a basic right, who should pay for health insurance, and what system for that payment is most fair and equitable.

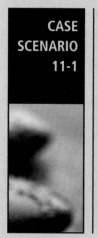

CASE SCENARIO 11-1

Ms. Percy takes her two children, Jolie and Kyle, to the emergency room for Jolie's stubborn rash and Kyle's asthma attacks. The children do not get regular physical examinations, or booster shots of immunizations. The hospital bills continue to increase, for the most part, unpaid. You are working in the Emergency Department when Kyle comes in with another asthma attack.

CASE ANALYSIS

1. How can you assist Ms. Percy to determine if the children are eligible for the SCHIP program in your state?

2. What are your state's eligibility requirements?

3. What has your Emergency Department done to assist people such as Ms. Percy to learn about SCHIP?

SUPPLEMENTAL SECURITY INCOME (SSI) BENEFITS

General tax revenues, apart from those set aside for Social Security, are used to provide services for individuals with special needs or conditions. Such needs include blindness, disabilities, and age. States provide additional financial assistance to these individuals and their families to meet their care needs. Individuals eligible for SSI benefits are usually also eligible for Medicaid based on formulas determined by federal and state guidelines. As a result, SSI benefit eligibility is a function of state of residence and cannot be assumed to be either similar or portable to another state. In some states, eligible children are covered under the state's SCHIP program for health insurance, with other benefits determined separately.

OTHER PUBLIC FUNDING SOURCES

The majority of health insurance in the United States is provided by private insurers through employers and through the federally sponsored Medicare and Medicaid programs. However, governmental entities also provide health insurance for other groups. Some of these programs are mentioned here. Details are kept brief, but are presented to illustrate once again the range and complexity of health care insurance and illustrate the difficulty in introducing reforms. Plans were introduced to meet the specific needs of groups and there is no uniformity in coverage, management, or governmental unit responsible for oversight. There is no uniform standard for the benefits, or for the cost of care—or insurance premiums—for beneficiaries.

The Federal Employees Health Benefit Program (FEHBP)

Health care benefits are provided for all permanent civilian employees of the United States government. A fee-for-service plan is offered, but managed competition has introduced variability into the system; there is no uniformity in coverage across sectors and employees have choices from ten or even more plans, depending upon where they work. Some plans are regional, others are national. Federal employees are eligible for health care coverage within 60 days of employment. Premiums vary from plan to plan, and employees can select among differing options for level of coverage and pay accordingly. The government employer pays up to 75% of the plan premium based on a formula set by law (www.opm.gov). Some workers have a higher percentage paid because of collective bargaining agreements they have negotiated with the federal government. An example of a group that uses such collective bargaining is postal workers. Members of Congress are all eligible for this health care coverage, and their eligibility is life-long. Another feature of the federal employee plan is that the portion of their pay that covers their health insurance is not taxed, so they realize additional financial benefits. Further details can be found on the Web sites http://www.opm.gov and http://www.federaldaily.com. Follow the links to the handbooks that describe employee health insurance benefits.

Military Health Services System (MHSS)

The U.S. Department of Defense provides medical insurance coverage for the active duty and retired members of all branches of the armed services. While the first priority of the military health system is for war-related care, the system must also meet needs during peacetime operations. The need to provide care in an increasingly expensive and technological health care system lead to a situation in which the demand for health care began to exceed the ability of the existing system to deliver that care. As the direct result, the design of the military health plan was altered in 1997, introducing options within an HMO model (Military Report, 2007).

The military health plan is called TRICARE. All active duty military personnel are automatically enrolled in the most basic TRICARE. Family enrollment is not automatic; the military person must take steps to enroll family members. There are three different options under TRICARE, each with fees and deductibles. Options are selected by military personnel depending upon the geographic location of a military provider, individual and family needs, and other cost and accessibility factors. See the Web page http://www.militaryreport.com and follow the link to the brochure for further program details.

Veterans Health Care Eligibility Act

In 1996, Congress enacted the Veterans Health Care Eligibility Act, to be administered by the Department of Veterans Affairs. This action provided a medical benefits package for all enrolled veterans, including preventive and primary care as well as inpatient and outpatient services. Veterans returning from active duty may be eligible for free, federally funded medical, hospital, and home care for all illnesses of injuries related to their service. This coverage does not apply to such events as colds, prior disorders, or injuries clearly not related to service. There is no dental coverage.

Coverage for veterans is determined by a complex system of eligibility. Categories were determined based on variables such as discharge status, length of service, disabilities (and the permanence of those disabilities), income, and whether injuries were acquired in the line of duty. Eight (8) priority groups were established, each with varying eligibility and enrollment requirements. Additionally, there are "specialized projects," categories that created particular service-related health care conditions. Examples of such specialized projects include victims of Agent Orange, Gulf War Syndrome, radiation after-effects, and blindness suffered in the line of duty.

Regardless of the priority group into which a veteran is categorized, the Veterans Health Service provides hospital care and out patient care "as needed." Eligibility is also subject to lack of any other health insurance, including Medicare and Medicaid. Regional access to care is an issue, as is availability of services for all veterans who would like to take advantage of their benefits. Further information and updates are available at http://www.military.gov and http://www.VA.gov. Follow the links for health benefits.

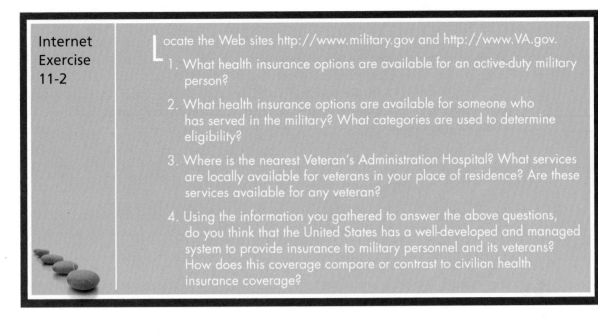

Internet Exercise 11-2

Locate the Web sites http://www.military.gov and http://www.VA.gov.

1. What health insurance options are available for an active-duty military person?

2. What health insurance options are available for someone who has served in the military? What categories are used to determine eligibility?

3. Where is the nearest Veteran's Administration Hospital? What services are locally available for veterans in your place of residence? Are these services available for any veteran?

4. Using the information you gathered to answer the above questions, do you think that the United States has a well-developed and managed system to provide insurance to military personnel and its veterans? How does this coverage compare or contrast to civilian health insurance coverage?

Indian Health Service (IHS)

The Indian Health Service (IHS) is a part of the U.S. Department of Health and Human Services (DHHS). Since 1955, the federal government has assumed responsibility for providing health care for American Indians and Alaska Natives. Prior to 1955, these health services were provided by the Bureau of Indian Affairs. Although the Bureau of Indian Affairs still exists, it was determined that raising health care standards for American natives would be best served by transferring responsibility to the entity devoted to health and the provision of health services.

The Indian Health Service operates hospitals, clinics, and health stations and provides comprehensive services for American Indians and Alaska Natives. American Indians and Alaska natives are members of sovereign nations, and are also citizens of the United States. However, even though they are not citizens of the states in which they reside, they are eligible for state-provided services. The Indian Health Service provides a set of comprehensive, parallel health care services for residents of reservations.

The IHS is headquartered in Rockville, Maryland, and operates 12 area offices, which function as administrative units. Most of these area offices are located in the western states. Anyone who is a member of a recognized tribe or a descendent of such a member is eligible for coverage under the IHS. To better picture the extent of the IHS programming needs, there are 560 federally recognized tribes, living mostly on reservations and in rural communities in 35 states. The HIS operates 33 hospitals, 59 health centers, and at least 50 health stations. In addition, there are 34 American-Indian health projects located in urban areas. The National Council of Chief Clinical Consultants, which resides in New York City, provides medical specialty support and consultation. Thus, the complexity and wide range of required services challenges the system to provide outreach, and preventive and therapeutic measures. In addition, the IHS works closely with tribal members to provide culturally acceptable care. Special initiatives to do so include incorporating traditional tribal medicine, elder care, and attending to the particular health care challenges existing within this population. Further information about the Indian Health Services can be obtained on the Web site http://www.info.ihs.gov.

Mental Health Services

Health insurance is designed to cover medical problems. Even though many mental health disorders are biological in origin, behavioral health problems are not covered in the same way as are physical health problems.

Historically, health insurance plans offered no coverage for psychiatric/mental health/substance-abuse conditions. Today, the gap in coverage has been lessened, but true parity for mental illnesses remains an illusive goal. (Note that the term "mental illness" includes disorders of "alcohol and substance abuse," and further, that "mental health" and/or "behavioral health" have all but replaced the term "psychiatric" when referring to diagnostic categories or diseases.)

Parity

The 1993 movement toward managed care (as compared to the traditional fee-for-service payment model) raised questions regarding **parity**, or equivalence, of insurance coverage for mental health conditions. According to the National Alliance for the Mentally Ill, parity requires an attitude and concomitant action, in this case insurance coverage, for mental illness as a disease just like any other disease. Parity is not a mandate for certain treatments or services, but rather, a coverage condition (National Alliance for the Mentally Ill, Mental Health Insurance Coverage, A Guide to State Parity Law, 2007). That is, if insurance coverage is offered for mental illness, limits and conditions should be the same as for anything else that the policy covers.

A few years later, in 1996, the Mental Health Parity Act (MHPA) was enacted; it has been renewed every year since that date. This federal legislation introduced the first step toward ensuring coverage for mental health and substance abuse problems by requiring that employers with over 50 employees must provide the same annual and life-time dollar limits for mental health conditions as they do for medical/surgical conditions (AACAP, Mental Health Parity Legislation 2007; National Alliance for the Mentally Ill, Mental Health Insurance Coverage: A Guide to State Parity Law, 2007). Note that there were major gaps in the mandated coverage. First, any employer with fewer than 50 employees was not required to provide coverage for mental illness. Second, the mandate stated that policies had to provide the same limits in annual and life-time. However, this did not mean that other limits could not be put into place. Policies providing mental health coverage typically limit the number of inpatient days and outpatient visits, and many also limit the amount that they pay per day or visit. An example of typical policy benefits is coverage for 20 inpatient days and 30 outpatient visits, with great variation in co-payments and deductibles depending on the many factors that determine what a particular policy offers for a particular group or individual. Policies could be "managed" in the same way as policies pertaining to physical illnesses—networks, preferred providers, and/or exclusion of services not deemed medically necessary.

The MHPA did provide a source of momentum, spurring state legislation for mental health coverage for their citizens. Prior to 1996, only 5 states had any legislation regarding mental health insurance parity; in 2007, 34 states had such legislation (National Alliance for the Mentally Ill, Mental Health Insurance Coverage: A guide to State Parity Law, 2007). State-mandated coverage offers some improvement over the federal requirements. However, just as in Medicare and Medicaid policies, states have discretion in mandates for coverage. One illustration: states have the option of defining what is considered a mental illness. A state can offer comprehensive coverage, that is, cover all diagnoses listed in the Diagnostic and Statistical Manual of the American Psychiatric Association (DSM). On the other hand, states can also limit coverage requirements to coverage for certain disorders (O'Sullivan & Krauss, 2007). For example, anorexia and attention deficit hyperactivity disorder (ADHD) are both included in the DSM, but are not required to be included in insurance policies as mental illnesses in some states.

In 1999, the Federal Employees Health Benefits Program (FEHBP) was modified to include mental health coverage. That coverage began in 2001. In 2003, both the U.S. House and Senate introduced the Paul Wellstone Mental Health Equitable Treatment Act. This bill was modeled on the provisions included in the FEHBP plan: mental health provisions equivalent to the plan's other health benefits and prohibited caps, limits on access, or other restrictions that made treatment options or costs different from those for physical illness. In 2007, this legislation was still pending.

The primary argument against requiring full parity for mental illness contends that the cost for such coverage is prohibitive. In particular, insurance companies claim that extending coverage to include mental health would be too costly. Spending more to provide care would then drive up premiums and make insurance less affordable. Insurers further claim that if individuals are offered more coverage, they will demand more services as the out-of-pocket cost for care decreases. And, insurers insist that they should not pay for treatment of illnesses that they claim are not truly illnesses (O'Sullivan & Krauss, 2007). However, data from the Department of Human Health and Services indicate that health care premiums in states that do offer mental health parity increase by an average of only 1% (U.S. Department of Health and Human Services, The Costs and Effects of Parity, 2007). In addition, untreated mental illnesses produce hidden costs such as losses in worker productivity. In the United States, an estimated $79 billion is lost each year in wages and productivity as the result of untreated mental illnesses (Kessler, 2005).

Many individuals in need of mental health services seek treatment in primary-care settings. Primary care providers are not experts in mental health treatment modalities, but many prescribe psychiatric medications. It is unclear how effective treatment in primary-care settings is compared to full psychiatric services. However, advances in psychopharmacology, cognitive-behavioral therapy, and other forms of psychotherapy have produced outcomes on par with those of treatment of chronic medical conditions (O'Sullivan & Krauss, 2007).

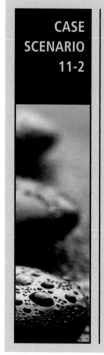

CASE SCENARIO 11-2

Devone Ellison was recently diagnosed by his pediatrician as having a childhood depressive disorder. His school teacher had asked his parents to seek an evaluation by Devone's pediatrician because his school performance and social interactions were both suffering by his lack of affect. His parents assume that since the school system referred them to Devone's pediatrician and the pediatrician made a referral to a psychologist, that the treatment for Devone's condition is covered by their medical insurance.

CASE ANALYSIS

1. In your state, would childhood depression be considered as a mental illness for insurance purposes?

2. How would you counsel Mr. & Mrs. Ellison as they proceed to seek treatment for Devone?

3. What if Devone had been diagnosed with Attention Deficit Hyperactivity Disorder? Would your state consider ADHD as a mental illness for insurance purposes?

4. When schools are involved in assessment, evaluation of student performance, and making treatment recommendations, is there a blurring of lines between the educational and the health care systems? Which bears the burden of cost for diagnosis and/or treatment?

The Uninsured

The number of people without health care insurance rose to over 47 million in 2006, an increase that the Census Bureau attributed to the loss of employer-supported coverage. Average premium costs have been increasing, averaging 7.7% per year since 1999 (Centers for Disease Control, Health Insurance Coverage: Estimates from the National Health Interview Survey, 2004; Kaiser Family Foundation, Health Care Costs: A Primer, 2007).

As the number of uninsured increases, some states have implemented plans to require or offer health insurance for their citizens. Other states have programs or laws to help small employers provide medical insurance. Some states cover more children under SCHIP than the federal government requires. In New York, the governor suggested raising the income limit to 400% of poverty level, up from 250%. (In 2006, a family of four is considered to be in poverty with an annual income of less $20,650). At issue is the fact that states are facing a shortfall in federal funding to provide for the uninsured, resulting in the possibility that some children may lose coverage (*New York Times*, "States and U.S. at Odds on Aid for Uninsured," February 13, 2007).

And, some states have addressed the needs of the largest growing segment of the uninsured population, young adults. Young adults may have been covered under their parents' plans or SCHIP, but may no longer be eligible for such coverage simply due to their age. Some states are using tobacco settlement money to fund such programs. Other states tax employers who do not provide health benefits for their workers.

However, the federal government has argued that states are straying from the intents and purposes of SCHIP by extending federal limits or going beyond federal guidelines and allowing parents or childless adults to enroll in state-sponsored health insurance programs. The argument is that the SCHIP program was created to cover poor children. The counter argument, made particularly by the State of Wisconsin, is that by covering more poor adults, more poor children will be covered (*New York Times*, "States and U.S. at Odds on Aid for Uninsured," February 13, 2007).

SUMMARY

This chapter has discussed the history and evolution of American health care insurance, the way in which most health care is paid for in the United States. That history traces the changes that have occurred in methods of payment for health care, illustrating the role of social and political factors that influenced the type of payment models that did evolve. The role of private industries, the federal government, and state governments in the development and provision of health care to Americans was described. Examples of the various models of health insurance coverage are given. The complexity of the mixed public/private model of health care insurance that has evolved in the United States illustrates why changes to that system are so difficult to enact.

Nursing has been a relatively absent party in the developments in health care insurance. It is important for nurses, individually and collectively, to change this absent, invisible status. The nursing profession itself has been shaped by the same factors that have impacted the payment systems for health care. The shift from hospital care to community-based care is one striking example of how an insurance model, namely managed care, altered the practice of nursing.

The current challenges to the health care delivery system primarily focus on financing and payment for care in an environment in which there is rapid technological advances and increasing cost for care. Nurses who are concerned about the quality of patient care must also be concerned about how health care is paid for. It is time for nurses to join in the discussions and debates, bringing a perspective that includes knowledge of the health care delivery system, as well as extensive knowledge of patient care. These combined knowledge bases will offer more powerful tools for change than either approach alone. It is time for nurses to accept this challenge, become involved, and impact the next stages in payment for health care.

The nursing profession cannot afford to sit on the sidelines as issues are discussed and plans are presented to solve the dilemmas presented by the existing health insurance conundrum. In its first ever analysis of the world's health systems, the World Health Organization (WHO) ranked the United States #37 out of 191 countries, using WHO standards (World Health Organization, World Health Organization Assesses the World's Health Systems, June 21, 2000). Evidence and outcomes are the rationale for professional practice. The outcomes of our health system and methods for paying for health care should stand under the same analysis and scrutiny as does our day-to-day professional activity. Nurses need to understand the system in which they work, and decide that it is an important part of their professional role to challenge and to influence the structure and the outcomes of that system.

It is the mark of great people to treat trifles as trifles and important matters as important.

–Doris Lessing

REFERENCES

American Academy of Child & Adolescent Psychiatry. (2007). *Mental health parity legislation approved in senate committee!*. Retrieved April 15, 2009, from http://www.aacap.org/cs/legislative_action_110th_congress/mental_health_parity_legislation_approved_in_senate_committee

Barr, D. A. (2007). *Introduction to U.S. health care policy: The organization, financing, and delivery of health care in America* (2nd ed.). Baltimore, MD: The Johns Hopkins University Press.

Cohen, R., & Martinez, M. (2005). *Health insurance coverage: Estimates from the national health interview survey, 2004*. Retrieved April 15, 2009, from http://www.cdc.gov/nchs/data/nhis/earlyrelease/insur200506.pdf

Centers for Medicare & Medicaid Services, Department of Health and Human Services. (2006). *Brief summaries of Medicare and Medicaid: Title XVIII and title XIX of the Social Security Act*. Retrieved April 15, 2009, from http://cms.hhs.gov/MedicareProgramRatesStats/downloads/MedicareMedicaidSummaries 2006.pdf

Forbes (2006). *CEO compensation*. Retrieved April 15, 2009, from http://www.forbes.com/lists/2006/12/Rank_1.html

Hicks, L. L., Stallmeyer, J. J., & Coleman, J. R. (1993). *Role of the nurse in managed care*. Washington, DC: American Nurses Publishing.

Indian Health Service. (2007). *IHS fact sheets*. Retrieved April 15, 2009, from http://info.ihs.gov

The Kaiser Family Foundation. (2009). *Health care costs: A primer, key information on health care costs and their impact*. Retrieved April 15, 2009, from http://www.kff.org/insurance/upload/7670_02.pdf

The Kaiser Family Foundation. (2009). *Medicare: The Medicare prescription drug benefit—updated version*. Retrieved April 15, 2009, from http://www.kff.org/medicare/upload/7044-09.pdf

The Kaiser Family Foundation. (2007). *Medicare: A primer*. Retrieved April 15, 2009, from http://www.kff.org/medicare/upload/7615.pdf

Kessler, R. C., Berglund, P., Demler, O., Jin, R., Merikangas, K. R., & Walters, E. E. (2005). Lifetime prevalence and age-of-onset distributions of DSM-IV disorders in the national comorbidity survey replication. *Archives of General Psychiatry, 62*(6), 593–602.

Kongstvedt, P. R. (1995). *Essentials of managed health care*. Gaithersburg, MD: Aspen Publishers, Inc.

Lee, C. (2007). Rise in cost of employer-paid health insurance slows. *The Washington Post*. Retrieved April 15, 2009, from http://www.washingtonpost.com/wp-dyn/content/article/2007/09/11/AR2007091100666.html

Military Report. (2007). *TRICARE: Your military health plan*. Retrieved July 31, 2007, from http://www.militaryreport.com/tricarebrochure.htm

National Alliance on Mental Illness. (2007). *Mental health insurance coverage: A guide to state parity law*. Retrieved April 15, 2009, from http://www.nami.org/Content/ContentGroups/Policy/Issues_Spotlights/Parity1/Mental_Health_Insurance_Coverage_A_Guide_to_State_Parity_Law1.htm

O'SULLIVAN, C. K., & Krauss, J. B. (2007). True mental health parity: A long-overdue public health policy. *American Journal of Nursing, 107*(1), 77–79.

PEAR, R., & Hernandez, R. (2007). States and U.S. at odds on aid for uninsured. *The New York Times.* Retrieved April 15, 2009, from http://www.nytimes.com/2007/02/13/us/13insure.html

SACK, K. (2007). Many eligible for child health plan have no idea. *The New York Times.* Retrieved April 15, 2009, from http://www.nytimes.com/2007/08/22/health/policy/22insure.html?_r=1

STARR, P. (1982). *The social transformation of American medicine: The rise of a sovereign profession and the making of a vast industry.* New York: Basic Books.

U.S. DEPARTMENT OF HEALTH AND HUMAN SERVICES, Substance Abuse and Mental Health Services Administration. (2007). *The costs and effects of parity for mental health and substance abuse insurance benefits.* Retrieved April 15, 2009, from http://mentalhealth.samhsa.gov/publications/allpubs/mc99-80/Prtyfnix.asp

WORLD HEALTH ORGANIZATION. (2000). *World Health Organization assesses the world's health systems.* [Press Release]. Retrieved April 15, 2009, from http://www.who.int/inf-pr-2000/en/pr2000-44.html

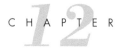

COST, ACCESS, AND QUALITY: CRITICAL HEALTH CARE ISSUES

AMY BARLOW BRITT
MSN, RN, CEN, Instructor, Riverside School of Health Careers

Life was simple before World War II. After that, we had systems.

–Grace Hopper

LEARNING OBJECTIVES

At the completion of the chapter, the learner should be able to do the following:

1. Describe the participants in the health care delivery system.
2. Compare health care issues from different participants' perspectives.
3. Analyze the factors associated with rising health care costs.
4. Discuss barriers to accessing health care.
5. Discuss factors that affect health care quality.
6. Analyze the use of rationing in health care today.
7. Evaluate strategies for nurses to use to address cost, access, and quality issues.

KEY TERMS

Core Measures
Disparities
Effectiveness
Gross Domestic
    Product (GDP)
High Deductible Health
    Plans (HDHP)
Health Indicators
Health Literacy
Healthy People 2010
Joint Commission
Medicaid

Medicare
Morbidity
Mortality
North American Nursing
    Diagnosis Association
    (NANDA)
Nursing Interventions
    Classification (NIC)
Nursing Outcomes
    Classification (NOC)
National Quality
    Forum (NQF)

Organisation for Economic
    Co-operation and
    Development (OECD)
Patient-Centered Care
Per Capita
Preventable Adverse Events
Rationing
State Children's Health
    Insurance Program (SCHIP)
Unlicensed Assistive
    Personnel (UAP)

INTRODUCTION

Ask someone what is wrong with the health care system today, and chances are they can describe a problem—probably more than one. Anyone involved in health care, either as a patient or a provider, can identify issues with the system. Americans believe health care is an important area of concern. In a recent survey, respondents were asked to identify the most critical issue facing the United States. Health care was identified as the most important issue, followed by the Iraq War, energy and gas prices, terrorism, the economy, education, and Social Security (Helman, Greenwald & Associates, & Fronstin, 2006). They were then asked to rate the quality of the health care system. A majority (59%) rated the current United States health care system negatively as either "poor" or "fair," primarily because of high costs.

There are signs that the health care delivery system is not as it should be. Information is distributed to patients on how to "stay safe" while being hospitalized. Patients are instructed to make sure the medications they are receiving are correct, and to make sure the nurse verifies their identity before administering them. Surgical patients must use a marker to write on themselves to confirm for the surgical team which part of the body is to be operated on. Also, it appears there are people "fleeing" our health care system. There is a growing segment of the travel industry known as "medical tourism." More Americans are traveling oversees to receive discounted medical care—primarily surgical procedures. Some residents close to the borders drive to Canada or Mexico for less expensive prescription medications.

The problems with health care delivery are the focus of much public scrutiny. There are Web sites and blogs for people to view and share negative health care experiences. Books are written on the subject, with such titles as *Sick, Health Care Meltdown,* and *Who Killed Health Care?* In 2007, filmmaker Michael Moore released "Sicko," a documentary containing dramatic personal stories illustrating the shortcomings of the United States' health care system. Private citizens are not the only ones discussing health care delivery. Politicians at all levels of government debate health care issues and proposed changes to the system. The apparent multitude of health care delivery problems are all in fact related to three fundamental issues: health care costs, access to health care, and health care quality.

PARTICIPANTS IN HEALTH CARE DELIVERY

The health care delivery system involves multiple participant groups. When it comes to these issues, everyone involved has a different point of view. Each participant group is influenced by their unique perspective, values, opinions, and beliefs. Participants define and describe health care issues from their vantage point. To better understand the issues of cost, access, and quality, it is necessary to first identify the participants in the system. Participants can be classified as patients, providers, or payers.

Patients

Patients are the largest group of participants in the health care system (Figure 12-1). The 2005 American Community Survey conducted by the United States Census Bureau (2005b) provides a profile of the country. In 2005, the United States population totaled 288.4 million people, with the population evenly divided between males (49%) and females (51%). There were 111.1 million households, with an average size of 2.6 people per household. Families comprised most households (67%). The majority of nonfamily households were people living alone. Twelve percent of the people living in the United States were born elsewhere. Among all citizens at least five years old, 19% spoke a language other than English at home. In terms of education, 84% of people 25 years and older had at least a high school education, and 27% had a bachelor's degree or higher.

The population continues to grow larger, and is projected to reach 392 million by 2050 (U. S. Census Bureau, 2007b) (Figure 12-2). Even though the size of the population is growing, it is not increasing as rapidly as in the past. Instead, the significant trends in population growth are related to aging and increasing diversity (U. S. Census Bureau, 2007b). As the baby boomers (the members of the population born between 1946 and 1964) age, the median age of the population

Figure 12-1
Patients comprise
the largest group
in health care.

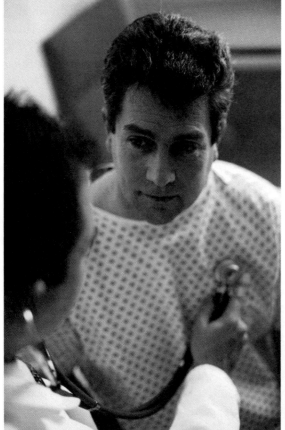

COURTESY OF PHOTODISC.

Figure 12-2
Projected
population growth
for the United
States. *(U.S. Census
Bureau, 2007B.)*

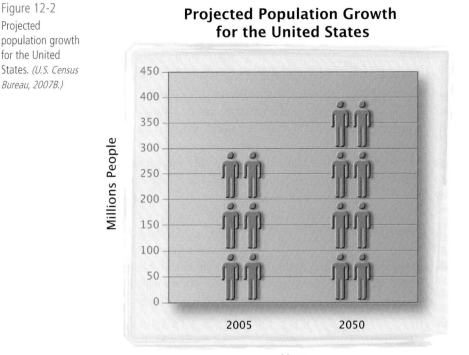

**Projected Population Growth
for the United States**

Year

will rise through about 2050. In 2005, the median age was 36.4 years, and 12% of the population was 65 years and older (U. S. Census Bureau, 2005b). The median age is expected to peak at 39.1 in 2035. The last of the baby boomers will turn 65 in 2029. At that time they will represent approximately 16% of the total population. Non-Hispanic white Americans are projected to be the slowest growing population group, while minority groups including Black; Asian and Pacific Islander; American Indian, Eskimo, and Aleut; and Hispanic Americans will experience the fastest growth rates. These changing demographics will present significant challenges to the health care system in the future.

The National Center for Health Statistics monitors health care utilization. In the past, patients received most of their care from hospital-based services. In recent years, however, there has been a shift towards providing more care in outpatient settings. As a result, hospital admissions and lengths of stay have decreased over time. The average length of stay in an acute-care hospital was 4.8 days in 2004, which is down from 7.5 days in 1980 (National Center for Health Statistics, 2006). Also, an increasing number of surgical procedures are being performed on patients, particularly those over age 65. As a result, inpatient care has become more intensive and complex.

Between 1995 and 2005, visits to primary care offices, surgical care offices, and outpatient departments increased by about 20% (Burt, McCaig, & Rechtsteiner, 2007). Visits to medical specialty offices increased by 37%, and the number of visits to emergency departments increased

7%. About 29% of all ambulatory care visits were for chronic diseases and 25% were for preventive care, including checkups, prenatal care, and postsurgical care. The majority of ambulatory care visits involved medication administration and management, with 71.3% of all visits having one or more medications prescribed (up by 10% since 1995). In 2004, the majority of Americans (45.8%) had between one and three outpatient contacts with the health care system each year (National Center for Health Statistics, 2006). An outpatient contact is defined as a visit to a physician's office, emergency department, or a home visit by a nurse or other health care professional. That same year, 24.6% of the population had between four and nine contacts, 16.1% had none, while 13.5% had ten or more.

The amount of disease prevention and early detection services provided in the community has increased (National Center for Health Statistics, 2006). For example, the percentage of children between the ages of 19 and 35 months of age that have been vaccinated was 82% in 2005, up from 74% in 1995. The percentage of adults age 18 and older receiving the flu vaccine in the past 12 months was 29.5% in 2004, up from 9.6% in 1989. Use of mammography has doubled among women over the age of 40. In 1987, only 29% received a mammogram compared to 69.5% in 2003.

Even though there is an increase in disease prevention and community-based care, a greater share of patients' money is still spent on hospital services (National Center for Health Statistics, 2006). In 2004, 37% of personal health care expenditures were for hospital care. Physician care represented 26% of personal health care expenditures, followed by prescription drugs (12%) and nursing home care (7%). The remaining 18% of personal health expenditures was spent for other personal health care, including visits to nonphysician medical providers, medical supplies, and other health services (Figure 12-3). Even though a lot of money is spent on hospital services, the share of total personal health care expenditures devoted to hospital care has declined by 9% since 1980, reflecting the shift in health care from inpatient to ambulatory care settings.

Usually there is strength in numbers. However, when it comes to health care some would argue patients are the least powerful of all the participant groups. Patients are generally uninformed consumers despite the overwhelming amount of health-related information that is available to

Figure 12-3
Personal Health
Expenditures.
*(National Center
for Health Care
Statistics, 2006.)*

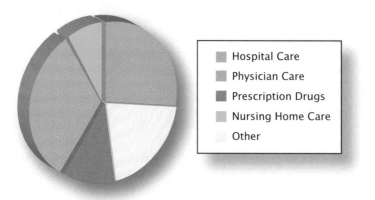

Personal Health Care Expenditures

Hospital Care
Physician Care
Prescription Drugs
Nursing Home Care
Other

the public. Patients lack the knowledge and expertise that health care providers have in order to use and apply this information to their health. This hinders their ability to advocate for themselves and to maneuver through the health care system efficiently. Another factor that limits patients' influence in health care is that they tend to not pay the full cost of their care. For many patients, some form of health insurance shares the cost. This means the general public does not have much purchasing power with which to negotiate their care.

Patients want access to quality health care that is affordable. They want to see providers they select, rather than be limited to providers selected for them by their health plan. Patients desire lower health insurance premiums and out-of-pocket expenses and prefer more access to the system. They think it is cumbersome and time-consuming to obtain authorizations or referrals before seeking treatment. Patients want to receive the best care possible, and would rather not have to wait for it.

Internet Exercise 12-1	Review a Web site that provides information to help patients become more informed consumers of health care, such as http://www.myhealthcaredollar.com.

1. What information is provided in this (these) Web site(s)?

2. What is/are the source(s) of the information?

3. How much of the information is based upon scientific research?

4. How much of the information is provided by special-interest groups?

5. Is the information easy to understand?

Providers

Health care providers consist of both individuals and organizations. Individual health care providers include nurses, physicians, pharmacists, therapists, and other health care practitioners. Registered nurses are the largest group of health care providers numbering over 2 million (National Center for Health Statistics, 2006). Despite the seemingly high numbers of nurses, the system is actually facing a shortage of nurses. It is projected that by 2020, the supply of registered nurses will satisfy only 64% of the demand (Health Resources and Services Administration, 2004). Even though nurses are the most prevalent providers, they are not the most influential providers politically. Currently the profession is still struggling with establishing a standard educational preparation for practice, as well as validating the important contributions of nursing to health care delivery.

Physicians are the second largest group of providers (Figure 12-4), numbering approximately 800,000 (National Center for Health Statistics, 2006). Approximately one-third of those are generalists, or primary care physicians (U.S. Department of Health and Human Resources, 2006). This includes family practice physicians, pediatricians, and internal medicine practitioners.

Figure 12-4
Physicians are the
second largest
group of health
care providers.

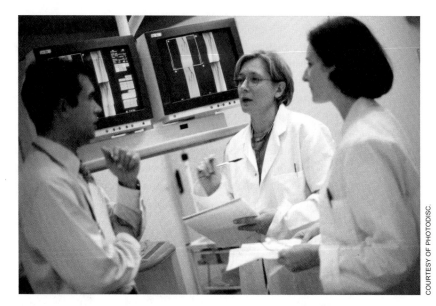

COURTESY OF PHOTODISC.

The remaining two-thirds of physicians are specialists. Like nursing, a shortage of physicians is forecasted, although it is not expected to be as severe (U.S. Department of Health and Human Services, 2006). A key trend contributing to the shortage of physicians is the increasing number of female physicians. In 2003–04, enrollment in medical school was 50% female, an increase from only 29% in 1980–81 (National Center for Health Statistics, 2006). Female physicians are more likely to choose nonsurgical specialties, spend fewer hours providing patient care, are less likely to practice in rural areas, and retire earlier than male physicians (U.S. Department of Health and Human Services, 2006). In addition to the overall shortage, there will continue to be a problem with physicians not being distributed evenly throughout the country to meet the population's needs. Currently, approximately 7,000 primary care physicians are currently needed in underserved areas (U.S. Department of Health and Human Services, 2006).

Pharmacists are the third largest group of health providers, numbering 196,000 in 2000 (National Center for Health Statistics, 2006). The role of the pharmacist in direct patient care is growing. More pharmacists are becoming involved in teaching patients about their medications, and not just dispensing them. Physical, occupational, and speech therapists have an integral role in patient care practicing in both inpatient and outpatient settings. Demand for their services is also expected to grow as the population ages.

New and different types of health practitioners continue to evolve to meet the system's needs. The numbers of massage therapists, medical assistants, and medical equipment preparers have grown significantly in recent years (National Center for Health Statistics, 2006). Additionally, many health care organizations are turning to the use of **unlicensed assistive personnel (UAP)** to fill the void created by the nursing shortage and to decrease labor costs (Kleinman & Saccomano, 2006). Unlicensed assistive personnel are trained to assist registered nurses in the provision of patient care activities as delegated by the nurse (American Nurses Association, 1992). The term is used to describe aides, orderlies, assistants, attendants, or technicians used to provide care. This presents a challenge for nursing as health care organizations utilize more of these workers to provide nursing-type care. This puts additional responsibilities on nurses of having to manage and evaluate the care unlicensed assistive personnel provide.

Health care organizations such as hospitals, rehabilitation, and long-term care facilities are places where direct patient care is provided. Over time, there has been a decline in the number of hospital beds (Figure 12-5), reflecting a shift towards outpatient care (National Center for Health Statistics, 2006). In 2004, there were approximately 5,759 hospitals in the United States with 955,768 beds at an occupancy rate of 68.9%. That same year there were 16,117 nursing homes with 1,744,258 beds and an occupancy rate of 82.7%.

Other organizations, such as medical supply and pharmaceutical companies, and accrediting organizations, participate in patient care indirectly. Medical supply and pharmaceutical companies have provided many technological advances to health care. However, these innovations come at high financial costs to the system. These organizations, particularly pharmaceutical companies, have come under scrutiny for the high cost of their products. For example, a new medication for a certain type of skin cancer was introduced in 2006 that costs over $7,000 for a month's supply. Most patients, even if insured, would have difficulty covering the cost of that medication. To compare how drug prices have changed, in the mid-1990s the cost of medications (per patient) to treat colon cancer was approximately $500. Today, the cost is about $250,000 (Fleck, 2006).

Figure 12-5

Over time, there has been a shift towards outpatient care and a decline in the number of hospital beds.

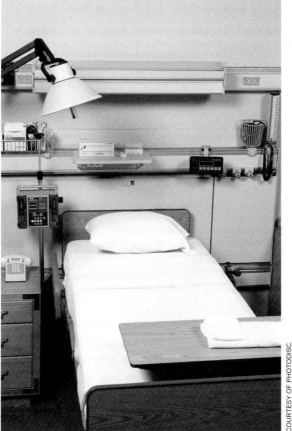

COURTESY OF PHOTODISC.

The **Joint Commission** (formerly The Joint Commission on Accreditation of Healthcare Organizations) is the leading accrediting agency for health care organizations. Quality reviews of health care organizations began in 1918, when the American College of Surgeons (ACS) conducted on-site inspections to determine if hospitals were meeting the "Minimum Standards for Hospitals," a one-page document published the previous year (http://www.jointcommission.org). The Joint Commission was formally established in 1951, when the ACS joined with the American College of Physicians, the American Hospital Association, the American Medical Association, and the Canadian Medical Association to create a separate organization dedicated to providing voluntary accreditation. It has evolved to become a very influential organization, since hospitals are accredited by the Joint Commission to participate in the Medicare and Medicaid programs.

Health care providers' expertise is the key to their influence in the system. Their services are fundamental to health care, and require a specialized knowledge base to perform. As a result, they have considerable power and authority. Providers want to be able to provide quality care that their patients can afford, without having to deal with excessive bureaucracy. Providers face constraints on their practice from insurance companies and regulatory agencies. Gone are the days when the patient and provider could maintain an exclusive relationship. The care provided to patients is usually influenced by outside parties. Providers believe these administrative requirements limit their autonomy, and interfere with their clinical decision-making. Providers are also concerned with over-regulation. For example, hospitals are directly regulated by over 25 different entities including state and local governments, the Food and Drug Administration, the Occupational Safety and Health Administration, the Joint Commission, and others (American Hospital Association, 2001). Providers are expected to meet the standards of these multiple outside agencies monitoring their care.

Writing Exercise 12-1	Consider your thoughts on health care delivery. Do you think health care is a right or a privilege? What is your philosophy of practice? How do you see the role of the nurse in today's health care system? What are your concerns about today's health care system?

Payers

Health care payers include taxpayers, insurance companies, and employers. The government is the leading payer for health care, funding several programs for specific populations (U.S. Census Bureau, 2005a) (Figure 12-6). **Medicare** is the federal program that provides health insurance for people 65 and older, and for people under 65 with long-term disabilities. The **Medicaid** program covers people with demonstrated financial need. It is administered at the state level, and may be known by different names in different states. Military health care includes TRICARE/

Plan:	Target Population:
Medicare	People 65 and older; under 65 with certain long-term disabilities
Medicaid	Eligible low-income individuals and families
SCHIP	Low-income children whose parents do not qualify for Medicaid
TRICARE/CHAMPUS	Active duty and retired members of the uniformed services, their families and survivors
CHAMPVA	Eligible veterans and their dependents and survivors
VA	Eligible veterans of the Armed Forces
HIS	Eligible American Indians

CHAMPUS (Civilian Health and Medical Program of the Uniformed Services), which provides care for active duty and retired members of the uniformed services, their families, and survivors. CHAMPVA (Civilian Health and Medical Program of the Department of Veterans Affairs) provides coverage for eligible veterans, their dependents, and survivors of veterans. The Department of Veterans Affairs (VA) provides coverage for veterans of the Armed Forces. The Indian Health Service (IHS) is a health care program through which the Department of Health and Human Services provides medical assistance to eligible American Indians at HIS facilities.

The **State Children's Health Insurance Program (SCHIP)** is the newest federal program. It was enacted in 1997 to provide health insurance for low-income children whose parents do not qualify for Medicaid, but who are unable to afford private insurance. Like Medicaid, SCHIP may be known by different names in different states. The federal government provides funds for the states to offer the program in one of three ways:

1. Increasing the number of children enrolled in Medicaid.
2. Developing a new, separate health insurance program.
3. Creating a combination of the two.

Currently, nine states and the District of Columbia operate Medicaid expansions, 18 states operate separate programs, and 23 states operate combination programs (SCHIP 101: What is the State Children's Health Insurance Program, and how does it work?, 2007).

Private health insurance is the next largest payer (Figure 12-7). It is obtained usually through a person's employer, or the employer of a family member. A small number of people purchase insurance themselves. In 2005, 68.5% of the nonelderly received health care coverage from their employer; only 9.2% purchased it themselves (U. S. Census Bureau, 2007a). Employer-based health insurance is a unique aspect of health care that is not found in other countries. In terms of costs, it is beneficial because buying insurance collectively can decrease the costs. However, small employers are frequently unable to afford it.

A significant portion of the population is uninsured. It is estimated that 15% of the population, or over 44 million people, do not have health insurance (U.S. Census Bureau, 2007a). There are multiple reasons why people are uninsured. Many people simply cannot afford it.

Figure 12-7
Sources of
Government-
Sponsored Health
Insurance and
Sources of Private
Health Insurance.
(U.S. Census Bureau.)

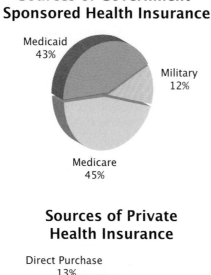

Sources of Government-Sponsored Health Insurance

Medicaid 43%

Military 12%

Medicare 45%

Sources of Private Health Insurance

Direct Purchase 13%

Employment–Based 87%

Health care costs have outpaced incomes and fewer businesses are offering health insurance (Kaiser Commission, 2006). Some people are in between employment, and very small percentages do not enroll in plans even though they are eligible. People are uninsured for different lengths of time. The gap between insurance coverage might only be a matter of weeks or months. Other patients may be without coverage for a year or more. They pay for health care themselves if they can afford it. These patients are at a disadvantage because they do not have the same purchasing and negotiating powers that insurers do. As a result, self-pay patients usually end up facing significantly higher rates for services.

Money drives the provision of health care. In general, if a treatment is reimbursable or paid for it is provided. For this reason, the payers seem to enjoy significant power in the current health care delivery system. They have implemented various cost-sharing and other mechanisms to attempt to control costs. However, they essentially dictate what they will pay for treatments. So care is generally reimbursed based upon amounts that the payers are willing to pay, not what the providers are willing to accept. Payers want to lower health care costs, and have control over how their money is spent.

Despite the apparent differences between participant groups and their perspective on health care delivery issues, there are actually key similarities in the problems they identify. The issues that participants identify are all fundamentally related to three areas: cost, access, and quality.

COST

Health care is very expensive, and it is getting more expensive each year. Currently, health care spending represents the largest part of the economy. The **Gross Domestic Product (GDP)** is the total spending on goods and services in the United States. The percentage of the GDP spent on health care has been rising steadily over the past 40 years (Goldman & Alpert, 2005) (Figure 12-8). In 1960, the amount spent on health care was slightly more than 5% of the total GDP. By 2002, that amount had tripled to about 15%. In terms of 2002 dollars, health care spending rose from $108 billion in 1960 to $1.6 trillion in 2002 (Goldman & Alpert, 2005).

Rising health care costs are not unique to the United States. The cost of health care is increasing around the world. The **Organisation for Economic Co-operation and Development (OECD)** is an international agency that studies political and social policies and collects statistics that describe the health of the world's population. According to the OECD in 2004, United States health care spending as a percentage of the GDP (15%) was the highest in the OECD—more than 6 percentage points higher than the average of 8.9% (OECD, 2006). The United States spends more on health care **per capita** (per person) than any other country. In 2004, the United States spent 6,100 United States Dollars (USD), more than twice the OECD average of 2,550 USD (OCED, 2006). At the same time, the United States utilizes fewer health care services than other

Figure 12-8
Health Care Spending as a Percentage of the GDP (1960–2002). (*Data from Goldman & Alpert, 2005.*)

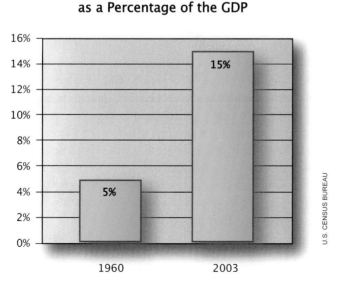

Health Care Spending as a Percentage of the GDP

countries, which implies that the price of health care is higher in the United States than in other countries (Goldman & Alpert, 2005).

Most of the money spent in the United States is on hospital services. In 2002, 53 cents of every dollar spent on health care was spent on hospital and physician services (Goldman & Alpart, 2005). Hospital costs are the most expensive component of the health care system. In 2004, total hospital costs (excluding physician expenses) rose to $295 billion—an increase of 21.9% from 2000 (Russo, Merrill, & Friedman, 2007). A key factor influencing this trend is the increase in the number of procedures performed on patients. In 2004, more than 60% of hospital stays involved some type of procedure. Procedures are usually associated with rising health care costs for several reasons: they are used to treat severely ill patients, the high costs of provider salaries, and the use of newer technologies and more expensive equipment.

Technological advances is one of several factors that contributes to rising health care costs. Health care technology is expensive. Technology and innovation is more widely available and more costly in the United States than in other countries (Bodenheimer, 2005b). Advances in technology usually improve quality, and also increase costs. Because the technology is available it tends to be used. Greater availability is associated with greater per capita use and higher spending on these services. For example, in the early 1990s magnetic resonance imaging (MRI) technology was new and relatively scarce (less than one site for every 100,000 persons in the United States) (Goldman & Alpert, 2005). In less than 10 years the number of sites had more than doubled, with a corresponding increase in the number of procedures performed. The laparoscopic cholecystectomy is another example of new technology that causes an increase in the number of procedures being performed (Bodenheimer, 2005b). A laparoscopic cholecystectomy is usually less expensive than an open cholecystectomy, however 60% more cholecystectomies (both laparoscopic and open) have been performed since the laparoscopic method was introduced.

Not all technology is used appropriately. Sometimes a new technology is not all it is touted as—sometimes the older way of doing something works just as well. Unlike many other developed nations, the United States does not have a uniform system to evaluate new technology (Bodenheimer, 2005b). Different participants in the system evaluate new technology—individual providers, organizations, and even payers. The evidence-based assessments compete with marketing and pressure from the manufacturers to determine the extent to which the technology is used. Of course, manufacturers are not the only ones that push the use of new technology. Patients tend to expect more advanced technology to be used. For example, implantable cardiac defibrillators are increasingly being used in an attempt to decrease the number of deaths from sudden fatal heart arrhythmias. In 2005, 162,000 of these devices were implanted in patients at a cost of approximately $40,000 per case (Fleck, 2006). It is projected by the year 2010, as many as 600,000 might be implanted at a cost of $24 billion per year. Many patients would argue that since these can save lives the cost is worth it. However, the criteria for implantation of these devices are not very specific, and consequently they never defibrillate 81% of the people who have had them for five years (Fleck, 2006).

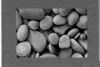

Several provider issues contribute to the increasing cost of health care. The types of physicians practicing in the United States, and the income they receive, increase the cost of health care (Bodenheimer, 2005c). The United States has more physician specialists than in other countries. Nations with more primary care practitioners have lower health care expenditures. Also, physicians in the United States charge more than their counterparts in other countries, and receive higher salaries. Physicians in the United States receive higher fees for similar services than do physicians in other countries. Physicians' income is three times higher in the United States than in the average nation that belongs to OECD. The ratio of average physician income to average employee compensation is 5.5 in the United States compared to 1.5 in the United Kingdom and Sweden.

Another provider factor that drives up cost is that health care providers tend to "corner the market"; that is, there is not a competitive market in health care (Bodenheimer, 2005a). Patients are not able to "shop around" and find the best provider at the lowest cost. In theory if patients could compare, physicians and hospitals would lower their fees to attract patients. There are several factors that limit a patient's ability to pick and choose providers. Most patients are restricted to certain providers who accept their health insurance. Also, since health insurance exists to protect patients from the financial disaster of serious illness, patients really do not need to shop for the lowest-priced services. Finally, different health conditions lead to widely differing costs. The patient is dependent upon the provider to diagnose the problem. For example, a patient with a headache could have a migraine or a brain tumor. A final provider issue that affects the cost of health care is the shortage of providers. Shortages are projected for most health care providers in large part because of the aging of the population. Salaries are rising to attract and retain certain providers such as nurses, which of course adds to the cost of health care.

Administrative costs and insurance also increase the expenses associated with health care. In 1999, administrative costs associated with health care totaled 24% of the total national expenditures on health care (Bodenheimer, 2005b). If the insurance system was simplified, billions of dollars could be saved. There are multiple insurance companies, and each offers different plans. Each insurer has different policies and procedures. Paperwork is abundant. Bureaucratic processes can be very cumbersome. Providers must hire staff in their offices dedicated to managing all of these tasks.

Two additional problems compounding the issue of rising costs are the inability to identify the true cost of health care and the aging population. First, it is difficult to identify the actual cost of health care. Organizations charge amounts for their services that may or may not reflect the true costs. Then there are multiple sources paying for health care, and they each pay different amounts. For example, a hospital may bill a patient $13,000 for a cesarean section. That patient's insurance company may have a contractual agreement for a reimbursement of $3,000. Another patient's insurance company may pay $4,000. A patient who does not have insurance would be billed for $13,000, unless other arrangements are made. The aging population is another concern. The amount spent on health care grows exponentially with age. People 65 and over spend about four times more than those under 65 (Goldman & Alpert, 2005). Medicare expenditures are projected to increase more than the projected revenues to fund the program (Davis & Collins, 2005–2006). Thus, it will become increasingly difficult to control costs as the baby boomers age.

ACCESS

A lot of money is spent on health care, but not everyone who needs the care will receive it. In the United States, adults receive only about half of the recommended health care services (Asch et al., 2006). The issue of access to health care is more than whether or not someone has insurance. There are multiple factors that affect access to care including financial, structural, and personal barriers.

Financial barriers to accessing health care include being uninsured, underinsured, or not having the means to cover services outside a health plan or insurance program (U.S. Department of Health and Human Services, 2000). Access to the system for these patients is through the emergency department, free clinics, and through regular providers with whom they can make financial arrangements. Over 40% of nonelderly uninsured adults have no regular source of health care (Kaiser Commission, 2006). It is estimated that **mortality** (death) could be reduced by 5 to 15% if the uninsured had continuous health insurance coverage (Kaiser Commission, 2006).

Another segment of the population is underinsured. These patients have health insurance, but the policies do not cover all of their costs. Some policies may have co-payments and deductibles that are too expensive for the policyholders. In some cases, pre-existing medical conditions are excluded. Some policies do not cover preventive care. Others may not cover certain types of services such as fertility treatments. Most policies have limitations on services such as prescription medications, outpatient services, and mental health services. Also, policies may be subject to lifetime maximum benefits. For example, children who receive an organ transplant must take costly medications to maintain the transplant. It is not unusual for these patients to find that after several years, their insurance will not pay for the medications any longer because they have reached a financial limit on their policy.

Having an insurance card does not guarantee access to care. It is not a gold card that a patient can use to obtain any services they need. In addition to the limitations of being underinsured, there are providers who simply do not accept certain insurances. Privately insured patients must usually see only providers in the plan's network. Patients who have Medicaid or Medicare may have to search for a provider who accepts it. Sometimes the provider accepts the insurance, but is not currently taking new patients with it. Patients frequently have to obtain referrals or authorizations for certain services, which may be declined. For certain medications or treatments, physicians may have to write a letter or fill out paperwork to justify the medical necessity of the treatment to the insurance company. The burden is frequently left to the patient to appeal any denials.

Structural barriers to health care access include the lack of providers or facilities to meet the population's needs as well as logistical barriers (U.S. Department of Health and Human Services, 2000). There are multiple parts of the country that are underserved by the medical community. Approximately 20% of Americans live in rural areas, yet only 9% of physicians practice there (AHRQ, 2005). Many rural hospitals are financially troubled, or have closed. Residents in these locations have limited access for even routine services. Research shows that rural Americans represent a population at risk for certain health **disparities**. These are differences that occur by gender, race or ethnicity, education or income, disability, geographic location, or sexual orientation (Office of Minority Health, 2007). Rural residents are more likely to be elderly, poor, in fair or poor health, have chronic health conditions, and die from heart disease (AHRQ, 2005). Relevant measures of rural health care are tracked in the National Healthcare Disparities Report. Patients face multiple logistical barriers to care. Patients frequently have to go to several sites for different aspects of their treatment. They may have to take off work to make appointments, which can be an added financial strain. Some patients have transportation issues, and must rely on family, friends, or public transportation to get to appointments.

Various personal barriers limit access to care (U.S. Department of Health and Human Services, 2000). Personal characteristics—race, ethnicity, age, and sex—all influence access and use of health care (Bronstein, Adams, & Florence, 2006). Research shows that patients who are women, older, members of racial and ethnic minorities, poorer, less educated, or uninsured have less access to care (Asch et al., 2006). Black persons have higher visit rates than white persons to hospital outpatient departments and emergency departments, but lower visit rates to office-based primary care and to surgical and medical specialists (Burt et al., 2007).

Cultural or spiritual differences and language barriers make it difficult for patients to access care. Prescribed treatments may conflict with a person's cultural or religious beliefs. For example, a patient may refuse medications because he or she believes in the healing power of home remedies. Patients with strict religious dietary guidelines may decline to be admitted to a hospital if they are going to be served traditional hospital food. Language barriers add challenges to caring for clients. Fortunately, the widespread availability of telephone-based interpreters can help to minimize communication issues. Some patients are reluctant to access care because of concerns about confidentiality or discrimination. A person who is HIV-positive may not seek treatment for fear of being treated differently by health care providers. Finally, people with disabilities may face environmental challenges when attempting to access different health care facilities.

Health literacy is another personal barrier that limits access to care. This term refers to a person's ability to understand their health care issues and effectively care for them in the health care system (Cutulli, 2007). Health literacy significantly affects health outcomes and costs. The ability to read is crucial to understanding self-care activities, including prescriptions, appointment cards, informed consent, and written instructions (Cutilli, 2007). Health literacy yields less frequent visits to care providers, shorter hospital stays, and lower health care costs (Speros, 2005). In fact, health literacy appears to be a stronger predictor of health status than socioeconomic status, age, or ethnic background. Inadequate health literacy is most prevalent among the elderly and those reporting poor health, which suggests that those with the greatest need for health care have the least ability to read and understand information needed to manage their own care (Speros, 2005). The increasing multicultural and multilingual diversity in the United States will present a challenge to this area.

QUALITY

One would expect that for all of the money the United States is spending on health care, the population would receive the highest quality care. According to the OECD (2006), that does not appear to be the case. In 2004, the life expectancy in the United States was 77.5 years, which is below the OECD average of 78.3 years. Infant mortality rates in the United States were 6.9 deaths per 1,000 live births in 2003, which is above the OECD average of 5.7. The countries with the lowest infant mortality rates are all below 3.5 deaths per 1,000 live births. Improvement in the near future does not appear likely. The United States is the OECD country with the highest obesity rates, which will have a substantial impact for future incidence of health problems.

In a recent study of health care in six countries (Australia, Canada, Germany, New Zealand, the United Kingdom, and the United States), the United States' health care system was ranked last (Davis et al., 2007). Several different areas were studied: Quality Care, Access, Efficiency, Equality, and Indicators of Healthy Lives. The United States did slightly better in some aspects of quality care. It ranked first on preventive care, and only next-to-last on coordinated care and patient-centered care (these are three of four aspects of quality care measured in this study). On all other measures, the United States ranked last.

In the United States, medical errors have become a prominent quality concern. In 1999, the Institute of Medicine (IOM) published a landmark study on medical errors that drew attention to the fact that **preventable adverse events**, or medical errors, are a leading cause of death in the United States (Kohn, Corrigan, & Donaldson, 1999). This has led to heightened awareness of the issue of health care quality. From its research, the IOM developed a multidimensional definition of health care quality that offers a new, comprehensive viewpoint of quality (Figure 12-9). Quality health care is: safe, effective, patient-centered, timely, efficient, and equitable (IOM, 2001). The IOM identified six specific aims for improvement based upon its definition of quality. The American Nurses Association (2005) endorses these six strategies to improve health care quality.

Health care should be delivered safely—when it is not, preventable adverse effects result (IOM, 2005). The definition of safe care is avoiding injuries to patients from the care that is intended to help them. It is naturally assumed if you technically do the right thing it will lead to the right patient outcome. However, safe care is not necessarily effective care. People should get the care they need and need the care they get. Together these concepts are referred to as **effectiveness**

Figure 12-9

Elements of Quality Health Care and Resulting Poor Outcomes. (*Data from IOM, 2001, and McGlynn, 2005.*)

Safe	→	medical errors or preventable adverse effects
Effective	→	under-used or over-used treatments
Patient-centered	→	unresponsive care
Timely	→	delayed care
Efficient	→	waste
Equitable	→	disparities

(IOM, 2005). If people do not get the care they need, the problem of under-use results. In a national study on health care quality, it was determined patients failed to receive needed services 46% of the time (McGlynn, 2005). The recommended care for managing chronic conditions was provided only 56% of the time. Preventive care met quality standards only 55% of the time, and recommended care for acute health problems was provided only 54% of the time. If people get care they do not need, the problem of overuse results. There are patients who receive interventions not expected to improve their health, and that may even be harmful. Many health care treatments lack evidence of their effectiveness. Early studies have shown that one-third of common surgical procedures may not benefit patients (McGlynn, 2005).

Patient-centered care is respectful of and responsive to individual patient preferences, needs, and values (IOM, 2005). It ensures that patient values guide all clinical decisions. Care that is not patient centered shows the health care system is not responsive to patients' needs and preferences. Timely care means reducing waits and the sometimes-harmful delays for both those who receive and those who give care. Efficiency in health care allows providers to avoid waste, including waste of equipment, supplies, ideas, and their energy. Equitable health care means providing care that does not vary in quantity because of personal characteristics such as gender, ethnicity, geographic location, and socioeconomic status. If equitable care is not provided, disparities are the result.

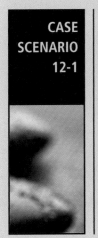

CASE SCENARIO 12-1

An uninsured man comes to the emergency department. He is diagnosed with a serious infection and needs to be admitted for IV antibiotics. He refuses because he says he cannot afford it, yet without the treatment he will suffer serious consequences and could die. He requests that he be allowed to stay at home, and come into the hospital every 12 hours to receive the IV antibiotic. The patient will receive the antibiotic in different locations of the hospital depending upon which location is open (the outpatient department during the day during the week, and the emergency department during the evening and on the weekends).

CASE ANALYSIS

1. How do the issues of cost and access appear in this patient situation?

2. How is this compromise plan beneficial to the patient?

3. What are the quality issues?

ADDRESSING THE ISSUES

The issues of cost, access, and quality are widely recognized for their impact on health. **Healthy People 2010**, the document that outlines the government's vision for the health of the nation, contains two overall goals for the United States to work towards for the year 2010 (U.S. Department of Health and Human Services, 2000) (Figure 12-10). The first goal is to increase the quality and years of healthy life. Obviously providing health care to the population can

Figure 12-10
Goals and Focus
Areas of Healthy
People 2010.
*(Source: U.S.
Department of
Health and Human
Services, 2000.)*

Goals: **Increase the quality and years of healthy life.** **Eliminate health disparities.**	
Focus Areas:	
1. Access to Quality Health Services	15. Injury and Violence Prevention
2. Arthritis, Osteoporosis, and Chronic Back Conditions	16. Maternal, Infant, and Child Health
3. Cancer	17. Medical Product Safety
4. Chronic Kidney Disease	18. Mental Health and Mental Disorders
5. Diabetes	19. Nutrition and Overweight
6. Disability and Secondary Conditions	20. Occupational Safety and Health
7. Educational and Community-Based	21. Oral Health Programs
8. Environmental Health	22. Physical Activity and Fitness
9. Family Planning	23. Public Health Infrastructure
10. Food Safety	24. Respiratory Diseases
11. Health Communication	25. Sexually Transmitted Diseases
12. Heart Disease and Stroke	26. Substance Abuse
13. HIV	27. Tobacco Use
14. Immunization and Infectious Diseases	28. Vision and Hearing

decrease **morbidity**, or disease and disability, as well as increase life expectancy. In order for this to occur, the population has to be able to afford health care and have access to it. Additionally, the interventions they receive have to be of good quality, that is, appropriate and therapeutic for the patients' condition.

The second goal of Healthy People 2010 is to eliminate health disparities. The expected growth and changes to the population will magnify the importance of addressing health disparities. Groups currently experiencing poorer health status are expected to grow as a proportion of the total population. The future health of the nation will be influenced substantially by improving the health of these groups. The Department of Health and Human Services is focusing on six areas in which racial and ethnic minorities experience serious disparities in health access and outcomes: infant mortality, cancer screening and management, cardiovascular disease, diabetes, HIV infection/AIDS, and immunizations. These were selected because they affect multiple groups at all life stages. Other conditions that disproportionately impact racial and ethnic minorities are mental health problems, hepatitis, syphilis, and tuberculosis.

Through Healthy People 2010, the government presents a comprehensive vision for improving the population's health. However, much work remains to be done. In order to meet the goals and objectives of Healthy People 2010, the United States must address the health care issues of cost, access, and quality. Progress towards meeting the goals and objectives of Healthy People 2010 is measured using **health indicators**. Health indicators describe measurable behaviors, environmental factors, or health system issues that affect health status. Access to health care is one of the health indicators in Healthy People 2010 (U.S. Department of Health and Human Services, 2000).

It is difficult to reach a consensus on the best solutions for health care problems. Since the issues of cost and access can be controversial, the most advances have been made in the area of quality. Politically it is much easier for different participants to support improved quality. The most research on health care quality to date is in the area of clinical effectiveness of treatments. Researchers in different professions are developing a growing body of literature on evidence-based practice. Another development in the area of health care quality is the practice of sharing the results of quality reviews with the public. This potentially will enable the patients to become more informed consumers of health care. At the same time, there are concerns that the most meaningful data are not being shared with patients. Also, there is the risk that data will be misunderstood or misinterpreted by the public.

The **Core Measures** program, developed by the Joint Commission, is a sizable effort to promote standardized, quality care in hospitals. Data are collected by hospitals on selected acute care (inpatient) populations including patients who are diagnosed with pneumonia, congestive heart failure, and myocardial infarctions, as well as surgical and obstetrical patients. Hospitals are expected to meet certain standards of care for these patients. For example, pneumonia patients are expected to have pulse oximetry checks, and the appropriate antibiotics administered soon after arrival. Patients with congestive heart failure are supposed to receive written instructions regarding their condition and how to manage it at home. The hospitals' data are made available to the public, so anyone can review a hospital's performance. Their performance also has financial consequences. The Joint Commission is in the process of finalizing how the results will be linked to reimbursement. Hospitals that do not meet the standards of care for these patients will risk losing money. So the stakes for hospitals are high—meet these quality standards, or risk negative publicity as well as decreased reimbursement.

Payers are also becoming involved in quality issues. The Leapfrog Group is a notable example of this. The Leapfrog Group is a consortium of major companies and other large health care purchasers whose mission is to trigger giant "leaps" forward in the safety, quality, and affordability of health care (http://www.leapfroggroup.org). This group believes that money speaks, and quality would improve if the payers recognized it and rewarded it. They are advocating for four safety practices that have overwhelming scientific support, are feasible to implement in the short term, and that consumers and purchasers can readily recognize and appreciate. The four practices are: the use of computer physician order entry, evidence-based hospital referral, intensive care unit staffing by physicians experienced in critical care medicine, and the Leapfrog Safe Practices Score, which measures the use of procedure to decrease the risk of medical errors.

Internet Exercise 12-2

Review the Web site http://www.leapfroggroup.org.

1. Compare the quality ratings for at least two hospitals near you.

2. How are the ratings computed?

3. Are the ratings explained clearly enough for a patient to understand?

4. What conclusions might a patient draw about the hospital(s)?

Finally, there is an integrated effort to improve health care quality. The **National Quality Forum (NQF)** is a private, nonprofit organization that is working to improve the quality of health care through the development of standards and methods to measure quality care (http://www.qualityforum.org). This organization is a product of the 1998 Presidential Advisory Commission on Consumer Protection and Quality in the Health Care Industry. According to the Web site, it is a public-private partnership with participation from numerous patients, providers, and payers. The organization has completed or continues the ongoing research and development of quality standards in multiple areas, including for different medical conditions such as cancer and diabetes. They are also working to measure nursing's contribution to health care quality through the development of nursing-specific indicators.

Writing Exercise 12-3

Review the issues with the health care system you identified in Writing Exercise 12-1. From the viewpoint of a patient, consider each issue. Identify a solution for each concern from the perspective of the patient. Now, try this from the perspective of a provider, and then from a payer. Did you identify a solution that would satisfy everyone?

Even though participants in health care delivery are concerned about the same issues—cost, access, and quality—it does not mean they all agree on the same solutions. In fact, frequently participants' solutions are in opposition. For example, everyone is concerned about the high cost of health care. Patients would lower premiums and out-of-pocket expenses. The patients' solution would mean either more money would have to be paid by insurers, or providers would receive less money for their services. This solution would not be supported by either of those groups. This example illustrates the roadblock to any meaningful reform in health care today. It is difficult to come up with a solution to these issues that satisfies everyone. Since no one can agree on a solution, not much is being done. Small fixes or patches appear here and there, but so far there has not been any significant changes to the system. As a result, the subject of health care rationing is becoming more relevant.

RATIONING

Everything in life is rationed—there is not a limitless supply of anything. If there is not enough of a particular resource, there must be some means of allocating it. Usually, resources are rationed by price (Bernstein, 2006). If more people want homes in a particular neighborhood than there are homes available, then the price of the homes goes up. If there are more homes available than interested buyers, then the prices of the homes declines. However, in health care it is difficult to use price as a means of **rationing** since most patients do not pay the entire cost of their care. So, simply increasing the price of a health care service does not lead to the usual amount of rationing.

Health care rationing is a pressing issue. The question is not whether or not rationing should occur, but instead what mechanism of rationing is the best (Bernstein, 2006). Rationing has been occurring in health care for some time as an outcome of the current delivery system. Two rationing methods that have stemmed from the current health care system include rationing based upon prices or cost of health care to the patient, and rationing by creating a hassle for the patient (Bernstein, 2006).

The use of co-payments and deductibles has been used for some time to force patients to share the cost and think carefully before utilizing health care services. Now, a new means of price rationing is emerging in the form of health savings accounts (Bernstein, 2006). These are for people who have **high deductible health plans (HDHP)**, with deductibles of generally at least $1,000 for an individual, or $2,000 for a family. The account owner and/or the employer contribute money tax-free into this account, which is then withdrawn tax-free and used to pay medical expenses. Theoretically, patients with this type of account will more carefully consider the price of a health care service before utilizing it (Bernstein, 2006). This will lead to either decreased utilization of health care services, and/or encourage shopping around. A possible negative outcome of these plans is that a patient may not get needed treatments because they do not want to or are not able to pay the costs.

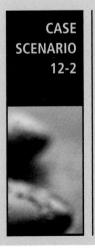

CASE SCENARIO 12-2

You are caring for a patient in the emergency department who has a severe headache and a dangerously high blood pressure reading. You determine he has several chronic health problems, and recently switched to a high-deductible health plan. He must meet a $1,000 deductible before his insurance plan will pay for his medical care. He has not seen his primary care physician for any follow-up because he did not want to pay for the visit.

CASE ANALYSIS

1. What are the issues in this scenario?

2. What educational needs does this patient have?

3. How you would approach the patient?

4. What information would you give the patient?

The second form of rationing that occurs is rationing by hassle (Bernstein, 2006). Patients cannot rapidly get the care they need; instead they must work to get it. Gatekeeping is a form of rationing by hassle. If a patient is in a health maintenance organization (HMO), they must first contact their primary care physician to get authorization for other services. Another example of rationing by hassle is when patients want a certain medication, and physicians must fill out forms to get authorization for the medication to be covered by insurance.

The idea of more overt rationing has been introduced. In 1994, Oregon was facing a budget crisis, and rather than decrease the number of enrollees or cut reimbursement to providers, a list was developed that prioritized health care treatments. When introduced, the list was perceived as rationing of health care. It was very controversial, and evoked national debates about the topic (but Oregon's health care initiative holds lessons for other states, March 2007). The list was formed through a process of community meetings, public opinion surveys on quality-of-life preferences, cost-benefit analyses, and medical outcomes research (Oberlander, Marmor, & Jacobs, 2001). Medical diagnoses and their corresponding treatments were then ranked according to their benefit. However, the list was not formulated completely on a scientific basis. Calculations were used, but the list was manipulated to satisfy different political interests (Oberlander et al., 2001). Once the list was complete, a line was drawn and conditions below it were not covered. For example, in 1999, the line was placed after diagnosis/treatment #574 of 743 (Oberlander et al., 2001). The first five non-covered diagnoses/treatments (#575–579) were: medical therapy for chronic anal fissure, complex prosthetics for broken dental appliances, medical and psychotherapy for impulse disorders, medical and surgical treatment for sexual dysfunction, and psychotherapy for sexual dysfunction.

Oregon's list did not end up the rationing tool as expected for several reasons. First, the line below which services may be denied is actually set quite low (Bodenheimer, 1997a). The total number of excluded services is relatively small with marginal medical value. In fact, the list only saved approximately 2% of costs during the first five years of the plan because so few treatments were denied (Oberlander et al., 2001). Providers also work around the list. Patients with co-morbidities are diagnosed with problems above the line, but still receive treatment for problems below the line (Oberlander et al., 2001). Finally, the list only has to be adhered to with the small percent (13%) of patients that are in the fee-for-service Medicaid program (Bodenheimer, 1997a). The rest of the enrollees (87%) are in managed-care plans that do actually provide care for treatments below the line.

The final version of Oregon's plan does not truly represent health care rationing. Oregon actually expanded benefits for its population rather than reducing them (Bodenheimer, 1997a). Because of the intense debate over rationing, ironically the developers of the plan were forced to define a minimum package of services that provided basic coverage for everyone (Fox & Leichter, 1993). As part of the plan more citizens became eligible for Medicaid, and the Medicaid program began covering services that were not previously included in its program. When it was first introduced the Oregon Health Plan was considered innovative; however, because of decreased funding and arbitrary cuts it now basically resembles other states' Medicaid programs (but Oregon's health care initiative holds lessons for other states, March 2007). No other state has attempted to copy Oregon's plan (Oberlander et al., 2001). At this point, overt rationing of health care is not accepted in the United States. This shows that despite significant problems with the health care system, the United States is not ready to make the difficult decisions necessary to address these problems. Any significant changes to the system are extremely difficult to enact because of special-interest groups fighting them.

Another well-known example of rationing occurred in 2004, when the United States experienced a shortage of flu vaccinations. The Centers for Disease Control (CDC) identified guidelines for rationing the available supply (Olick, 2005). Several special high-risk populations were identified, and were eligible to receive the vaccine. The CDC determined risk for infection, risk for serious illness, and risk for spreading infection to be the key factors for identifying candidates for vaccination. The controversy was lessened because the guidelines did not establish priorities among the high-risk populations, and were not done based upon ability to pay. Because of this experience, the CDC formed an ethics advisory panel to assist with the rationing of the flu vaccine and to set the groundwork for how to make future rationing decisions (Olick, 2005).

Rationing is a controversial topic that raises several important questions. Who makes the decisions regarding which treatments to ration? What are the criteria for identifying the patients who will receive the treatments? How do you avoid discrimination? How do you handle lifestyle-related health issues? At what point is it legitimate or ethical to ration health care to a patient because the patient is seen as having caused the health problem (Dimond, 2006)? This is an important question, as a majority of the leading causes of death are caused by lifestyle-related health problems. For example, do you deny a person who smokes the latest treatment for chronic lung disease? Again as the Oregon plan illustrates, the United States is not fully prepared to answer these and other tough questions that are required to implement rationing.

HEALTH CARE DELIVERY ISSUES AND THE IMPLICATIONS FOR NURSING

Nurses practice in every setting in which health care is delivered, and routinely face issues related to cost, access, and quality. Ironically, there is not much in the nursing literature about the profession's perspective on these subjects. Yet, there is significant opportunity for nurses to make a difference in these three areas.

Nurses manage patient resources, and have the potential to make a significant difference in terms of health care costs. This is particularly true in the hospital setting where a majority of nurses practice. For example, a significant amount of waste occurs in health care when supplies are ordered and not used. There are no national estimates of the amount of health care spending that can be attributed to waste (McGlynn, 2005). However, in one study, the use of six expensive and frequently used anesthesia drugs was studied over a one-year period in one hospital. The researchers compared the amount of medication ordered to the amount actually administered, and found that the total cost of unadministered drugs was $165,667, or 26% of what was spent on all drugs in the anesthesia department (McGlynn, 2005).

Providing nursing care represents a significant health care cost, but the exact financial impact is not readily known. Nursing is the only profession with 24-hour direct accountability for care of hospitalized patients (Welton, Fischer, Degrace, & Zone-Smith, 2006). Nursing labor costs are the main part of a hospital's budget. However, little is known about the relationship between the cost of nursing care and reimbursement (Welton et al., 2006). Nursing charges have generally been incorporated into room and board charges. However, actual nursing care and costs varies from patient to patient despite the room and board charges being the same. Researchers are in the process of developing and refining languages that label and describe the work nurses do. The **North American Nursing Diagnosis Association (NANDA)** taxonomy contains diagnostic labels used to identify patient problems. The **Nursing Interventions Classification (NIC)** describes nursing interventions, while the **Nursing Outcomes Classification (NOC)** labels patient outcomes. This type of research is a necessary step towards having a better understanding of the actual cost of nursing care and ultimately receiving direct reimbursement for it.

With regards to access to health care, nursing is well poised to address this issue. Nurses advocate for patients, and educate them regarding their options in the health care system. Nurses who work as case managers in particular have the chance to study and improve access to health care. Also, the concept of health literacy is becoming more prominent in the nursing literature. Nurses have multiple opportunities to improve the health literacy of their patients to help them access and maneuver more efficiently through the system (Figure 12-11).

The issue of quality in health care delivery is the one area in which nursing has made the most progress. The growth of research on evidence-based practice is apparent in the nursing literature.

Figure 12-11
Nurses can work to improve the health literacy of their clients.

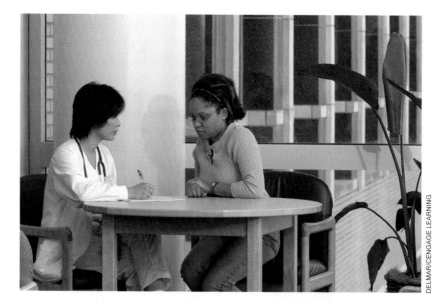

DELMAR/CENGAGE LEARNING

Nurse researchers are studying the profession's contributions to health care in order to demonstrate that nursing care and expertise contributes to positive patient outcomes. Researchers are also studying the correlation between the utilization of RNs versus lower skill mixes of providers and the impact on quality care. Nursing care provided by RNs is positively correlated with patient and employee satisfaction as well as clinical quality (Clark, Leddy, Drain, & Kaldenberg, 2007).

Nursing has the opportunity to make a difference in terms of providing safe care. Unfortunately the typical work environment for nurses contains multiple barriers to providing safe care. Several practices can help overcome these barriers (Kalisch & Aebersold, 2006). Start by creating a value-driven environment—make patient safety a priority. Encourage reporting of mistakes and consistently analyze mistakes and near-misses. Remove the fear of retribution when mistakes occur, and instead view them as learning opportunities. Foster resilience so that the staff can identify, address, and move forward from errors that occur. Look for the unexpected, and anticipate problems that could occur with a patient. When possible, simplify work processes and minimize interruptions. Create and promote teamwork among staff on the unit. At the same time, recognize expertise. Include nurses in the decision-making and administrative processes that govern patient care, since they are the hands-on providers of care.

Knowledge is key to addressing the issues of cost, access, and quality. Improving one's own knowledge is a necessary first step. Nurses should strive to be informed providers who understand the context in which they practice. Nurses must learn all they can about the health care delivery system, and stay up-to-date on current health care issues. Self-awareness is important for the nurse to practice ethically. Nurses can get involved at the organizational level to control costs, help facilitate access, and to facilitate quality improvement. In the community, nurses should keep up with local, state, and national issues. Membership in a professional organization is a good way to become politically active. The American Nurses Association is working for the creation of a health care system that is patient centered and provides equal access to safe, high-quality care for every citizen and resident in a cost-effective manner (American Nurses Association, 2005).

Nurses need to educate patients on these issues of cost, access, and quality. Nurses should strive to inform and empower patients. Learning more about health literacy, its pervasiveness in society, and its relationship to outcomes is essential (Speros, 2005). Nurses can shape the clinical environment to support the health of the less literate (Hixon, 2004). Walk through the clinical area and view it from the patient's perspective. Make sure enrollment forms are as simple as possible, and informed consent documents and other patient information are easy to read and understand. When working with patients create a nonjudgmental environment. Use tact, do not stigmatize—the goal is to individualize care based on the client's needs (Hixon, 2004). Also, use plain language (avoiding medical jargon), speak slowly, use pictures and visual images, limit the amount of information given in one encounter, and ask patients to recall what they have learned (Speros, 2005). On a broader level, nurses should advocate at the policy level against barriers to access and understanding of health information for vulnerable groups (Speros, 2005).

SUMMARY

There are multiple participants in the health care system that can be classified as either patients, providers, or payers. They all recognize that cost, access, and quality are the three key issues in health care today. However, the participants do not necessarily share the same viewpoint when it comes to resolving these issues. Incremental changes to the system occur, but so far no one participant group has been able to enact any significant reform to the system. As a result, health care rationing is emerging as a significant issue that needs to be addressed. Nurses are at the forefront of health care delivery and are well poised to address these three issues.

All easy problems have already been solved.

–Anonymous

REFERENCES

AGENCY FOR HEALTHCARE RESEARCH AND QUALITY. (2005). *2005 National healthcare disparities report.* Retrieved August 18, 2007, from http://www.ahrq.gov/qual/nhdr05/nhadr05.pdf

AMERICAN HOSPITAL ASSOCIATION. (2001). *The case for a better health system.* Retrieved June 7, 2007, from http://www.aha.org/aha/issues/CBHCS/index.html

AMERICAN NURSES ASSOCIATION. (1992). *Registered nurse utilization of unlicensed assistive personnel.* Retrieved July 16, 2007, from http://www.nursingworld.org/readroom/position/uap/uapuse.htm

AMERICAN NURSES ASSOCIATION. (2005). *ANA's health care agenda 2005.* Retrieved July 16, 2007, from http://www.nursingworld.org/readroom/anahca05.pdf

ASCH, S. M., Kerr, E. A., Keesey, J., Adams, J. L., Setodji, C. M., Malik, S., et al. (2006). Who is at greatest risk for receiving poor-quality health care? *New England Journal of Medicine, 354,* 1147–1156.

BERNSTEIN, J. (2006). Topics in medical economics: Health care rationing. *Journal of Bone and Joint Surgery, 88,* 2527–2532.

BODENHEIMER, T. (1997a). The Oregon health plan—Lessons for the nation (First of two parts). *NEJM, 337,* 651–655.

BODENHEIMER, T. (1997b). The Oregon health plan—Lessons for the nation (Second of two parts). *NEJM, 337,* 720–723.

BODENHEIMER, T. (2005a). High and rising health care costs. Part 1: Seeking an explanation. *Annals of Internal Medicine, 142,* 847–854.

BODENHEIMER, T. (2005b). High and rising health care costs. Part 2: Technologic innovation. *Annals of Internal Medicine, 142,* 932–936.

BODENHEIMER, T. (2005c). High and rising health care costs. Part 3: The role of health care providers. *Annals of Internal Medicine, 142,* 996–1002.

BRONSTEIN, J. M., Adams, E. K., & Florence, C. S. (2006). SCHIP structure and children's use of care. *Health Care Financing Review, 27,* 41–51.

But Oregon's Healthcare Initiative Holds Lessons For Other States. (March 2007). *Healthcare Financial Management*, 12–13.

Burt, C. W., McGaig, L. F., & Rechsteiner, E. A. (2007). Ambulatory medical care utilization estimates for 2005. *Advance data from vital and health statistics; number 388*. Hyattsville, MD: National Center for Health Statistics.

Clark, P., Leddy, K., Drain, M., & Kaldenberg, D. (2007). State nursing shortages and patient satisfaction: More RNs—better patient experiences. *Journal of Nursing Care Quality, 22*, 119–127.

Cohn, J. (2007). *Sick: The untold story of America's health care crisis—and the people who pay the price*. New York: HarperCollins Publishers.

Cutilli, C. C. (2007). Health literacy in geriatric patients: An integrative review of the literature. *Orthopaedic Nursing, 26*, 43–48.

Davis, K., & Collins, S. (Winter 2005–2006). Medicare at forty. *Health Care Financing Review, 25*(2), 53–62.

Davis, K., Schoen, C., Shoenbaum, S., Doty, M., Holmgren, J., Kriss, J., & Shea, K. (May 2007). *Mirror, mirror on comparative performance of American health care*. The Commonwealth Fund. Retrieved August 14, 2007, from http://www.commonwealthfund.org/publications/publications_show.htm

Dimond, B. (2006). Rights, resources, and health care. *Nursing Ethics, 13*, 335–336.

Goldman, D. P., & Alpert, A. E. (2005). Costs and insurance. In D. P. Goldman & E. A. McGlynn, (Eds.), *U.S. health care facts about cost, access, and quality*. Santa Monica, CA: RAND Corporation. Retrieved May 7, 2007, from http://www.rand.org/pubs/corporate_pubs/2005/RAND_CD484.1pdf

Fleck, L. M. (2006). The cost of caring: Who pays? Who profits? Who panders? *Hastings Center Report, 36*(3), 13–17.

Fox, D. M. & Leichter, H. M. (1993). The ups and downs of Oregon's rationing plan. *Health Affairs, 12*(2), 66–70.

Health Resources and Services Administration. (2004). *What is behind the HRSA's projected supply, demand, and shortage of registered nurses?* Retrieved July 21, 2007, from ftp://ftp.hrsa.gov/bhpr/workforce/behindshortage.pdf

Helman, R., Greenwald, M. & Associates, & Fronstin, P. (2006). 2006 Health Confidence Survey: Dissatisfaction with health care system doubles since 1998. *EBRI Notes, 27*(11), 2–10.

Herzlinger, R. (2007). *Who killed health care: America's $2 trillion medical problem and the consumer-driven cure*. New York: McGraw-Hill.

Hixon, A. L. (2004). Functional health literacy: Improving health outcomes. *American Family Physician, 69*, 2077–2078.

Institute of Medicine. (2001). *Crossing the quality chasm: A new health system for the 21st century*. Washington, DC: National Academy Press.

Kaiser Commission. (2006). *The uninsured and their access to health care*. Retrieved April 15, 2007, from http://www.kff.org/uninsured/1420.cfm

Kalisch, B., & Aebersold, M. (2006). Overcoming barriers to patient safety. *Nursing Economic$, 24*, 143–149.

Kleinman, C. S., & Saccomano, S. J. (2006). Registered nurses and unlicensed assistive personnel: An uneasy alliance. *Journal of Continuing Education in Nursing, 37*, 162–170.

Kohn, L. T., Corrigan, J. M., & Donaldson, M. S. (Eds.). (1999). *To err is human: Building a safer health system*. Washington, DC: National Academy Press.

Leapfrog Group. (2007). *Fact sheet*. Retrieved July 17, 2007, from http://www.leapfroggroup.org

LeBow, B. (2002). *Health care meltdown: Confronting the myths and fixing our failing system*. Boise, ID: JRI Press.

McGlynn, E. A. (2005). Quality of care. In D. P. Goldman & E. A. McGlynn (Eds.), *U.S. health care facts about cost, access, and quality*. Santa Monica, CA: RAND Corporation. Retrieved May 7, 2007, from http://www.rand.org/pubs/corporate_pubs/2005/RAND_CD484.1pdf

Moore, M. (Writer/Director). (2007). *Sicko* [motion picture]. United States: Dog Eat Dog Films.

National Center for Health Statistics. (2006). *Health, United States, 2006 with chartbook on trends in the health of Americans.* Hyattsville, MD: Author. Retrieved May 14, 2007, from http://www.cdc.gov/nichs/data/hus/hus06.pdf

National Quality Forum. (n.d.). Retrieved July 12, 2007, from http://www.qualityforum.org

Oberlander, J., Marmor, T., & Jacobs, L. (2001). Rationing medical care: Rhetoric and reality in the Oregon health plan. *CMAJ, 164,* 1583–1587.

Office of Minority Health. (2007). *Eliminating racial & ethnic health disparities.* Retrieved August 16, 2007, from http://www.cdc.gov/omh/AboutUs/disparities.htm

Olick, R. S. (2005). Ethics in public health: Rationing the flu vaccine. *Journal of Public Health Management Practice, 11,* 373–374.

Organisation for Economic Co-operation and Development. (2006). *OECD health data 2006: How does the United States compare.* Retrieved June 30, 2007, from http://www.oecd.org/topic/0,3373,en_2649_37407_1_1_1_1_374 07,00.html

Russo, C., Merrill, C., & Friedman, B. (April 2007). Procedures with the most rapidly increasing hospital costs, 2000–2004. *HCUP statistical brief #28.* Rockville, MD: Agency for Healthcare Research and Quality. Retrieved May 14, 2007, from http://www.hcup-us.ahrq.gov/reports/statbriefs.jsp

SCHIP 101: What is the State Children's Health Insurance Program, and how does it work? (June 2007). Retrieved August 12, 2007, from http://www.familiesusa.org/assets/pdfs/SCHIP-101.pdf

Speros, C. (2005). Health literacy: Concept analysis. *Journal of Advanced Nursing, 50,* 633–640.

United States Census Bureau. (2007a). *Current population survey 2005 and 2006 annual social and economic (ASEC) supplement.* Retrieved April 14, 2007, from http://www.census.gov/hhes/www/hlthing/usernote/usernote 3-21rev

United States Census Bureau. (2007b). *National population projections.* Retrieved July 15, 2007, from http://www.census.gov/population/www/pop-profile/natproj.html

United States Census Bureau. (2005a). *Health insurance.* Retrieved July 16, 2007, from http://www.census.gov/hhes/www/hlthins/hlthinstypes.html

United States Census Bureau. (2005b). *United States: Population and housing narrative profile: 2005.* Retrieved August 9, 2007, from http://factfinder.census.gov/

United States Department of Health and Human Services. (2006). *Physician supply and demand: Projections to 2030.* Retrieved August 3, 2007, from ftp://ftp.hrsa.gov/bhpr/workforce/PhysicianForecastingPaperFinal.pdf

United States Department of Health and Human Services. (2000). *Healthy People 2010: Understanding and improving health (2nd ed.).* Washington, DC: U.S. Government Printing Office.

Welton, J., Fishcer, M., DeGrace, S., & Zone-Smith, L. (2006). Hospital nursing costs, billing, and reimbursement. *Nursing Economic$, 24,* 239–262.

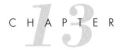

C H A P T E R

13

INFORMATION AND LIFE-LONG LEARNING

PAMELA SHERWILL-NAVARRO

MLS, AHIP, Librarian, Remington College of Nursing

Knowledge is of two kinds. We know a subject ourselves, or we know where we can find information on it.

–Samuel Johnson

LEARNING OBJECTIVES

At the completion of the chapter the learner should be able to do the following:

1. Explain the difference between popular press materials and professional literature.
2. List at least three different domain names and tell what they stand for.
3. Give an example of an information need that would be best answered by a textbook and one that would be best answered by a journal article.
4. Discuss the different journal publication types: case report, case series, cohort studies, clinical trials, randomized control trials, editorials, and news reports.
5. Compare and contrast systematic reviews and a meta-analysis.
6. Demonstrate how to search a database using advanced features such as subject headings, limiting, and field searching.
7. Formulate a search statement to answer an information need.
8. Define a federated search engine, or Meta search, and analyze the advantages and pitfalls of using one.
9. Create a searchable, evidence-based query.
10. Identify several ways of facilitating life-long learning.

KEY TERMS

Bibliographic Management
    Software
Case Reports
Case Series
CINAHL

Clinical Trials
Cochrane Database of
    Systematic Reviews
Databases
Evidence-Based Practice

Federated Search Engines
Magazines
Meta-Analysis
Peer Review
PICO

Professionalism   Refereed   Textbooks
Professional Journals   Search Engines   RSS
PubMed   Search Statements   Web sites
PsycInfo   Systematic Reviews   Wiki
Randomized Control Trials

INTRODUCTION

Since the 1960s, when libraries began to automate their catalogs, to the 1990s, many databases migrated from print format, to CD-ROMS, to the Internet. The types and amounts of information available have increased exponentially. Being able to search the vast number of Web sites, databases, journals, and library catalogs efficiently and to be able to quickly evaluate the results is necessary to avoid information overload. Knowing the major types of information, who produces them, where they are found, and what is the best type to answer a particular information need is the basis of information literacy (Figure 13-1). It is impossible to

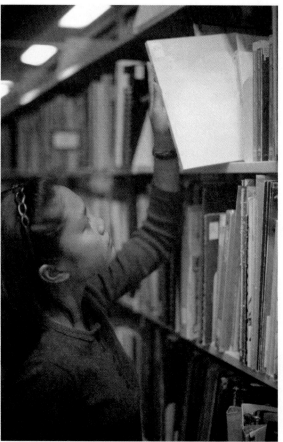

Figure 13-1
Information literacy means knowing the best types of information to answer a specific need, including who produces it and where it is located.

COURTESY OF PHOTODISC.

read everything published in the nursing and health care field, yet failure to read research and continue to develop your professional knowledge base will result in a failure to practice in a manner that is research- or evidence-based, current, and safe.

There is a lag between medical discoveries and the time it takes for those developments to be integrated into practice. The time lag has been estimated to be between ten and twenty years (*Translating research into practice (TRIP) — II, 2001*). More than 20,000 randomized control trials are published each year (Glasziou & Del Mar, 2003). It was estimated in 1993 that the amount of nursing literature doubles every five years (Weaver, 1993). Since that article was written in a pre-Internet world, that number is probably a very conservative estimate of how many articles are published annually. It is impossible to read all of the new nursing literature.

INFORMATION SOURCES

We are bombarded with many types of information. Information comes to us from radio, television, newspapers, magazines, e-mail, Web sites, professional publications, pod casts, conferences, Webinars (Web-based seminar), and colleagues. Depending upon the intended use for the information, sources may vary in relevance. Radio, television, newspapers, and magazines frequently cover medical and health care news, however these reports usually do not include the level of details necessary for professionals to evaluate and incorporate the information into their practice. Reports in the popular press may, however, be a starting point for selecting a topic that is of interest to you and your area of practice.

What is the difference between popular and professional press articles? Magazine articles are usually written by staff writers, not experts in the field. They frequently include interviews with subject experts in their story. These articles rarely include a bibliography or citation of sources used in writing the article. When sources are included they are frequently mentioned in the text without the complete citation. Such articles are not original reports of research. **Magazines** often have gloss color photographs rather than graphs, tables, diagrams, or charts in the articles. It is usually easy and convenient to purchase a current magazine issue at the grocery store, news stand, or other stores that sell magazines. Obtaining copies of professional journals without a subscription can be much more difficult, expensive, and sometimes impossible.

Newspapers may write articles that are brief summaries of articles just released in professional journals. While they frequently do not list the title, author, volume, and issue of the journal, with careful reading it is usually possible to locate the original report of the research. The name of the lead author is often listed, as is the title of the journal. Scanning the latest issue of the journal will often reveal the original article.

Articles published in **professional journals** are usually written by authors who are subject experts that conduct research related to the topic. Their professional affiliation is often identified within the article. These experts are not employed by the journals and are rarely financially compensated for writing an article. These articles usually contain a list of references and information that is cited within the text. Most professional journals contain a limited amount of advertising.

THE UBIQUITOUS WORLD WIDE WEB

The World Wide Web (WWW) has greatly increased the amount of information available to anyone with a computer and Internet connection (Figure 13-2). The Internet is a powerful medium because it can be accessed by people all over the world. It is an accessible medium due to the fact that anyone with a HTML (hyper text markup language) editor, access to a Web server, and minimal skills can create and post a Web page about any topic, and then the page can be viewed by people the world over. Some of these pages look very amateurish and not very believable, while others are slick and professionally done. There is no formal or informal mechanism to verify or evaluate Web sites prior to posting. It can be a case of buyer beware.

An Internet address, called IP address or Internet Protocol address, is the unique address that each device connected to the Internet is assigned. While it is not actually a physical address, it is the virtual equalivant of a street address. However, while specific Internet providers can be identified, the name of the owner or operator of individual computers is not readily available. **Web sites** also have addresses. These addresses can tell you something about a Web site, the server or domain name, and the type of site that it is (Figure 13-3). Some Web sites begin with "www"

Figure 13-2
The World Wide Web has given people all over the world unprecedented access to information, but it also allows anyone, anywhere to post anything they want, leading to a wide range of quality and accuracy in the information available. When out on the Web, "buyer beware."

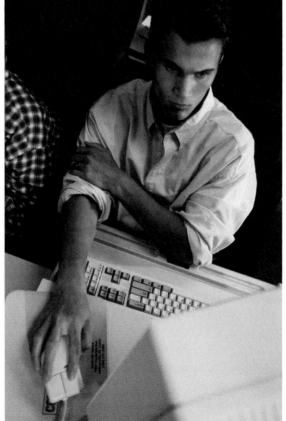

COURTESY OF PHOTODISC.

Figure 13-3
Parts of an
Internet Address.

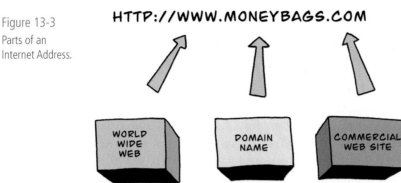

while others do not. Originally servers were named according to the function they performed. A server beginning with "www" meant that it hosted Web sites. However, it is not necessary to begin an Internet address with "www." There are some other initials used in Internet addresses, such as "HTTP" or Hyper Text Transfer Protocol. This is a communication protocol or file type, similar to ".doc" used to identify Microsoft Word files. Internet addresses that appear to be written in words are actually read by computers as strings of numbers (128.227.69.241). To see your IP addresses go to: http://www.ip-adress.com/, then click on the IP Tracer or Locator for more information. The words seen in addresses are like nicknames, which are easier to remember than the numbers. An address such as http://www.Yahoo.com is only meaningful as an address because it has been assigned to the actual IP address, 66.94.234.13. The part of an address after the "www" is called the domain or host name. It is often the name of the company, product, or something usually memorable. The ending of an IP address can tell you something about the type of organization or company that has created or commissioned the site. The system is not as pure as it was originally, but it can still provide some information about the Web site. Web addresses ending in "com" are often commercial, "edu" are educational organizations, "gov" are U.S. government sites, "net" can be anything, and sites ending in "mil" are military Web sites.

SO MANY CHOICES: WHAT DO YOU PICK?

The main types of information sources are professional journals in either print or electronic format, **textbooks** in print or electronic format, Web sites, popular press publications, newspapers, and colleagues. There is often a particular source best designed to answer your specific need. Before beginning the search think about the type of information that you need. When you are looking for established laboratory values, descriptions of diseases, adverse effects of medications, or recommended dosages, then the best source for information is usually a book in print or electronic format. Books take several years to write, edit, publish, or distribute, so they are usually the best resource for these types of factual information. These days it is not unusual for reference and textbooks to be published in both print and electronic format.

Articles in professional journals that report original reports of research provide access to the latest research or information on a subject. When looking for the most recent information on diagnosis, therapy or research on a topic, articles from professional journals are the best source for current and authoritative information. They publish to disseminate the results of their research and to add to the knowledge base of the profession. The article types included are: case reports, case series, cohort studies, clinical trials, randomized control trials, review articles, guidelines, and systematic reviews. Remember that not all research or evidence is created equally. Professional journals are published on varying schedules. Some major publications, such as *JAMA, Nursing Times,* and the *New England Journal of Medicine,* are published weekly. Other journals are published monthly, bimonthly, or quarterly. Whatever the publication schedule of a journal is, it is a quicker cycle than for books.

A **case report** is written about a single individual. It presents detailed diagnosis, treatment, and follow-up information about that individual. While the information is usually quite detailed, it is not very generalizable since it is based upon one person. Case series are similar. A **case series** is a report of a small group of individuals diagnosed with the same disease and given the same treatment. Both of these are basically descriptive studies of very small groups and are not experimental in design. Their applicability to changing practice is minimal due the inability to generalize from such small samples. Frequently clinicians write case reports or case series when they treat unusual conditions or presentations.

Clinical trials are most frequently used in the development of new medications and drugs or in determining optimum dosing and treatment schedules. Clinical trials have several stages: I, II, III, and IV. Phase I clinical trials enroll a small group of subjects to test an experimental treatment for safety, dosage, and possible side effects. In phase II clinical trials, a larger group of subjects is used to determine if the experimental treatment is effective and if further study should be conducted. In phase III clinical trials, large groups of subjects are enrolled to measure effectiveness, monitor adverse effects, and compare the effectiveness to current treatments used. Once a treatment has been approved and is being marketed, phase IV, post-marketing studies are done. The purpose of this phase is to obtain additional information about the risks or benefits and how to best use it (National Library of Medicine, 2007). **Randomized control trials** are studies that separate the similar subjects into groups randomly. When a trial is described as blinded, the investigators do not know which group is the experimental group (receiving the new treatment), and which group is the control group receiving the standard treatment.

A review article is a summary and review of the current literature on a topic. When beginning research on a topic, these can be an excellent starting point. They provide background information and a summary of the topic. Review articles usually have extensive bibliographies, another good source of additional resources. **Systematic reviews** are different than review articles. Properly done, they are preplanned and extensive. Researchers often begin with a specific, clinically relevant question. Then they search appropriate **databases** to identify all relevant research studies about the subject. All of these studies are individually evaluated to determine if the methodology and quality of the research meets the authors' predetermined standards for the systematic review. If the authors use statistics to combine the results of the multiple studies, then the article may also be a **meta-analysis.** Systematic reviews focus on randomized control trials. Cochrane Systematic Reviews are the most widely known collection of systematic reviews.

The final publication type is a clinical practice guideline. Clinical practice guidelines are statements about practice developed by experts. They are developed to assist both health care professionals and patients by presenting recommendations or strategies to assist in decision making in regards to diagnosis of and therapy for certain health conditions. These guidelines may be developed by professional societies, governmental agencies, or health care organizations. Clinical practice guidelines are based upon research evidence and expert opinions. They are regularly reviewed and revised as available research and evidence becomes available.

Another feature of many but not all professional journals is the **peer review** process. Peer review is a blinded review process that articles go through prior to being accepted for publication. Popular press or magazine articles are typically reviewed by the internal editorial staff. When authors submit articles to a journal that is peer reviewed (also sometimes called **refereed**), identifying information such as author and institutional names are removed, and the manuscript is sent to several experts on the subject. The experts read and review the article, and then make recommendations for acceptance or rejection. The expert reviewers may recommend changes to the article, suggesting additional information to be added, sections to be revised, or that statements be verified by citations.

Web sites often provide the most up-to-date information about professional organizations, news items, or online continuing education. Most journals are now offered in print and online format, with the online format being available quicker than the print journal is delivered. Many of these resources are not freely available and access is regulated by institutional affiliation and what products they purchase. Online journals, books, and databases are costly items. They are the electronic equal of the print publications.

Colleagues can be very knowledgeable, but it is important to determine if they are the best source for the information needed. They are human and may not remember details. They may not want to admit that they do not know something, or they may unwittingly provide incorrect information. How do you determine the source of their information? Research has shown, however, that colleagues are the most frequent source used to answer information needs (Tannery, Wessel, Epstein, & Gadd, 2007).

FINDING INFORMATION ONLINE

Search engines are used to find information online. There are a variety of them, and you may already have a favorite. Search engines take the search terms that you enter and run an algorithm to locate pages related to those terms. Since they do not all use the same algorithm, they do not locate the same sites. Search engines are amazing. They quickly sort through millions of pages in seconds and retrieve your results. Sometimes they do a better job than other times. All search engines rank the retrieved results, which is done using their unique algorithms, which may incorporate fees paid by Web sites to the search engine company. How the algorithms work are carefully guarded secrets. Not all of the World Wide Web is accessible. The portion that is searchable is called the visible Web, and the inaccessible portion is called the invisible Web. An example of the invisible Web would be material located on a company's internal Intranet, or Web pages that require subscriptions to view, such as journals or databases that are not freely accessible. Sometimes pages are part of the invisible Web because the files are of a type not searched by the Web spiders and Web robots that index the Web. Due to the enormous size of the World Wide Web, it would be impossible for humans to manually search it efficiently. Instead programs are written that methodically visit Web pages and create an electronic copy that the search engine indexes. The indexing of hundreds of thousands of Web pages is how GOOGLE can deliver 30,000 results in mere seconds. Web page designers are constantly trying to learn how to maximize the number of search engines that identify their page and to increase the rankings of their pages. Sometimes Web page owners pay fees to search engine companies to rank their site higher than other sites, or fees are paid every time someone clicks on the Web page link from the search results. The next time you use a search engine, notice the number of commercial Web sites on the top or side of the results screen. If you are interested in learning more about how search engines work, go to http://www.searchenginewatch.com or http://computer.howstuffworks.com/search-engine.htm.

OTHER INTERNET RESOURCES

Internet Exercise 13-1 should demonstrate that while there is a great deal of information available on the Internet, not all of it is relevant and not all of it is quality information. The Internet has also developed into a platform to deliver databases and full text journals and books. Some of these resources are freely available, and others are available only to subscribers who purchase access. There are some excellent resources available free of charge, but there is a great deal more that is available for a fee. These resources are time consuming and costly to produce, with the creator or owner charging users to offset their costs or to make a profit. Often the high-quality free products are developed by government agencies, universities, or professional associations. The National Library of Medicine is a leader in providing quality resources to anyone with an

Internet Exercise 13-1	Select one of the following terms and run a search for it in all of the listed search engines. List the number of results and then scan the first three pages of results and rate the relevance as poor, fair, good, or excellent.

Nursing history, nursing theory, treatment of diabetes, nursing process, or nursing education.

1. Google.com	# results _____	Ratings – poor fair good excellent
2. Scholar.google.com	# results _____	Ratings – poor fair good excellent
2. Ask.com	# results _____	Ratings – poor fair good excellent
3. Yahoo.com	# results _____	Ratings – poor fair good excellent
4. Msdewey.com	# results _____	Ratings – poor fair good excellent
5. Dogpile.com	# results _____	Ratings – poor fair good excellent

Internet connection without charge. To view the collection of databases and resources produced by the National Library of medicine go to http://gateway.nlm.nih.gov.

Database Resources

The databases used most frequently by nurses are CINAHL, Medline, PsycInfo, and Cochrane Database of Systematic Reviews. **CINAHL,** or the Cumulated Index to Nursing and Allied Health Literature, is the primary nursing database. It indexes many nursing journals, books, book chapters, continuing-education resources, computer programs, dissertations, and other materials. **PubMed,** the public version of Medline, is produced by the National Library of Medicine. This is an enormous database that currently contains more than 18,000,000 citations. It indexes the literature of the medical, biomedical, nursing, dentistry, and health administration fields, as well as the history of medicine literature. The database contains citations from 70 languages and covers from the 1950s to the present. **PsycInfo** is the primary index to the literature of psychology, and covers this literature from the 1800s to the present. This database contains over 2.5 million records. The **Cochrane Database of Systematic Reviews** is a relatively new database developed in the late 1990s. This small, specialized database indexes systematic reviews that are written and continually updated by members of the Cochrane Collaboration group. The systematic reviews in the Cochrane Database are often regarded as very high quality due to the rigor with which they are created and maintained. Each group has a specific clinical question for which they monitor the literature and reports of research, and they revise their recommendations as the results of research increases the knowledge base. Some examples of systematic reviews from the Cochrane database are: Vitamin C for preventing and treating the common cold; Strategies for increasing the participation of women in community breast cancer screening; Protein supplementation of human milk for promoting growth in preterm infants; and relaxation therapies for the management of primary hypertension in adults.

Medline

Medline is available in many formats from a variety of database producers. The contents of the database are the same because the database information is produced by the National Library of Medicine and then sold to database producers to upload into their format. PubMed is the free public interface for the Medline database. Medline traces its history back to the print indexes produced by John Shaw Billings from the Library of the Surgeon General's Office of the army in the 1800s (Garrison & Hasse, 1915). That library eventually developed into the National Library of Medicine. Dr. Billings began to index medical articles with the assistance of army clerks. The clerks copied the article titles, and Dr. Billings or his assistant would add one or two appropriate subject headings. Dr. Billings's collection of index cards formed the basis for the print index, *Index Medicus,* produced later by the National Library of Medicine (Figure 13-4). This is the humble beginning of the world's largest biomedical database, MEDLINE (Garrison & Hasse, 1915).

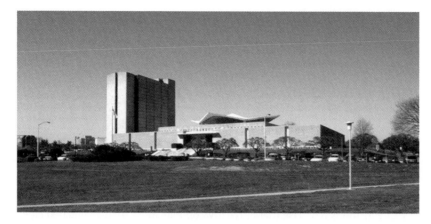

Figure 13-4

This 1999 photograph depicts the National Library of Medicine (NLM), located on the campus of the National Institutes of Health in Bethesda, Maryland. It is the world's largest medical library, collecting materials and providing information and research services in all areas of biomedicine and health care. The NLM's MedlinePlus™ online database can help consumers find information on health topics of all kinds, including diseases, wellness, hospitals, physicians, and pharmaceuticals. NLM also coordinates the National Network of Libraries of Medicine, which provides health care professionals and the public equal access to biomedical and health care information resources. *(Courtesy of CDC/Dr. Edwin P. Ewing, Jr.)*

The print index was an important development in making medical literature accessible to researchers. Journal article citations were entered into the print format of *Index Medicus* with two subject headings. If you were searching for articles on diabetes you would go to the alphabetical index for diabetes. There you would find a list of article citations that were about diabetes. However, if you were looking for articles that combined diabetes and cardiovascular disease it was much more cumbersome. You would have to look up both topics and, based on the words in the title listed under both subject headings, attempt to determine if any articles would be useful. These indexes were printed quarterly and then cumulated into annuals. Each year would need to be searched separately. The amount of medical articles published annually began to strain this manual system of the 1950s. In 1964 with a grant of $3 million from the National Heart Institute, the process of indexing, organizing, storing, and preparing camera-ready pages was greatly accelerated. At this time the number of subject headings assigned to each article was increased from two to ten (Zipser, 1998). Eventually the process of producing the indexes developed into MEDLARS (Medical Literature Analysis and Retrieval System). Medline (MEDLARS online) was the only database to run on this system. While this system was a great improvement, it took three weeks from search request until the results were received. Written requests were mailed to the National Library of Medicine, where specially trained librarians performed the search and then mailed the resulting list of citations to the requestor. Searching the literature has definitely improved since that time.

In June of 1997, the National Library of Medicine announced that MEDLINE would be available free of charge using the PubMed interface on the World Wide Web. Since that time the system has been improved to better meet the needs of the searchers. These improvements became necessary as the amount of material published has accumulated and increased exponentially. Today there are over 18 million citations indexed in Medline.

To search PubMed go to http://www.pubmed.gov. There are several databases that can be searched using this interface; however, PubMed is most relevant for nursing information. The other databases cover such topics as genomes, structures, proteins, and nucleotides. Anyone with an Internet connection is able to search the database and view abstracts when available. The amount of full text that is available depends upon electronic journal subscriptions available via your institution. There is a small amount of free full text available through PubMed Central, which is the U.S. National Library of Medicine's digital archive of biomedical and life science journals. Unfortunately at this time there is a very limited amount of nursing journals in this archive. Journal publishers are commercial companies seeking to make a profit, so free access is limited. PubMed also provides links to open-access journals that are freely accessible but not stored in PubMed Central. Links to full text within PubMed are provided by publishers, so not every article that is available in electronic format is included. If your institution does not have subscription access to an article that is available electronically, many will provide access to articles for a fee. These fees may be high, so if you have access to a medical or health sciences library, contact them for assistance first. Articles can usually be borrowed from another medical or hospital library either without charge or at a lower cost than charged by the publishers.

CINAHL

There is no free access available for CINAHL. It is available only via subscriptions. Beginning in 2008 this database will only be available from EBSCO. This database is the primary nursing database. The subject headings are based upon the Medical Subject Heading used in Medline/PubMed, but additions were made to address nursing concerns such as conceptual frameworks, nursing classification systems, and levels of nursing education. This database covers the literature from 1982 to the present. If your information need is for citations about the nursing process, nursing theory, conceptual frameworks, nursing education, or anything that is uniquely about nursing, then CINAHL should be your first choice for a database to search.

CINAHL indexes journal articles, book chapters, computer programs, continuing-education material, and dissertations to name a few of the formats. This database also indexes most state nursing journals. This is another database that uses a controlled vocabulary or subject headings to index the entries. Using this makes searching much more precise, and it reduced the amount of irrelevant citations. CINAHL indexes the nursing and allied health literature from 1982 to the present.

PsycInfo

If your area of interest or specialty is psych or mental health nursing, then the PsycInfo database will be a useful resource. This resource indexes journal articles, reports, dissertations, book chapters, and books in the discipline of psychology. Journal indexing begins in 1806 and goes to the present. Citations from articles in thirty-five languages are included. The subject coverage is clinical, nonclinical, and experimental psychology. PsycInfo is also indexed by subject heading: however, the subject headings are much broader than either CINAHL or PubMed subject headings. It also lacks the subheadings used by CINAHL or PubMed. The lack of subheadings makes it more difficult to focus on specific aspects of a subject. PsycInfo is only available via commercial databases. There are several companies that produce interfaces of PsycInfo.

Cochrane Database of Systematic Reviews

Cochrane Systematic Reviews are often referred to as the "Cadillac" of systematic reviews. This is because they are developed according to a specific protocol and standards. Each multinational group develops a specific clinical question, determines which databases would contain the best resources to answer the question, evaluates the studies identified according to a predetermined standard, and develops a structured abstract on the clinical question that it is researching. The majority of the clinical questions deal with therapy and diagnosis. The structured abstracts may be as long as one hundred pages. Development of these systematic reviews is very involved and requires assistance from groups of people. Another factor that separates these systematic reviews from others is that regular searches of the literature occur to identify new research applicable to the research question, which is then evaluated according to the pre-established criteria. If the new research changes the recommendations of the review, the reviews are amended to reflect the new information. Sometimes if the changes are substantial, the review may be retitled or even withdrawn. Cochrane Systematic Reviews are only available in electronic format, and the older systematic reviews are not archived. The reviews are a continually moving target that follows the evidence or research. The database is updated quarterly. These systematic reviews are very comprehensive and may be as long as one hundred pages (Negrini, Minozzi, Taricco, Ziliani, & Zaina, 2007).

The Cochrane Database of Systematic Reviews is a commercial database; however, the database can be searched and an abstract and plain-language summary may be viewed free of charge. Currently there is not a nursing group, but the establishment of one is under discussion. If your institution does not have access to this database and you need the complete systematic review, you can purchase it from the database company. This database does not use a controlled vocabulary; it is strictly text-word searchable. When searching this resource it is important to use synonyms to locate all relevant reviews. However, using text words for searches can increase the amount of irrelevant reviews retrieved. To search this database, if you do not have access to it from your institution, go to http://www.cochrane.org/reviews.

Other Nursing Databases and Indexes

There are several relatively new nursing databases available. One is Mosby's Nursing Index, which indexes over 2,500 titles of peer-reviewed journals, trade publications, and electronic resources. The subject headings are based upon the terms used in EMBASE, a European medical index. Recent comparisons between Mosby's Nursing Index and CINAHL showed that there are more than 800 titles in CINAHL that are not included in the Mosby product. Librarians that have executed searches on the same topics in both CINAHL and Mosby's Nursing Index have stated that at this time CINAHL is retrieving more relevant results (Jacobs, 2007).

Proquest Nursing and Allied Health Source is another database that institutions frequently have available for nursing students. This product indexes only about 620 titles, with 580 of them in full text. Coverage in this database begins in 1986, which is later than CINAHL or PubMED. Proquest contains full text, and that is one of the primary reasons that libraries purchase it. However, recent changes in contracts with journal publishers have reduced the percentage of journals that are nursing related and increased the amount of allied health titles. There is a thesaurus associated with the database, but it is a broad one used across disciplines and databases and not specific to nursing, as is CINAHL's.

IT IS PRINTED SO IT MUST BE SO

Research and reference material is not all created equally. There is a difference in the accuracy, authority, objectivity, content, and the currency of materials. While these elements should be considered when reading any health-related book, newspaper article, and journal or magazine article, it is especially true when reading Web pages. Theoretically the peer-review process that many journals and texts undergo ensures a certain level of quality and confidence in the material. However, with Web pages there is not a universal review process, so there should be a healthy amount of skepticism when accessing them.

The first step in evaluating resources, both print and online, is to determine the source or authorship of the materials. Books from reputable publishers and journals from legitimate societies or organizations can be considered authoritative. When these same publications appear in electronic versions they are still from the same authoritative sources. Frequently access to these online sources is sold as the equivalent to the print version. These types of materials undergo the process of peer review, which should verify the accuracy, authority, objectivity, content, and currency of the materials at the time of publication. It is important to note the copyright or publication date of texts and articles; they were current when they were published, but the information may not still be current or standard of practice years after publication.

When reading health information from unknown sources, especially Web sites, evaluation of the information is necessary. There are five main elements that you should examine: accuracy, authority, objectivity, currency, and coverage (see Table 13-1). When checking the accuracy of a site, attempt to identify the site author and look for contact information. What was the purpose of the Web page? Is the author qualified to write on the subject? What is the authority of the Web material? Are author or contributor credentials listed? Is it a ".com," ".edu," ".gov," or ".net" site? What was the purpose of designing the site? Is it a national organization disseminating information, or a commercial site providing biased information to market a product? Is the information complete and current? How long ago was the Web page updated? How easy is the site to use? Does it require that you download or purchase programs to use it? Web sites can be abandoned; still available but no longer relevant. Sites are

Table 13-1 Web Page Evaluation

Characteristic	Definition/Interpretation
AUTHORITY	Who is responsible for the page? What are their qualifications and credentials? Can you verify authorship and/or credentials? What is the domain name?
ACCURACY	Are sources listed for factual information? How is the spelling, grammar? Is there consistency within the Web site? Is the author qualified to write on the topic? Who owns or is represented by the Web site?
OBJECTIVITY	What are the goals or objectives? Are they stated? Is the information detailed? Is it factual or opinion? Who is the potential audience?
CONTENT	What is the focus of the site? Are links complementary to the site theme? Is there a balance of text and graphics? Is the material cited correctly? Is the information free? Does it require special software?
CURRENCY	When was it produced? Has it been updated (check the footer)? Is the information current? Are the links dead or alive?

developed for a variety of purposes. They may be created as a personal or vanity page, for promotion or advertising of a product, to disseminate new or current information, to provide a forum for interests or hobbies, for advocating for points of view, for instructing or teaching, to register for courses, products, or information, and finally for entertainment. One of the first steps in evaluating a Web site is to determine its purpose. Knowing your information need will help you to determine if the purpose is complimentary or conflicting to your information search. Web sites are created by a variety of people with a variety of Web-page designing skills. For that reason information that could be useful in evaluating them, such as authorship, credentials or qualifications of the information provider, date of creation, and even contact information, may be missing or difficult to locate. This omission may be either intentional or accidental. Web sites that are not from known entities should be regarded with healthy skepticism. There are Internet domain names that utilize their similarity to known resources, creating the illusion that they are something that they are not. The official Web site of the U.S. White House and current president is http://www.whitehouse.gov. There is also a Web site http://www.whitehouse.com. Three little letters, but a big difference in content. The official White House Web site has news and information about presidential speeches, policies, and news releases. The Whitehouse.com site does not provide information on the site owners. It has news items related to current events, videos of government official's speeches, and an online poll that you can respond to.

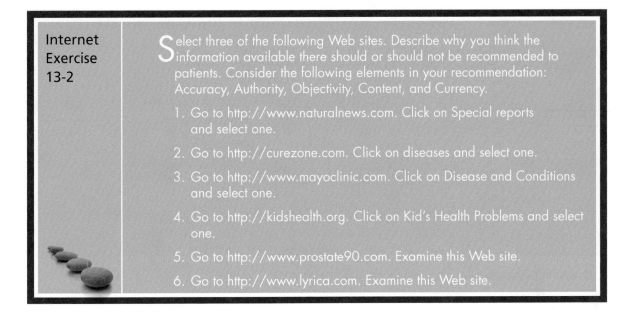

Internet Exercise 13-2

Select three of the following Web sites. Describe why you think the information available there should or should not be recommended to patients. Consider the following elements in your recommendation: Accuracy, Authority, Objectivity, Content, and Currency.

1. Go to http://www.naturalnews.com. Click on Special reports and select one.

2. Go to http://curezone.com. Click on diseases and select one.

3. Go to http://www.mayoclinic.com. Click on Disease and Conditions and select one.

4. Go to http://kidshealth.org. Click on Kid's Health Problems and select one.

5. Go to http://www.prostate90.com. Examine this Web site.

6. Go to http://www.lyrica.com. Examine this Web site.

HOW TO SEARCH LIKE A PRO

Librarians and other experienced searchers approach the process differently than novice or inexperienced searchers. When approaching a new Internet search engine or database, there are some common elements that experienced searchers seek. If these tools are not readily available, they will quickly check the help section to locate them. The tools increase the precision of searching by reducing irrelevant hits and increase the likelihood of finding what you need. Some of the tools function slightly differently in various environments but produce similar results.

In the Beginning

Before librarians or experienced searchers begin a search, they usually contemplate the subject in which they are interested. Librarians searching the literature to identify research about "the most successful method of promoting smoking cessation for cardiac patients from these choices: individual counseling, support groups, or written educational materials" would first identify the main concepts.

The main concepts would be *smoking cessation, counseling, support groups,* and *written educational materials.* Next they would need to decide if the process of cardiac patients quitting smoking is different than any other group of people. Often there are additional elements needed to focus the search that are not concepts but limits. Some of these limits might be research articles, review articles, various age groups, language of the articles, or publication date. Limits are added later and are not included in the initial search.

In the following **search statements**, decide what you think the main concepts are and underline them.

Example: Does the daily administration of 500 mg of vitamin C to adolescents reduce the incidence of the common cold?

1. How can pregnancy in teens be prevented?

2. If every person over the age of 50 is administered a flu shot, how would that affect the annual death rate due to respiratory infection in that age group?

3. What does the research say about health-care workers wearing artificial nails and bacterial transmission in hospitals?

4. Does the use of pill sorters/boxes increase medication compliance in the elderly who are prescribed multiple medications?

Boolean Operators: And, Or, Not

Combining terms allows you to do searches that contain multiple concepts. There are various ways to combine terms, and it is important to use the correct term to obtain the desired outcome. The combining terms "and," "or," and "not" are known as Boolean operators. The most commonly used Boolean operator is "and." It allows unrelated or unlike concepts to be searched simultaneously to identify articles that contain both concepts. Using "and" narrows a search and reduces the number of items retrieved. Combining terms with "or" usually broadens a search and increases the amount of retrieval. However, if you use "or" to combine search sets, duplicates will be removed. The connector "not" excludes terms from the retrieval.

If these concepts are still unclear, consider peanut butter and jelly sandwiches (see Figure 13-5). If you ask someone to make a peanut butter *and* jelly sandwich, they will put both peanut butter and jelly on the bread. If you ask them to make peanut butter *or* jelly sandwich, they might use only peanut butter, or jelly, or they might include both. When you order a sandwich with peanut butter and *not* jelly, or the reverse jelly and *not* peanut butter, you will only get the one that you want and not the other.

Truncation

Truncation is a tool that quickly allows you to add multiple forms of a word to a text or key-word search. When a text-word search is performed the search engine looks for the exact match to the search terms. It does not include alternative forms of the terms. Truncation allows alternate forms to be included without having to list them individually. The symbol for truncation varies some among databases, but it is often a "*." Sometimes it is a "!" or a "$." If "child*" is entered, it will retrieve hits on child, child's, children, and childhood to name a few.

Figure 13-5
Boolean Operators.

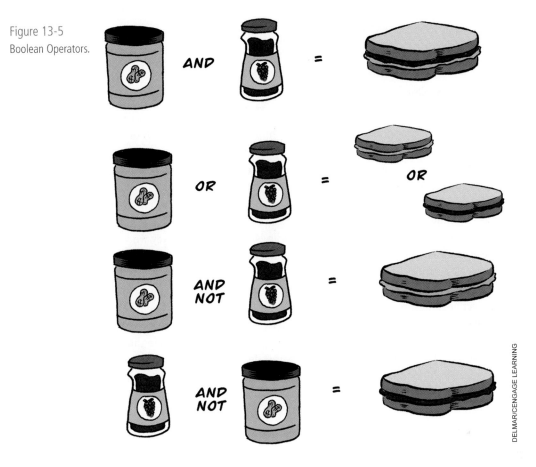

DELMAR/CENGAGE LEARNING

Limits

Databases that have a limits or refinement feature allow the searcher to restrict the search results to records containing certain elements. While the elements vary by database, some common limits are language of publication, publication date, and full text. PubMed provides limits to publication types, age groups, human or animal studies, articles with abstracts, gender, journal subsets, or individual fields. CINAHL offers similar choices, but it does not index animal studies, so that limit is not available. CINAHL also provides the searcher the ability to limit the results to articles reporting the results of research.

Searching in a Field

Databases that index articles take the information such as author, publication date, journal name, author(s) name, volume, issue, article tile, subject headings, and other elements and place them in individual tagged fields. These fields are then searchable. This can be very useful when attempting to locate an article when the information available about the article is partial or incomplete.

Key Word vs. Subject Searching

Key-word searching allows the searcher to enter any words or groups of words for the database to search. The database structure determines which fields are searched when key words are entered. Key-word searching looks for matches to the word or words entered; it does not evaluate the relationship of the term(s) to the focus of the article. When multiple terms are entered in a key-word search, the search engine determines that the words are present but not that they are related in the article. Key-word searching can be a good way to begin a search, especially if you are unable to identify relevant subject headings. Searching with key words frequently identifies more citations than searching with subject headings; however, there is a greater possibility that there will be more irrelevant citations.

Anyone who has used the yellow pages has had experience using a controlled vocabulary or subject headings. When looking for a place to buy a new car, you begin in the "c" section for car dealers. There may be a "see" reference that says to also see automobile dealers. The term "automobile dealers" is the subject heading for the concept of a business that sells new cars. When you turn to that section the entries will be car dealers and nothing else. Using subject headings makes searching more efficient and precise because it groups similar information together. In databases such as PubMed and CINAHL using subject headings also allows subheadings to be added, which focuses the search on specific aspects such as diagnosis, prevention, and control, adverse effects, education, or other areas.

Stop Words

Stop words are very common words that are ignored in a search statement because, while they help the searcher to make sense of the query, they do not add anything of value to the search. They are filtered out of the search. Many databases and search engines actually have a list of specific stop words that will be ignored. These are the words that searchers use to define the relationship between the search key words. They are common words that do not improve search results. The list of stop words varies by database, but usually includes articles, prepositions, helping verbs, and pronouns. Table 13-2 lists some common words ignored by many database or search engines.

More Equals Less

When doing a search, it is normal to want to include every possible term, especially when an initial search fails to retrieve results. If a search on one term is unsuccessful, inexperienced

Table 13-2 Stop Words Commonly Ignored by Search Engines and Databases

a	between	had	now	the
about	both	hardly	of	there
after	but	has	often	they
again	by	have	oh	this
against	came	he	ok	very
all	can	here	said	was
almost	cannot	how	same	we
also	certain	if	seem	were
always	could	in	seen	what
an	etc	into	several	when
and	do	is	shall	where
any	does	it	she	while
are	during	mainly	should	who
as	each	make	significantly	whose
at	either	many	similar	why
be	else	might	slightly	with
before	ever	necessary	to	
became	every	none	than	
because	for	not	that	

searchers will often add more terms or more specific terms. For example if a search on the terms "nursing education" does not retrieve results, adding the term undergraduate will only narrow the search and will still not retrieve additional results. To broaden the search, remove terms or substitute more general terms.

FEDERATED OR META SEARCH ENGINES

There is a relatively new type of search engine that searches multiple databases or Internet search engines simultaneously. These search engines are called meta or **federated search engines.** Here are some Internet meta search engines to try.

- http://clusty.com
- http://www.dogpile.com
- http://surfwax.com
- http://www.mamma.com

Meta Internet search engines will search multiple search engines using the same text words. Theoretically this might seem to be a time saver; however, due to the fact that search engines are not created equally and work on different algorithms, the quality of the results may be disappointing. There will also be some duplication in the Web sites retrieved but it will not be complete. Another potential pitfall is the fact that not all search engines use the same method of portraying the Boolean operator used for "anding" sets, some use "and" while others use "+." For searchers that frequently utilize the advanced features of a search engine, a meta search engine may not provide results that are as relevant.

Search engines that are able to search more than one online database simultaneously are similar to a meta search engine but are usually referred to as federated search engines. This is becoming a popular feature promoted by libraries. The concept is intriguing and appealing as a time-saving mechanism, but there are some caveats. First, not all databases are designed to be cross searchable. Second, if you are a sophisticated searcher, you know that databases have different controlled vocabulary and search refinements that allow the searcher to customize the results to what they are looking for. Cross searching with a federated search engine will lose the power of individual databases' tools. However, when the searcher is still in the early stages of the search process and still selecting or refining the topic, it can be a quick way to survey which database may have the most information on the topic or what type of information on the topic is available. Most federated search engines are commercial products purchased by libraries. Some popular library federated search engines that you may have used are:

- Metalib http://www.exlibrisgroup.com. Select the products tab and click on metalib.
- Serials Solution http://www.serialssolutions.com. Select Serials Solution 360.
- Science.gov http://www.science.gov.

BIBLIOGRAPHIC MANAGEMENT SOFTWARE: A VIRTUAL FILE CABINET

If you frequently search databases and have piles of articles or searches, **bibliographic management software** might be of interest. Bibliographic software is actually a database that is specially designed for saving citations and formatting. This type of software also assists in creating a bibliography in multiple writing styles such as American Psychological Association (APA), Modern Language Association (MLA), Chicago and others. There are a number of these products on the market. The newest type of bibliographic software is Web based. Previously they were programs loaded on individual PCs. Some of the more popular bibliographic software programs are: EndNote, ProCite, Reference Manager, RefWorks, and EndNote Web. These products are wonderful time savers, but it is necessary to scan the document and check the results, which sometimes require minor corrections.

EVIDENCE-BASED PRACTICE

Research is constantly being conducted and new developments occur daily. During the course of your education to become a nurse you will be taught and will learn many things. However, it was impossible for your instructors to teach you everything. As a health care professional you have chosen to enter a profession that is constantly changing and evolving. As researchers discover new and better ways of diagnosing, preventing, and treating illness and providing care for patients, the knowledge base expands and the previous standard of care will adjust. In order to provide the best, safest, and evidence-based care it is your responsibility to monitor developments and changes in your area of practice. This task may seem overwhelming, but it does not need to be.

Developing an Evidence-Based Practice

Now that you are overwhelmed with information and wondering how you can possibly keep up with changes in the profession, let us examine some tools available to make it manageable. First, remember that you do not need to read everything that is printed about nursing, medicine, or health care. Second, once you have graduated and secured a professional position, that position will define your area of specialization and that is where your focus should be.

Many databases have the feature that allows you to save searches that are either automatically run at specific intervals or run when you manually choose to. PubMed from the National Library of Medicine has a feature they call "My NCBI." My NCBI has two major functions. It allows you to save complex search strategies with limits. The searches can be automatically run on a schedule that you determine and e-mailed to you, or My NCBI allows you to run the search when you choose, to see only what is new for that topic. Using My NCBI requires free and simple registration. Your search strategies are saved on the National Library of medicine servers and not your computer, so they can be accessed from any computer with Internet access. My NCBI also allows you to save collections of citations. These features can be very useful when you have identified questions or problems that you need in order to follow new developments or research.

CINAHL and PsycInfo via the EBSCO platform also allows you to create an account and save searches that can be accessed and re-run when you wish. There are several other databases on the EBSCO platform that utilize this feature. Utilizing this can save you time and make it easy to stay current on topics of interest with a minimum of time and effort. Check the databases that you use to determine if a similar feature is available.

Searchable Evidence-Based Queries

Developing searchable evidence-based questions is the first step in the process. There are several nursing models of evidence-based practice. All of them are based upon the original Evidence-Based Medicine model developed by David Sackett in 1996. His definition, the most widely quoted, is:

> "Evidence based medicine is the conscientious, explicit, and judicious use of current best evidence in making decisions about the care of individual patients. The practice of evidence based medicine means integrating individual clinical expertise with the best available external clinical evidence from systematic research. By individual clinical expertise we mean the proficiency and judgment that individual clinicians acquire through clinical experience and clinical practice. Increased expertise is reflected in many ways, but especially in more effective and efficient diagnosis and in the more thoughtful identification and compassionate use of individual patients' predicaments, rights, and preferences in making clinical decisions about their care. By best available external clinical evidence we mean clinically relevant research, often from the basic sciences of medicine, but especially from patient centered clinical research into the accuracy and precision of diagnostic tests (including the clinical examination), the power of prognostic markers, and the efficacy and safety of therapeutic, rehabilitative, and preventive regimens. External clinical evidence both invalidates previously accepted diagnostic tests and treatments and replaces them with new ones that are more powerful, more accurate, more efficacious, and safer" (Sackett, Straus, Richardson, & Rosenberg, 1996, pp. 7–8).

Becoming an evidence-based practice is much more involved that this brief description; entire books have been written about it. Graduate-level nursing programs present the topic in great detail. Developing the ability to turn information queries into a searchable, evidence-based, practitioner format is only the first step towards becoming an evidence-based practitioner.

PICO: Developing EBP Searchable Questions

The mnemonic **PICO** is very useful when developing evidence-based-practice (EBP) questions. The "P" stands for patient or problem, the "I" for intervention, the "C" for comparison, and the "O" is for the desired outcome (Sackett, Straus, Richardson, & Rosenberg, 1996).

Here is an example of a PICO question. In elderly patients with stage-3 decubitus ulcers, are hydrogel dressings more effective (quicker healing with fewer complications) than regular dressings in healing these ulcers? The patient or population group is elderly patients with stage-3 decubitus ulcers. Hydrogel dressings is the intervention that is being investigated. The comparison is between hydrogel and standard dry dressings. The desired outcome is quicker healing and less-adverse effects.

Writing
Exercise
13-2

Take the following clinical situations and create a PICO for each one using the table.

PATIENTS OR PROBLEM	
INTERVENTION	
COMPARISON	
OUTCOME	

1. As a nurse in an intensive care unit you are concerned with the amount of ventilator-acquired pneumonia that patients contract. You have heard that oral care can reduce incidence of pneumonia in this group of patients. Turn this information need into a PICO question.

2. You are a nurse in a neonatal intensive care unit. You are always interested in identifying additional interventions that will assist your little patients to grow and thrive. Recently you read an article about kangaroo care and wonder if there is research about its use with this population. Create a PICO with this information need.

3. You are a nurse in a geriatric practice. Many of the patients take multiple prescriptions each day. They sometimes forget to take their medications or take them irregularly. You wonder if the use of compartmentalized pill boxes will increase medication compliance. Develop a PICO for this information need.

4. While in nursing school you were taught to insert IV needles with the bevel up. Several of the nurses that you work with consistently insert them bevel down. You want to determine if this is incorrect or if research has determined if it makes a difference. Write a PICO for this.

5. You are a nurse on a pediatric medical–surgical floor. You have noticed several nurses and nursing assistants are inconsistent in where they take a patient's blood pressure. Sometimes they attach the cuff to the right arm, sometimes the left, and sometimes they will apply the blood pressure cuff to one or the other leg. You want to research if this practice is a sound clinical practice or if it should be done consistently, and if it affects the readings. Take this information need and develop a PICO statement about it.

LIFE-LONG LEARNING, CONTINUING EDUCATION

Many, but not all, states require nurses to acquire continuing-education credits in order to renew their licenses. The Internet can be one method of acquire continuing education credits. Over the years, the continuing education available on the Internet has increased in both the amount and the variety. The cost varies depending upon the provider, and there is even some that is available without charge. Sometimes it is even possible to find continuing-education courses that are required by specific states for licensure.

Here are some nursing continuing-education sites to examine (Before registering and completing any continuing-education courses be sure to check that the course will be accepted by your state's board of nursing. Any Internet search engine will identify additional sites.):

- http://www.nurseceu.com
- http://www.nursingceu.com
- http://nursingworld.org/ce/cehome.cfm
- http://www.nursingcenter.com/prodev/ce_online.asp

Web 2.0 Tools

When the World Wide Web became a graphical interface it was a collection of Web sites. Over time different types of platforms developed, and a subtle shift occurred in the late 1990s and early 2000s. These applications attempt to provide virtual social networking, collaboration, wikis, and online sharing. The term "Web 2.0" was developed in 2004 by O'Reilly Media to acknowledge the shift in purpose. Prior to coining the title "Web 2.0," no one realized that the early Web was called "Web 1.0." Some of these new Web tools can be helpful in maintaining current professional knowledge with minimum time and effort. To learn more about some of the Web 2.0 sites that are available read this article, http://web2magazine.blogspot.com, and click on Web 2.0 sites on the right sidebar.

Blogs, RSS Feeds, Wikis, and More

Some of the new Web 2.0 tools will not be useful in maintaining **professionalism** and facilitating learning. There are many, and more develop each day, so only a select few will be discussed. The term "blog" is short for Web log. A blog is an online diary. Sometimes blogs are a next-generation bulletin board that allows anyone to contribute, and sometimes they are individual efforts. Often they are an online form of a journal or diary. Frequently blogs are created for a particular interest or subject and are an online discussion of that subject. They are public Web pages that express private thoughts, ideas, or opinions. Knowing the credentials and expertise of bloggers can determine how much credibility or belief you invest in the postings. Typically information is posted in reverse-chronological order, or last in, first out. The very popular Web site My Space is actually a blog. When blogs first appeared on the Web, bloggers, people who write blogs, needed to code their postings using HTML, an Internet language. Now there are

Web sites such as My Space, Blog.com, Blogger.com, livejournal.com, Yahoo360.com, and many more that have simplified the process, which makes blogging possible for anyone. A recent search of http://blogspace.google.com on the topic of nursing identified sites on travel nursing, legal issues related to nursing, student news from nursing programs, health care news, and nursing home staffing. Taking the time to log on to blogs regularly on the chance that there have been new postings does not seem an efficient way of following topics of interest. Another Web 2.0 development called **RSS**, or really simple syndication, automates the process of notifying subscribers of updates by e-mail notifications, or subscribers can log on to a RSS reader or aggregator, where new postings from all the blogs you are subscribed to are stored for you. If an aggregator is used, notices of the postings are saved until you log on and read them. There are several RSS readers. RSS readers may be Web based, or they may be software that is installed on an individual computer (see Figure 13-6). **Wikis** are Web sites that allow collaborative editing of its content and structure by users. A good example of a wiki is http://www.wikipedia.org, an international online encyclopedia with hundreds of thousands of user-created entries.

If you are overwhelmed with Web 2.0 technologies there are some less-techie options that are convenient, easy, and free. Some services will send you e-mails with summaries of the latest nursing news and research. It takes only minutes to skim the e-mails and then to read only what is of interest. While there might occasionally be some overlap of information from these services, they are not identical.

Nurse Linx is a service for nurses from MD Linx. There are several different divisions at MD Linx, Nurse Linx, NP Linx, Dentist Linx, Pharmacist Linx, PA Linx, and Med Student Linx. When you register you select the division or divisions to which you wish to subscribe. They monitor the major journals for each profession and send a daily e-mail with summaries of approximately five current articles. They provide a summary to the full text of the articles, but access to the full text may require a subscription or pay-per-view access. Occasionally the article is freely available, and then it will link to the full text. To sign up for Nurse Linx go to https://www.mdlinx.com. Select nursing from the list of specialties on the left sidebar.

Figure 13-6
RSS Readers.

PC-Based RSS Readers	**Web-Based RSS Readers**
Akregator http://akregator.kde.org	BlogLines http://www.bloglines.com
BlogBridge http://www.blogbridge.com	GoogleReader http://www.bloglines.com
FeedDemon http://www.newsgator.com/Individuals/ FeedDemon/Default.aspx	GoogleNews http://www.bloglines.com
RSSOwl http://www.rssowl.org	Netvibes http://www.netvibes.com
NetNewsWire http://www.rssowl.org	Feed each other http://feedeachother.com

The American Nurses Association has developed an e-mail service that is called ANA SmartBrief. This is another free service that automatically e-mails you daily. The messages are short, so it is easy to skim and read only what is of interest. Membership in the American Nurses Association is not required to subscribe. This service aggregates news items that may be of interest to nurses. Register at http://www.smartbrief.com/ana.

Medscape, another free service, focuses on primary health care providers and has a section for nurse practitioners. They send weekly e-mails that link back to the free, full text at their Web site. Medscape offers medical and health news, free CME credit, patient information, review articles, selected full-text journals, and more. This is a site that provides a broad variety of information. Subscription to Medscape is free and registration is easy (http://www.medscape.com).

Electronic Table-of-Contents Services

Historically if you wanted to survey the current literature in the key journals of your field or areas of interest, you would scan the table of contents of each journal and then flip to any article of interest and read it. Now there is a different way to accomplish this. Many journals now produce electronic tables of contents. They can be e-mailed to you automatically or, if the journal produces an RSS feed, you can access it via a feed reader such as Bloglines, Google Reader, or others whenever you wish. A journal subscription is not required to access the table of contents or article abstracts. Unless the journal is open access and freely available, accessing the full text requires either a subscription or affiliation with an institution that has a subscription. To determine if a journal provides electronic table of content service go to the journal's Web site and look for a link to e-mail alerts or table of contents. If you prefer to use the RSS feed, look for a button that says RSS Feed. The journal Western Journal of Nursing Research is a good example—to investigate this service go to the Web site: http://wjn.sagepub.com. This type of service works best when you do have electronic access to the full text of the articles.

Social Bookmarking

Social bookmarking is a Web 2.0 concept developed in the late 1990s. Previously, people saved their bookmarks or favorites on their own computers. This could be a problem when a new computer was purchased, the hard drive crashed, or when you were working on a different computer and trying to remember a Web address. Social bookmarking is a different way of saving and accessing favorite Web sites via the Web. In 2003 Del.icio.us, a widely used bookmarking site came online and allowed users to tag their saved links. Tagging allows users to add tags or metadata to each saved site. These tags are actually key words selected by the user to identify or file the Web pages. There are no right or wrong tags as long as what the key word selected is helpful to the individual user in organizing and locating specific sites or types of sites. If a user is interested in gardening, sailing, and nursing and uses one of those tags to identify each of their saved Web sites, then all of their Web sites would be grouped under one of those topics. Additional descriptors can be added to further identify sites. For example if someone saves flower gardening and vegetable gardening Web sites, tagging them as "gardening—flower" or "gardening—vegetable" makes locating a particular site quicker and easier. The tags are key words selected by each user, so the same site may have very different words depending upon their interests and why they selected the site. Another feature of social bookmarking is that one's saved set of Web addresses can be shared by others looking for sites on similar topics. Sites that you save are marked with the number of other people who have also saved the site. This feature can assist you in finding more Web sites on a subject because you have identified others interested in the same site. Social bookmarking sites also allow you to share your list of Web sites with others or to keep your saved bookmarks private. This method locates sites that have been selected by another human rather than a computer bot or spider.

Some social bookmarking sites:

- General: http://del.icio.us
- Scientist: http://www.connotea.org
- General: http://www.simpy.com
- Physicians: http://www.peerclip.com

SUMMARY

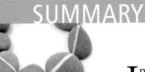

In this chapter the differences between popular and professional publications were discussed. Types of Web sites and the purposes for creating them were presented, along with basic Web site evaluation techniques. Learners should now be able to determine the type of resource that is best for answering particular types of questions or information needs. Comparisons between databases and Web sites and the value of both were presented. Databases useful for nurses were introduced and subject coverage was described. Basics of database functions were presented. A review of primary research studies, level of evidence, and an introduction to developing **evidence-based practice** questions for research were covered. Web 2.0 tools to develop professionalism and life-long learning were described.

Be careful about reading health books. You may die of a misprint.

–Mark Twain

REFERENCES

GARRISON, F. H., & HASSE, A. R. (1915). *John Shaw Billings: A memoir.* New York: G. P. Putnam's Sons.

GLASZIOU, P., & Del Mar, C. (2003). *Evidence-based medicine workbook: Finding and applying the best evidence to improve patient care.* London: BMJ Publishing Group.

JACOBS, S. K. (2007). *Comparison of CINAHL and Mosby's Nursing Index.*

NATIONAL LIBRARY OF MEDICINE. (2007). *Clinical trials. Gov.* Retrieved November 3, 2007, from http://clinicaltrials.gov

NEGRINI, S., Minozzi, S., Taricco, M., Ziliani, V., & Zaina, F. (2007). A systematic review of physical and rehabilitation medicine topics as developed by the Cochrane Collaboration. *Europa Medicophysica, 43*(3), 381–390.

SACKETT, D. L., Straus, S. E., Richardson, W. S., & Rosenberg, W. (1996). *Evidence based practice: How to practice and teach EBM.* Edinburgh: Churchill Livingstone.

TANNERY, N. H., Wessel, C. B., Epstein, B. A., & Gadd, C. S. (2007). Hospital nurses' use of knowledge-based information resources. *Nursing Outlook, 5*(1), 15–19. DOI:10.1016/j.Outlook.2006.04.006.

TRANSLATING RESEARCH INTO PRACTICE (TRIP) – II. (2001). (Fact Sheet No. 01-P017). Rockville, MD: Agency for Heatlhcare Research and Quality. Retrieved November 2, 2007 from http://www.ahrq.gov/research/trip2fac.pdf

WEAVER, S. M. (1993). Information literacy: Educating for life-long learning. *Nurse Educator, 18*(4), 30–32.

ZIPSER, J. (1998). *MEDLINE to PubMed and beyond.* Retrieved November 3, 2007, from http://www.nlm.nih.gov/bsd/historypresentation.html

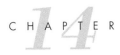

EVIDENCE-BASED PRACTICE

MAUREEN C. CREEGAN

Ed.D., RN Director and Professor, Division of Nursing, Dominican College

Tell me and I'll forget. Show me and I'll remember. Involve me and I'll understand.

–Confucius

LEARNING OBJECTIVES

At the completion of the chapter, the learner should be able to do the following:

1. Describe the evolution of evidence-based practice (EBP).
2. State the influence of critical thinking and ethical reasoning on clinical decision making.
3. Identify components of an EBP system.
4. Compare and contrast research utilization and EBP.
5. Define integrative review, systematic review, meta-analysis, and meta-synthesis.
6. Explain the difference between meta-analysis and meta-synthesis.
7. Differentiate among types of evidence: quantitative versus qualitative, intervention studies, and outcomes research.
8. Describe the future of nursing in an EBP environment.

KEY TERMS

Clinical Decision Making
Clinical Practice Guidelines
Critical Thinking
Evidence-Based
  Medicine (EBM)
Evidence-Based
  Nursing (EBN)
Evidence-Based
  Practice (EBP)

Evidence Hierarchy
Integrative Review
Intervention Research
Iowa Model of EBP
Meta-Analysis
Meta-Synthesis
Outcomes Research
PICO

Qualitative Research
Quantitative Research
Research Utilization
Risk/Benefit Ratio
Stetler Model
Systematic Review
Ways of Knowing

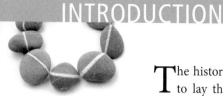

INTRODUCTION

The history of nursing is replete with examples of men and women who worked tirelessly to lay the foundation that defines today's nursing profession. By forging ahead boldly with their ideas, example, and action, pioneering nurses planted the seeds of **evidenced-based practice (EBP)** (Creegan, 2007). Rapid clinical advances and the knowledge explosion are reframing the health care arena. Cultural sensitivity, and personal, esthetic, empirical, and ethical **ways of knowing,** which help shape the **clinical decision making** that affects bedside care and system-wide operations, are basic to the evidence-based practice movement. Concern for patient welfare, knowledge, and clinical expertise are driving nurses to seek best practices that ensure patient safety and satisfactory health outcomes.

The EBP movement has stirred debate and hatched a cadre of critics, who indict EBP as a cookie-cutter approach to treatment that limits choices and fails to incorporate individual differences (Freshwater, 2004; Hasnain-Wynia, 2006; Mitchell, 2004). Proponents hail the approach as delivering the best possible care to the greatest number of people while monitoring cost in a limited-resources environment.

The purpose of this chapter is to describe the evolution of evidence-based practice, appraise the various sources of evidence, take the path to find the evidence, and offer strategies to move from evidence to action. The EBP journey has begun and health care disciplines are seeing their way clear to a new, more accountable era in health care.

THE EVOLUTION OF EVIDENCE-BASED PRACTICE

Health care experts advocate the use of scientifically based evidence to assure implementation of best practices. Before clinicians can make intelligent, well-reasoned decisions, they must develop sound critical thinking and ethical reasoning abilities.

Critical Thinking and Evidence-Based Practice

What nurses believe and think informs their contributions to health care, and how they think and subsequently act are based on the development of **critical thinking** and ethical reasoning abilities. "Critical thinking is the art of analyzing and evaluating thinking with a view to improving it…in short it is self-directed, self-disciplined, self-monitored, and self-corrective…" (Paul & Elder, 2007a, p. 4). Learning how to think analytically and reflectively helps us tackle problems and make intelligent, well-reasoned decisions. Well-reasoned decisions require conscious thought, inquisitiveness, analysis, and creativity, which are attributes of critical thinkers. Paul and Elder (2007a) list some universal intellectual standards that apply to quality thinking. To understand the basis of EBP, a clear understanding of critical thinking and how it influences decision making is essential.

Intellectual Standards for Critical Thinking

According to Paul and Elder (2007a, p.10), "…clarity is the gateway standard." Clear decision making depends on identifying and stating problems clearly, succinctly, and accurately. Reasoned decisions should be based on information that is reliable, consistent, and accurate. Precision involves questions related to details and specifics. Have you examined all aspects of a problem and collected all the information that will inform a reasoned decision? Precision means being specific in assembling information about a problem, as well as looking at information that gives more detail about the circumstances surrounding the problem. Relevance speaks to the importance of a problem. Did you examine all the information connected to the problem? Did you carefully review all aspects of importance prior to making your decision? Depth and breadth mean that you examine problems thoroughly and look at complex, individual situations that may affect your decisions. Skillful critical thinking is at the core of EBP. Arriving at well-reasoned conclusions is based on formulating good questions, searching through relevant information, thinking open-mindedly, looking at standards, testing out possible solutions, and collaborating with other disciplines to incorporate the best evidence into daily practice (Paul & Elder, 2007, p. 4). Cultivated thinkers take into account the various ways of knowing and assimilate them into their personal and intellectual lives. Carper (1978) described the various ways of knowing, which have implications for integrating intellectual standards and cultivating high-level thinking skills essential for EBP.

Ways of Knowing

In her seminal work, Carper (1978) conceptualized the fundamental patterns of knowing in nursing and designated them empirical, esthetic, and personal knowledge in nursing and ethics, the component of moral knowledge in nursing.

Empirical knowing is obtained by systematic collection of information with intent to objectively describe, explain, and predict phenomena. Nursing science has evolved to include a high degree of empirical knowledge, which is based on deductive reasoning and is factual in nature. Clarity, precision, and accuracy are thought processes that underpin empirical knowledge.

Esthetic knowing includes the creative process of discovery, of perceiving the individual behaviors of others, and designing and providing nursing care that is unique to individuals. It is not the practice of manual or technical skills, but is deeply associated with the knowledge gained by communicating with patients and feeling their experience of health and illness through empathy. Relevance, depth, and breadth are thinking processes that underpin esthetic knowledge.

Personal knowing is described as "subjective, concrete, and existential…" (Carper, 1978, p. 20). It includes recognizing the uniqueness of others, their differences and complexities, and their right to choose treatment alternatives. Depth and breadth are essential thinking processes in the quest for personal knowledge.

Ethical knowing, simply put, is questioning right from wrong. Although codes and standards (American Nurses Association [ANA], 2001) exist to help with ethical decision making, the notion of obligation intertwines with the right thing to do. Moral choices and actions to be taken are enmeshed and ethical codes guide thinking, but do not provide answers to many complex health care decisions. Relevance, depth, and breadth are thinking processes that help to develop ethical knowledge. Ethical knowing includes elements of ethical reasoning. "Whenever we think…we use ideas and theories to interpret data, facts, and experiences in order to answer questions, solve problems, and resolve issues" (Paul & Elder, 2006, p.3). To pose important questions that have relevance to patients, nurses' reasoning must be both critical and ethical. Figures 14-1 and 14-2 show the elements of thought and their relationship to the universal structures of thought.

Why is reasoned thinking important? Why spend time discussing our need to think more clearly? The essence of EBP is better patient outcomes. Best practices and improved patient outcomes will not occur without clear and reasoned thinking. How do we separate quality information from poor information? How do we know what really benefits patients? Critical thinking, which includes ways of knowing, development of key thought processes, and ethical reasoning, enables us to analyze and make sense of information. The way we assimilate information to make the best decisions in the practice world depends on highly developed reasoned thought.

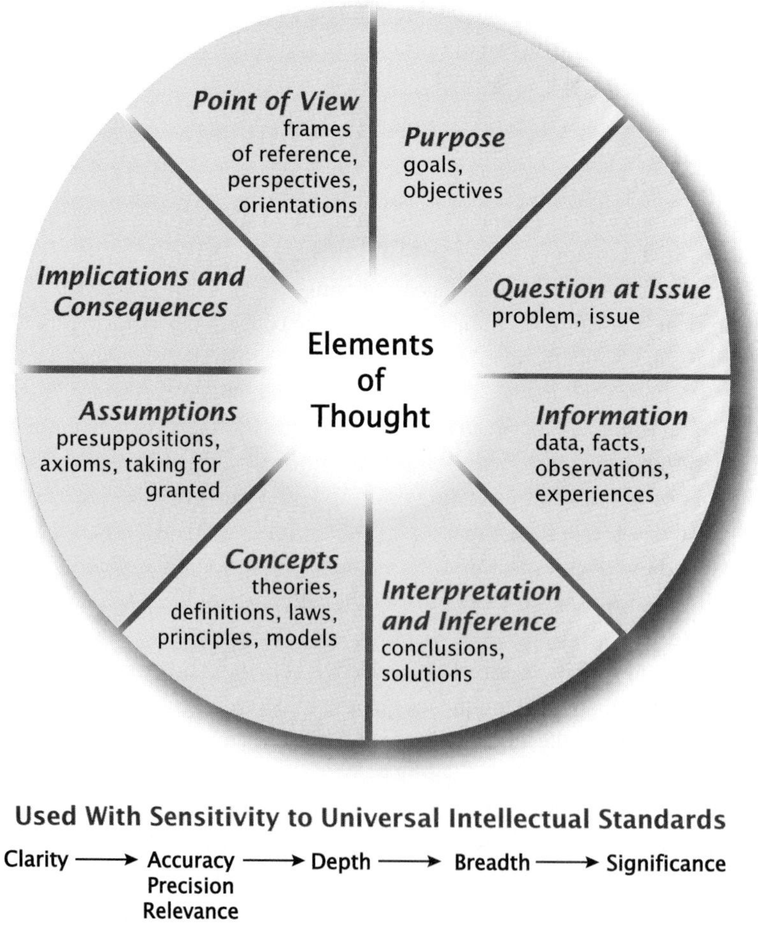

Figure 14-1
The Elements of Thought.
(*Reproduced with permission from Paul, R. P. & Elder, E. (2007), The miniature guide to critical thinking: Concepts and tools. Dillon Beach, CA: The Foundation for Critical Thinking. http://www. criticalthinking.org.*)

Point of View frames of reference, perspectives, orientations

Purpose goals, objectives

Implications and Consequences

Elements of Thought

Question at Issue problem, issue

Assumptions presuppositions, axioms, taking for granted

Information data, facts, observations, experiences

Concepts theories, definitions, laws, principles, models

Interpretation and Inference conclusions, solutions

Used With Sensitivity to Universal Intellectual Standards

Clarity ⟶ Accuracy Precision Relevance ⟶ Depth ⟶ Breadth ⟶ Significance

Figure 14-2
To analyze
thinking we must
learn to identify
and question
its elemental
structures.
*(Reproduced with
permission from Paul,
R. P. & Elder, E. (2006).
The Thinker's Guide to
Analytical Thinking.
Dillon Beach, CA: The
Foundation for Critical
Thinking. http://www.
criticalthinking.org.)*

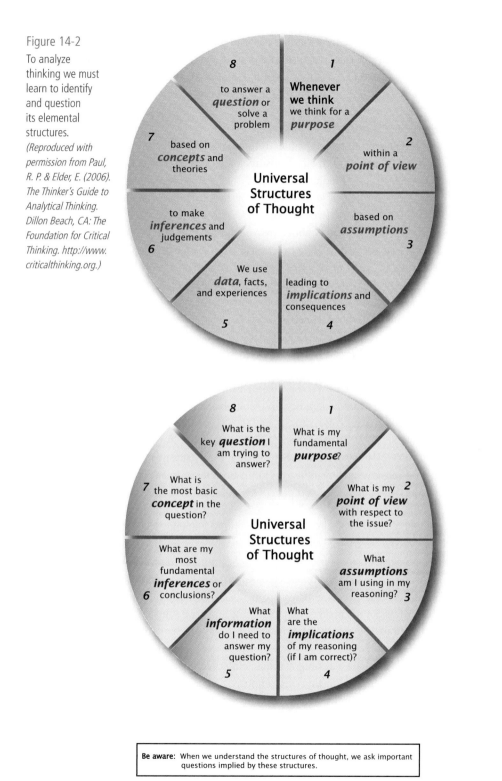

Be aware: When we understand the structures of thought, we ask important questions implied by these structures.

"All information is based on data, information and evidence. Restrict your claims to those supported by the data you have…and make sure that all information used is clear, accurate and relevant to the question at issue…" (Elder & Paul, 2006, p. 9). In summary, reasoned, ethical thinking is substantive critical thinking and is the cornerstone of evidence-based practice.

What Is Evidence-Based Practice?

The conscientious integration of patient values and preferences, and clinical expertise, with the best available research information to effect positive patient outcomes is known as evidenced-based practice (EBP) (Institute of Medicine [IOM], 2001). During the 1950s and 1960s, Dr. Archie Cochrane, a British epidemiologist, wrote extensively about using evidence from randomized controlled trials (RCTs). Dr. Cochrane decried the dearth of systematic evidence available to physicians to make the best decisions about treatments for patients. As a result of his work, the Cochrane Center was formed in 1993 in Oxford, UK. The Cochrane Collaboration, which currently has centers all over the world, provides systematic reviews of the effects of health care interventions on populations (Cochrane Collaboration, 2005, http://www.cochrane.org).

Sackett and colleagues (1996, p. 71) defined the movement called **evidence-based medicine (EBM)** as "…integrating individual expertise with the best available external evidence from systematic research." Guyatt and Rennie (2002) wrote the *Users' Guides to the Medical Literature: A Manual for Evidence Based Practice*, which provided a guide to the literature on diagnosis, treatment, prognosis, and systematic reviews. **Clinical practice guidelines** were also generated. Because of the work of these pioneers, the idea of EBM flourished and expanded to include collaboration among health care disciplines. Evidence-based practice advanced from EBM to include **evidence-based nursing (EBN).**

In 1994, the American Nurses Association (ANA) created the National Database of Nursing Quality Indicators (NDNQI) to discover links between empirical data and patient outcomes. NDNQI has proposed nursing-sensitive quality indicators for in-hospital care. The indicators include prevalence of pressure sores, in-patient falls, and patient-centered outcome measures like failure to rescue, which is an indicator of mortality among surgical patients with serious surgical complications (Clarke & Aiken, 2003). The University of Kansas School of Nursing (KUSON) and the Midwest Research Institute (MRI) were selected to house the national center and begin research and data collection on nursing-sensitive quality indicators. Pilot studies conducted by a number of state nursing associations laid the foundation for the initial database built by KUSON and MRI. Nursing-sensitive quality indicators reflect the impact of nursing care on hospitalized patients. The indicators are composed of structure, process, and outcomes of nursing care and are defined as follows:

1. Structure describes the supply of nurses, the skill mix, and nurses' level of education.
2. Process indicators measure assessment, nursing interventions, and job satisfaction.
3. Outcomes are patient indicators that show improvement in response to nursing care (e.g., pressure ulcers, falls, infections, drug events) (http://www.nursingquality.org).

Today's evidence-based practice movement has evolved from a medical orientation, to include nursing and allied health. Interdisciplinary groups of health professionals are committed to improve outcomes and provide consistent, cost-effective, quality care with quality evidence at its foundation (Finkelman & Kenner, 2007; Long, 2003).

Infrastructures as well as health care personnel are challenged to redesign better health care systems. The *Quality Chasm Report* (IOM, 2001) identified ten important rules to guide system redesign and focus on better patient outcomes. One of the ten rules included evidence-based decision making. The committee called for a number of initiatives. Among their recommendations were: improve interdisciplinary communication and collaboration; institute procedures that assure patient safety; encourage patients to take ownership of their health information and make informed decisions; provide patients access to their medical records; and, improve patient outcomes by providing care based on the best scientific evidence available. In 2003, the IOM identified five competencies based on patient need. The competencies stipulated that all health professionals provide patient-centered care; work as interdisciplinary team members to provide the various levels of expertise needed by patients; employ evidence-based practice to ensure that patients understand their illnesses and know how to care for themselves; apply quality improvement methods to continuously record patient progress; and, use informatics to search, retrieve, update, and monitor patient records to track outcomes of care (IOM, 2003b). Clearly, these five competencies are interrelated.

Writing Exercise 14-1	The Institute of Medicine Reports have framed health care for the 21st century. The reports on safety call for improving patient safety, which is defined as "freedom from accidental injury." Discuss how you would assure patient safety on a hospital unit. Write a short paragraph about keeping patients safe. Include at least three critical principles that nurses are implementing to assure patient safety in the practice environment. Refer to *To Err is Human: Building a Safer Health System* (IOM, 1999) (http://www.iom.edu/report.asp?id=5575). For an EBP environment to flourish, an overhaul of educational curricula and system infrastructures must occur.

REFRAMING EDUCATION

Nursing education has been slow to adopt changes mandated by the 21st-century health care system. As Em Bevis reportedly said, curriculum change is, "…akin to moving a cemetery" (Bargagliotti & Lancaster, 2007, p. 158). Nursing service leaders and nursing faculty responded to IOM initiatives and joined together to provide a model that will guide curriculum development and help prepare nursing students to deliver safe, quality care (Cronenwett, et al., 2007). The Quality and Safety Education for Nurses (QSEN) project, funded by the Robert Wood Johnson Foundation, convened to formulate competencies for prelicensure graduates. The knowledge, skills, and attitudes (KSA) needed by future nurses focus on patient-centered care, interdisciplinary collaboration and teamwork, evidence-based practice, quality improvement, and nursing informatics (Cronenwett, et al., 2007). KSAs appropriate to prelicensure nursing education at diploma, associate, and baccalaureate levels were outlined, as the team acknowledged that all nurses must be prepared to provide quality care. The educators determined that *all* undergraduates must understand the difference between opinion and empirical evidence, incorporate values and cultural differences when planning care, and critique evidence for applicability to practice. The committee found that *all* nursing programs "…[did not]…go beyond basic scientific understanding…and were perceived to be lacking in sufficient KSAs [that undergird EBP]."

(Cronenwett, et al., p.129). The QSEN group concluded that nursing curriculum for a new age in health care must incorporate research evidence, patient values and preferences, and engage in continuous improvement practices based on evaluation of patient outcomes. Figure 14-3 lists one example of the recommended KSAs to integrate EBP in clinical practice.

What opportunities are available to learners to search, evaluate, and apply evidence? What research competencies do learners need? How must faculty restructure curriculum to emphasize patient-centered, collaborative care, and integrate quality improvement learning activities? First and foremost, faculty and clinicians must nurture in learners a spirit of inquiry and self-reflection.

Figure 14-3
Knowledge, Skills
and Attitudes to
Integrate Evidence-
Based Practice in
Clinical Practice.

Knowledge	Skills	Attitudes
Demonstrate knowledge of basic scientific methods and processes	Participate effectively in appropriate data collection and other research activities	Appreciate strengths and weaknesses of scientific bases for practice
Describe EBP to include the components of research evidence, clinical expertise and patient/family values	Adhere to Institutional Review Board (IRB) guidelines	Value the need for ethical conduct of research and quality improvement
	Base individualized care plan on patient values, clinical expertise and evidence	Value the concept of EBP as integral to determining best clinical practice
Differentiate clinical opinion from research and evidence summaries	Read original research and evidence reports related to area of practice	Appreciate the importance of regularly reading relevant professional journals
Describe reliable sources for locating evidence reports and clinical practice guidelines	Locate evidence reports related to clinical practice topics and guidelines	
Explain the role of evidence in determining best clinical practice	Participate in structuring the work environment to facilitate integration of new evidence into standards of practice	Value the need for continuous improvement in clinical practice based on new knowledge
Describe how the strength and relevance of available evidence influences the choice of interventions in provision of patient-centered care	Question rationale for routine approaches to care that result in less-than-desired outcomes or adverse events	
Discriminate between valid and invalid reasons for modifying evidence-based clinical practice based on clinical expertise or patient/family preferences	Consult with clinical experts before deciding to deviate from evidence-based protocols	Acknowledge own limitations in knowledge and clinical expertise before determining when to deviate from evidence-based best practices

Having a personal philosophy that includes ways of knowing and how EBP processes intertwine with fundamental patterns of knowing is essential. Mentoring nursing students in EBP and encouraging a spirit of discovery and inquisitiveness will motivate them to implement EBP and evaluate what is best for patients (Cronenwett, et al., 2007; Day, 2007; Fineout-Overholt & Johnston, 2006). Faculty and clinicians who foster EBP create adoption of EBP practices by other colleagues (Melnyk, et al., 2004). Revised research courses should include the following content/activities:

1. Exercises to identify pressing clinical questions.
2. Computer access and basic literacy to help learners track down the best information in a timely, efficient manner.
3. Collaborative experiences with librarians, who explain and assist with electronic access and retrieval.
4. Opportunities to critically appraise data sources and choose among the best available, with the goal of effecting positive changes in patients, systems, and policies.
5. Partnering learners with quantitative and qualitative researchers and clinicians to learn and appreciate research methodology and its application to practice settings.
6. Engaging learners in measurement of outcomes to evaluate the effectiveness of nursing interventions.

These changes "…should facilitate learning for the practical purpose of improving patient care versus simply an intellectual exercise" (Fineout-Overholt & Johnston, 2006, p. 195). Add to these new approaches collaborative exchange among disciplines, and learners will be prepared to participate in the EBP environment (Fineout-Overholt & Johnston, 2006; Levin & Feldman, 2006a; Sherwood & Drenkard, 2007).

System Overhaul

Strong leadership in health care organizations is necessary to make EBP happen (Aiken, Clarke, Sloane, Sochalski, & Silber, 2002; Block & Le Grazie, 2006; Daniels, 2007; Hamilton, Jacob, Koch, & Quammen, 2004; Matter, 2006; McCaughan, Thompson, Cullum, Sheldon, Trevor, & Thompson, 2002; Rafferty, Maben, West, & Robinson, 2005; Redman, 2005; Winch, Henderson, & Creedy, 2005). Visionary leaders actively engage employees in the organizational environment. The International Council of Nurses (2005) reported effects of management practices on nurses. Particularly noted was the need to include employees in organizational decision-making. Providing nurses with clinical evidence at the point of care is the aim of an EBP program. Information technology (IT) enables access to the best evidence. Studies report concrete evidence that automated systems decrease follow-up time with the hospital pharmacy, enhance implementation of protocols because they generate consultation orders immediately on admission of patients, and make clinical best practices available with one strike of a key (Hamilton, Jacob, Koch, & Quammen, 2004). For example, a pilot program that integrated evidence-based knowledge into the electronic health record (EHR) was initiated by PinnacleHealth, a four-hospital health system in Harrisburg, PA. (Matter, 2006).

The idea behind this project was to increase communication among nurses and provide application of evidence-based knowledge to common problems encountered by nurses in everyday practice. The pilot involved connecting the computer IT care planning and documentation screens to the evidence, which enabled nurses to locate current research findings. As a result, patient care plans reflected the most current, best protocols available for effecting beneficial outcomes on certain measures. The nursing-sensitive performance measures selected were fall prevention, smoking cessation, pain management, and pressure ulcer prevention. At completion, the pilot program allowed for customized care plans that could be accessed at the bedside. As a result nurses were empowered by the shift "…from executing orders to managing patient problems, from task-based documentation to knowledge-based decision-making…critical thinking and collaboration between staff and advanced practice nurses [was substantially elevated]." (Matter, p. 36). The Institute for Healthcare Improvement (IHI), in partnership with several organizations, formed the Surgical Care Improvement Project (SCIP) to reduce morbidity and mortality among hospital in-patients. SCIP has developed several evidence-based interventions to reduce complications from blood clots, pneumonia, and infections. The IHI and SCIP are committed to the 5 Million Lives Campaign (2006–2008) to reduce medical morbidity and mortality in hospitals across the country (http://www.ihi.org).

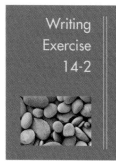

Writing Exercise 14-2

Surgical site infections (SSI) account for 14–16% of hospital-acquired (iatrogenic) infections (Daniels, 2007). You are working on a surgical unit and are assigned to prep your patient for the operating room (OR). Based on the evidence, list two (2) pre-op measures you will take to help reduce surgical site infection. Base your answer on recommendations from the Surgical Care Improvement Project (SCIP) (http://www.medqic.org/scip).

Creating systems that translate research findings into practice is a challenge. Nevertheless, the challenge continues to be met with the emergence of several EBP models. Several system models explain the steps and processes in EBP. Two models, which were developed by nurses as a framework for nursing **research utilization (RU)** and evolved into EBP, are discussed here. The Stetler Model of Research Utilization (Stetler, 2001) and the Iowa Model of Research in Practice (Titler, Kleiber, Steelman, Rakel, Boudreau, Everett, et al., 2001) include components of EBP. First, it is important to understand the differences between research utilization and EBP.

Research Utilization and EBP

Research utilization is the synthesis and application of research results to solve clinical problems and change existing practice (Burns & Grove, 2005; Di Censo, Guyatt, & Ciliska, 2005; Melnyk & Fineout-Overholt, 2005; Polit & Beck, 2008). Evidence-based practice synthesizes the highest quality empirical research within the context of diversity and patient values to change practice and improve patient outcomes. Rogers's theory of diffusion of innovations (1995) provides a framework for research utilization in practice settings.

Planned change is never easy, but the process of diffusing knowledge as proposed by Rogers gives direction to thought processes, and outlines actions that facilitate an EBP environment. In Rogers's view, diffusion and dissemination of knowledge are synonymous. Guided by development of ideas, communication, and timelines, planned innovation can be implemented by like-minded individuals who envision better patient outcomes. Theoretically, systems that embrace ideas and open channels of communication among interested people set ideas in motion and formulate a plan to try them out. For example, nurses and administrators in a hospital are a social system driven by a common goal to provide high-quality, cost-controlled services to consumers. The group works on problem-solving as part of the innovation-to-decision process. The ultimate goal is to provide patient care based on research (Titler, 2007).

The **Stetler Model** (Stetler, 2001), originally crafted as an RU framework for individuals and organizations, evolved into a model for EBP program development (Figure 14.4). The Stetler framework helps nurses inform education, direct clinical decision-making, and create or change policy. The steps in the process are: 1) preparation, 2) validation, 3) clinical decision making/comparative evaluation, 4) translation, and 5) evaluation. A brief overview of the phases follows.

Preparation

This phase includes identifying the nature and scope of the problem. Problems can be practice related, managerial in nature, or policy issues that need revision. The next step is to form a committee of agency stakeholders to tackle several questions. What is the purpose for implementing the change? Will the change improve the practice of nurses? Will patients benefit from the change/innovation? Will the organization as a whole benefit? Will the cost to implement be manageable? How will the change/innovation affect interaction with external constituents/agencies? These are some of the questions to be asked and answered before initiating any change.

For example, a hospital is thinking about implementing a Comprehensive Physician Order Entry (CPOE) management system to improve patient safety. A committee of stakeholders identifies the most pressing problem as improved patient safety through better medication management. The group discusses various CPOE packages that include physician data entry, medical record keeping, and medication management. Members conduct a comprehensive literature review about medication errors and patient safety. The committee identifies increased safety as the most beneficial outcome for patients. The literature shows that medication errors decrease with a coding method of patient identification and recording. The **risk/benefit ratio** is weighed as well as expenditures to purchase computer equipment and train staff. To assure successful acceptance of the new system, the preparation phase requires careful examination of internal and external influences. The decision arrived at must be a collaborative one with all stakeholders on board.

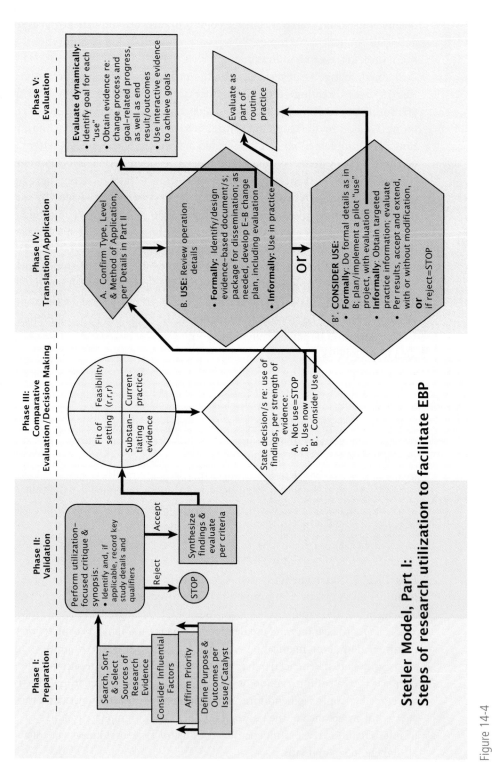

Figure 14-4

Stetler Model, Part I: Steps of research utilization to facilitate EBP. *(Reprinted from Nursing Outlook, 49, Stetler, C., Updating the Stetler Model of research utilization to facilitate evidence-based practice, 272–279, (2001), with permission from Elsevier.)*

Validation

This is the second phase in the Stetler Model and involves a critical look at the literature that either supports or negates the innovation. In our example of increasing patient safety through instituting a medication management system, the committee examines the evidence. What does the research show? Is the evidence strongly in favor of implementing a medication management system? Do several studies consistently demonstrate decreased medication errors? Because the CPOE system is a costly venture, and patient safety is a priority, the committee weighs the evidence, and finds the evidence supports purchase of a medication management system as the first move toward safety outcomes for patients.

Clinical Decision-Making/Comparative Evaluation

This third phase of the process follows acceptance of the plan to move forward with the new procedure. In our example, the hospital must adapt to the new procedure. In other words, the goodness-of-fit is important. This phase involves the three Rs: risk, resources, and readiness (Burns & Grove, 2005). Will the staff buy into the system? Will the hospital offer computer training to prepare the staff to comfortably work in the system? What additional resources will be needed? Assuming that the hospital committee in our example has weighed in on the evidence and examined the benefits and risks to patients, a decision is made to implement the medication system on one unit.

Translation

This phase means applying the findings to practice. In our example, the medication system is piloted on one unit. This pilot unit will be monitored for staff productivity, efficiency, patient outcomes, and cost savings. The idea is to evaluate the workings of the new procedure and correct any kinks in the operation before system-wide implementation begins. How is the staff working with the new system? Are there sufficient resources to support the system? During this phase the hospital will collect information about patient satisfaction and outcomes of care, i.e., what is the medication error rate on this unit? The unit data will then be examined, and a decision made to move forward or cancel implementation of the medication management system as a hospital-wide project.

Evaluation

The final phase involves the system-wide impact of the innovation on hospital personnel and patient outcomes. What are the overall benefits to patients, hospital, and staff? Is staff comfortable with the new system? After reviewing patient records, do the data show accurate, consistent recording of medications? Does the system facilitate and support better use of staff time? What do patients say about the new system? These are some of the questions asked during the evaluation phase.

Stetler's framework is comprehensive yet succinct, and can be used by individual nurses or tailored to suit development of EBP programs in multiple-practice settings. The **Iowa Model** (Figure 14-5) is another interesting approach that diagrams processes and procedures to follow in crafting an EBP program in organizations.

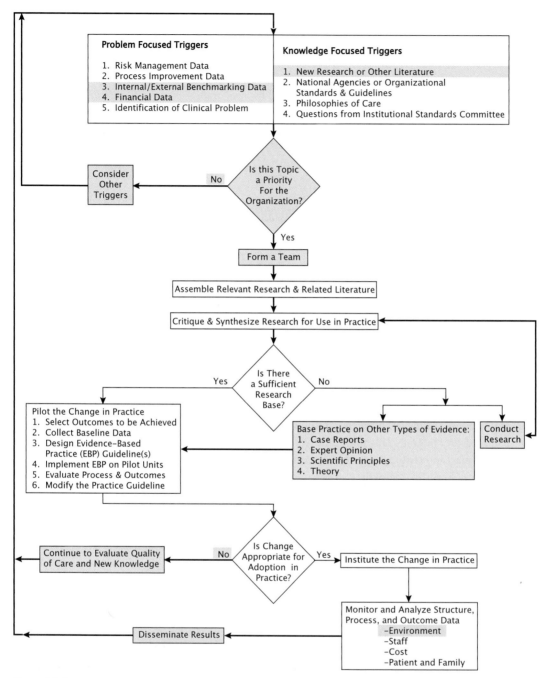

Figure 14-5

The Iowa model of research-based practice to promote quality care. Diamond = decision point; heavy lines = new feedback loop; shaded areas = new terminology and action steps. *(Courtesy of Marita Titler, PhD, RN, FAAN. Reprinted from* Critical Care Nursing Clinics of North America, *13, Titler, M. G., Kleiber, C., Steelman, V. J., Rakel, B. A., Boudreau, G., Everett, L. Q., et al. The Iowa model of evidence-based practice to promote quality care, 497–509, Copyright Elsevier (2001).)*

Developed by nurses in a university hospital environment, the Iowa model describes problem-focused and knowledge-focused triggers (Titler, et al., 2001). Triggers set off thoughts or actions that initiate change. Problem-focused triggers may come from risk management information, benchmarking procedures, or financial data. Knowledge-focused triggers may come from internal organizational committees, external professional standards and organizations, or new research findings. Is the trigger a priority for the organization? If yes, then a committee is formed to conduct a rigorous and relevant critique of the literature that will either support or refute the trigger.

If there is insufficient research on a topic, the trigger may be abandoned, or the clinical facility may decide to conduct research on the topic. As well, goodness-of-fit is an important concept in the Iowa Model, and piloting the innovation is an essential step preliminary to adopting any change in practice. The Iowa model includes formulating and modifying practice guidelines according to results of pilot data, as well as monitoring outcomes of care. In the final step, changes in practice should be widely disseminated among colleagues to institute best practices (Titler, 2007). If the model is followed and the agency monitors changes in practice, then an EBP system is in place.

THE PATH TO EVIDENCE

Formulating the right questions and examining a variety of sources sets us on the path to uncovering the evidence (Johnston & Fineout-Overholt, 2005). The notion of evidence-based practice refers to the integration of the best research evidence, clinical expertise, and patient values in making decisions about the care of individual patients (Burns & Grove, 2005; DiCenso, Guyatt, & Ciliska, 2005; IOM, 2001; Levin & Feldman, 2006b; Molloch & O'Grady, 2008; Polit & Beck, 2008). Nursing knowledge is acquired in many ways. In the past, nurses relied on tradition and communicated acceptable behaviors to colleagues new to the field. Nursing has a rich history, yet many traditional practices continue without accuracy or support of nursing research. Tradition states "this is the way we have always done it" and this statement is unacceptable in today's EBP environment. Equally unacceptable is the trial-and-error method. This strategy uses multiple methods until the "right one" appears to work. Because of trial and error, patients may be subjected to adverse events. Authority is another way of transmitting nursing knowledge. Nurses with years of experience in nursing are often seen as experts and wield position power. However, position power does not define expertise. Nurses who practice from a research knowledge base are authorities in practice and should influence the practice of others. Integrating knowledge from other disciplines has enriched nursing practice (AACN, 1999). However, practicing nursing solely from the perspective of another discipline clouds the vision of nursing as a distinct discipline. Nurses who practice in the medical model, and attend to diagnosis and treatment of disease, sacrifice prevention and health-promotion activities. Using knowledge from other disciplines expands understanding of humans and their nature. However, information obtained exclusively from other disciplines cannot answer questions particular to nursing and nursing practice.

Today's nurse is part of a unique discipline that integrates social, natural, and physical sciences. The 21st century nurse practices in a EBP arena where scientific evidence guides practice and challenges old ways. Because trial and error can cause detrimental patient outcomes, nursing actions should follow current, scientifically based best practices to improve the quality of care delivered.

APPRAISING THE EVIDENCE

Several experts in the field of EBP have come together to rate the quality of evidence. Evaluating the strength of the evidence is important because it provides clinicians with a framework for guiding their decisions.

Evidence Hierarchy

The strength of scientific evidence is rated using a grading system, also called a **hierarchy** or taxonomy. The hierarchy situates randomized controlled trials (RCTs) at the pinnacle and places expert opinion at the base (DiCenso, Guyatt, & Ciliska, 2005; Melnyk & Overholt, 2005; Polit & Beck, 2008; Sackett, 2000). Although all levels of evidence are valued, the rigor of the design positions each in the hierarchy (see Figure 14-6).

Figure 14-6
Steps in the
Evidence Hierarchy.

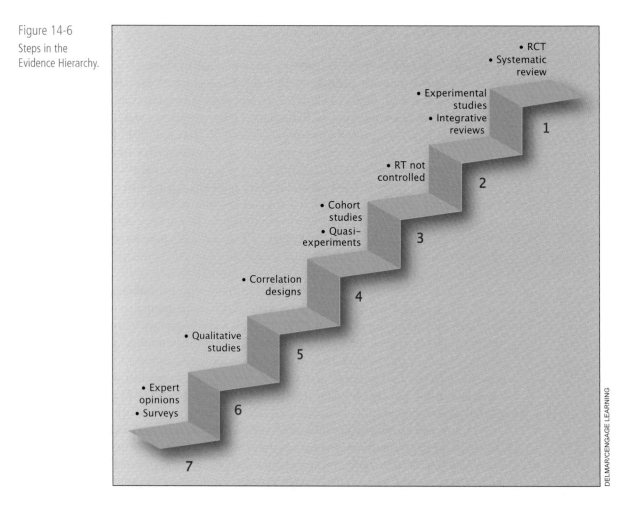

DELMAR/CENGAGE LEARNING

RCTs are the gold standard of EBP, because the results of several trials that include large randomized samples of subjects are reliable and valid, making generalizability possible across multiple populations. Cause-and-effect relationships are established with large randomized samples and control of confounding variables. The results of a well-designed study strengthen the findings and increase the likelihood of generalizability and applicability to clinical practice.

Critical appraisal of the literature and synthesis of research findings are sophisticated tasks that should be performed by expert researchers who are familiar with different types of reviews and when to use the appropriate one. The following section discusses the types of reviews conducted by experts in the field of EBP.

Types of Reviews

Integrative reviews identify, analyze, and synthesize results from independent empirical studies, and summarize conclusions on a particular topic (Beyea & Nicoll, 1998; Burns & Grove, 2005). The American Association of Colleges of Nursing (AACN) includes integrative reviews as part of the scholarship of integration, which is defined as "…writings that use concepts and original works from nursing and other disciplines in creating new patterns, placing knowledge in a larger context, or illuminating the data in a more meaningful way…" (AACN, 1999, p. 7). The *Annual Review of Nursing Research* is a good example of published integrative reviews on a number of nursing topics.

Systematic review is a rigorous process conducted by experts who identify, analyze, and synthesize research studies on a specific question to draw conclusions about the worth of the data (Melnyk & Fineout-Overholt, 2005; Polit & Beck, 2008). RCTs provide the majority of rigorous evidence on which practice is based (Fain, 2004; Melnyk & Fineout-Overholt, 2005; Sackett, et al., 1996; Sackett, 2000; Stevens, 2001). High-quality studies on a topic must satisfy certain criteria in order to be included in empirical systematic reviews. Researchers set the inclusion/exclusion criteria before they conduct a systematic review. Systematic reviewers scour volumes of information available on a topic, analyze and synthesize the information, and package the conclusions as a summary of the best evidence. Systematic reviews of **quantitative research** or empirical studies include a technique called **meta-analysis.** Meta-analysis is a process that summarizes results of multiple similar quantitative studies and provides a summary statistic that measures the single effect of an intervention across multiple studies (Fain, 2004; Melnyk & Fineout-Overholt, 2005; Polit & Beck, 2008). Objectivity is the major advantage of meta-analysis, as it is conducted on summarized findings of studies and contributes to the strength of the evidence (Fain, 2004). Meta-analysis is performed on RCTs of high quality to provide the best evidence for making decisions about how to treat patients. In meta-analysis, if the effective size of the intervention is acceptable, or of clinical significance, the information becomes a framework for best practice, and evolves into a clinical guideline (Levin & Vetter, 2007). The Cochrane Collaboration provides results of systematic reviews (http://www.cochrane.org) and AHRQ provides clinical guidelines based on results of meta-analysis of systematic reviews. To understand the procedures involved in systematic review and meta-analysis, the following section discusses the process.

Examples of Systematic Reviews

A systematic review of the role of exercise in patients with Type 2 diabetes concluded that exercise did not influence morbidity and mortality, but did lower A1C blood levels, adiposity, and triglyceride levels. The researchers—meta-analysts—reviewed several databases, among them the Cochrane Central Register of Controlled Trials (CENTRAL), Medline, and EMBASE. Bibliographies were also manually searched. To meet inclusion criteria for the systematic review, the researchers examined clinical trials that compared aerobic fitness training of any type and progressive fitness training with no exercise in persons with Type 2 diabetes. In the case of treating a newly diagnosed patient disinclined to take medication, the evidence strongly suggested treatment with oral hypoglycemic agents, coupled with exercise and diet. Exercise alone did not improve quality of life, nor decrease mortality from diabetes (Cayley, 2007).

In another systematic review, estimates of the advantages and disadvantages of breast screening mammography were identified in the literature. The result of a PubMed systematic search of the question, "How should physicians counsel women about mammography?" revealed that for every two thousand women screened throughout ten years, only one would have her life prolonged, and ten healthy women would be treated unnecessarily as a result of screening. After systematic review and meta-analysis, the effect of the mammography screening intervention was found to be inconclusive. The result: no recommendation was made to change screening practices because the effect size was too small to show whether screening mammography did more harm than good (Potter, 2007).

Similarly, nurses at the Northern Navajo Medical Center in Shiprock, New Mexico, asked the question, "Does bathing with chlorhexidine (CHG) preoperatively prevent risk of post-surgical site infection (SSI)?" The nurses reviewed a meta-analysis of RCTs that used several thousand preoperative patients at various hospital sites. The studies compared the use of CHG with bar soap, placebo, and no washing. Results from the Cochrane Database of Systematic Reviews revealed that although surgical antiseptic soap is commonly used, it is no more effective than any other wash in reducing post SSI. On the basis of their systematic review of the literature, nurses in Navajo Medical Center decided that CHG as a preoperative prep would no longer be used on their surgical patients (Elkins, et al., 2007).

These examples of systematic reviews show that clinicians are investigating and answering relevant, pressing clinical questions. After evaluating systematic reviews and meta-analysis of high-quality empirical studies, clinicians make their decisions with the goal of providing quality, cost-effective care. Subsequently, clinical guidelines are formulated based on the findings of systematic reviews.

The Agency for Healthcare Research and Quality (AHRQ) is a repository of clinical guidelines. The Agency evaluates evidence on the basis of three domains: quality, quantity, and consistency. Quality describes overall research design, analysis, sample selection, measurement, and confounding biases. Quantity includes the numbers of studies that have evaluated the same question, sample size across all studies, magnitude of treatment effects, and the relative risk/odds ratio. Consistency means that numerous studies with similar or different designs reach similar conclusions (AHRQ http://www.ahrq.gov; Melnyk & Fineout-Overholt, 2005, 2002). AHRQ brings together experts who use the three domains as a framework for developing clinical guidelines. Nurses should frequently visit the AHRQ Web site for updates and new guidelines.

In contrast to meta-analysis, **meta-synthesis** is conducted by qualitative researchers who study and generate theory, explore lived experiences of individuals, or examine cultural ideas or developments. One definition of meta-synthesis suggested that it is "...the breaking down of findings, examining them, discovering the essential features and, in some way combining phenomena in a transformed whole" (Schreiber, Crooks, & Stern, 1997, p. 314). "Statistical integration" used in meta-analysis is inappropriate for qualitative studies (Polit & Beck, 2008, p. 665). Skilled qualitative researchers conduct meta-synthesis and follow similar steps to those followed by quantitative meta-analysts. However, subjectivity of the meta-synthesis method is in sharp contrast to the objectivity of meta-analysis. In meta-synthesis, the reviewers may make subjective decisions about the data, which may be based on personal preferences. Subsequently, the reviewers may draw different conclusions from the data. Objectivity is further decreased because no statistical calculations are performed across qualitative studies. Nevertheless, meta-synthesis is a valuable approach to integrating qualitative findings and addressing the complex variations people exhibit. Suffice it to say, qualitative researchers are wrestling with the ways to conduct meta-synthesis (Finfgeld, 2003; Sandelowski, Docherty, & Emden; 1997; Schreiber, Crooks, & Stern, 1997; Thorne, Jensen, Kearney, Noblit, & Sandelowski, 2004).

A discussion of several ways to generate evidence, including quantitative, qualitative, intervention, and outcomes approaches follows.

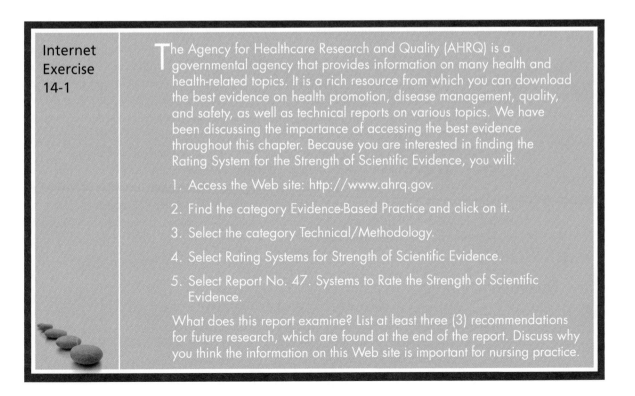

Internet Exercise 14-1

The Agency for Healthcare Research and Quality (AHRQ) is a governmental agency that provides information on many health and health-related topics. It is a rich resource from which you can download the best evidence on health promotion, disease management, quality, and safety, as well as technical reports on various topics. We have been discussing the importance of accessing the best evidence throughout this chapter. Because you are interested in finding the Rating System for the Strength of Scientific Evidence, you will:

1. Access the Web site: http://www.ahrq.gov.

2. Find the category Evidence-Based Practice and click on it.

3. Select the category Technical/Methodology.

4. Select Rating Systems for Strength of Scientific Evidence.

5. Select Report No. 47. Systems to Rate the Strength of Scientific Evidence.

What does this report examine? List at least three (3) recommendations for future research, which are found at the end of the report. Discuss why you think the information on this Web site is important for nursing practice.

APPROACHES TO GENERATING EVIDENCE

There are a number of approaches to generating evidence. Choosing an approach depends on the personal preference of the researcher and the question, problem, or issue of interest. A well-formulated question will set the stage for the research design.

Quantitative Approach

Quantitative researchers use numbers to describe data and report findings. The empirical or quantitative researcher objectively measures variables with the goal of establishing facts and allowing prediction of outcomes. For example, quantitative researchers might investigate:

1. What factors influence smoking behaviors in adolescent youth?
2. Which treatment for rheumatoid arthritis is more effective?
3. What lifestyle and demographic factors are associated with a higher incidence of coronary artery disease (CAD)?

Hallmarks of good quantitative design are large sample sizes, subjects selected at random, and control over competing variables. How the sample is selected has a profound effect on the outcomes of a study. Randomization increases representativeness of a sample because each member of the sample has an equal chance of selection and inclusion. Control over extraneous variables guarantees that the intervention, or treatment, is solely responsible for the outcome. Statistical analysis is conducted, and inferences are drawn from the results. Some RCTs are longitudinal studies that include large numbers of participants who are randomly selected and studied over long periods of time. As previously discussed, RCTs are the premier standard of quantitative or empirical research. Recall our discussion about Chlorhexidine (CHG) as an antiseptic presurgical scrub. After systematic review and meta-analysis, the nurses at Navajo Medical Center concluded that any wash would do since no specific wash prevented surgical site infection (SSI) (Elkins, et al.). This is an example of quantitative research, which has been subject to systematic review and meta-analysis.

In summary, quantitative research, also called empirical research, has three components: control, randomization, and treatment. The most recognized high-quality quantitative research is the RCT because it satisfies these three criteria. Results of these trials are subject to systematic review and meta-analysis. If, after meta-analysis, the data are found to be clinically significant, clinical guidelines may be formulated.

Qualitative Approach

Qualitative research is conducted to identify themes and patterns, record the lived experiences of subjects, and generate and modify theories (Patten, 2005; Polit & Beck, 2008). The goal of most qualitative research is to understand individuals' perceptions of phenomena as it exists for them in the context of their environment. Rich descriptions of human complexity and differences are hallmarks of qualitative work. There are no independent and dependent variables, and manipulation and control are rarely used. Small groups of persons who meet preset criteria are sought and selected for participation in studies about their culture, values, and perceptions. There are several ways to conduct qualitative research, and in-depth discussion of these designs is beyond the scope of this chapter. To understand the relevance of qualitative findings to the development of a comprehensive EBP program, a brief review of grounded theory, ethnography, and phenomenology follows.

Grounded Theory

Generating and modifying theory falls under the umbrella of grounded theory research. The main concern of the participants/subjects emerges from the data. In this realm, the qualitative researcher collects information via observations and interviews. Next the researcher analyzes the information observed and/or recorded to find patterns or recurring themes. In other words, the grounded theory method used by the qualitative researcher generates information that is grounded, or embedded, in the observations or words of the interviewee. The approach is cyclical in that "…researchers collect the data, categorize them, describe the emerging central phenomena, and then recycle earlier steps" (Polit & Beck, 2008, p. 230).

Ethnography

Rooted in anthropology, ethnography is the study of behaviors and practices of various cultures. Ethnographers conduct field studies and write rich descriptive reports about their observations. Typically, ethnographers become immersed in the culture under study and become the "researcher as instrument" (Polit & Beck, 2008, p. 225). Behaviors of cultures, objects used by individuals in a particular culture, and how members communicate are of interest to ethnographers. Diaries, journals, and other sources of information about the culture are examined. In-depth interviews and observations are also conducted to obtain detailed information.

Phenomenology

Phenomenologists explore the truths about reality that are evident in the everyday lived experience of individuals. Suffering, pain, and living with chronic illness are some topics of interest to nurse phenomenologists, who examine perceptions of subjects as a way to acquire knowledge about humans (Polit & Beck, 2008; Patten, 2005). In-depth conversations with subjects and introspective reflection are hallmarks of the method. Phenomenological studies involve small groups of participants whose insights help us understand the human condition.

Grounded theory, ethnography, and phenomenology are three qualitative methods that offer rich data and insight into human behavior. Qualitative researchers are said to be interested in human science. They are concerned with individual differences that affect patient responses to situations and events, and directly influence either recovery from acute illness or adaptation to chronic illness. When information is sparse on a topic, the qualitative approach is favored. For example, when the Severe Acute Respiratory Syndrome (SARS) outbreak occurred, little was known about it. Interviewing survivors and asking them broad questions about how they felt, what they ate, where they were, and what they were doing at the time they fell ill supplied rich descriptive data for an otherwise nonexistent database.

New topics for investigation are constantly emerging and lend themselves to qualitative study, as little is known about them. Domestic terrorism and online instruction as an educational method are two more examples ripe for qualitative research because they are areas where research is in its infancy (Patten, 2005).

Collection of information, from which patterns or themes emerge, gives direction to initial treatment. For example, Schoofs (2001) conducted a qualitative research study about interference with daily life and activities as experienced by women with secondary Sjogren's syndrome (SS), an autoimmune cluster of symptoms of rheumatoid arthritis and systemic lupus erythematosis. Women with secondary Sjogren's Syndrome, ages 27 to 83, were asked how they managed to cope with their symptoms on a daily basis. The researcher used the grounded theory method to generate a theory of hope. The 4-H Model of Living, with four categories of helping, hindering, hoping, and hurting, emerged (Figure 14-7).

Figure 14-7
The 4-H Model.
(Reprinted from Journal of Professional Nursing, *17, Schoofs, N., Seeing the glass half full: Living with Sjogren's Syndrome, 194–202, (2001), with permission from Elsevier.)*

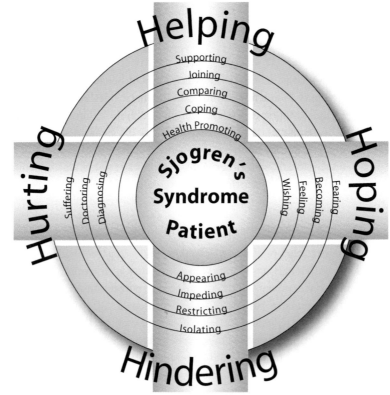

The 4-H Model

The lived experience of a sample of patients across the age spectrum, who live with SS every day, is important for nurses to read and understand in order to provide unique care to persons suffering from this chronic illness. Living with Sjogren's is a journey of ups and downs, similar to other journeys of patients with chronic illnesses.

Findings from qualitative studies, like the one just discussed, could be subject to meta-synthesis with a vision of developing ways to help women cope with chronic debilitating disease. New patterns and themes on the topic of chronic disease may emerge and offer insight into chronic illness management, an important concern for nurses and other health care providers in the 21st century and beyond.

In summary, EBP involves both quantitative and qualitative approaches. Studying the human condition is important, as the quantitative approach alone does not work in health care or in any other environment where humans flourish. The most beneficial, comprehensive clinical decision making places the patient at the focal point and includes understanding diversity within the context of individual values and culture. If nurses truly want to deliver patient-centered, evidence-based care, then both randomized trials and patient perceptions of care must drive care delivery. To value both quantitative and qualitative research is to provide the best evidence for the practice of nursing.

Intervention Approach

Intervention research is of particular interest to nurses because the findings move from "causal connection to causal explanation" (Burns & Grove, p. 312). The focus becomes one of seeking and identifying what interventions work, why they work, and to what extent they work to benefit populations. The thrust of intervention studies is to establish a scientific basis for nursing actions, and to ultimately generate evidence for nursing care. Intervention research may include both qualitative and quantitative approaches to determine the effectiveness of outcomes. Since intervention research may incorporate the collection of both qualitative and quantitative data, composition of the study team should include experts in both approaches.

Intervention research requires thorough planning for successful implementation and involvement of a variety of interested stakeholders. Also important is pilot testing the intervention to note its effects, or to identify snags in implementation at an early stage. Some interventions are still applied because of tradition, trial and error, authority, and expert opinion. The intervention should be evidence-based, incorporate clinical expertise, and integrate best practices, which may be found in a comprehensive literature search.

Nurses provide many different treatments and therapies to improve patient care. Determining the effectiveness of interventions on patient outcomes is essential. For example, a smoking cessation program may include several different treatment modalities and teaching protocols. Nurses may help patients with stress reduction, medication management, and avoidance of certain beverages they associate with smoking, to help patients control their urge to smoke. Efforts by nurses to prevent or reduce complications through deliberate actions are ripe areas for intervention research. What worked—and what didn't—is important to measure, so that the methods and interventions in the smoking cessation program may be refined or eliminated.

Evaluating the benefits or harms of care provided to patients is the essence of intervention research. Expanding teams of investigators to multiple locations, with diverse sample populations and consistent application of interventions, will create a database that has far-reaching implications for evidence-based practice (Department of Health and Human Services [DHHS], 2001; IOM, 2001; Magyary, Whitney, & Brown, 2006; Sidani & Braden, 1998; Smedley, Stith, & Nelson, 2003).

Outcomes Approach

Outcomes research focuses on changes that occur as a result of interventions. Interventions may aim to improve health care services, point-of-care at the bedside, or health of populations. The Institute of Medicine (IOM) has issued several reports calling for patient-centered care, safety, quality outcomes, improved information technology infrastructures, interdisciplinary collaboration, and integration of best evidence at the point-of-care (IOM, 1999, 2001, 2003a, 2003b, 2004, 2007; Smedley, et al., 2003). Several exemplars committed to improving patient outcomes are underway.

Exemplars of Outcomes Research

The Quality and Safety Education for Nurses (QSEN) project is one exemplar. Members of this project group included educators who formulated competencies for undergraduate nursing students. As a result of their work, recommendations were made to ensure that all nursing undergraduates understand the differences between opinion and empirical evidence, incorporate values and cultural differences in care situations, and critically appraise the evidence for applicability to practice. The proposed new-age curriculum includes research evidence, patient values and preferences, engagement of physicians, nurses and allied health disciplines in collaborative care, and continuous evaluation of patient outcomes (Barnsteiner, Disch, Hill, Mayer, & Moore, 2007).

Another exemplar, launched in 2003, is the Transforming Care at the Bedside (TCAB) initiative sponsored by the Robert Wood Johnson foundation in collaboration with the Institute for Healthcare Improvement (http://www.IHI.org). Designed to measure how nurses' contributions affect the safety and quality of patient care, TCAB explores hospital organizational efficiency, ways to reduce errors, and fiscal survival as applied to the standard hospital unit.

Indicators of Quality

Organizations are also involved in supporting outcomes research. The National Quality Forum (NQF), a not-for-profit, public-private organization established in 1999, is committed to a national strategy focused on improving patient outcomes and workforce productivity while containing health care costs (NQF, 2006) (http://www.qualityforum.org). The NQF has published over 200 consensus standards reached as the result of work among health care organizations, professionals, labor unions, health plans, and many other constituencies. The standards are measurable and publicly reported as indicators of quality.

The National Database of Nursing Quality Indicators (NDNQI) has submitted nursing-sensitive quality indicators to NQF. Consensus standards on four of those nursing-sensitive quality indicators are endorsed by NQF: patient falls; physical restraints; staff mix of RNs,

LPNs, and unlicensed assistive personnel (UAP); and, nursing care hours provided per patient day. The NQF is a work in progress and the NDNQI continues to analyze data provided by member hospitals and submit information to NQF for creation of consensus standards.

Outcomes research is also concerned with aggregates. "The momentum propelling outcomes research comes…from policymakers, insurers, and the public" (Burns & Grove, p. 273), who are interested in providing cost-effective care based on the risks and benefits to consumers and the health care industry at large.

Aggregate evidence drives the health care system, and outcomes research looks at findings of both quantitative and qualitative studies to identify problems and begin to seek solutions and improve care of populations. For example, the U.S. has the highest percentage of citizens who lack insurance coverage—roughly 16%, or 47 million uninsured—compared to citizens of the United Kingdom, Australia, Germany, and New Zealand, whose numbers of uninsured are negligible (Governance Institute, 2007; Lockee & Stepnick, 2007). Many uninsured persons use emergency rooms for point-of-care services, which are said to escalate health care costs. Why do people seek care for nonurgent conditions in emergency rooms (ERs) (Koziol-McLain, Price, Weiss, Quinn, & Honigman, 2000)? Health care access and the plight of the uninsured are ripe areas for outcomes research that may inform policy and increase cost-effective care.

GENERATING THE EVIDENCE

Health care providers pose many interesting, pressing questions and seek evidence-based answers. What should health care providers tell patients with Type 2 diabetes about the role of exercise (Cayley, 2007)? Does the use of chlorhexidine (CHG) presurgical prep reduce surgical site infection (SSI) in postsurgery patients (Elkins, et al.)? Why do patients use emergency rooms for point-of-care access (Koziol-McLain, et al., 2000)? Essential to beginning a search for evidence, is forming a clear and concise question.

PICO and PS Development

The **PICO** method begins with asking the pressing, or burning, question. Next the nurse or health care team identifies the population (P) affected; describes the proposed intervention (I); cites the comparison (C) group, status quo, or current standard for comparison; and states the outcome(s) (O) of the intervention (Melnyk & Fineout-Overholt, 2002, 2005; Stone, 2002). This format is used to formulate questions measured quantitatively. The method used to construct qualitative questions is somewhat different and suggests naming the population (P) affected and the situation (S), condition, or experiences the researcher wants to explore (DiCenso, Guyatt, & Ciliska, 2005; Polit & Beck, 2008). Figure 14-8 shows examples one and two in the PICO format, and question three using the PS format.

In all cases, PICO or PS gives direction to pursuing the evidence. Once the question is formulated, a search of the literature follows. Studies are examined according to the quality of the findings. At this point, it is important to form a team of experts to scour the literature for relevant information on a topic. Quantitative and qualitative experts will review studies for evidence in their

Figure 14-8
Clinical questions
using PICO and
PS formats.

1. Does the use of chlorhexidine (CHG) as a pre-operative prep reduce the risk of surgical site infection (SSI) as compared to the use of no special soap?
   P = surgical patients
   I = CHG prep used preoperatively
   C = regular or no soap used preoperatively
   O = reduction in risk of SSI

2. What is the impact of exercise on Type 2 diabetes?
   P = patients with Type 2 diabetes.
   I = exercise in patients with Type 2 diabetes
   C = no exercise in patients with Type 2 diabetes
   O = benefit of exercise decreasing morbidity and mortality in diabetics.

3. Why do patients use emergency rooms for treatment of non-urgent conditions?
   P = insured and uninsured persons who use emergency rooms for non-urgent conditions.
   S = What conditions, experiences or circumstances make people use ERs for non-urgent illness?

DELMAR/CENGAGE LEARNING

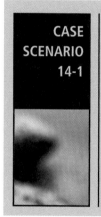

CASE SCENARIO 14-1

Despite medical advances, the common cold persists as one of the most frequent illnesses. Mrs. Harris visits the ambulatory care center with symptoms of the common cold. She has lost time from work and has a cough, nasal congestion, and an overall feeling of general malaise. You are interested in the use of various remedies to alleviate symptoms. Zinc has been used as a remedy for many years. Does taking oral zinc or nasal zinc effectively reduce the symptoms of the common cold in adults? Which delivery method works best?

CASE ANALYSIS

1. Write the question in PICO format.

2. Search CINAHL and locate a systematic review on zinc and the common cold.

3. Based on your findings, what recommendations would you make to Mrs. Harris?

respective areas. Single physiological studies, cohort studies, case studies, and other designs in the evidence hierarchy are reviewed, as well as bibliographies found at the end of current articles.

Finding the Evidence

A major challenge to access the best evidence is library support. Health sciences librarians are critical to identifying and retrieving electronic information for nurses (Fain, 2004; Klem & Weiss, 2005; Levin, 2007). Practicing nurses may have limited access to full-text articles and interlibrary loan. Accessing, retrieving, and appraising the evidence is a major challenge. Use of online evidence has been associated with the nursing role and both managerial and organizational support (Gosling, Westbrook, & Spencer, 2004). Partnering with health science centers and universities are suggestions to remedy the access problem, as well as provide the necessary electronic resources and library support to nurses at the point of care (Levin, 2007).

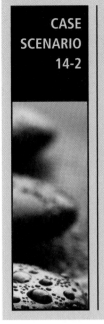

CASE SCENARIO 14-2

Mr. Rodriquez, a 54-year-old elementary school teacher, comes to the clinic complaining of fatigue, excessive thirst, and weight loss. The advanced practice nurse performs a history and physical, and orders blood work including a lipid profile and HgA1c. Because Mr. Rodriquez is diagnosed with diabetes, his immediate care management is a priority. Mr. Rodriquez will have to make a number of lifestyle changes. Several members of the health care team will manage the care of Mr. Rodriquez. He must be taught to monitor his glucose, watch his intake, and exercise, among other things.

CASE ANALYSIS

1. The nurse practitioner will coordinate an interdisciplinary team to manage his care. Name at least two members who will participate. Describe information that each will contribute to Mr. Rodriquez's care.

2. Search one database to find a clinical guideline on diabetes, exercise, and glycemic control.

3. Mr. Rodriquez has access to a personal computer. After discussing symptom management and follow-up care, you provide your e-mail address for further questions. Suggest a database that Mr. Rodriquez can access to find information about living with diabetes.

Resources to Find the Evidence

The American College of Physicians Journal Club (http://www.acponline.com) publishes interpretations and summaries of single articles based on criteria established by the reviewer. This resource is helpful when you need to access high-quality information quickly. Also helpful are two other resources: The National Guideline Clearinghouse (NGC), which provides access to a collection of clinical guidelines http://www.guideline.gov; and the Agency for Healthcare Research and Quality (AHRQ), which provides guidelines compiled by members of evidence-based practice centers (EPC). AHRQ guidelines are formed as a result of consensus by experts and are disseminated in the public domain; the NGC is a repository of guidelines from many organizations and, as such, may be subject to bias.

Evidence Databases

Sackett and colleagues (2000, pp. 30, 32) suggested "...burn [your] textbooks...and invest in databases...." Electronic databases provide access to a volume of evidence that has only recently been available to health care professionals. The accelerated pace of information technology is largely responsible for our ability to seek out and provide the best evidence. The following list is neither mutually exclusive nor exhaustive; however, it does offer a number of databases from which to choose to begin a search.

EBMR (Evidence-Based Medicine Reviews) by OVID technologies, (http://www.ovid.com), includes links to the Cochrane Database of Systemic Reviews, Evidence-Based Nursing (EBN), HealthSTAR, Joanna Briggs Institute, and MEDLINE (Fain, 2004; Melnyk & Fineholt, 2005; Sackett, 2000). Figure 14.9 presents an overview of selected resources.

Figure 14-9
Selected
Databases
for Evidence-
Based Topics.

1. Evidence Based Medicine Reviews (EBMR) Overall, this is the best database because it combines several electronic databases including most of the ones listed here.

2. Best Evidence (BE) indexes systematic reviews and individual studies based on explicit criteria for science and merit.

3. Evidence-Based Nursing (EBN) (http://www.ebn.bmjjournals.com/misc/about.shtml) summarizes the findings from traditional journals including only the best evidence of clinical relevance to nurses. It is a quarterly publication of the British Medical Journal and provides commentary on studies from several international journals.

4. Healthstar (HealthSTAR) focuses on different aspects of health care delivery. Material from books, book chapters, government documents and technical reports, as well as journals of clinical and non-clinical topics in health care may be found in this data base. The database may be accessed through the Library of Medicine. (http://www.nlm.nih.gov/).

5. MEDLINE/PubMed (http://www.ncbi.nlm.nih.gov/PubMed) is available on line and CD-ROM. Index Medicus and the International Nursing Index may be accessed through MEDLINE. It is by far the largest biomedical research database and includes biological and physical science literature as well as the humanities. Since it features over 12 million references, MEDLINE presents a maze of information and finding your exact topic may be difficult.

6. Cumulative Index of Nursing and Allied Health (CINAHL) (http://www.cinahl.com) has over 2 million references and includes nursing articles, books and journals and information on allied health and biomedicine.

7. Joanna Briggs Institute (JBI) is based in Adelaide, Australia with a connection to collaborators throughout the world. The group produces systematic reviews and information on topics of interest to nurses. (http://www.joannabriggs.edu.au/pubs/best_practice.php)

8. COCHRANE LIBRARY (http://www.cochrane.org) contains several databases, among them: the database of Systematic Reviews, data base of Abstracts and Reviews of Effectiveness, the Cochrane Central Register of Controlled Trials, the Cochrane Review of Methodology, the National Health Service Economic Evaluation database, and the Health Technology Assessment database. Its full-text, regularly updated systematic reviews are prepared by international members of the Cochrane Collaboration, and are widely accessed for the best evidence.

Posing the right question, using the PICO system, and scouring databases for studies that support or refute your actions, are ways to begin evidence-based inquiry. Critically appraising the literature means analyzing and synthesizing material included on the steps of the hierarchy ladder. The move from evidence to action occurs when best practices are formulated based on preferences and values of patients as well as on synthesized findings.

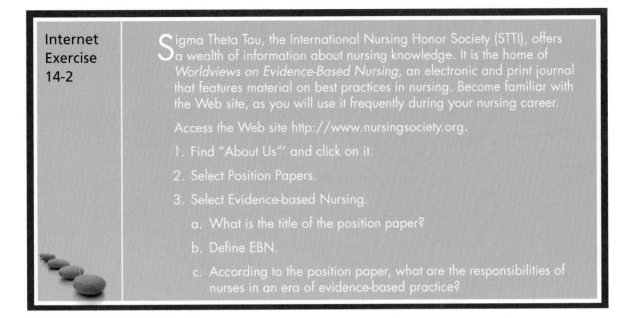

Internet Exercise 14-2

Sigma Theta Tau, the International Nursing Honor Society (STTI), offers a wealth of information about nursing knowledge. It is the home of *Worldviews on Evidence-Based Nursing,* an electronic and print journal that features material on best practices in nursing. Become familiar with the Web site, as you will use it frequently during your nursing career.

Access the Web site http://www.nursingsociety.org.

1. Find "About Us"' and click on it.

2. Select Position Papers.

3. Select Evidence-based Nursing.

   a. What is the title of the position paper?

   b. Define EBN.

   c. According to the position paper, what are the responsibilities of nurses in an era of evidence-based practice?

FROM EVIDENCE TO ACTION

Integrating research into everyday practice is critical to obtaining the best patient outcomes. Most important is knowing "…what to do…how to do it…[and] who in the multidisciplinary team is best suited to do it, and finally that the systems and processes exist to undertake it correctly" (Kitson, 2000, p. 459). Several studies provide nurses with information about their competencies, skill development, and overall knowledge of evidence-based practice. Other studies suggest that nurses' primary concern should be revision of systems and processes that elevate patient safety.

Deterrents to Evidence-Based Nursing Practice

Lack of time and access to electronic information at the point of care are two areas cited by nurses as deterrents to implementation of evidence-based practice (Fineout-Overholt & Johnston, 2006). Nurses must have time to access, read, and evaluate research, otherwise the best patient care will not occur. Professional literature is not readily available in the workplace, as electronic data support and librarians in hospitals are not readily available. In previous pilot studies using random samples of RNs and advanced practice nurses in Louisiana and New York, researchers found that only a small percentage were familiar with evidence-based practice, and only about 20% of all nurses surveyed accessed MEDLINE or CINAHL (Pravikoff, Pierce, & Tanner, 2003). Expanding this research to include a wider geographic representation of nurses across the U.S. was necessary to identify patterns. Researchers mailed 3,000 surveys to a random sample obtained from the national Sample Survey of Registered Nurses in the Pacific Northwest to: 1) identify RNs' perceptions of the importance of evidence-based practice to care delivery; 2) determine the ease with which RNs could access and find relevant information; and, 3) determine the institutional supports needed to make an evidence-based practice environment happen. Results indicated that approximately 58% of RNs did not use research reports to support their practice; 76% never searched CINAHL; and 58% never searched MEDLINE (Pravikoff, et al, 2005). Of particular note was the fact that respondents did not value research, and indicated that their work environments did not perceive research as practical in the real world. (Pravikoff, et al, 2005). The educational level of this group of 768 RN respondents was primarily diploma and associates degree, and the majority graduated prior to 1984.

A similar study, with a smaller sample, was conducted electronically by Sigma Theta Tau International (STTI). Surveys were e-mailed to 565 RNs to inquire about EBP. The sample was randomly selected from three marketing lists and was considered representative with 95% confidence. The findings showed improved knowledge concerning EBP, particularly among those who had graduated within the last five years (STTI, 2006). The level of familiarity with EBP had risen to 76%, but the appraisal and analysis of research evidence posed the greatest challenge for these RNs. Valuing research, reading, and understanding and synthesizing evidence continues to be a concern for nurses in clinical practice (Alspach, 2006; Jolley, 2002; Pravikoff, et al., 2003; Pravikoff, et al., 2005; STTI, 2006).

Insufficient numbers of staff, and education of nurses—particularly registered nurses—is frequently cited as impeding delivery of high-quality care (Aiken, Clarke, Cheung, Sloane, & Silber, 2003; IOM, 2001, 2003a, 2003b; IOM, 2004; Kitson, 2000; Needleman, Buerhaus, Mattke, Stewart, & Zelevinsky, 2002; Pravikoff, Tanner, & Pierce, 2005; Tourangeau, et al., 2006). Creating an evidence-based practice environment means using appropriate levels of nursing personnel. Rethinking how we use our nursing workforce and particularly examining the expanding role of nurses on the health care team are critical elements to delivery of quality, safe, evidence-based care (Algase, 2006; Henry, 2006; Kitson, 2000).

Education-Practice Gap

Registered nurses may be assigned to patients according to level of expertise, and various patient complexities. For example, as the predictability and instability of patient populations rises, so should the complement of registered nurses (Aiken, et al., 2003; Kitson, 2000; Tourangeau, et al., 2006). The most expert nurses should be found in primary-care settings engaged in health promotion; for those employed in hospitals, intensive-care areas should be staffed by expert nurses who are responsible for patients with unstable, highly volatile profiles. The notion of stability-volatility infers increased knowledge, which is supported by research on mortality and failure-to-rescue statistics in places where baccalaureate nurses are employed. Recent study findings indicated that improved patient outcomes occurred when higher proportions of baccalaureate nurses cared for medical and surgical patients with serious complications (Aiken, et al., 2003; Tourangeau, et al., 2006). Higher use of protocols to guide patient care indicated an increase in survival rates of hospitalized patients, a new finding that supports the importance of using evidence-based practice guidelines. (Tourangeau, et al., 2006, p. 41). Findings also indicated that knowledge was more important than experience in caring for complex patients (Aiken, et al., 2003; Daniels, 2007; Tourangeau, et al, 2006).

FUTURE INITIATIVES

Sigma Theta Tau International (STTI, 2005), and other organizations, support the use of evidence and integrate EBP policy into their associations. Most associations provide educational materials, access to informational Internet sites, support and promote conferences on EBP, and sponsor special-interest groups (Holleman, Eliens, van Vliet, and van Achterberg, 2006).

Several strategies, including journal clubs, devising PICO questions, conducting EBP rounds at clinical sites, and developing research competencies, are good ways to foster implementation of evidence-based practice.

SUMMARY

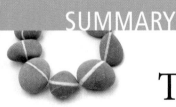

The nursing community is faced with increasing responsibility for providing safe, cost-effective, quality care and must consider the evidence from the top down—systematic reviews to expert opinion—in creating the protocols and guidelines essential in making positive changes in practice. Critical thinking, ways of knowing, and ethical reasoning undergird sound clinical practice and are fundamental to system models that facilitate EBP. Patient values, appreciation of cultural differences, and listening to the lived experiences of patients provide rich information on which to craft clinical protocols. Identifying the pressing clinical questions and how to formulate them and use the library and online databases to ferret out information is essential for today's practicing professional nurse.

The challenge for today and the future is to teach nurses to collect and use evidence to create practice guidelines and improve patient outcomes. In addition, how nurses evaluate their performance as well as outcomes of care are important action-oriented competencies that guarantee checks and balances in the health care system. The skills and competencies of nurses grounded in principles of evidence-based practice will meet the needs of the human condition. It is, after all, the combination of human science and empiricism that directs how nurses respond to people's needs.

Knowing is not enough; we must apply. Willing is not enough; we must do.

–Johann Wolfgang von Goethe

REFERENCES

AGENCY FOR HEALTHCARE RESEARCH AND QUALITY (AHRQ). (2002). *Systems to rate the strength of scientific evidence.* File Inventory, Evidence Report/TechnologyAssessment No. 47. AHRQ Publication No. 02-E016. Rockville, MD: AHRQ. Retrieved from http://ahrq.gov/clinic/strevinv.htm

AIKEN, L., Clarke, S. P., Cheung, R. B., Sloane, D. M., & Silber, J. H. (2003). Educational levels of hospital nurses and surgical patient mortality. *Journal American Medical Association [JAMA], 290,* 1617–1623.

AIKEN, L., Clarke, S. P., Sloane, D. M., Sochalski, J., & Silber, J. H. (2002). Hospital nurse staffing and patient mortality, nurse burnout, and job dissatisfaction. *Journal American Medical Association, 288,* 1987–1993.

ALGASE, D. L. (2006). What's so critical about evidence-based nursing practice? *Research and Theory for Nursing Practice: An International Journal, 20,* 99–100.

ALSPACH, G. (2006). Nurses' use and understanding of evidence-based practice: Some preliminary evidence. *Critical Care Nurse, 26,* 11–12.

AMERICAN ASSOCIATION OF COLLEGES OF NURSING. [AACN]. (2006). *Position statement on nursing research.* Washington, DC: Author.

AMERICAN ASSOCIATION OF COLLEGES OF NURSING [AACN]. (1999). *Position statement on defining scholarship for the discipline of nursing.* Washington, DC: Author.

AMERICAN NURSES ASSOCIATION. (2001). *Code of ethics with interpretive statements.* Kansas City, MO: Author.

BARGAGLIOTTI, L. A., & Lancaster, J. (2007). Quality and safety education in nursing: More than new wine in old skins. *Nursing Outlook, 55,* 156–158.

BARNSTEINER, J. H., Disch, J. M., Hall, L., Mayer, D., & Moore, S. M. (2007). Promoting inter-professional education. *Nursing Outlook, 55,* 144–150.

BEYEA, S. C., & Nicoll, L. H. (1998). Writing an integrative review. *Association of Operating Room Nurses [AORN] Journal, 67,* 877–880.

BLOCK, L. M., & Le Grazie, B. A. (2006). Don't get lost in translation. *Nursing Management, 37,* 37–40.

BURNS, N., & Grove, S. K. (2005). *The practice of nursing research: Conduct, critique, and utilization* (5th ed.). New York: Elsevier.

CARPER, B. A. (1978). Fundamental patterns of knowing in nursing. *Advances in Nursing Science, 1,* 13–24.

CAYLEY, W. E. (2007). Cochrane for Clinicians. The role of exercise in patients with type 2 diabetes. *American Family Physician, 75*(3). Retrieved October 19, 2007, from http://www.aafp.org/afp/20070201/cochrane.html

CLARKE, S. P., & Aiken, L. H. (2003). Failure to rescue. *American Journal of Nursing, 103,* 42–47.

CREEGAN, M. C. (2007). From practice to professionalism: The struggle within. In K. Polifko (Ed.), *Concepts of the nursing profession.* Clifton Park, NY: Delmar, Cengage Learning

CRONENWETT, L., Sherwood, G., Barnsteiner, J., Disch, J., Johnson, J., Mitchell, P., et al. (2007). Quality and safety education for nurses. *Nursing Outlook, 55,* 122–131.

DANIELS, S. M. (2007August). Protecting patients from harm: Improving hospital care for surgical patients. *Nursing 2007,* 36–41.

DAY, L., & Smith, E. L. (2007). Integrating quality and safety content into clinical teaching in the acute care setting. *Nursing Outlook, 55,* 138–143.

DEPARTMENT OF HEATH AND HUMAN SERVICES [DHHS]. *New Freedom Commission on Mental Health. Achieving the promise: Transforming mental health care in America. Final Report.*

Publication No. SMA-03-3832. Rockville, MD: Author.

Di Censo, A., Guyatt, G., & Ciliska, D. (2005). *Evidence-based nursing: A guide to clinical practice.* St. Louis, MO: Elsevier.

Elder, E., & Paul, R. P. (2006). *The thinker's guide to analytical thinking.* Dillon Beach, CA: The Foundation for Critical Thinking.

Elkins, M., Diswood, L., Phoenix, L., Hodgins, D., Accountius, D., & Verbus, R. (2007). Shiprock Service Unit's methods for adoption of an evidence-based nursing model. *The Indian Health Service (HIS) Primary Care Provider, 32*(8), 227–231.

Fain, J. A. (2004). *Reading, understanding, and applying nursing research.* Philadelphia: F. A. Davis.

Fineout-Overholt, E., & Johnston, L. (2006). Teaching EBP: Implementation of evidence: Moving from evidence to action. *Worldviews on Evidence-Based Nursing, 3,* 194–200.

Finfgeld, D. (2003). Metasynthesis: The state of the art—so far. *Qualitative Health Research, 13,* 893–904.

Finkelman, A., & Kenner, C. (2007). *Teaching IOM: Implications of the Institute of Medicine reports for nursing education.* Silver Spring, MD: ANA.

Freshwater, D. (2004). Aesthetics and evidence-based practice in nursing: An oxymoron? *International Journal of Human Caring, 8,* 8–12.

Gosling, A. S., Westbrook, J. I., & Spencer, R. (2004). Nurses' use of online clinical evidence. *Journal of Advanced Nursing, 47,* 201–211.

Guyatt, G., & Rennie, D. (2002). *Users' guides to the medical literature.* American Medical Association: AMA.

Hamilton, C., Jacob, J. M., Koch, S., & Quammen, R. L. (2003). Automate best practices with electronic healthcare records. *Nursing Management, 35,* 40.

Hasnain-Wynia, R. (2006). Is evidence-based medicine patient-centered and is patient-centered care evidence-based? *Health Services Research, 41,* 1–8.

Henry, B. (2006). Quality of care, health systems errors, and nurses. *Journal of Advanced Nursing, 56,* 219.

Holliman, G., Eliens, A., van Vliet, M., & van Achterberg, T. (2005). Promotion of evidence-based practice by professional nursing associations: Literature review. *Journal of Advanced Nursing, 53,* 702–709.

Institute of Medicine. (1999). *To err is human: Building a safer health system.* Washington, DC: Author and National Academies Press.

Institute of Medicine. (2001). *Crossing the quality chasm: A new health system for the 21ˢᵗ century.* Washington, DC: National Academies Press.

Institute of Medicine. (2003a). *Keeping patients safe: Transforming the work environment of nurses.* Washington, DC: National Academies Press.

Institute of Medicine. (2003b). *Health professions education: A bridge to quality.* Washington, DC: National Academies Press.

Institute of Medicine. (2004). *Keeping patients safe: Transforming the work environment for nurses.* Washington, DC: National Academies Press.

Institute of Medicine. (2007). Advancing quality improvement research: Challenges and opportunities—Workshop summary, Board on Health Care Services. Washington, DC: National Academies Press.

Johnston, L., & Fineholt-Overholt, E. (2005). Teaching EBP: Getting from Zero to one. Moving from recognizing and admitting uncertainties to asking searchable, answerable questions. *Worldviews on Evidence-Based Nursing, 2,* 98–102.

Johnston, L., & Fineout-Overholt, E. (2006). Teaching EBP: The critical step of critically appraising the literature. *Worldviews on Evidence-Based Nursing, 3,* 44–46.

JOLLEY, S. (2002). Raising research awareness: A strategy for nurses. *Nursing Standard, 16,* 33–39.

KITSON, A. (2000). Toward evidence-based quality improvement: Perspectives from nursing practice. *International Journal for Quality in Health Care, 12,* 459–464.

KLEM, M. L., & Weiss, P. M. (2005). Evidence-based resources and the role of librarians in developing evidence-based practice curricula. *Journal of Professional Nursing, 21,* 380–387.

KOZIOL-MCLAIN, J., Price, D. W., Weiss, B., Quinn, A., & Honigman, B. (2000). Seeking care for non-urgent medical conditions in the emergency department: Through the eyes of the patient. *Journal of Emergency Nursing, 26,* 554–563.

LEVIN, R. (2007). Developing the infrastructure to support EBP: It takes a library. *Research and Theory for Nursing Practice: An International Journal, 21,* 77–79.

LEVIN, R. F., & Vetter, M. J. (2007). Evidence-based practice: A guide to negotiate the clinical practice guideline maze. *Research and Theory for Nursing Practice: An International Journal, 21,* 5–9.

LEVIN, R. F., & Feldman, H. R. (2006a). Teaching evidence-based practice: Starting with the learner. *Research and Theory for Nursing Practice: An International Journal, 20,* 269–272.

LEVIN, R. F., & Feldman, H. R. (2006b). The EBP controversy: Misconception, misunderstanding, or myth. *Research and Theory for Nursing Practice: An International Journal, 20,* 183–186.

LOCKEE, C., & Stepnick, L. (2007 August). Healthcare: It's a global issue. *BoardRoom Press, 18* (4), 5–9.

LONG, K. A. (2003). The Institute of Medicine Report. Health Professions education: A bridge

to quality. *Policy, Politics, & Nursing Practice, 4,* 259–262.

MAGYARY, D., Whitney, J. D., & Brown. M. A. (2006). Advancing practice inquiry: Research foundations of the practice doctorate in nursing. *Nursing Outlook, 54,* 139–151.

MATTER, S. (2006). Empower nurses with evidence-based knowledge. *Nursing Management, 37,* 34–37.

MCCAUGHAN, D., Thompson, C., Cullum, N., Sheldon, T., Trevor, A., & Thompson, D. (2002). Acute care nurses perceptions to barriers to using research information in clinical decision making. *Journal of Advanced Nursing, 39,* 46–60.

MELYNK, B. M., & Fineout-Overholt, E. (2002). Key steps in evidence-based practice: Asking compelling clinical questions and searching for the best evidence. *Pediatric Nursing, 28,* 262–263, 266.

MELNYK, B. M., & Fineout-Overholt, E. (2005). *Evidence-based practice in nursing and healthcare.* Philadelphia: Lippincott, Williams & Wilkins.

MELNYK, B. M., Fineout-Overholt, E., Feinstein, N., Li, H. S., Small, L., Wilcox, L., et al. (2004). Nurses perceived knowledge, beliefs, skills, and needs regarding evidence-based practice: Implications for accelerating the paradigm shift. *Worldviews on Evidence-Based Nursing, 1,* 185–193.

MITCHELL, G. J. (1999). Evidence-based practice: Critique and alternative view. *Nursing Science Quarterly, 12,* 30–35.

MOLLOCH, D., & Porter-O'Grady, T. (2008). *Evidence-based nursing practice.* New York: Jones & Bartlett.

NEEDLEMAN, J., Buerhaus, P., Mattke, S., Stewart, M., & Zelevinsky, K. (2002). Nurse staffing levels and the quality of care in hospitals. *New England Journal of Medicine, 346,* 1715.

PATTEN, M. (2005). *Understanding research methods* (5th ed.). Glendale, CA: Pyrczak.

PAUL, R. P., & Elder, E. (2007). *The miniature guide to critical thinking: Concepts and tools.* Dillon Beach, CA: The Foundation for Critical Thinking.

PAUL, R. P., & Elder, E. (2003). *The miniature guide to understanding the foundations of ethical reasoning.* Dillon Beach, CA: The Foundation for Critical Thinking.

POLIT, D. F., & Beck, C. T. (2008). *Nursing research: Generating and assessing evidence for nursing practice* (8th ed.). New York: Lippincott, Williams & Wilkins.

POTTER, M. B. (2007). Cochrane for Clinicians. Counseling women about mammography: Benefits vs. harms. *American Family Physician, 76*(5). Retrieved October 18, 2007, from http://www.aafp.org/afp/20070901/cochrane.html

PRAVIKOFF, D. S., Pierce, S., & Tanner, A. (2003). Are nurses ready for evidence-based practice? *American Journal of Nursing 103,* 95–96.

PRAVIKOFF, D. S., Tanner, A. B., & Pierce, S. T. (2005). Readiness of U.S. nurses for evidence-based practice. *American Journal of Nursing, 105,* 40–51.

RAFFERTY, A. M., Maben, J., West, E., & Robinson, D. (2005). *What makes a good employer?* Geneva, Switzerland: International Council of Nurses (ICN). Retrieved November 11, 2007, from http://www.icn.ch/global/#3

REDMAN, R. W. (2005). Improving practice environments based on best management practices. *Research and Theory for Nursing Practice: An International Journal, 19,* 213–215.

ROGERS, E. M. (1995). *Diffusion of innovations* (4th ed.). New York: Free Press.

SACKETT, D. L., Rosenberg, W., Muir Gray, J. A., Haynes, R., & Richardson, W. (1996). Evidence-based medicine: What it is and what it isn't. *British Medical Journal, 312,* 71–72.

SACKETT, D. L., Strauss, S. E., Richardson, W. S., Rosenberg, W., & Haynes, R. B. (2000). *Evidence-based medicine: How to teach and practice EBM* (2nd ed.). Edinburgh, Scotland: Churchill Livingston.

SANDELOWSKI, M., Docherty, S., & Emden, C. (1997). Qualitative metasynthesis: Issues and techniques. *Research in Nursing and Health, 20,* 365–371.

SCHOOFS, N. (2001). Seeing the glass half full: Living with Sjogren's Syndrome. *Journal of Professional Nursing, 17,* 194–202.

SCHREIBER, R., Crooks, D., & Stern, P. N. (1997). Qualitative meta-analysis. In J. M. Morse (Ed.), *Completing a qualitative project* (pp. 311–326). Thousand Oaks: CA: Sage.

SHERWOOD, G., & Drenkard, K. (2007). Quality and safety curricula in nursing education. *Nursing Outlook, 55,* 151–155.

SIDANI, S., & Braden, C. J. (1998). *Evaluating nursing interventions: A theory-driven approach.* London: Sage.

SIGMA THETA TAU INTERNATIONAL. (2006). *EBP study: Summary of findings.* Available at http://www.nursing knowledge.org/go/study

SIGMA THETA TAU INTERNATIONAL. (2005). *Position paper on evidence-based nursing.* Available at http://www.nursingsociety.org/research/main.html1#ebp

SMEDLEY, B., Stith, A., & Nelson, A. (2003). *Unequal treatment: Confronting racial and ethnic disparities in healthcare.* Washington, DC: Institute of Medicine.

STETLER, C. (2001). Updating the Stetler Model of research utilization to facilitate evidence-based practice. *Nursing Outlook, 49,* 272–279.

STEVENS, K. R. (2001). Systematic reviews: The heart of evidence-based practice. *AACN Clinical Issues: Advanced Practice in Acute and Critical Care, 12,* 529–538.

STONE, P. (2002). Popping the PICO question in research and evidence-based practice. *Applied Nursing Research, 16,* 197–198.

THORNE, S., Jensen, L., Kearney, M., Noblit, G., & Sandelowski, M. (2004). Qualitative metasynthesis: Reflections on methodological orientation and ideological agenda. *Qualitative Health Research, 14,* 1342–1365.

TITLER, M. (2007). Translating research into practice. *American Journal of Nursing, 107* supplement, 26–33.

TITLER, M. G., Kleiber, C., Steelman, V. J., Rakel, B. A., Boudreau, G., Everett, L. Q., et al. (2001). The Iowa model of evidence-based practice to promote quality care. *Critical Care Nursing Clinics of North America, 13,* 497–509.

TOURANGEAU, A. E., Doran, D. M., Hall, M. L., Pallas, L. O., Pringle, D., Tu, J. V., et al. (2006). Impact of hospital nursing care on 30-day mortality for acute medical patients. *Journal of Advanced Nursing, 57,* 32–44.

WINCH, S., Henderson, A., & Creedy, D. (2005). Read, think, do!: A method for fitting research evidence into practice. *Journal of Advanced Nursing, 50,* 20–26.

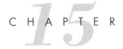

C H A P T E R

15

TRENDS IN WORKPLACE SAFETY

NANCY NIVISION MENZEL

PhD, RN, PHCNS-BC, COHN-S, CNE, Associate Professor, University of Nevada, Las Vegas, School of Nursing

We ought to show peculiar zeal in taking precautions for workers' safety, so that they may work at their chosen calling without loss of health.

–Bernardino Ramazzini

LEARNING OBJECTIVES

At the completion of the chapter, the learner should be able to do the following:

1. Describe the nurse/patient dyad in health and safety.
2. Recognize at least four workplace hazards found in health care settings.
3. Compare and contrast control strategies for hazards found in health care settings.
4. Identify laws that regulate workplace health and safety.
5. Evaluate prospective workplaces for health and safety risks and protection.

KEY TERMS

Accident (Workplace)
Acute Health Effect
Chronic Health Effect
Dose
Employee Health Nurse
Epidemiology
Ergonomics
Exposure
Health Hazard
Hierarchy of Controls
Industrial Hygienist
Material Safety Data Sheet

National Institute for
   Occupational Safety and
   Health (NIOSH)
Noise
Occupational and
   Environmental
   Health Nurse
Occupational Safety and
   Health Administration
   (OSHA)
Occupational Safety
   and Health Act

Personal Protective
   Equipment (PPE)
Respirator
Risk
Route of Exposure
Safety Professional
Toxicity
Workers' Compensation
   Insurance
Workplace Violence

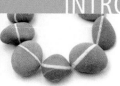

INTRODUCTION

As early as the 1700s, back pain and infections were noted as common among wet nurses and midwives, considered the precursors of modern nurses (Ramazzini, 1713). Despite this early recognition that nursing could be hazardous to the health of its practitioners, nurses were socialized to put the safety of the patient ahead of their own, most likely beginning with the example set by Florence Nightingale as she labored under hazardous conditions in Turkey, near the Crimean War front. She may have contracted brucellosis there, which is thought to have resulted in her lifelong disability upon returning from the war zone (Young, 1995). Nursing's origins in religious orders may also be responsible for some of the selfless culture, as nuns gave up worldly comforts to provide care to the sick. However, times have changed. With the nursing shortage, there has been increasing recognition that preservation of the health of the nursing workforce is vital to maintaining an adequate supply of these highly knowledgeable caregivers. As today's new nurses face the prospect of having to work more years before retirement than the generations that preceded them, they too must take steps to preserve their health and work capacity.

Hospital employee health departments once focused almost exclusively on activities designed to protect patients from infections transmitted by care providers. They screened for tuberculosis and ensured that measles, mumps, and rubella vaccinations were current. In a paradigm shift precipitated by a push from national blood-borne pathogens legislation in 1991, hospitals began to offer hepatitis B vaccine to protect their employees from infections transmitted by patients. Today, in response to requirements of external regulatory agencies and good business practices, most hospitals have begun advanced health and safety programs to ensure their direct patient caregivers are protected from known hazards.

From the aspect of safety, the nurse and patient/client are a dyad; the health of one affects the other. For example, the more dependent a patient, the more physical effort the nurse must expend to assist with mobility and positioning. At the same time, if the nurse is fatigued and in pain from a musculoskeletal disorder, he or she is less likely to provide assistance that requires use of overworked muscles. So, it is time to give up the expectation that nurses must sacrifice their health by putting themselves in harm's way; the best way to assist patients is for nurses to work in a healthy work environment (Figure 15-1).

HEALTH CARE WORKFORCE TRENDS AND SAFETY

Nursing involves heavy physical labor, yet unlike other physically demanding jobs such as firefighting, manual labor, and transportation, the workforce is predominantly composed of women (Figure 15-2). In a national sample of nurses in 2004, men were found to comprise only 5.7% of the workforce, an insignificant increase over the 2000 percentage of 5.4% (Health Resources and Services Administration, 2005). Based on the long history of nursing as a female occupation, it is unlikely that men will enter the profession in larger numbers in the immediate future. In addition, the nursing workforce is aging, with an average age of 46.8

Figure 15-1

Nurses shouldn't sacrifice their own health in the line of duty, but should focus on creating and participating in a healthy work environment.

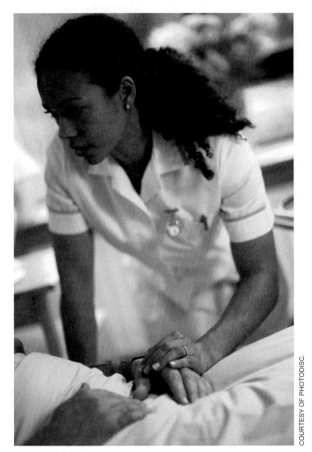

COURTESY OF PHOTODISC.

years in 2004, compared to 42.3 years in 1996 (Health Resources and Services Administration, 2005). The trajectory of increasing age is projected to continue. Most women are not as physically strong as men (particularly in the upper body), and all persons lose strength as they age. Both of these factors affect the ability of older females to perform the essential physical functions of nursing.

Against this background of an aging, predominantly female nurse workforce are superimposed trends for increasing patient acuity, increasing patient obesity, and decreasing per capita ratios of RNs. Americans are living longer than ever, while at the same time requiring more medical care as they age. With hospital stays shortened as a result of insurer cost-control measures, average patient acuity has risen, which increases the workload of nurses. One risk to caregiver health and safety is the increased weight of patients, who are, on average, heavier than ever, with an increase in obesity prevalence from 15.0% to 32.9% in the past twenty-five years (Centers for Disease Control and Prevention, 2007). At the same time, the supply of nurses has been unable to keep up with increasing demand, forcing nurses to work longer hours in inadequately staffed workplaces (American Nurses Association, 2008). This increases their exposure to job hazards, such as handling and moving heavier patients.

Figure 15-2
Nursing is a physically demanding job with a workforce composed predominantly of women. As the workforce ages, the physical demands of the profession may become a challenge.

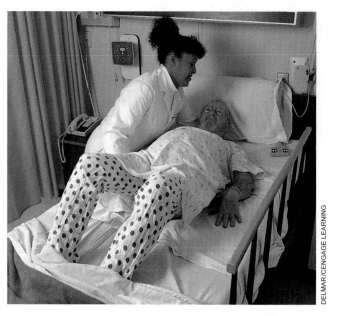

DELMAR/CENGAGE LEARNING

NURSE INJURY STATISTICS

The U.S. Department of Labor, Bureau of Labor Statistics (BLS) extrapolates statistics for worker injuries from injury logs kept at sample private employer workplaces. (The data exclude local, state, and federal government employees.) The 2006 statistics for nature of injury or illness involving days away from work for registered nurses (RNs) show strains/sprains to be the most frequent category (Table 15-1). In fact, RNs ranked fifth worst on a list of occupations with the most musculoskeletal disorders (MSDs) (U.S. Department of Labor, 2007a).

The BLS injury statistics may appear lower than expected. One reason is that BLS does not include occupation-specific data for injuries or illnesses that do not involve medical treatment or time away from work, leaving only speculation as to the total number. In addition, nurses have been found to under-report workplace injuries for a number of reasons (Brown, et al., 2005).

Table 15-1 RN Nature of Injury/Illness Involving Days Away From Work, 2006

Nature	Sprains, strains	Bruises	Fractures	Cuts, punctures	Heat burns	Chemical burns
Number	11,460	1,980	1,100	400	50	30

Source: BLS (U.S. Department of Labor, 2007b)

By comparing BLS statistics against insurance claims for work-related injuries and illnesses, several studies have found extensive under-reporting in all occupations (U.S. House of Representatives, 2008). The size of this discrepancy becomes apparent when considering that the **National Institute for Occupational Safety and Health (NIOSH),** the federal agency that conducts research on occupational hazards and their prevention, estimates that between 600,000 and 800,000 needle sticks occur annually in hospitals (NIOSH, 2000), yet BLS reported only 400 cuts/punctures involving days away from work in 2006.

HAZARDS OF HEALTH CARE ENVIRONMENTS

Any setting where nurses deliver care presents hazards to both the nurse and the client, whether it is a simple environment, such as a home, or a complex environment, such as an operating room or intensive care unit. A **health hazard** is "an agent or chemical substance for which there is scientific evidence to show that exposure may cause adverse health outcomes in susceptible employees who may be exposed" (Hatch, 2008, p. 168). Hazards that threaten the health of nurses fall into five main categories (Table 15-2).

Table 15-2 Categories of Hazards

Hazard	Definition	Health Care Example
BIOLOGICAL	Living organisms, such as bacteria, viruses, molds, or parasites	Blood-borne pathogens, vaccine-preventable communicable diseases
CHEMICAL	Any element, chemical compound, or mixture of elements or compounds; can be in a dust/particulate, fume, mist, liquid, vapor, or gas form	Latex, chemotherapeutic agents, disinfectants
MECHANICAL/ BIOMECHANICAL	Interface between worker and work space, work requirements, or equipment and the body mechanics required	Manual handling, poorly designed or laid out work spaces (ICUs, homes)
PHYSICAL	A force or agent that may damage the body	Ionizing radiation, noise
PSYCHOSOCIAL	A work factor or environment that causes disruption to a person's psychological or social well-being	Workplace violence, shift work, stress

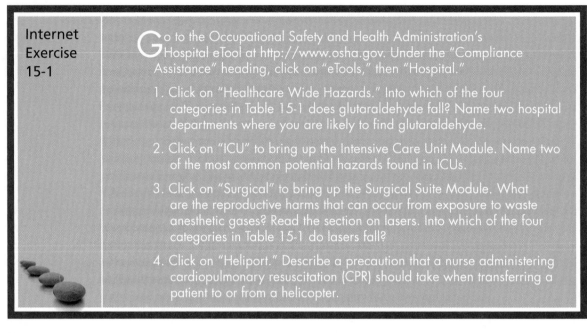

Internet Exercise 15-1

Go to the Occupational Safety and Health Administration's Hospital eTool at http://www.osha.gov. Under the "Compliance Assistance" heading, click on "eTools," then "Hospital."

1. Click on "Healthcare Wide Hazards." Into which of the four categories in Table 15-1 does glutaraldehyde fall? Name two hospital departments where you are likely to find glutaraldehyde.

2. Click on "ICU" to bring up the Intensive Care Unit Module. Name two of the most common potential hazards found in ICUs.

3. Click on "Surgical" to bring up the Surgical Suite Module. What are the reproductive harms that can occur from exposure to waste anesthetic gases? Read the section on lasers. Into which of the four categories in Table 15-1 do lasers fall?

4. Click on "Heliport." Describe a precaution that a nurse administering cardiopulmonary resuscitation (CPR) should take when transferring a patient to or from a helicopter.

Exposure Concepts

By now you are starting to see that there are many hazards facing nurses in the work environment. But how likely is it that one or more of these hazards will actually cause harm? In other words, what is the **risk** (the likelihood that harm will occur)? For that, consider the concepts of toxicity, exposure, and dose. These terms are used most often in the context of chemical hazards but can be applied to other types of hazards as well.

Toxicity is the degree of potential harm of the hazard. Although all chemicals are harmful to humans at some level (even H_2O), some chemicals are more toxic than others. The most toxic chemicals are labeled poisons. The potential of other agents to cause harm varies. For example, **noise** is hazardous to hearing only when it exceeds a certain intensity; the louder it is, the more hazardous. The risk from lifting a patient varies with patient weight and other factors.

Exposure is the opportunity to receive a dose; a **dose** is the actual amount of the chemical (or other hazard) received. Just because a nurse is exposed to a hazard does not mean that he or she received a dose. For example, nurses working in a helicopter are exposed to hazardous noise levels, but if they are wearing adequate noise attenuation devices (e.g., muffs), they are protected from receiving a harmful "dose" of noise to their hearing organs.

Epidemiology is the study of the distribution and determinants of a disease or condition in a population. So far, we have discussed only agent (hazard) and environmental (exposure) factors. In the epidemiological triangle (Figure 15-3), a third factor comes into play: the host. That means you! Some individual factors that affect risk are age, gender, physical condition and size, allergic tendencies, smoking, alcohol use, medication use, and current diseases. For example,

Figure 15-3
Epidemiologic
Triangle.

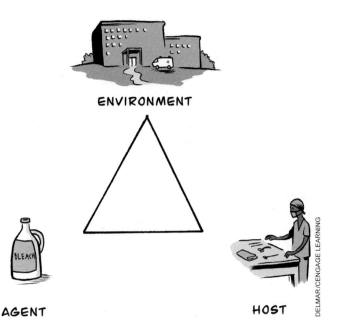

ENVIRONMENT

AGENT

HOST

DELMAR/CENGAGE LEARNING

a nurse with cirrhosis secondary to chronic hepatitis B will show toxic effects from exposure to chemicals detoxified through the liver (such as solvents) at lower doses than someone with normal hepatic function.

For chemical and biologic hazards, it is important to understand the **route of exposure** (i.e., how they enter the body). The main routes are inhalation, skin absorption, and ingestion. Exposure through the skin (including the conjunctiva of the eye and other mucous membranes) can occur from direct surface contact or through injection/puncture.

Another concept needed to understand health hazards is the type of adverse effect produced: acute or chronic. An **acute health effect** is an immediate untoward response to a single high dose of a chemical or other toxin; it is easily linked to the suspect agent. For example, a nurse who is wiping down a counter with a bleach solution inadvertently splashes some in her eye and reports pain and burning at the site. A **chronic health effect** is a delayed reaction that may occur after prolonged, low-level exposures and is harder to link to the suspect agent because of the passage of time and the possibility that other factors produced the adverse effect. For example, most hospital nurses work in shifts over many years. Although repeated disruptions in sleep patterns have been associated with a higher incidence of peptic ulcers, coronary heart disease, and poor pregnancy outcomes (Knutsson, 2003), it is more difficult to link these adverse outcomes to shift work, given their multifactorial etiology.

Allergic reactions have features of both acute and chronic effects. For example, some nurses may develop an irritant contact dermatitis from using latex gloves (acute effect). Others may use latex gloves and handle latex medical devices for many years with no adverse health effects. However, they may become sensitized over time to the allergy-causing proteins (antigens) in natural rubber latex and a subsequent latex exposure triggers an allergic response, including hives, asthma, other respiratory problems, or shock. This allergy persists (chronic effect).

CASE SCENARIO 15-1

Roberta (35 years old) and Sarah (26 years old) are RNs who graduated from the same university a few years ago and are now working in an out-patient oncology clinic where they administer antineoplastic drugs (ANDs) by infusion. They frequently administer cyclophosphamide (Cytoxan), which is a known carcinogen, cytotoxic agent, and reproductive health hazard, with exposure most common by skin contact or from inhalation. Roberta often takes shortcuts with safety precautions when preparing, administering, and disposing of ANDs, while Sarah is more deliberate, always preparing solutions in a laminar air-flow hood, wearing gloves, laboratory coat, eye protection, and mask when handling ANDs or patients' urine, and thoroughly washing her hands after each drug or patient contact. Sarah comes to work one day and tells Roberta the good news, that she and her husband are expecting a baby. Although Roberta is happy for her friend, she wonders aloud why she and her husband have been unable to conceive after a year of trying.

CASE ANALYSIS

1. Have both RNs been exposed to ANDs (i.e., had the opportunity to receive a dose)? How likely is it is that Roberta received a dose of ANDs? How likely is it that Sarah did? Explain your reasoning.

2. What are some possible host factors in this situation that could intensify the harm of any dose received?

3. Because difficulty conceiving is a known adverse health effect associated with Cytoxan, would you characterize Roberta's infertility as a possible acute or chronic effect? Why? What might be some other possible causes of her infertility?

4. If you were Sarah, how might you respond to Roberta's concern about her inability to conceive?

Hazard Controls

The good news about workplace exposures is that employers and workers can recognize, control, and avoid them. Industrial hygienists, safety professionals, and occupational and environmental health nurses have had specialized education and experience in evaluating and controlling workplace hazards. Among other skills, **industrial hygienists** have expertise in monitoring work environments for levels of hazardous chemicals and recommending ways to make sure the levels are reduced to safe limits. **Safety professionals** have expertise in accident prevention. A **workplace accident** is an unwanted event that results in injury or death. Despite the common misconception that accidents are unforeseen or unpredictable, the contrary is true. In theory, all accidents are preventable; in practice, however, the goal is preventing as many accidents as practicable. **Occupational and environmental health nurses** are focused on preserving the health of worker populations through primary and secondary prevention interventions. The goal of primary prevention is blocking the injury or illness from ever occurring; for example, vaccinations. Secondary prevention involves screening and early treatment for detected conditions; for example, skin testing for tuberculosis. In hospital settings, occupational health nurses are often called **employee health nurses.** Practitioners in each of these disciplines may be certified, indicated by the initials CIH (Certified Industrial Hygienist), CSP (Certified Safety Professional), or COHN/COHN-S (Certified Occupational Health Nurse/Specialist).

The **Occupational Safety and Health Administration (OSHA)** is the federal agency that is charged with protecting most employees from workplace hazards through regulation and inspection. Although OSHA has regulations covering many occupational health hazards, it does not specifically regulate others hazards, such as manual handling. However, Section 5a of the **Occupational Safety and Health Act of 1970** (OSH Act) states that employers have a general duty to provide a workplace "free from recognized hazards that are causing or are likely to cause death or serious physical harm to his employees" ("Occupational Safety and Health Act," 1990) by controlling all recognizable hazards, whether or not OSHA has a specific regulation covering them. Once hazards have been identified by a thorough workplace assessment, the employer (through the committee, department, or individuals it has designated responsible for workplace health and safety) follows a **hierarchy of controls** to reduce the risk of exposure and harm. The hierarchy of controls ranks strategies by their degree of effectiveness, with preference given to those near the top of the list (Table 15-3).

Table 15-3 Hierarchy of Controls

Control	Definition	Health Care Example
Hazard elimination/substitution	The hazard is completely eliminated or less hazardous chemicals, equipment, or process is substituted	Replacing mercury sphygmomanometers with aneroid ones Substituting a less toxic disinfectant for a more toxic one
Engineering	Blocking hazards from reaching the worker; don't depend on worker effort	Safer needle devices, such as ones with self-retracting needles Negative pressure isolation rooms for tuberculosis patients to prevent contaminated air from escaping
Work practices	Worker behaviors that reduce risk of exposure	Hand washing after patient contact Prohibiting eating or smoking where chemicals or biohazards are present
Administrative	Management control of work performance to reduce the risk of exposure	Reducing shift lengths from 12 to 8 hours Prohibiting mandatory overtime
Personal protective equipment (PPE)	Equipment designed to be a barrier between the worker and the hazard; least effective method because it relies on worker effort to use it	Providing face shields, goggles, masks, gloves, and gowns

Personal protective equipment (PPE) is a last resort because it relies on the worker to use it, it may not be available or in good working order, and is subject to failure (e.g., torn gloves).

COMMON HAZARDS IN HEALTH CARE

No matter the work setting, nurses are exposed to many hazards in common. These include the following.

Biologic Hazards

Blood-borne pathogens are the infectious agents to which nurses are most often exposed, due to the prevalence of blood and body fluids in their work environments. Although hepatitis B, hepatitis C, and the human immunodeficiency virus (HIV) are the best known of the blood-borne pathogens, syphilis, malaria, brucellosis, Creutzfeldt-Jakob disease, leptospirosis, and other lesser known diseases are also transmitted through blood and body fluid contact. Of these three main infectious risks, hepatitis B is the most easily contracted through occupational contact with blood or body fluids, with 6% to 30% of unvaccinated health care workers infected after a single needle stick (NIOSH, 2000).

Occupational exposure can occur through injury by contaminated sharps or contact with potentially infectious material to the eyes, mouth, mucous membranes, or nonintact skin. In addition to blood, the body fluids and tissues listed in Figure 15-4 are considered potentially infectious.

Blood-borne pathogens are not the only infectious agents to which nurses are exposed. Nurses may come into contact with patients or visitors who may have rubeola, mumps, rubella, chickenpox, pertussis, SARS, influenza, tuberculosis, or other easily transmissible diseases.

The nurse's work environment, whether institutional or in homes, may contain pathogenic and allergenic molds, which produce toxic chemicals called mycotoxins. Toxic molds grow on damp ceilings or interior walls, particularly in older facilities.

Prevention and Control

Workplace exposure to blood-borne pathogens is controlled by OSHA, through its Blood-borne Pathogens Standard (OSHA, 1991) and through a federal law ("Needlestick Safety and Prevention Act," 2000). These regulations mandate engineering controls through the use of safer needle devices, work practice controls (e.g., standard or universal precautions), and administrative controls (e.g., offering free hepatitis B vaccination to exposed employees, use of biohazard labels), as well as the provision and use of PPE, such as gloves. The standard also mandates employers to compose and follow an exposure control plan and to provide testing, treatment, and follow-up for health care employees who have suffered an accident that carries with it the potential for infection, such as skin puncture with a contaminated sharp.

Vaccination and periodic screening can prevent or provide early detection for many infectious diseases. However, nurses should always wash their hands after every patient contact and use PPE (including respirators) when caring for known or potentially infected patients.

Figure 15-4
Potentially
Infectious Body
Fluids and Tissues.
(Data from OSHA,
1991, Section
1910.1030b.)

semen
vaginal secretions
cerebrospinal fluid
synovial fluid
pleural fluid
pericardial fluid
peritoneal fluid
amniotic fluid
saliva in dental procedures
any body fluid that is visibly contaminated with blood
all body fluids in situations where it is difficult or impossible to differentiate between body fluids
any unfixed tissue or organ (other than intact skin) from a human (living or dead)
HIV-containing cell or tissue cultures, organ cultures, and HIV- or HBV-containing culture medium or other solutions
blood, organs, or other tissues from experimental animals infected with HIV or HBV

Respirators provide a barrier between the nurse's breathing zone and harmful agents. There are different types of respirators for different hazards (e.g., bacteria, chemicals, dust), but the N-95 disposable particulate respirator is the one most commonly used in hospitals to provide basic protection against *mycobacterium tuberculosis* and other infectious agents. Note that not all surgical masks are N-95 rated. Powered air purifying respirators provide even more protection but are bulky, noisy, and difficulty to work in.

The best protection against inhalation of mold toxins is elimination by reporting areas of moisture-discolored ceiling tiles or walls and respiratory symptoms (e.g., wheezing) or allergic symptoms (e.g., itchy eyes) associated with working in suspect areas. When working in a potentially contaminated home, alert the residents to the problem and consider wearing a particulate respirator when providing services in that setting.

Chemical

The most common chemical hazard nurses face is from handling, preparing, administering, or disposing hazardous drugs (ones that have been shown to cause cancer, reproductive toxicity, birth defects, or acute harm to health). While calculated amounts of drugs are intentionally given to willing patients to produce a beneficial effect, the exposure of nurses to these drugs is involuntary and unintended, with no therapeutic intent and an unknown dose. The American Society of Hospital Pharmacists has defined drugs with occupational hazards as ones with any of the following four characteristics, each of which alone makes a drug hazardous:

- Genotoxicity
- Carcinogenicity
- Teratogenicity or fertility impairment
- Serious organ or other toxic manifestation at low doses in experimental animals or treated patients (OSHA, n.d.)

Examples of drugs that are classified as hazardous are cyclosporin, fluorouracil, mercaptopurine, and vincristine. Drugs delivered by aerosol, such as pentamidine, pose an inhalation risk to the nurse (OSHA, n.d.). Hazardous drugs are not the only chemical exposures for nurses. They also work with or around disinfectants, sterilizing agents, mercury, and waste anesthetic gases.

Prevention and Control

While most chemical exposures (particularly drugs) cannot be eliminated, it is sometimes possible to substitute less toxic products for disinfectants. Engineering controls include hoods for preparing drugs and other types of ventilation. Work practice controls are important to prevent adverse health effects from chemical exposures. Safe handling procedures are described in every chemical's **Material Safety Data Sheet** (MSDS), which your employer must make immediately available to you, under the requirements of OSHA's Hazard Communication Standard ("Right to Know"). The MSDS contains sections that describe spill or leak procedures, protection information/control measures, and special precautions. Administrative controls include chemical safety training that OSHA requires your employer to provide upon hire. OSHA also recommends that health care employers develop a written Hazardous Drug Safety and Health Plan that includes standard operating procedures, engineering controls, periodic medical monitoring, and designation of an individual or entity responsible for drug safety in the facility (OSHA, n.d.). Lastly, personal protective equipment in the form of eye protection, protective clothing, and gloves are useful in preventing skin and mucous membrane contact.

Latex, defined as natural rubber latex and products made from dry natural rubber, is ubiquitous in hospitals and poses risks not only to nurses but also to patients, both of whom can develop severe allergic responses to contact. (See Table 15-4.) About 10% of health care workers are thought to be allergic to latex (American Nurses Association, 1996).

Once latex allergy has occurred, there is no treatment other than complete removal from latex exposure. This can end a nurse's career. The American Latex Allergy Association provides information for those with latex allergy at http://www.latexallergyresources.org.

NIOSH recommends several control strategies to reduce exposure to latex and thereby reduce sensitization.

Table 15-4 Latex Containing Products

Emergency Equipment	Hospital Supplies
Blood pressure cuffs Stethoscopes Disposable gloves Oral and nasal airways Endotracheal tubes Tourniquets Intravenous tubing Syringes Electrode pads	Anesthesia masks Catheters Wound drains Injection ports Rubber tops of multidose vials Dental dams
Personal Protective Equipment	**Household Objects**
Gloves Surgical masks Goggles Respirators Rubber aprons	Automobile tires Motorcycle and bicycle Handgrips Carpeting Swimming goggles Racquet handles Shoe soles Expandable fabric (waistbands) Dishwashing gloves Hot water bottles Condoms Diaphragms Balloons Pacifiers Baby bottle nipples
Office Supplies	
Rubber bands Erasers	

Source: NIOSH, 1997

- Substitution: use nonlatex gloves when there is no contact with infectious materials, such as when cleaning; use powder-free, reduced-protein latex gloves when there is contact with infectious materials.
- Work practices: thorough hand washing when removing latex gloves, ensuring there is good housekeeping to remove latex-containing dust from the workplace, using only non-oil-based skin care products while at work. Become familiar with the signs and symptoms of latex allergy and report them to the employee health nurse or supervisor. Remove yourself from further exposure if you develop latex allergy.
- Administrative: attend latex allergy training programs in your institution.

Note that gloves labeled "hypoallergenic" are not necessarily low in latex allergens. The label simply means that the product is low in certain skin irritating chemicals used in manufacture.

Mechanical/Biomechanical Hazards

Musculoskeletal disorders (MSDs) disable more nurses every year than any other condition. MSDs are disorders of the muscles, nerves, ligaments, and joints (e.g., low back pain, shoulder strain). Other terms include soft tissue injuries, overexertion injuries, sprains/strains, and cumulative trauma disorders. These disorders usually result from repeated microtrauma to the musculoskeletal system, but can occur after performing a single hazardous task. Stress and job dissatisfaction appear to heighten the biomechanical load. Nurses experience MSDs from moving and handling loads in excess of their physiologic capacity. The risk factors for MSDs in patient care include the weight of load lifted or handled, the frequency of the lift, and awkward postures. Examples of the most hazardous tasks are:

- Lateral transfers (bed to stretcher, stretcher to x-ray table, bed to scale)
- Vertical transfers (bed to chair, wheelchair to toilet, floor to bed or chair)
- Bathing/dressing patient in bed
- Applying anti-embolism stockings
- Making an occupied bed
- Pushing/pulling an occupied bed or stretcher ("road trips")
- Repositioning a patient (side to side, up in bed or up in wheelchair)
- Feeding a bedridden patient
- Changing an absorbent pad

For the past 50 years, most nursing schools have instructed students to use body mechanics to lift or move patients; however, there is no evidence to support body mechanics, an out-of-date method for lifting objects, as an effective strategy to protect caregivers from manual handling injuries. Most patients (except babies) exceed the NIOSH-recommended maximum safe lift weight of 35 pounds (Waters, 2007). Most nurses dangerously overestimate their physical abilities and underestimate the risk when lifting, repositioning, or transferring an adult patient. For a patient weighing 200 pounds, even four caregivers are not sufficient to reduce the load lifted to a safe level. The same nurse who would refuse to slide a 100-pound bag of rice from a shelf to a shopping cart will attempt to transfer a 200-pound patient from bed to stretcher without a moment's hesitation.

A mechanical hazard is workplace design or layout. Many hospitals were built before the proliferation of medical equipment that exists today, resulting in work spaces for nurses that are inadequate to allow free movement without suffering bumps and bruises or requiring awkward postures to provide nursing care. Cluttered environments can cause slips, trips, and falls not only for the nurse but for the patient as well. In addition, many hospital units have long corridors with no place for nurses to sit except at the central nurses' station. Walking long distances over a twelve-hour shift can lead to fatigue and musculoskeletal pain and may affect the quality of care due to the barrier posed by the time it takes for the nurse to travel between resources and the point of care.

Prevention and Control

Health care **ergonomics** is the science of fitting the job to the worker by reducing the risk factors associated with performing patient care tasks. Using the hierarchy of controls, the first focus is on eliminating manual handling. Examples include patient beds that convert to chairs, which eliminate the need to transfer a patient in and out of bed; beds with built in scales; special sheets that prevent patients from sliding down; and powered beds or stretchers, which eliminate the need to push or pull an occupied bed/stretcher. When manual handling cannot be eliminated, the next level of control is engineering in the form of safe patient handling equipment (Nelson, Motacki, & Menzel, 2008). There are many modern lifting and moving aids available, including height-adjustable beds to bring the patient to the caregiver's hip level, friction-reducing devices to help lateral transfers of patients (bed to stretcher), powered full-body sling lifts that move dependent patients from bed to chair or bathroom (Figure 15-5), powered sit-to-stand lifts that assist patients to rise from bed and be wheeled to the bathroom, and gait belts with handles that reduce the injury risk to both nurse and patient from an unexpected loss of balance when ambulating with assistance. Also available are specialized pieces of equipment designed to handle and move bariatric (morbidly obese) patients. In addition, there are engineering modifications that

Figure 15-5
Example of a ceiling-mounted lift that provides for nurse safety and patient security during transfers into and out of bed. Ceiling-mounted equipment increases the likelihood that a nurse will use it, while at the same time reducing room clutter and solving storage problems (Nelson, Motacki, & Menzel, 2008). *(Courtesy of SureHands Lift & Care Systems, Pine Island, New York.)*

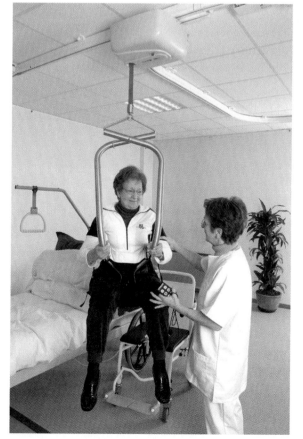

can be made to existing equipment, such as replacing the wheels on medication and laundry carts to make them easier to push and turn or removing friction-increasing carpet in patient care areas.

In the absence of any federal ergonomics law, several states have passed their own safe patient handling legislation, including Maryland, Minnesota, New Jersey, Rhode Island, Texas, and Washington, with pilot projects underway or bills pending in several other states. Whether or not a nurse's employer is required by law to comply, as a matter of good policy it should have a safe patient handling or ergonomics program. Elements include: 1) a risk assessment for the work environment, 2) purchase of appropriate equipment in consultation with employees, 3) regular equipment maintenance, 4) a nonpunitive safe lifting policy, and 5) regular staff training on equipment use. The key to MSD protection is assessing patients' lifting needs in a systematic fashion (using the algorithms described below) and selecting and using the correct assistive equipment.

Home health nurses have more limited options if the client does not own safe patient handling equipment or aids. Transferring completely dependent clients in home environments is made more difficult by room clutter and few people to assist. Home health agencies can furnish their nurses with lightweight friction-reducing devices that are portable and useful for repositioning in bed.

Nurses should not attempt to lift or move a patient who exceeds their physical capacity to do so and, instead, seek guidance from a supervisor. As always, nurses must use infection control techniques when using the same equipment on multiple patients.

Engineering control suggestions for cluttered rooms include replacing floor-based equipment with wall- or ceiling-mounted equipment (e.g., wall-supplied oxygen, ceiling-mounted

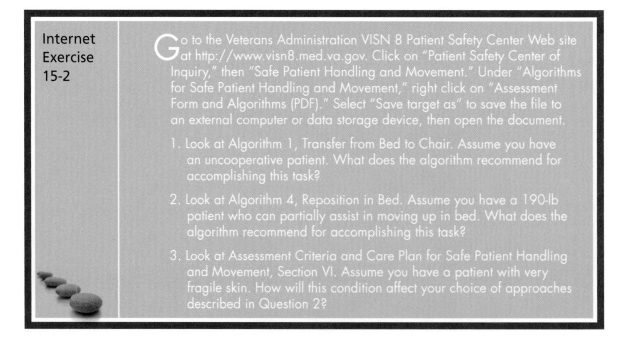

Internet Exercise 15-2

Go to the Veterans Administration VISN 8 Patient Safety Center Web site at http://www.visn8.med.va.gov. Click on "Patient Safety Center of Inquiry," then "Safe Patient Handling and Movement." Under "Algorithms for Safe Patient Handling and Movement," right click on "Assessment Form and Algorithms (PDF)." Select "Save target as" to save the file to an external computer or data storage device, then open the document.

1. Look at Algorithm 1, Transfer from Bed to Chair. Assume you have an uncooperative patient. What does the algorithm recommend for accomplishing this task?

2. Look at Algorithm 4, Reposition in Bed. Assume you have a 190-lb patient who can partially assist in moving up in bed. What does the algorithm recommend for accomplishing this task?

3. Look at Assessment Criteria and Care Plan for Safe Patient Handling and Movement, Section VI. Assume you have a patient with very fragile skin. How will this condition affect your choice of approaches described in Question 2?

intravenous hooks, and full-body sling lifts), removing one or more beds from multi-patient rooms, and remodeling. For the fatigue caused by long hours standing, engineering control strategies include constructing a sitting nook midway down the corridor to allow nurses to rest periodically, and improved communication, observation, and monitoring systems to reduce the need to walk to remote patient rooms while still assuring patient visualization and verbal contact. A work practice control is making sure that the most dependent patients are placed closest to the nurses' station. Inviting nurses to have a seat at the table when new facilities are being planned to make sure the architects include ergonomic designs is an effective administrative control.

Physical Hazards (Radiation, Lasers, Gas under Pressure)

Exposure to radiation and lasers is possible in most health care environments. Radiation is used in a variety of diagnostic procedures, from simple X-rays of body parts to complex imaging in Computed Axial Tomography (CAT) scans. In addition, radioactive materials are used in diagnostic imaging and in some types of cancer treatment. Lasers are used in operating rooms. The risk of unintended exposure can be substantial, depending on the work environment. Nurses may receive a dose of ionizing radiation when portable X-ray devices are used in multi-bed ICUs without walls or in operating rooms, for example. OSHA has summarized the health effects of radiation and lasers in health care environments (Table 15-5).

In addition to radiation, nurses are also subject to injury from the physical hazard of compressed gases in tanks under pressure, which can explode or leak. Such an event constitutes a chemical exposure as well.

Prevention and Control

Because the control of radiation hazards is complex, nurses should ask their supervisor who is responsible for it and then find out what precautions are being taken to protect workers. For example, proper inspection and periodic maintenance of X-ray equipment is a key factor in radiation safety. When you know that X-rays will be used in your vicinity, leave the area, if possible; if you are assisting with the X-ray procedure, request a well-fitting lead apron as PPE.

Physical Hazards (Noise)

Ear-damaging noise in certain health care environments, such as helicopter transport, is obvious. However, lower-level noise has hazards as well. Noise pressure is measured in A-weighted decibels, abbreviated as dB(A), with higher numbers indicating higher threat to the auditory system that may result in a permanent, irreversible hearing impairment when the dose received is above a certain threshold for intensity and length of exposure. For comparison purposes, a whisper is 35 dB(A), a piano 80 dB(A), and a rock concert 110 dB(A) (Frenzilli, et al., 2004). Noise above 85 dB(A) for 8 hours is damaging to the ear (World Health Organization, 2001).

Table 15-5 Radiation and Laser Hazards in Health Care

Agent Use or Exposure	Health Effects
LASER Used in the operating rooms for excision and cauterization of tissue. Class 3b and 4 lasers are most often used. Exposure usually occurs from unintentional operation or when proper controls are not in effect. The high electrical energy used to generate the beam is a potential shock hazard. The smoke plume during a surgical procedure and the laser's reaction to certain explosive or flammable agents also present hazards in the operating room.	**Acute:** From direct beam exposure, burns to skin and eyes possibly resulting in blindness. Chemical by-products in the smoke plume may cause irritation to the eyes, nose, and throat, and nausea (see OSHA Hazard Information Bulletins). Biological and inert particulates can also be found in the smoke plume but these have not been well studied for their effects. **Chronic:** Unknown.
IONIZING RADIATION Portable and fixed X-ray machines are used for diagnostic procedures. Exposure occurs when unprotected employees are near a machine in operation. The degree of exposure depends on the amount of radiation, the duration of exposure, the distance from the source, and the type of shielding in place. Kits containing radioactive isotopes or specimens and excreta of humans and animals who have received radionucleotides may pose a hazard. Exposure may also result from handling of radioactive spills (29 CFR 1910.1096).	Effects of radiation exposure are somatic (body) or genetic (offspring) in nature. **Acute:** Erythema and dermatitis. Large whole-body exposures cause nausea, vomiting, diarrhea, weakness, and death. **Chronic:** Skin cancer and bone marrow suppression. Genetic effects may lead to congenital defects in the employee's offspring.
MAGNETIC RADIATION Magnetic resonance instrumentation.	No conclusive effects are documented.
ULTRAVIOLET RADIATION Ultraviolet lamps are sometimes used in biological safety cabinets.	**Acute:** Skin burns, damage to the eye. **Chronic:** No documented effects other than cataracts.

Source: OSHA, n.d.

However, noise below 85 dB(A) is not without other adverse health effects. Such noise levels in hospitals cause stress to both patients and staff, as Florence Nightingale noted in 1859: "Unnecessary noise, then, is the most cruel absence of care which can be inflicted either on sick or well" (Nightingale, 1914, p. 61). Hospital noise has been associated with headaches, irritability, delayed wound healing, and increased pain perception (Biley, 1994). ICUs, operating rooms, emergency departments, and nurseries are a few of the hospital areas where bothersome noise levels have been identified. Noise above 70 dB(A) causes annoyance. A recent study found a noise level of 73 dB(A) at the triage area of a large urban hospital's emergency department (Orellana, Busch-Vishniac, & West, 2007). In the nurse/ patient safety dyad, high background noise levels affects both. Nurses report that the most disturbing noises are those that carry a message that action is required, such as monitor alarms (Buelow, 2001).

The general din found in hospital units (running water, flushing toilets, alarms, equipment operation, multiple conversations, ringing telephones, buzzing pagers, drawers shutting, garbage cans closing, noisy shoes) contributes to communication difficulties among staff members and between patients and nurses, and also interferes with the acoustic parts of physical assessment, such as listening to heart and lung sounds with a stethoscope.

Prevention and Control

A sign of excessive noise levels in your work area is difficulty communicating with other staff members or patients without raising your voice to be heard. The first step would be to request from your supervisor that an industrial hygienist or safety professional assess your work area for noise through the use of a sound level meter. If noise levels at or above 85 dB(A) are found, your employer may be subject to OSHA's Occupational Noise Exposure Standard, which requires engineering, administrative, and PPE controls to reduce the hazard and periodic hearing tests, among other provisions. If the ambient noise levels are below 85 dB(A) but above 70 dB(A), your unit or employer should consider methods to reduce stressful background noise. Controls include elimination (e.g., buying quieter equipment), engineering (e.g., isolating either the sound source or the sound recipient by closing patient doors, turning down alarm volumes), work practice controls (e.g., having staff wear soft-soled shoes, limiting telephone calls at the front of the nurses' station), administrative (e.g., enforcing quiet hours when patients are trying to sleep), or as a last resort, PPE (ear plugs or muffs). Because the latter not only reduce noise but also impair communication, noise attenuation devices have very limited applicability in health care.

Psychosocial

The most widely recognized psychosocial hazard for nurses is stress. NIOSH defines job stress as "the harmful physical and emotional responses that occur when the requirements of the job do not match the capabilities, resources, or needs of the worker. Job stress can lead to poor health and even injury" (NIOSH, 1999, Section "What is Job Stress?").

It doesn't matter if the demand is caused by pleasant or unpleasant things; if the nurse perceives the demand as more than he or she can handle with available resources, then the mind and body interpret this demand as stress (Figure 15-6). Although a certain amount of stress is thought to be beneficial (eustress), too much stress has been linked to physiological reactions that, if continued, can cause harm, such as excessive secretion of cortisol. Nurses may try to handle excessive stress with negative coping behaviors, such as smoking, drinking alcoholic beverages, or overeating.

Figure 15-6
Demands that exceed the nurse's available resources are perceived by the mind and body as stress.

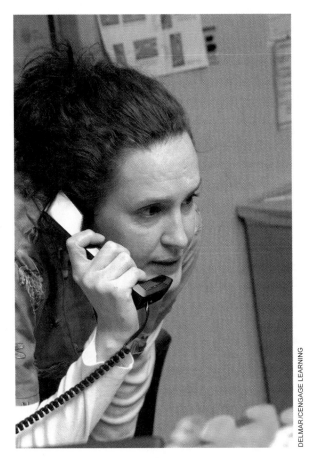

DELMAR/CENGAGE LEARNING

In the epidemiological triangle, host factors are thought to be important in determining the threat of harm from stress. Some individuals appear to be more resilient than others and either don't perceive high stress in most situations or handle stressful situations more easily.

Job-related (environmental) stressors in nursing include dealing with sick and dying patients, heavy workloads due to understaffing, shift work, mandatory overtime, interpersonal conflicts, organizational restructuring, job insecurity, lack of peer support, and low job control. Finally, host factors influence the effects of stress as well. Nurses are subject to stress in their personal lives as well, which can reduce their ability to handle job stress. NIOSH has modeled the effect of these factors on the risk of harm from stress (Figure 15-7). While some stress is deflected and some passes through the host without effect, some of it increases the risk of adverse outcomes.

The early warning signs of stress include headaches, sleep disturbances, difficulty concentrating, short temper, upset stomach, and low morale. High stress levels have been linked to the incidence of medical errors and workplace injuries. Chronic stress is thought to play a role in the development of cardiovascular disease, mental health disorders, and musculoskeletal disorders (NIOSH, 1999).

Figure 15-7
Stress Model.
*(Source: NIOSH
(National Institute for
Occupational Safety
and Health), 1999.)*

NIOSH Model of Job Stress

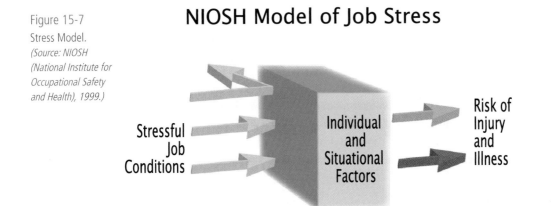

Prevention and Control

Although it is unrealistic to think that employers can eliminate stress from a health care setting, management can use administrative controls to reduce stress levels through organizational change. Possible actions include:

- Taking into consideration employees' outside job demands and responsibilities when putting together schedules
- Providing sufficient RN staffing for patient acuity levels (nurse/patient ratios)
- Instituting a shared governance organizational model, with nurses having a say in management decisions and policies
- Supporting autonomy in nursing practice

Another administrative control is offering Employee Assistance Programs (EAPs), which provide connections to stress management resources. Some employers offer on-site stress management classes as well.

Writing
Exercise
15-1

Assess your ability to handle stress. In nursing, what do you find are the most stressful situations? For example, do you function well during an emergency situation? What about when an adult or pediatric patient dies? Have you found communicating with instructors, supervisors, patients, or their family members to be stressful? Do you function better under stress or when surroundings are calm? What symptoms do you experience when you perceive you are stressed? Will your self-assessed stress capacity influence where you will seek work after graduation (e.g., emergency department versus geriatric out-patient clinic)? What stress management techniques have you tried and which work best for you?

On a personal level, there are steps you can take to manage stress. One of the most effective stress management techniques is getting adequate physical activity. Even very busy people can find the time in their workdays for a little exercise. If your employer doesn't offer a place to exercise or a gym membership, you can build in some refreshing activity by parking at the furthest end of the parking lot, taking the stairs up to and down from the work area, and building in a walk as part of your meal break. Limiting your work hours by resisting the temptation to work more than one job, getting adequate sleep, and eating nutritious food will also reduce stress and tension.

Internet Exercise 15-3

Watch the NIOSH streaming video *Working with Stress* at http://www.cdc.gov/NIOSH. Under "Spotlights," click on "Stress at Work," then "NIOSH Books and Videos." Click on "Working with Stress Video."

1. What does NIOSH state is the most effective way to prevent/reduce stress—stress management education or organizational change?

2. What are some consequences to the organization from high stress levels in its workers?

Another psychosocial and physical stressor is **workplace violence,** all too prevalent in hospitals and other health care settings. In 2000, 48% of all nonfatal injuries from occupational assaults and violent acts occurred in health care and social services (OSHA, 2004). Nurses are at high risk, with 24.8 victimizations per 1,000 nurses annually; psychiatric nurses are at the highest risk (State of New Jersey Public Health Services Branch, n.d.).

After psychiatric registered nurse Jill Dangler was assaulted by a patient, she described the attack.

> After attempting to strangle me, he repeatedly punched my face causing my head to hit the wall at each blow. He repeatedly kicked all my body parts as I lay on the floor. It was another patient who heard the sounds of the attack and intervened to save my life (Testimony before the New York State Occupational Safety & Health Hazard Abatement Board, June 24, 2003, p. 2).

Against a background of escalating societal crime, drug use, and inability to access health care services, increasing violence in health care facilities is a worrisome trend. Environmental risk factors include the following factors (NIOSH, 2002; OSHA, 2004):

- The prevalence of handguns and other weapons among patients, their families, or friends.
- The increasing use of hospitals by police and the criminal justice system for criminal holds and the care of acutely disturbed, violent individuals.
- The increasing number of acute and chronic mentally ill patients being released from hospitals without follow-up care.
- The availability of drugs or money at hospitals, clinics, and pharmacies, making them likely robbery targets.

- Long waits in emergency or clinic areas that lead to client frustration over an inability to obtain needed services promptly.
- The increasing presence of gang members, drug or alcohol abusers, trauma patients, or distraught family members.
- Low staffing levels during times of increased activity such as mealtimes, visiting times, and when staff are transporting patients.
- Isolated work with clients during examinations or treatment.
- Solo work, often in remote locations with no backup or way to get assistance, such as communication devices or alarm systems.
- Lack of staff training in recognizing and managing escalating hostile and assaultive behavior.
- Poorly lit parking areas.
- Inadequate security.
- Unrestricted movement of the public in health care facilities.

Assaults are physical attacks or threats of attack (verbal or behavioral) (NIOSH, 2002). While violence in non-health care work places is usually related to robbery by strangers, assaults on hospital workers are most often at the hands of patients or their family members. However, worker-on-worker and criminal-intent violence also occur. The highest risk areas for violence are psychiatric units, emergency departments, waiting rooms, and geriatric units. Staff shortages increase the risk of assaults (Tuller, 2008).

The health effects of violence include physical and psychological injuries. (See Figure 15-8.) In the past, nurses accepted aggressive acts by patients as part of their job, but as awareness has increased that nurses should not have to tolerate this, reports of violence have risen, and consequently more workplaces are taking steps to control it by improving security.

Figure 15-8
Physical injuries to a nurse who was assaulted by a psychiatric patient. *(Courtesy of Catheline Seguin, RN.)*

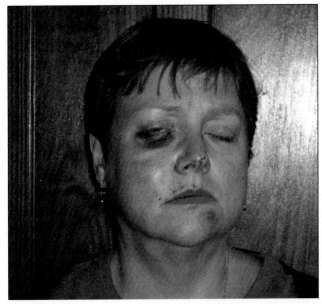

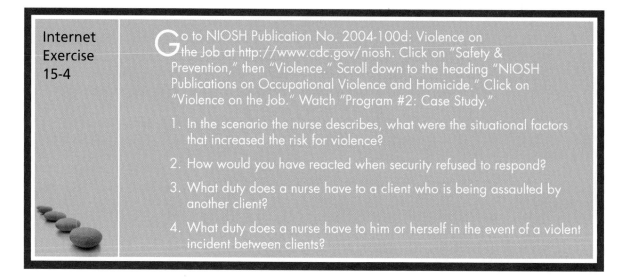

Internet Exercise 15-4

Go to NIOSH Publication No. 2004-100d: Violence on the Job at http://www.cdc.gov/niosh. Click on "Safety & Prevention," then "Violence." Scroll down to the heading "NIOSH Publications on Occupational Violence and Homicide." Click on "Violence on the Job." Watch "Program #2: Case Study."

1. In the scenario the nurse describes, what were the situational factors that increased the risk for violence?

2. How would you have reacted when security refused to respond?

3. What duty does a nurse have to a client who is being assaulted by another client?

4. What duty does a nurse have to him or herself in the event of a violent incident between clients?

Prevention and Control

Health care employers can best protect nurses through a combination of elimination, engineering, administrative, and work practice controls included in a workplace violence prevention program. At a minimum, OSHA recommends that this program include management commitment and employee involvement, as well as the following elements (Occupational Safety and Health Administration, 2004):

- Zero tolerance policy for workplace violence
- Nonpunitive reporting of incidents and near incidents of violence
- Investigation of all incidents of victimization
- Comprehensive security plan, including engineering controls such as locks, alarms, panic buttons, and video surveillance
- Assignment of responsibility for violence reduction to a knowledgeable individual or team with adequate resources
- Putting employee safety on the same level of importance as patient safety
- Employee training
- Prompt medical and psychological care for victims
- Periodic evaluation of program effectiveness

Although PPE might be possible (e.g., bullet-proof vests for emergency department workers), it is neither practical nor recommended. Although there are no evidence-based techniques to intervene with an individual at risk of losing control, the nurse can learn to recognize signs that violence might be imminent. Warning signs include increasing agitation (both verbal and physical), apparent hallucinations, and evidence of intoxication (drugs or alcohol). When these signs are present, the nurse should avoid increasing any conflict and withdraw to a safe area to call for security assistance. The nurse should never allow a potentially violent individual to block a quick escape.

CASE SCENARIO 15-2

A receptionist working at a hospital-based, out-patient medical clinic was required to collect insurance co-payment from patients seeking care. At the reception window, the clinic had posted large signs describing its right to withhold service for nonpayment, a step it had taken recently after its chief financial officer discovered the magnitude of co-payment bad debt. A couple entered the waiting room, with the husband approaching the reception window to sign in for his wife. When the receptionist asked him for the $20 co-payment, he said he had neither money nor a credit card. The receptionist advised him of the clinic's policy and offered to reschedule the appointment. At this point, the man began to yell, demanding to see a supervisor. The receptionist asked him to keep his voice down while she called for the nurse manager. The nurse entered the waiting room and positioned herself between the reception window and the pacing, agitated man. She then pointed to the sign and reiterated the clinic's policy. Upon hearing this, the man lunged at the nurse, grabbed her by the throat, and pushed her to the ground, where he began kicking her repeatedly. By the time the receptionist could telephone hospital security to request their assistance, the nurse had suffered facial fractures, a concussion, and a dislocated shoulder. Security guards escorted the man and his wife to the clinic exit. The nurse later tried to file a police report of the assault, but the police refused to accept it, stating that the incident was a job issue between the nurse and her employer.

CASE ANALYSIS

1. What were the risk factors for violence in this case? Was violence predictable?

2. What are some engineering controls that might have spared the nurse or reduced the harm from the assault?

3. What actions could the nurse have taken to reduce her risk of being in harm's way?

4. Do nurses have a legal right to file assault charges against a violent client or coworker? What could the nurse do after being turned away by the police?

Work Schedules

Commonly, nurses in hospitals are required to work either rotating or permanent shifts, extended hours (12- to 16-hour shifts), and overtime. Studies have shown that those working 12-hour shifts have increased fatigue and decreased performance after the 9th hour, with adverse consequences for both nurse and patient (NIOSH, 2004). These ill effects are compounded when 12-hour shifts are combined with work weeks exceeding 40 hours. A government report on hazards in the work environments of nurses found that long work shifts posed one of the most serious threats to patient safety and recommended that state regulatory agencies prohibit work days longer than 12 hours and work weeks exceeding 60 hours (Page, 2004).

Shift work (schedules outside the hours of 6 a.m. to 6 p.m.) has additional risks. Hospital nurses usually work "day shift" (7 a.m. to 7 p.m.) or "night shift" (7 p.m. to 7 a.m.), with some nominal time included for breaks during the shift. However, it is not unusual to see shifts beginning as early as 4 a.m. to provide additional coverage during morning meal times. Adverse health outcomes for shift workers include sleep disturbances, poor pregnancy outcomes, and gastrointestinal and cardiovascular disorders (Levy, Wegman, Baron, & Sokas, 2006). Workers older than 45 are particularly susceptible to the ill effects of shift work.

Prevention and Control

Residential health care facilities, such as hospitals and nursing homes, must provide services 24 hours a day, 7 days a week, which means they have to require their employees to work around the clock. Although elimination or engineering controls are not possible, there are several administrative and work practice controls that can lessen the harm from extended schedules and shift work. These include having adequate backup nurse staffing resources to avoid mandatory overtime, limiting voluntary overtime to 12 hours a day and 60 hours a week, rotating shifts clockwise, restricting consecutive night shifts to no more than 3, and providing nap times during night shifts.

Although there is no PPE for the hazards of extended hours or shift work, the nurse can take steps to reduce the ill effects of these stressors by getting adequate rest between work periods (sleep hygiene). Night-shift workers face challenges getting to sleep because they leave work in full daylight, which is an environmental trigger for wakefulness. Preparing a bedroom with light-blocking curtains and silencing telephone ringers will help to limit sleep interruptions, but family responsibilities such as child care may require the nurse to split rest periods into short naps.

WORKPLACE SAFETY LAWS AND REGULATIONS

This chapter has repeatedly referenced OSHA, the U.S. Department of Labor enforcement agency for the OSH Act. However, federal OSHA does not regulate all health care workplaces. When the OSH Act was passed in 1970, states were given a choice of setting up an OSHA-approved state plan or relying solely on federal OSHA. Twenty-four states, Puerto Rico, and the Virgin Islands chose state plans and have adopted their own standards and enforcement policies that are at least as stringent as federal OSHA. They may also promulgate regulations that are even stricter than federal OSHA. For example, California (CalOSHA) has passed and enforces several such regulations. Federal employees (e.g., the Veterans Administration) in all states are covered by federal OSHA. For information on federal OSHA standards that apply to health care, go to http://www.osha.gov. Under the heading "Compliance Assistance," click on "Quick Start," then "Health Care."

Public employees in states that are under federal OSHA plans are not covered by OSHA. Most federal OSHA states have state agencies that provide some occupational health and safety protection for their public employees. However, Florida (a federal OSHA state), in 1999, abolished the agency that had previously protected the health and safety of its public employees. This means that nurses employed by public health care facilities in Florida are not protected by OSHA regulations and have no agency (other than their employer) to which to report workplace hazards and request inspection and remediation.

Nurses working for employers covered by OSHA have certain rights. OSHA spells these rights out in its poster "Job Safety and Health: It's the Law!" (see Figure 15-9).

In addition to the rights listed on the poster (Figure 15-9), the OSH Act gives workers the right to refuse work that they believe puts them in "imminent danger." Imminent danger means there is an immediate threat of death or serious physical harm. In health care, such a situation might arise if a supervisor asked a nurse to restrain an armed, violent patient, for example. In that situation, for workplaces under OSHA control, the nurse would have a right to refuse to carry out the assignment. Refusing assignments may result in disciplinary action, including dismissal, but that risk may be preferable to risk of bodily harm.

Virtually all states and jurisdictions require employers to provide **workers' compensation insurance** coverage for injuries and illnesses that arise out of and in the course of employment. While there is a federal workers' compensation system that covers federal employees, each state or jurisdiction has its own workers' compensation laws. Provisions vary from state to state, but all are no-fault insurance. That is, the employee gives up the right to sue the employer for workplace injuries and illnesses in return for the employer providing immediate medical care and wage replacement (after a waiting period). Employers cannot deny benefits based on employee negligence, although some states have passed laws that reduce benefits if employees are found to have refused to use safety devices, or that deny benefits if the employee is under the influence of illicit drugs or alcohol. The cost of workers' compensation insurance is in direct proportion to an employer's accident frequency and severity, giving employers a financial incentive to improve workplace safety.

Workers' compensation wage replacement is set at a percentage of a worker's weekly wage, up to a predetermined maximum amount and, although tax free, rarely provides buying power equivalent to the preinjury wage. The purpose of this wage reduction is to encourage the injured employee to return to work in full- or modified-duty capacity.

Despite the intent of the workers' compensation insurance system to reduce lawsuits after workplace accidents, in reality it has become one of the most heavily litigated areas of employment law (Menzel, 2006). Although workers' compensation insurance provides nurses with some benefits in the event of workplace injury, the best strategy for a long and productive career is to avoid injury and illness altogether by recognizing workplace hazards and taking protective steps.

The Joint Commission (formerly known as the Joint Commission on Accreditation of Healthcare Organizations, or JCAHO) has increasingly embraced the safety of hospital caregivers as well as patients. It has incorporated worker safety into its environment of care regulations, validating once again the nurse/patient safety dyad. The Joint Commission has great power to improve nurse safety because accreditation is required for health care institutions to receive reimbursement from federal and state governments and insurers.

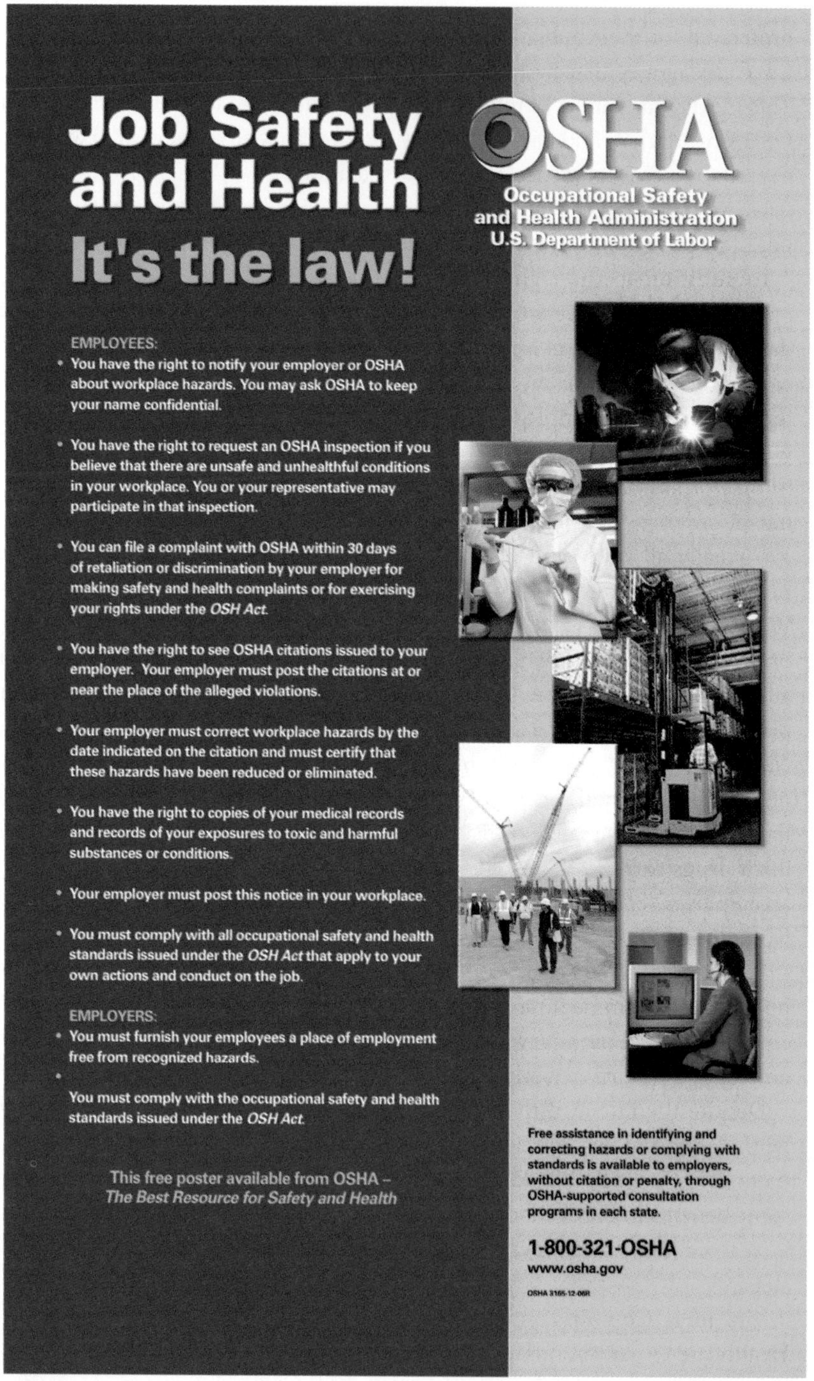

Figure 15-9
OSHA Job Safety
and Health Poster.
(Courtesy of OSHA.)

Although not all nurses are members, unions are another force for improving workplace health and safety. Through collective bargaining, unions can require employers to put in safety improvements, such as programs to protect against MSDs, infectious diseases, and workplace violence. Unions are also a force for getting state and federal safety regulations passed, as politicians wish to please large voting blocs. For other examples, go to the UAN (United American Nurses, AFL-CIO) Web site at http://www.uannurse.org/hs/index.html. The American Nurses Association and its nonunion state constituencies, as well as independent state nurses associations, are another force for workplace safety through legislative lobbying and workplace advocacy programs.

Getting Involved in Workplace Safety

Nurses should make it their business to get involved in improving workplace safety by volunteering to serve on their employers' safety or accreditation committees. If an employer is unwilling to address obvious hazards brought to its attention, nurses can report such violations to OSHA (in covered workplaces). OSHA is required to respond promptly.

OSHA requires employers to record workplace accidents and injuries that meet certain criteria for severity and post the log in an employee area from February through April of each year. Nurses should make a point to review the types of injuries, the number of lost days, and the areas in which these injuries occurred to get a better sense of uncontrolled hazards in their workplace and to request improved protection from the employer.

Considering that RNs constitute the largest number of health professionals, nurses can influence the passage of health and safety regulations by writing their legislators to demand they take action and making political contributions to those that do.

Elements of Safe Work Environments (What to Ask Before You Accept a Position)

New nursing graduates tend to focus most on clinical specialty, bonuses, and salary packages when looking for their first job. It's exciting to think of finally earning money and having some autonomy in practice. But salary and bonuses will mean little if you are injured on the job. Some facilities have to offer higher pay than others to attract nurses to replace those who have left due to poor working conditions or injury. Figure 15-10 is a list of questions the newly graduated nurses should ask before accepting any job offer, no matter how tempting the starting pay.

It is entirely likely that the nurse recruiter or human resources professional will not know the answer to all of these questions immediately. The facility's representative should promise to find answers to these questions and get back to you. If he or she does not offer to do this or becomes defensive, seek employment elsewhere. It's a seller's market for RNs. You don't want to wind up as a casualty, but as a nurse who has a long and safe career.

1. Is the workplace protected by OSHA? If yes, is it covered by a State Plan or Federal OSHA? If no, what state or local regulations protect employee health and safety?

2. Is there an occupational/employee health department on site? If yes, what services does it offer? If no, where do employees receive periodic screening and care? Does the facility offer any wellness services, such as gym membership? Does the facility offer modified duty for injured RNs?

3. Is there mandatory overtime? Is there a limit to the number of hours per day that staff can be required to work? Are rotating shifts required? If yes, how many night shifts in a row are routinely scheduled?

4. How many workplace injuries and illnesses occurred last year on _____ (name of unit)? In the facility? What were the top three types (e.g., strains/sprains, punctures) and causes (e.g., lifting, contaminated sharp) of injury/illness?

5. Does the facility have a health and safety committee? If yes, how often does it meet? What authority and resources does it have? What are its duties? Describe its last accomplishment.

6. Does the facility have a written program for protection from workplace violence? How many assaults were reported last year? What security services does the facility offer? Is the facility in a high-crime area?

7. Does the facility have a written health care ergonomics program? What are the number and type of patient handling assistive devices available on my preferred unit? Did the employees participate in deciding what equipment to purchase? Will I receive training in equipment operation? Are there adequate areas for me to sit during my work shift?

8. Does the facility have a Hazardous Drug Safety and Health Plan? Is there a radiation safety officer?

9. When was the last time the organization surveyed employees for stress levels? In the past two years, what steps has the organization taken to reduce workplace stress?

10. What health and safety training programs are offered during orientation? For which of these topics is there a training program?

   - chemical safety
   - hazardous drug safety
   - blood-borne pathogens protection
   - radiation safety
   - workers' compensation
   - safe patient handling and movement

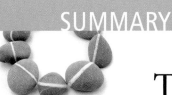

Writing Exercise 15-2

You are considering job offers from two hospitals, A and B, both in cities about an hour from your nursing program. Hospital A is offering you a chance to work in the emergency department (your first choice), a $5,000 sign-on bonus, and a slightly higher salary than Hospital B. Hospital B requires all new nursing graduates to work with a mentor for the first year on a medical-surgical floor and offers relocation assistance up to $2,000, but no sign-on bonus. In response to workplace safety questions you asked the recruiters, Hospital A reveals that its workplace violence protection program is in the planning stage in response to three separate incidents of gun violence in its emergency department last year. The Hospital A recruiter assures you that its plan will be operational in the coming year. It has no radiation safety officer but is exploring the need for one. Hospital B reports that it has had a comprehensive workplace violence protection program in place for the past seven years. Its medical-surgical units reported no assaults last year. It also has a written radiation safety plan and a full-time radiation safety officer.

1. Which employer would you choose? What are the risks and benefits you considered to arrive at this decision?

2. If you choose to work at Hospital A, what steps could you take to improve the health and safety of your environment? What safety guarantees could you ask for before accepting the job?

SUMMARY

To provide the best care to their patients, nurses must protect their own health and safety first. Nurses face a variety of threats to their personal health in hospitals, nursing homes, and community settings. Being aware of the risks allows nurses to take protective actions. Based on national injury statistics, the biggest threat to nurses' musculoskeletal health is manual patient handling. Nurses (and their employers) must incorporate patient handling technology to reduce biomechanical hazards.

Due to the nature of their work, nurses must contend with biological, chemical, physical, and psychosocial hazards as well. Although OSHA regulates some of these hazards (e.g., blood-borne pathogens, chemicals, radiation), it does not regulate others (e.g., stress, violence, shift work), highlighting the need for nurses to monitor their work environments and demand that their employers institute effective safety measures. Resources available to assist nurses in ensuring a safe work environment include federal and state regulators, professional nursing organizations, labor unions, and health-care facility credentialing organizations.

The first step on the path to maintaining an injury-free nursing career is choosing an employer based not only on the immediate benefits, but also on the employer's commitment to protecting its most valuable resource: its workforce. There is strong evidence of effectiveness underlying the prevention and control strategies in this chapter. During recruitment, a potential employer should be able to point to its accomplishments in protecting nurses from known hazards, reassuring new nurses that the employer will take good care of them so that they can take good care of their patients.

Health Care Without Harm is an international coalition of over 460 organizations in more than 50 countries, working to transform the health care sector so it is no longer a source of harm to people and the environment.

–*From the Health Care Without Harm Web site (http://www.noharm.org/us)*

REFERENCES

AMERICAN NURSES ASSOCIATION. (1996). *Latex allergy: Protect yourself, protect your patients.* Retrieved July 31, 2007, from http://www.nursingworld.org/osh/wp7.htm#3

AMERICAN NURSES ASSOCIATION. (2008). *Safe staffing saves lives.* Retrieved July 18, 2008, from http://www.safestaffingsaveslives.org

BILEY, F. C. (1994). Effects of noise in hospitals. *British Journal of Nursing, 3*, 110–113.

BROWN, J. G., Trinkoff, A., Rempher, K., McPhaul, K., Brady, B., Lipscomb, J., et al. (2005). Nurses' inclination to report work-related injuries: organizational, work-group, and individual factors associated with reporting. *AAOHN Journal, 53*, 213–217.

BUELOW, M. (2001). Noise level measurements in four Phoenix emergency departments. *Journal of Emergency Nursing, 27*, 23–26.

CENTERS FOR DISEASE CONTROL AND PREVENTION. (2007). *Overweight and obesity.* Retrieved July 28, 2007, from http://www.cdc.gov/nccdphp/dnpa/obesity/index.htm

FRENZILLI, G., Lenzi, P., Scarcelli, V., Fornai, F., Pellegrini, A., Soldani, P., et al. (2004). Effects of loud noise exposure on DNA integrity in rat adrenal gland. *Environmental Health Perspectives, 117*, 1671–1672.

HATCH, M. (2008). Working safely with drugs and other substances. In D. Fell-Carlson (Ed.), *Working safely in health care* (p. 168). Clifton Park, NY: Delmar, Cengage Learning.

HEALTH RESOURCES AND SERVICES ADMINISTRATION. (2005). *The Registered Nurse population: National sample survey of Registered Nurses: Preliminary findings.* Retrieved July 28, 2007, from http://bhpr.hrsa.gov/healthworkforce/reports/rnpopulation/preliminaryfindings.htm

KNUTSSON, A. (2003). Health disorders of shift workers. *Occupational Medicine (London), 53*, 103–108.

Levy, B. S., Wegman, D. H., Baron, S. L., & Sokas, R. K. (Eds.). (2006). *Occupational and environmental health* (5th ed.). Philadelphia: Lippincott, Williams & Wilkins.

Menzel, N. (2006). *Workers' comp from a to z: A "how-to" guide with forms.* Beverly Farms, MA: OEM Press.

Needlestick Safety and Prevention Act. (2000). *Public Law*, 106–430.

Nelson, A. L., Motacki, K., & Menzel, N. (Eds.). (2008). *The illustrated guide to safe patient handling and movement.* New York: Springer.

Nightingale, F. (1914). *Notes on nursing.* London, UK: Harrison & Sons.

NIOSH. (1997). *NIOSH alert: Preventing allergic reactions to natural rubber latex in the workplace.* Retrieved July 30, 2007, from http://www.cdc.gov/Niosh/latexalt.html

NIOSH. (1999). *NIOSH publication no. 99–101: Stress … at work.* Retrieved July 31, 2007, from http://www.cdc.gov/niosh/stresswk.html

NIOSH. (2000). *NIOSH Publication No. 2000–108: NIOSH alert: Preventing needlestick injuries in health care settings.* Retrieved July 29, 2007, from http://www.cdc.gov/niosh/2000–108.html

NIOSH. (2002). *DHHS (NIOSH) Publication No. 2002–101: Violence: Occupational hazards in hospitals.* Retrieved July 31, 2007, from http://www.cdc.gov/niosh/2002-101.html

NIOSH. (2004). *NIOSH Publication No. 2004–143: Overtime and extended work shifts: Recent findings on illnesses, injuries, and health behaviors.* Retrieved August 4, 2007, from http://0-www.cdc.gov.mill1.sjlibrary.org/niosh/docs/2004-143/

Occupational Safety and Health Act, Sec. 5a. (1970). *Public Law*, 91–596.

Orellana, D., Busch-Vishniac, I. J., & West, J. E. (2007). Noise in the adult emergency department of Johns Hopkins Hospital. *Journal of the Acoustic Society of America, 121,* 1996–1999.

OSHA. (1991). *Bloodborne pathogens - 1910.1030.* Retrieved April 3, 2009, from http://www.osha.gov

OSHA. (2004). *Guidelines for preventing workplace violence for health care and social services workers.* Retrieved August 2, 2007, from http://www.osha.gov/Publications/OSHA3148/osha3148.html

OSHA. (n.d.). *OSHA technical manual. Hospital investigations: Health hazards.* Retrieved July 31, 2007, from http://www.osha.gov/dts/osta/otm/otm_vi/otm_vi_1.html

Page, A. (Ed.). (2004). *Keeping patients safe: Transforming the work environment of nurses.* Washington, DC: Institute of Medicine, National Academies Press.

Ramazzini, B. (1713). *De morbis artificum diatriba [Diseases of workers].* Chicago: University of Chicago Press.

State of New Jersey Public Health Services Branch. (n.d.). *Workplace violence and prevention in New Jersey hospital emergency departments.* Retrieved August 4, 2007, from http://www.state.nj.us/health/eoh/survweb/documents/njhospsec_rpt.pdf

Tuller, D. (2008, July 8). Nurses step up efforts to protect against attacks. *The New York Times.* Retrieved July 12, 2008, from http://www.nytimes.com

U.S. Department of Labor, Bureau of Labor Statistics. (2007a). *Nonfatal occupational injuries and illnesses requiring days away from work, 2007.* Retrieved July 13, 2008, from http://www.bls.gov/iif/oshwc/osh/case/osnr0029.pdf

U.S. Department of Labor, Bureau of Labor Statistics. (2007b). *Table R9. Number of nonfatal occupational injuries and illnesses involving days away from work by occupation and selected natures of injury or illness, 2006.* Retrieved July 13, 2008, from http://www.bls.gov/iif/oshwc/osh/case/ostb1801.pdf

U.S. HOUSE OF REPRESENTATIVES. (2008). *Hidden tragedy: Underreporting of workplace injuries and illnesses.* Retrieved July 13, 2008, from http://edlabor.house.gov/publications/20080619Workp laceInjuriesReport.pdf

WATERS, T. R. (2007). When is it safe to manually lift a patient? *American Journal of Nursing, 107*(8), 53–58; quiz 59.

WORLD HEALTH ORGANIZATION. (2001). *Occupational and community noise.* Retrieved July 31, 2007, from http://www.who.int/mediacentre/factsheets/fs258/en/

YOUNG, D. A. B. (1995). Florence Nightingale's fever. *British Medical Journal, 311,* 1697–1700.

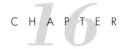

THE SUCCESSFUL MENTOR/MENTEE RELATIONSHIP

SHERYL L. CURTIS

MSN, ARNP, Clinical Assistant Professor, University of Florida, College of Nursing

A wise man learns by the experience of others. An ordinary man learns by his own experience. A fool learns by nobody's experience.

–Anonymous

LEARNING OBJECTIVES

At the completion of the chapter, the learner should be able to do the following.

1. Identify qualities and characteristics of an effective mentor.
2. Describe effective strategies for a successful mentoring relationship.
3. Analyze factors that affect the mentoring relationship.
4. Identify stages of the mentoring relationship.
5. Discuss the benefits of the development of mentoring relationships for both individual nurses and the health care system as a whole.

KEY TERMS

Mentee	Mentoring Gap	Organizational Culture
Mentor	Mentoring Relationship	Protégé
Mentoring	Novice	

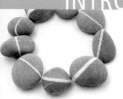

INTRODUCTION

Can you imagine a sailor beginning a long voyage across the ocean without a compass or navigational tools? In many ways, beginning a new career in nursing is much like setting sail on a very exciting, but precarious, journey. It is a journey that has been very much anticipated, with many expectations for the destinations ahead. Unfortunately, there are many opportunities to run aground in uncharted waters, to be overwhelmed by the storms of life, to become lost and find oneself at an undesired destination, or to helplessly drift along without the benefit of favorable winds. But, with proper use of the compass as a guide, one could also find oneself at the chosen destination with few delays, or perhaps at an even more desirable location that was previously thought to be too difficult to navigate.

Having the benefit of a **mentoring relationship** can offer just the kind of guidance that can be so necessary for navigating the sometimes treacherous waters of a new career. Promoting patterns of mentoring relationships within the discipline of nursing has been found to encourage scholarship and standards of excellence (Carroll, 2004). Dreher and Cox (1996) found that people who are mentored well have greater advancement opportunities, make better salaries, and in general feel that their jobs are more satisfying. In this chapter we will explore in depth the ways in which a successful mentoring relationship can impact a nurse's career, we will analyze factors that both positively and negatively affect **mentoring**, and also discuss ways in which mentoring benefits the nursing community as a whole and the organizations within which nurses work (see Figure 16-1).

Figure 16-1
Mentoring can have a positive impact on a nurse's career, and it can benefit the nursing community as a whole.

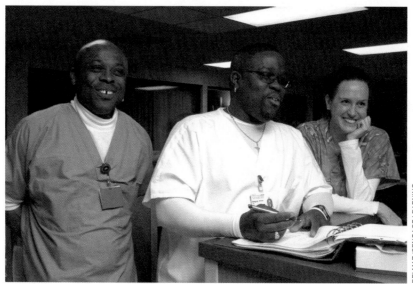

DELMAR/CENGAGE LEARNING

EXPLORING THE HISTORICAL RELEVANCE OF MENTORING

Although mentoring as a concept is relatively new to nursing (McKinely, 2004), it has been studied, taught, and utilized in the business community for many years. In fact, Stewart and Krueger (1996) reported that mentoring did not appear in the nursing literature until the late 1970s. It is currently a more frequently utilized career development tool (Gordon, 2000) and, as early as the mid-nineties, Walsh and Clements (1995) reported that 83% of influential nurses who practice in the United States have been mentored.

The word **mentor** has its origins in Greek mythology and was first mentioned in Homer's *The Odyssey.* According to the myth, Mentor was an old friend of King Odysseus who had entrusted him with the safety of his household, including his son Telemachus, while he was required to sail to Troy to fight in the Trojan War. The goddess of wisdom, Athena, who wanted to help young Telemachus, would often disguise herself as Mentor in order to be able to give guidance and wise counsel to Telemachus, helping him in his quest to find his father. As the word has evolved, mentor has come to mean a wise, experienced, and trusted advisor to someone wanting to develop professionally (Thorpe & Kalischuk, 2003; Cameron-Jones & O'Hara, 1996).

Famous **mentor–mentee** relationships have been well documented in historical accounts, literature, and the media. Medieval guild masters were concerned with not only the acquisition of skills by their apprentices, but also with the formation of their values and beliefs. Thomas Jefferson provided support and guidance to Merriweather Lewis in his preparations for his journey of exploration and scientific discovery in the uncharted regions of the western territories as described in *The Journals of Lewis and Clark* (DeVoto, 1997). Some of the other well-known, documented mentoring relationships, both real and fictional, have been Socrates and Plato, Merlin and his guidance of young King Arthur, Sherlock Holmes and Watson, Yoda and young Luke Skywalker in the *Star Wars* series, more recently Professor Albus Dumbledore to Harry Potter, and of course who could forget the beloved Spider, Charlotte, helping and guiding a bewildered Wilbur the pig in the classic *Charlotte's Web.*

Florence Nightingale, one of the most influential nurses of our time, also had many well-documented mentoring relationships with her former students (Lorentzon & Brown, 2003). One such student was Rachel Williams, with whom Nightingale had kept an active correspondence. In 1876, prior to Williams's appointment as reforming matron of St. Mary's Hospital, Nightingale advised her to proceed with caution and "not frighten doctors by starting at once any proposal to reform the nursing system or to have a training school" (Lorentzon & Brown, 2003, p. 269). Williams was also counseled in reference to her relationship with Dr. Sievking, an influential member of the Board of Governors: "St. Mary's is his primary object—the proposition of the training school would have to come from him" (Lorentzon & Brown, 2003, p. 269). Nightingale was integral in the preparation of Williams for this role by offering her emotional support, advice, and inspiration throughout their long-standing correspondence with each other.

MENTORING DEFINED

As defined by Lois Zachary (2005), "mentoring is best described as a reciprocal and collaborative learning relationship between two (or more) individuals who share mutual responsibility and accountability for helping a mentee work toward achievement of clear and mutually defined learning goals" (p. 3). In a mentoring relationship, learning is the vital process, purpose, and outcome of that relationship. Building, maintaining, and encouraging a relationship of mutual accountability and responsibility is essential to keeping this learning focused and on track (Zachary, 2005).

A mentor is someone with experience, usually, but not always, older, who is able to assist a mentee with personal, career, and professional development (Horton, 2003). The mentoring relationship can be formal, but is more often an informal relationship that had been formed mutually by both the mentor and the mentee. Hom (2003) describes it as a "role that an individual assumes in order to assist someone to grow and learn through transference of expertise" (p. 39). Mentoring is about investing your time, energy, personal knowledge, and values to support and promote the professional development of another (McKinley, 2004). Stewart and Krueger (1996) defined mentoring in nursing as a progression of education and learning that is encompassed within a long-term, personal, reciprocal relationship that develops between two nurses who are at different levels of expertise, who have different personalities and credentials, and who typically have generational differences. "Many, if not most, nursing leaders believe their careers benefited from mentors who took an interest in them" (Smith, McAllister, & Crawford, 2001, p. 102).

Many terms have been used interchangeably within the context of mentoring. "Coach," "preceptor," "teacher," and "instructor" have all been used to describe mentoring, but there are some very basic differences among these terms. As defined by Carolyn Hope Smeltzer (2002), a coach is someone who "provides an objective analysis and professional advice" (p. 501). This is usually a structured, formal relationship involving training, encouragement, and problem solving. A preceptor is usually assigned by an organization to instruct a new employee or a student in the policies, procedures, and expectations of the organization and to indoctrinate them into the organizational culture. The preceptor is usually determined to be a person of experience and maturity with good interpersonal skills. It is a formal relationship, very job specific, and takes place within a predetermined, finite length of time (Hom, 2003). A teacher or instructor is someone with expertise and knowledge in a given discipline charged with the teaching and instruction of students needing this information and these skills to progress in their chosen field. This is a predominately formal, structured relationship, but often a teacher not only shares information, but also can share values and can have the ability to influence pupils.

THEORETICAL FRAMEWORKS FOR MENTORING

Having a foundation based on theoretical frameworks can be invaluable in guiding the successful mentor–mentee relationship (Carroll, 2004). One such framework that can be utilized throughout the relationship is Parse's (1998) *Human Becoming Theory*. Emphasizing the creative process of unfolding as a nurse, rather than determining a list of stages and the interventions required for each particular stage, is the focus underpinning this theory. "Human becoming theory invites new nurses to imagine the nurses they want to become and mentors to help new nurses move in the direction of their choice" (Carroll, 2004, p. 319). Parse (2002) talks of mentoring as "a moment to moment process that arises in the beliefs and values that come up between an experienced professional and **novice**" (p. 97).

For any nurse entering a new career, from the new graduate to the experienced nurse changing careers or responsibilities, the task of developing the technical, psychosocial, and perhaps clinical skills required of the new position can be overwhelming and both physically and mentally taxing. Mentors to these nurses need to be aware of the enormous amount of emotional and mental support that is required as these nurses try to achieve competency and skill acquisition in their new careers. Patricia Benner studied how nurses develop skills, proficiency, and critical thinking in order to help those given the task of guiding these nurses through this process. Benner's (2001) novice-to-expert theory recognizes five levels of nursing skill acquisition and demonstrates a continuum in the development of proficiency in nursing from the new novice to the expert professional. This theory has been incorporated in the theoretical framework of many successful mentoring programs and highlights just how much emotional and mental output is necessary for someone to develop competency in the field of nursing (Hom, 2003).

Another theory that has been utilized in mentoring programs is Kanter's (1977) theory of organizational empowerment. This theory was initially utilized in business settings and was based on Kanter's in-depth study of a large American corporation. It has since been utilized extensively in health care settings. Kanter postulated that one's perceived access to empowerment structures (information, resources, opportunities, and support systems) was related directly to personal attitudes and behaviors in the organizational setting. An empowered work environment can provide access to these empowerment structures, thus facilitating and stimulating the growth and development of those who work within this environment (Nedd, Galindo-Ciocon, & Belgrave, 2006). One means of encouraging these empowered work environments is through the implementation of programs where mentoring is the mechanism utilized to provide less-experienced nurses with the empowerment tools of opportunity, resources, information, and support.

CHARACTERISTICS AND RESPONSIBILITIES OF SUCCESSFUL MENTORS

Mentoring is not just for a select few members of the profession; anyone who has the experience, enthusiasm, and interest in the career development of another can participate in a mentoring relationship. However, there are some qualities that a mentor should possess to ensure the success of this relationship (Figure 16-2).

A good mentor should possess knowledge, leadership skills, relevant experience, and have a sense of self-confidence and comfort in their role. Owens and Patton (2003) describe this person as someone who is at a point of strength in their career and a role model that is worthy of both observation and emulation, and who embodies everything that someone just beginning a career would aspire to. A mentor should also possess good interpersonal skills, including the ability to listen to and motivate others (Kay & Hinds, 2002). They must be available both physically and

Figure 16-2
While anyone who is experienced and interested in the career development of another colleague can be a mentor, there are some qualities such as knowledge, leadership skills, and self-confidence and comfort in their role, among others, that help ensure a successful mentoring relationship.

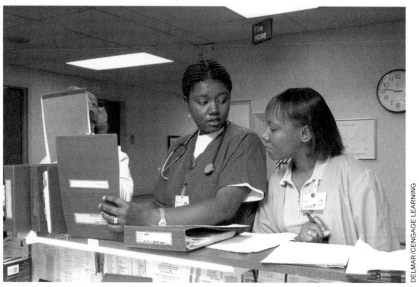

DELMAR/CENGAGE LEARNING

emotionally for their mentee to give advice, career counseling, and encouragement. They should be nonjudgmental and able to create an atmosphere of trust that gives the novice a chance to test boundaries and grow in a safe environment. A mentor should also feel free to share their dreams and professional values, helping to instill a sense of vision and direction in their protégée. They should encourage independent thinking, provide opportunities for their mentee to excel, and have high, but achievable, expectations.

The ultimate goal of a mentor should be that of helping their mentee reach their full potential by helping them to recognize their own personal strengths and weaknesses, by encouraging them to stretch and challenge themselves, by monitoring and evaluating their achievement of goals, and by identifying troublesome areas that may be impeding professional progress (Roman, 2001). Mentors are the "eye openers, door openers, idea bouncers, and problem solvers" (Horton, 2003, p. 191). But most importantly, mentors will often develop bonds with their protégées that create a sense of connection with them that fosters the commitment to invest the time and energy required for a successful and mutually rewarding mentoring relationship (Roberts, 2003).

Writing
Exercise
16-1

Think about the environment in which you presently work or have had clinical experiences. How diverse is this environment, and what have been some of the interactions, both positive and negative, that you have witnessed between your coworkers? Do you feel that a higher degree of diversity in a group of people represents more overall benefits to both individuals and the organization, or more challenges? How do you feel diversity can affect someone's ability to mentor or be mentored by another? Write down your thoughts on this and be prepared to discuss in class.

CHARACTERISTICS OF SUCCESSFUL MENTEES

The art of mentoring is a very dynamic process and a mentoring relationship is often, but not always, initiated by the mentor. Those entering a new career in nursing, whether it be that of novice staff nurse, nursing manager, or even a new faculty role, should be keenly aware of the benefits that a mentor could impart to the progression of their career and actively seek out those who could potentially provide mentoring to them. As nurses begin to consider those peers that they might want to develop a mentoring relationship with, they also need to be aware that certain personality traits, general characteristics, and attitudes may increase their appeal to prospective mentors and also enhance their ability to be mentored.

For a mentoring relationship to be successful, mentees must be able to effectively assess their own needs, determine and articulate their specific goals, know their own unique strengths and talents, and have a realistic understanding of the limits of the relationship. Mentees need to be open to receiving help and constructive criticism, and willing to ask for assistance or guidance (Sherwen, 2003). Nurses that are most likely to thrive and grow professionally under the guidance and support of a mentor are those nurses who have good listening and observation skills, who are able to effectively utilize feedback, who are open to different learning processes, who are not afraid to fail or take risks, and who are willing to make good use of the opportunities provided by their mentor. Also those who are active, assertive learners and who can demonstrate confidence in their ability to share ideas, opinions, and thoughts tend to obtain greater benefits from the mentoring process (Grindel, 2003).

Characteristics that are found to be attractive to potential mentors are those of motivation, professionalism, strong self-identity, willingness to take initiative, a passion for work, and a sense of commitment to career. It is also of benefit for the mentee to develop and demonstrate trust-building behaviors such as speaking firmly and frankly, confidence, asking appropriate questions, consistency, avoidance of being overly critical or judgmental, and respecting others as unique individuals.

Writing Exercise 16-2	As in many other professions, evaluation is an integral component of the nursing process. The exercise of self-evaluation is also very important in any situation where growth and maturation are required to advance professionally. Examine yourself and write down those qualities that you possess that would make you a good candidate for mentoring and those that would represent some challenges for a potential mentor. Also write down the aspects of your personality that would facilitate your ability to mentor a colleague now or in the future.

Many factors can affect the development and quality of a mentoring relationship, but those seeking this relationship should realize that mentoring is a two-way street, and that they must be willing to actively participate in the process, making a commitment to developing and changing themselves. They must form a partnership with their mentors to take full advantage of all the relationships have to offer.

MENTORING STAGES/PHASES

For most of us, change has become a constant in our fast-paced, hectic, technology-infatu-ated world. There are also many well-defined, expected patterns of change and progression in our lives—the changing of the seasons, the growth and development of a child, the educa-tion process, the achievement of major milestones in our lives such as graduation, marriage, or beginning that first job. For it to be effective and successful, the mentoring process, too, must evolve through a series of progressions or phases of development with the end goal being the transition of the mentee to an independent, productive, confident member of the organization.

Kram (1991) theorized that the mentoring relationship has four stages (see Figure 16-3). The first stage is "initiation" or the beginning of the relationship. Next is the "cultivation" stage, where the relationship grows and develops. The third stage is the "separation" stage, where the mentee begins to become more independent. Finally is the stage of "redefinition," when the relationship is either terminated or matures into a friendship.

Fox, et al., (1992) described three phases of mentoring: "recognition and development," "emerging independence," and "letting go" (see Figure 16-4). In the first phase, "recognition and development," both the mentor and **protégé** recognize the need for and begin their mentoring relationship. They will "size each other up," establish mutual expectations for and commitment to the relationship, and develop trust and respect. This phase represents the greatest "cost" to the mentor in terms of time, resources, and emotional energy. In the next phase, "emerging independence," the mentor uses his or her power base, status, and experience to enhance the learning experience of the novice. The novice benefits from self-discovery, awareness of newly acquired competence, and the continued encouragement and emotional support of the mentor. The mentor begins to see the "fruits of his or her labors" as the protégé continues to develop skills, self-confidence, and independence. The last phase, "letting go," is the final phase of the mentoring process, where the major task of this phase is the realignment of the relationship or its termination.

Figure 16-3
Kram's Four Stages of the Mentoring Relationship. *(Data from Kram, 1991.)*

Kram's 4 Stages of the Mentoring Relationship

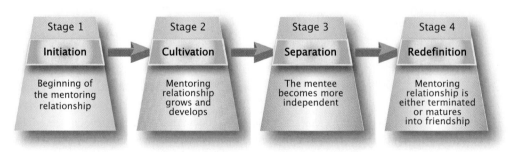

Stage 1	Stage 2	Stage 3	Stage 4
Initiation	Cultivation	Separation	Redefinition
Beginning of the mentoring relationship	Mentoring relationship grows and develops	The mentee becomes more independent	Mentoring relationship is either terminated or matures into friendship

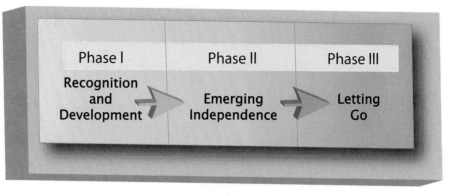

Figure 16-4
Fox, Rothrock,
and Skelton's
Three Phases of
the Mentoring
Relationship. *(Data
from Fox, et al., 1992.)*

Kochan and Trimble (2000) concluded that the process of mentoring has four distinct stages (see Figure 16-5). The first stage is "laying the groundwork," where both individuals decide that they want to be involved in the mentoring process and begin to asses their needs and define their goals. The second stage is the "warm-up" stage. In this stage both mentor and mentee begin to define the terms of their relationship. They next enter the "working" stage of the relationship, which involves the ongoing process of mentoring. The final stage is "long-term status," where there is an assessment of the relationship as to whether the goals of the relationship have been met, and whether the relationship should be continued or terminated.

Even though all of these authors express differing terms for the progression of the mentoring relationship, they all seem to agree that the goal of the relationship should be the development of the novice into an independent, successfully functioning member of the organization. Many of these successful dyads go on to become good friends, colleagues, and even develop comentoring relationships.

Internet
Exercise
16-1

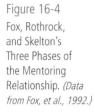

Do an Internet search for mentoring programs offered by different health organizations both in this country and internationally. Compare and contrast the goals, the method of enrollment, the communication mechanisms, and the overall structure of the various programs. Here are some examples of Web sites pertaining to nurse mentorship programs (go to each Web site and type in "mentoring" in the search box): UC Davis Health System: http://www.ucdmc.ucdavis.edu; Australian Rural Nurses and Midwives: http://arnm.asn.au; University of Virginia Health System: http://www.healthsystem.virginia.edu.

Figure 16-5
Kochan and
Trimble's Four
Distinct Stages
of the Mentoring
Relationship. *(Data
from Kochan and
Trimble, 2000.)*

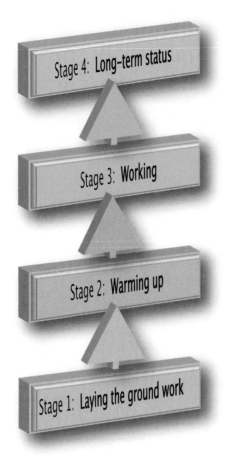

MENTORING FUNCTIONS AND STRATEGIES

With the reality of nursing shortages looming on the horizon and for some organizations already becoming a familiar struggle, the concept of mentoring is getting a second look as a potential tool to increase nurse retention and job satisfaction. In the evaluation of the relevance of mentoring in the attainment of these goals, it is important to discuss some of the functions of a mentoring relationship and to examine the strategies that help create a successful relationship.

Sharing the significant priorities of the job and the profession with their protégés is an important role of the mentor. They must guide and support them toward leadership roles and in doing so provide help, advice, and encouragement throughout the process. They must increasingly challenge the mentee to attain their goals and in the process spark the acquisition of new skills and build on internal strengths (Cullen & Luna, 1994). The concept of mentoring as having three critical characteristics in the form of a structural role, an organizational role, and a career development relationship was illustrated by Yoder (1990).

Pinkerton (2003) identified two elements of a mentoring relationship, the career function and the psychosocial function. Coaching, challenging, stimulating, protecting, sponsorship, skills acquisition, exposure and visibility, and faith in the potential of their protégé are all components of the career function of mentoring. The psychosocial function entails counseling, promoting confidence, nonjudgmental acceptance, role modeling, identity clarification, role development, and friendship.

Development of a protégé's career is one of the primary goals of a mentor. By smoothing the path, stimulating and supporting them, and facilitating both their personal and professional growth, the mentor is integral in expediting the mentee's ability to function in their new role. The mentor must also be able to help their mentee to fully utilize and capitalize on their strengths while recognizing, overcoming, and compensating for their areas of weakness.

Socialization of the mentee into the **organizational culture** is another very important function of a mentor (Figure 16-6). Most organizations have their own sets of rules, both written and unwritten, their own particular language, goals and values shared by the organizational members, social taboos and perhaps some "sacred cows," and an infrastructure of networking and communication that could be very confusing and foreign to someone new to the organization. A new member in an organization can also have a very small power base. By utilizing a mentor's

Figure 16-6

An important function of a mentor is helping to socialize the mentee into the organizational culture.

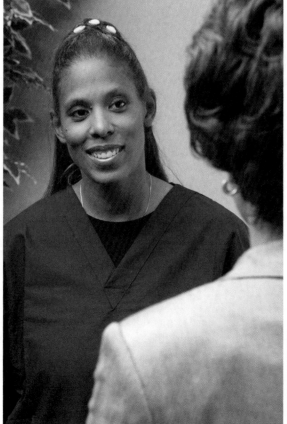

DELMAR/CENGAGE LEARNING

"reflected power" and expert guidance, mentees are able to survive the challenges and overcome the barriers to their acceptance into the organization. Helping to establish a networking system for their mentees and introducing them to influential colleagues are other ways in which a mentor can help advance the careers of their protégé. Greene and Puetzer (2002) found that good mentoring relationships can affect all areas of a mentee's career, and that through role modeling, the mentor can also promote a sense of pride and respect for the profession of nursing.

Mentoring has been predominately viewed as a very spontaneous, informal relationship that develops between two people, offering the satisfaction of helping in the development of another person for the one, and the career benefits provided for the other. But as for any good and effective relationship, there are strategies for mentoring that, if used, can determine the success of the relationship. The two parties must first develop mutual goals and then periodically reevaluate them as the relationship evolves. There must be dedicated time given to the relationship and steps should be taken to allow for frequent contact, utilizing communication means that are both accessible and convenient for both individuals. The mentor needs to be knowledgeable in the principles of adult learning and the concepts of a process-oriented relationship (Grindel, 2003). Lastly, no successful mentoring relationship can be sustained without an atmosphere of mutual trust and assurance of confidentiality.

THE SUCCESSFUL MENTORING RELATIONSHIP

Stewart and Krueger (1996), after an extensive review of current literature, concluded that the concept of a mentoring relationship included six essential attributes: a teaching-learning process; a reciprocity or mutuality; a career development relationship; a knowledge or competence difference between novice and expert; a time duration of several years; and a resonating phenomenon resulting in those who have been mentored mentoring others. Young and Perrewe (2000) developed a model that examines the relationships of formally assigned mentors and their mentees in a corporate organizational structure. They examined five factors that they believed affected the development and maintenance of a mentoring relationship. These factors were individual characteristics, relationship factors, environmental factors, career factors, and relationship type. They felt that the individual characteristics that most affected the mentoring relationship were individual learning styles and the skill of the mentor.

Typically, most people will present information in the learning style in which they are most comfortable unless they make an effort to discern their student's particular learning style. Adult learners generally fall into one or a combination of three distinct learning styles; auditory learners; kinesthetic or tactile learners; and visual learners (Hom, 2003). Auditory learners comprise about 20–30% of adults. They learn best if material is presented in a lecture format or with case situations discussed. Kinesthetic/tactile learners make up about 30–50% of adults. They do best in situations where learning involves their whole body such as role playing, simulation, and hands-on learning with return demonstration. The visual learners represent about 30–40% of adults. They want to visualize the learning process and feel most comfortable with videos, handouts, flip charts, and diagrams (Hom, 2003). Having compatible teaching/learning styles plays an important role in the mutual satisfaction of the mentoring experience.

The skills and comfort level of the mentor can have a significant impact on whether or not the goals of the relationship are achieved. Personality traits and habits in a mentor can have a definite adverse affect on a relationship. Mentors who break their promises, lack structure in their teaching, are poor communicators, have little consistency in their decision making, have difficulty investing time in the relationship, and are either overprotective or have unrealistic expectations tend to cause feelings of frustration and discontent in their mentees. With the utilization of metaphor, Nancy Busen and Joan Engbretson (1999) explored some "toxic" mentoring relationships. These were the "sculptor" approach, the "show-biz mom," and the "master-slave" metaphor. In the "sculptor" approach the mentor attempts to mold the protégé into a newer version of themselves and does not take into account that the protégé is a separate individual with a mind of their own, refusing to acknowledge any mutuality that would normally exist in a positive mentoring relationship. In the "show-biz mom" relationship, the mentor attempts to control the protégé and often becomes quite enmeshed in the relationship, becoming overbearing, smothering, and often inappropriate in their actions. The protégé very often needs to physically and emotionally break free of the relationship to be able to progress on their own career path. The last metaphor is that of "master-slave." In this relationship, the mentor, in a superior position of unchallenged power, attempts to totally control the experience of the protégé. The protégé is seen as a means of achieving the mentor's goals and career aspirations, usually with little regard to the protégé's own needs. This relationship can often be abusive, with the protégé continuing in it for fear of reprisal (Busen & Engbretson, 1999). In fact, many times ineffective mentors are a product of poor mentoring relationships themselves. Other characteristics that can have a bearing on the relationship and the compatibility of both persons involved are the individual's locus of control, self-esteem, need for power and control, need for achievement, the degree of altruism present, and the ability to communicate with each other (Young & Perrewe, 2000).

The unique backgrounds and experiences of the individuals, their attraction to each other, their level of commitment to the relationship, their personal and professional interests, and the degree that generational differences affect the alliance are all relationship factors that can determine whether or not the partnership continues until the mutual goals are achieved, or sours and becomes disagreeable to the extent that the relationship ends. For a mentoring relationship to be mutually satisfying there must be a level of trust such that both the protégé and the mentor can share in not only the successes, but also in the challenges and shortcomings that they may face. For this to happen there must be healthy self-esteem, mutual respect, and the ability to openly communicate on the part of both parties (Stewart & Krueger, 1996). A capacity for accepting and working with diverse cultures and an understanding of and skills in dealing with the generation gap are also very valuable traits for a mentor to posses.

In many workplaces there are now four different generations of nurses all working side by side with each other. Nurses who grew up in different time periods may have varying work ethics, values, and career expectations that can play a role in how they react or respond to various work-related situations (Kupperschmidt, 2000). They also tend to communicate in very different ways.

Nurses who were born in the aftermath of the Great Depression (1922–1945) are considered "traditional" or "veteran" nurses. They typically tend to respect authority, like to conform, and value logic. They tend to be hard workers, frugal, and loyal to organizations and managers (Kupperschmidt, 2000). They have usually been raised in traditional, nuclear families and most are not skilled in or comfortable working with newer technologies. Their leadership style tends to be directive, commanding, and controlling in nature and they like to work individually. Respect for their work is a motivating factor.

Nurses born in the Baby-Boom generation (1946–1964) are for the most part optimists and believe in involvement both in the community and their workplace. They usually have a strong work ethic and commitment to an organization. They can be idealists and workaholics who will value challenge and self-fulfillment in their careers, and can harbor a distrust of authority figures (Kupperschmidt, 2000). They are more likely to come from families who have been involved in divorce. Their leadership style is very consensual and collegial and they tend to be team players who love to have meetings. Feeling valued and needed can be motivating factors for these nurses.

Generation-Xers or "millennial" (1965–1980) nurses like to strike a balance in their life between their work and play time. They value their time off and tend to want flexibility in their schedules. They view the opportunity for skills acquisition and ways to increase their market-ability as vitally more important than a sense of loyalty to an organization. They tend to prefer "teamwork, experiential activities, and more involvement in their learning" (Billings, Skiba, & Connors, 2005, p. 130). Many of these nurses came from families where both parents worked or single-parent households, and quite a few had experiences as "latch-key" children. Their leadership style focuses on the equality of each individual and how each one brings their own set of strengths to the workplace. They tend to be multitaskers who are very comfortable with technology, and in fact view it as a necessity.

The last generation of nurses is the Generation-Y (1981–2000) nurses, who typically tend to be representative of the new graduate nurses. They tend to be very confident, good at mul-titasking, realistic, and social. They are usually very goal-oriented, entrepreneurial, and also comfortable with technology. They tend to view work as a means to an end and tend to have a participative style of interacting, and thus enjoy working on group projects. Many of these nurses have grown up in very diverse and blended families and tend to value balance in their life. They typically do not do well with delayed gratification and are most satisfied if they have immediate rewards for their efforts.

Having as many as four different generations of nurses in one organization, all working side by side, can present some substantial challenges (Figure 16-7). McKinley (2004) has described a phenomenon, termed a **mentoring gap,** wherein more-experienced nurses take the attitude that they have seen and done it all while working with younger nurses. They resent younger nurses who may disagree with them, often labeling them as cocky and arrogant for speaking up. Younger nurses may not respect the opinions of older nurses, feeling that they lack creativity and innovation and are outdated in their thinking. These attitudes may anger older nurses, as they do not feel valued or respected. Being aware of and knowledgeable about generational diversity can help mentors view these differences in attitudes and behaviors from a perspective that allows them to bridge this "mentoring gap."

The amount of organization support, the presence of adequate resources, and the types of reward structures, both formal and informal, are all environmental factors that can play a role in how successful mentoring is within an organization. Zachary (2000) looked at an organization's "mentoring culture" and discussed indicators of this within an organization. Some of these indicators were: the accountability of an organization toward mentoring; infrastructure in place to support mentoring programs; demand for mentoring; a common mentoring language; role

Figure 16-7

Four Generations of Nurses Working Together Side by Side in an Organization. The dynamics of these four groups shift as different groups interact with one or more of the other groups, which can also impact mentoring relationships.

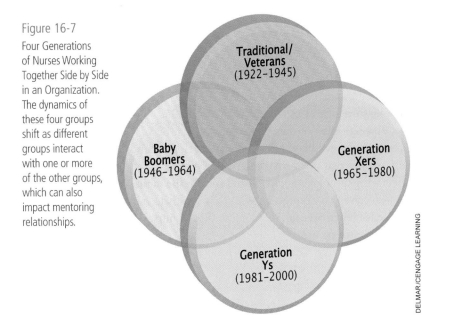

DELMAR/CENGAGE LEARNING

modeling; the presence of safety nets, including the expectations of privacy and confidentiality in the relationship; multiple venues for mentoring; and adequate training and education programs for potential mentors. Zachary (2000) also explored how the alignment of mentoring programs within an organization was reflected in the organization's goals and mission statement, and the degree to which mentoring was valued by the organization.

How important both mentors and mentees view the process in career development, and the amount of time, effort, and commitment that is willing to be made by both parties, are some career factors that affect the mentoring relationship. Finally, the relationship type, as well as the methods of communication, are influential in the development of the mentoring partnership. Mentoring can be either formal and structured, with these relationships usually having some organizational involvement, or informal and spontaneous. Whatever the relationship type, it is extremely important for its success to have frequent, consistent communication between the two individuals involved in the relationship. This communication can occur via telephone, e-mail, or correspondence if a face-to-face relationship is not always possible (Grindel, 2003).

Writing Exercise 16-3

We have explored how mentoring relationships are formed and some of the factors influencing the success of these relationships. Think back to any time in your past experience that you have been involved in a mentoring relationship or perhaps have witnessed this relationship in others. Do you feel that this relationship was successful and benefited both parties? Provide a written description of the environment and context in which this relationship developed, and the factors that either contributed to the success of it or were barriers to its progression. Be prepared to discuss this in class.

MENTORING A DIVERSE NEW GENERATION

Typically, when most nurses think of mentoring, they think of the new graduate nurse. But, as nurses advance and grow in their careers, they will be presented with many different opportunities to be mentored by and to mentor others. There may be opportunities to advance into a nurse manager role, to return to school, to become an educator, or to take on a more advanced nursing role. Through each of these transitions, it can be very important to have a strong mentoring relationship to facilitate the process of developing into this new role. Upon exploration of the various roles that mentoring can play in nursing, it becomes readily apparent that while basic mentoring principles and strategies remain the same across groups, certain populations of nurses also have some unique needs. New graduate nurses, minority nurses, nursing faculty, and nurse leaders/managers represent groups of nurses that need some special considerations during the mentoring process.

The New Graduate

A new graduate's first experience working as a nurse can be one of the most stressful and challenging of their career (Greggs-McQuilkin, 2004). They can also be dealing with generational differences in their relationships with their new colleagues (Green & Puetzer, 2002). Very often these new graduates are experiencing "reality shock" and are trying to integrate the values taught in school with the realities of practice. New graduates can benefit from strong role models who share their values and can guide and nurture them through this initiation into practice. Effective mentoring of these new graduate nurses has been proven to greatly decrease the costs to health care organizations by decreasing the amount of time required for the orientation process and improving retention rates (Greggs-McQuilkin, 2004). Respect and active listening are very important when working with new graduates. Interruptions, physical distractions, and anticipation of a reply are all deterrents when communicating with a novice nurse. Maintaining good eye contact and paraphrasing a mentee's thoughts and ideas are good strategies for building a strong, nurturing relationship. It is very important that mentors are ever vigilant for feelings of negativity, superiority, or a desire to manipulate, and that they control these feelings and foster open-mindedness, tolerance for new ideas, encouragement, and patience in dealing with their new protégées.

The Minority Nurse

The face of America is becoming increasingly culturally diverse and the workplace, including the health care environment, is beginning to reflect this at dizzying rates. However, the nursing workforce continues to lag behind the rest of the country, with minority nurses continuing to be underrepresented. Recruitment and retention of these minority nurses is becoming of greater importance to health care organizations, and mentoring programs for minority nurses are gaining more and more popularity. Mentoring is "a key component in building a diverse workplace focused on the development of multicultural leaders" (Washington, Erickson, & Ditomassi, 2004,

p. 167). Mentors can help assist minority nurses in understanding the cultural landscape of an organization, teaching them networking skills and helping them to maintain their sense of self-worth and personal identity. To adequately mentor minorities, individuals must possess good coping and communication skills. They need to be able to help minority nurses to navigate the intricacies of an organization's culture while at the same time having a perspective on how that nurse's particular culture and ethnic background might influence their reactions to situations.

Washington, Erikson, & Ditomassi (2004) discuss their "Five C's" of effective mentoring strategies for minority nurses (see Figure 16-8). They are "Candor, Compromise, Confidence, Complexity, and Champion" (p, 168). Candor is the ability to be honest about issues such as bias or concerns related to loss of ethnic identity, while maintaining an atmosphere of trust and inclusion. Compromise is teaching the minority nurse to develop the art of not "winning the battle while losing the war" and instructing them in effective problem solving and negotiation skills. Confidence is the concept of preserving the minority nurse's ethnic and cultural individuality, while at the same time encouraging them to work as a valued member of the team. Complexity is the acknowledgment that cultural and diversity issues have strong historical roots, and can be highly emotional. It is crucial that the mentor be able to establish a trusting relationship such that these issues can be worked through and dealt with in a constructive manner. Finally, Champion represents the idea that the mentor will become the minority nurse's advocate and supporter, providing opportunities for personal growth and career advancement.

Some goals for the minority nurse to achieve would be to discover how to be assertive in confronting issues as opposed to demonstrating avoidance or passive-aggressive behaviors, to be able to ascertain if there are "hidden agendas" in feedback that is received, to become skilled at negotiation, to learn to develop cross-cultural relationships, and to learn effective strategies for dealing with intra-cultural conflicts.

Figure 16-8
Washington, Erikson, & Ditomassi's (2004) Five C's of Effective Mentoring Strategies for Minority Nurses.

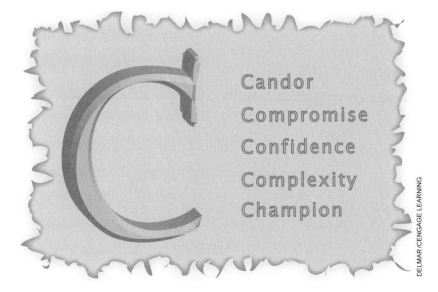

Candor
Compromise
Confidence
Complexity
Champion

DELMAR/CENGAGE LEARNING

New Nursing Faculty

New faculty are often overwhelmed with the stresses of meeting the needs of students, the education system, work expectations, and meeting obligations to professional organizations that they are involved in. Nursing colleges are currently examining how the mentoring of junior faculty can help with retention and foster excellence in teaching. Mentoring by senior faculty members can help junior faculty members to prioritize activities, learn organizational skills, and evaluate their own learning needs. Senior faculty can provide opportunities for junior faculty to gain new knowledge, stretch and challenge them mentally, and participate in activities that can strengthen their curriculum vitae. Senior faculty can help promote team building and socialize newer faculty into the culture of the college organization (Horton, 2003).

To be successful mentors, senior faculty members should be aware of the policies and procedures of their particular educational organization. They should anticipate and be prepared to deal with mistakes that will be made by junior faculty, offering support, guidance, and role-modeling appropriate responses to situations. Senior faculty need to provide ongoing, constructive feedback and to help junior faculty develop teaching strategies, discover methods to improve their knowledge of subject matter, and to help them in identifying available resources.

Novice Nursing Leaders

Traditionally those nurses who have excelled in the clinical setting have been the ones that have been encouraged to transition to leadership and management positions. Very often these same nurses who possessed such excellent clinical skills would have had little if any management training or skills. They would find that they had gone from a position of expert knowledge in their clinical area to one of being a virtual novice at the skills required for effective management (Gershenson, Moravick, Sellman, & Somerville, 2004). They typically have not had any formal orientation to the role and many times would find themselves feeling overwhelmed, frustrated, and inadequate, and ultimately then fail in this role.

New managers need to develop new models for practice to help them thrive in this role. They need to move from a task-oriented to a skill-oriented pathway of career development. They need to look at not only short-term goals, but at the long-term view or "big picture," and they will have to begin to evaluate the needs of the whole unit at the possible expense of individual needs and desires. Being able to function in this role requires much planning, as there are constant interruptions and distractions and the new nurse manager must develop skills in prioritization, conflict resolution, budget management, staff motivation, and effective communication.

Mentoring can be crucial to the development of a nurse manager and leader, and organizations would have much to gain by having mentors for these novice leaders. These mentors can ultimately decrease costs by minimizing management turnover, increasing staff satisfaction, and improving unit efficiency through effective management. They can prepare new leaders by identifying appropriate learning opportunities, serving as resources and guiding them through many of the multiple challenges of management. Mentors need to be aware that these new managers, as adult learners, have the ability to diagnose, plan, implement, and evaluate their own learning. They are usually self-motivated and self-directed, but need guidance on how to achieve their goals.

New nurse managers can have several different mentors, each to facilitate growth in different areas of their role. New managers should seek out mentors who have similar philosophies and goals, and realize that it can also be advantageous to have a mentor both inside of the organization and external to it (Grindel, 2003). An effective mentor can help a novice manager acquire the skills and qualities necessary for good leadership, such as integrity, the ability to network and work collaboratively, political sensitivity and candor, management, team building, and communication and organizational skills (Gershenson, et al., 2004).

CASE SCENARIO 16-1

You have been working as a staff nurse on a busy orthopedic floor for the past five years. Finally, after working many schedules of "off shifts" over the years, you have enough seniority to work your preferred shift, which is three twelve-hour day shifts per week. This schedule has been working very well for you and it has been much easier for you in dealing with family obligations. You also are aware that a charge nurse position will become available in the next six months or so, and you are very interested in it. There has been an increased shortage of nurses in your area and your hospital has decided to hire a group of new nurse graduates from the Philippines to increase staffing. You have heard rumors that their starting hire salary is equivalent to what you are now receiving and you find this troubling, as you have not gotten a raise for the past three years because of the hospital's budget shortfalls. One day your nurse manager pulls you aside and asks you to participate in a new nurse mentoring program for the nurses from the Philippines. You would have to change to a Monday-through-Friday evening-shift schedule and would not receive any extra pay for this, but your nurse manager does state that this would demonstrate maturity and leadership on your part, two traits that she admires highly. You feel that taking on this role would increase your chances of securing the charge nurse position and with some hesitation agree to be a mentor.

CASE ANALYSIS

1. You may experience some negative emotions in this situation that could potentially adversely affect your mentoring relationship. Describe some actions that you could take to proactively deal with these emotions.

2. The nurses that you are mentoring are not only new graduates, but also from a foreign country. Describe how their learning and mentoring needs might differ from those of a newly hired, experienced nurse from this country.

3. List some strategies that you feel might be beneficial in mentoring these nurses.

4. The addition of these nurses increases the diversity on this floor. Develop some creative plans and ideas for fostering a mentoring culture on this floor.

BENEFITS OF MENTORING

The benefits of mentoring relationships are numerous from organizational, professional, and personal perspectives. Based on predicted population reports, the U.S. Department of Health and Human Services (2002) reports that it anticipates that the national nursing deficit is expected to be about 29%, or approximately one million nurses, by 2020. From an organizational standpoint, mentoring can decrease attrition, which has been shown to increase costs to an organization and decrease the morale of remaining members. Mentoring can enhance the quality, creativity, and productivity of members, while at the same time decreasing boredom and stagnation (Grindel, 2003). An organization that fosters a work environment based on a mentoring culture increases the job satisfaction of its members and has been shown to improve retention rates (Grindel, 2003).

CASE SCENARIO 16-2

You have been working on a very busy medical-surgical floor for the past three years. You have noticed an extremely high turnover rate on your unit since you have begun work there. In fact, there are very few of the nursing staff that you originally began working with who still work on your floor. You have also observed that the morale of the nursing staff has begun to be affected, with an increase in the number of sick calls, constant pleas to work overtime, and very little teamwork during working hours or socialization of any kind after. The hospital management has also begun to take note, as this has become a hospital-wide issue and is felt to be adversely effecting patient satisfaction and ultimately hospital revenues. After hiring a consultant and examining the problem extensively, the hospital management has decided to create a mentoring program as one solution to the high rate of turnover with the nursing staff. Your nursing supervisor has asked you to be part of a task force charged with the development and implementation of a mentoring program for nursing.

CASE ANALYSIS

1. In the development of this program, what theoretical framework do you feel would be most relevant and applicable to the situation at hand?

2. What are some of the factors, unique to both the hospital as a whole and also to the individual units, that you would need to consider while developing this program?

3. What are some strategies that you would utilize to foster a mentoring culture in your hospital? How might those strategies differ from unit to unit?

4. What will be the role that nursing management plays in the implementation of this program? Hospital administration?

5. Explore and discuss some different approaches for disseminating information on the implementation of this program to the nursing staff.

6. What tools will you use to evaluate the effectiveness of this program and why?

From a professional level, nurses that have been mentored have been shown to have higher earnings, increased confidence and self-esteem, increased opportunities for promotion, and are generally more prepared for leadership roles (Grindel, 2003). They do not have to "reinvent the wheel" as they can learn from mistakes that mentors have made in the past and made their mentees aware of. Mentoring also strengthens the nursing profession by developing new leaders and building a professional culture among nurses. Nurses who are mentored tend to then go on and in turn mentor others. It has been documented that Rachel Williams, who was mentored by Florence Nightingale, went on to also mentor several protégés (Lorentzon & Brown, 2003).

Lastly, mentoring can have very profound rewards for both the mentee and the mentor. There can be personal and professional growth for both individuals from the stimulation and challenge of the relationship. Mentors can also gain insights into their own goals and experience career revitalization and satisfaction from peer and organizational recognition of their efforts.

SUMMARY

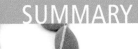

As today's health care environment becomes more complex, diverse, and ever changing, nursing leaders are needed now more than ever. Nurses are expected to function in roles that require ever-greater clinical and cultural competence and need experienced, reliable mentors to guide them (Smith, McAllister, & Crawford, 2001). "The mentoring process encourages development of leadership skills, advancing the protégés vision not only for individual success, but also for the future of nursing as a profession" (Owens & Patton, 2003, p. 43). In this chapter, we have explored various aspects of the mentoring process, including characteristics of mentors and those that they mentor, the functions of a mentoring relationship, factors that affect these relationships, and strategies for successful mentoring. Potential mentors need to be aware that effective and successful mentoring requires time, effort, and education. Developing good mentoring skills and strategies can do much to enhance and enrich the mentoring relationship, regardless of the situation in which mentoring occurs. Providing novice nurses with good mentors can go a long way in changing attitudes and nursing's appetite for "eating its young." Establishing a mentoring environment and culture will help to nurture nurses and facilitate healthy growth. Nurses on all levels must begin to recognize and comprehend the complex interconnections among leadership, organization culture, and the achievement of effective mentoring programs. This will enable nurses to begin to create empowering, innovative, and vibrant cultures that foster and nurture mentoring (Bally, 2007). This in turn can help organizations begin to deal with and correct some of the issues that have led to the current nursing shortage. The nursing profession and individual nurses can experience many benefits from involvement in mentoring relationships and programs. Mentoring is an ongoing, dynamic partnership that not only prepares individuals for their career paths, but also instills in them the desire to return the favor by mentoring others, which thus ultimately strengthens the nursing profession.

I choose to risk my significance,
To live so that which came to me as seed
Goes to the next as blossom
And that which came to me as blossom,
Goes on as fruit.

–Dawna Markova

REFERENCES

BALLY, J. M. (2007). The role of nursing leadership in creating a mentoring culture in acute care environments. *Nursing Economics, 25*(3), 143–148.

BENNER, P. (2001). *From novice to expert: Excellence and power in clinical nursing practice.* Upper Saddle River, NJ: Prentice Hall Health.

BILLINGS, D. M., Skiba, D. J., & Connors, H. R. (2005). Best practices in web-based courses: Generational differences across undergraduate and graduate nursing students. *Journal of Professional Nursing, 21*(2), 126–133.

BUSEN, N. H., & Engebretson, J. (1999). Mentoring in advanced practice nursing: The use of metaphor in concept exploration. *The Internet Journal of Advanced Nursing Practice, 2*(2). Retrieved March 9, 2008, from http://www.ispub.com/ostia/index.php?xmlFilePath=journals/ijanp/vol2n2/mentoring.xml

CAMERON-JONES, M., & O'Hara, P. (1996). Three decisions about nurse mentoring. *Journal of Nursing Management, 4,* 225–230.

CARROLL, K. (2004). Mentoring: A human becoming perspective. *Nursing Science Quarterly, 17*(4), 318–322.

CULLEN, D. L., & Luna, G. (1994). Mentoring: A valuable tool for professional development. *AARC Times, 18*(7), 34–35, 66.

DEVOTO, B. (Ed.). (1997). *The Journals of Lewis and Clark.* Boston: Houghton Mifflin Company.

DREHER, G. F., & Cox, T. H. (1996). Race, gender, and opportunity: A study of compensation attainment and the establishment of mentoring relationships. *Journal of Applied Psychology, 81*(3), 297–308.

FOX, V. J., Rothrock, J. C., & Skelton, M. (1992). The mentoring relationship. *American Operating Room Nurse Journal, 56,* 858–867.

GERSHENSON, T. A., Moravick, D. A., Sellman, E., & Somerville, S. (2004). Expert to novice: A nurse leader's evolution. *Nursing Management, 35*(6), 49–52.

GORDON, P. A. (2000). The road to success with a mentor. *Journal of Vascular Nursing, 18*(1), 30–33.

GREENE, T. M., & Puetzer, M. (2002). The value of mentoring: A strategic approach to retention and recruitment. *Journal of Nursing Care Quality, 17*(1), 63–70.

GREGGS-MCQUILKIN, D. (2004). Mentoring really matters: Motivate and mentor a colleague. *Medsurg Nursing, 13*(4), 209, 266.

GRINDEL, C. G. (2003). Mentoring managers. *Nephrology Nursing Journal, 30*(5), 517–522.

HOM, E. M. (2003). Coaching and mentoring new graduates entering perinatal nursing practice. *Journal of Perinatal and Neonatal Nursing, 17*(1), 35–49.

Horton, B. J. (2003). The importance of mentoring in recruiting and retaining junior faculty. *AANA Journal, 71*(3), 189–195.

Kanter, R. M. (1977). *Men and women of the corporation.* New York: Basic Books.

Kay, D., & Hinds, R. (2002). *A practical guide to mentoring.* Oxford, UK: How To Books.

Kochan, F. K., & Trimble, S. B. (2000). From mentoring to co-mentoring: Establishing collaborative relationships. *Theory into Practice, 39*(1), 65–76.

Kram, K. E. (1991). *Mentoring at work: Developing relationships in organizational life.* Glenview, IL: Scott Foresman.

Kupperschmidt, B. (2000). Multigenerational employees: Strategies for effective management. *Health Care Manager, 19*(1), 65–76.

Lorentzon, M., & Brown, K. (2003). Florence Nightingale as 'mentor of matrons': Correspondence with Rachel Williams at St. Mary's Hospital. *Journal of Nursing Management, 11,* 266–274.

McKinley, M. G. (2004). Mentoring matters: Creating, connecting, empowering. *American Association of Critical-Care Nurses, 15*(2), 205–214.

Nedd, N., Galindo-Ciocon, & Belgrave, G. (2006). Guided growth intervention: From novice to expert through a mentoring program. *Journal of Nursing Care Quality, 21*(1), 20–23.

Owens, J. K., & Patton, J. G. (2003). Take a chance on nursing mentorships: Enhance leadership with this win-win strategy. *Nursing Education Perspectives, 24*(4), 19–20.

Parse, R. R. (1998). *The human becoming school of thought: A perspective for nurses and other health professionals.* Thousand Oaks, CA: Sage.

Parse, R. R. (2002). Mentoring moments. *Nursing Science Quarterly, 15,* 97.

Pinkerton, S. E. (2003). Mentoring new graduates. *Nursing Economics, 21*(4), 202–203.

Roberts, D. (2003). Mentoring: The future of nursing. *MedicalSurgical Nursing, 12*(3), 143.

Roman, M. (2001). Mentors, mentoring. *Medical Surgical Nursing, 10*(2), 57, 59.

Sherwen, L. N. (2003). Finding a mentor: What every nursing student should know. *Nursing News, 27*(3), 16.

Smeltzer, C. H. (2002). The benefits of executive coaching. *Journal of Nursing Administration, 32*(10), 501–502.

Smith, L. S., McAllister, L. E., & Crawford, C. S. (2001). Mentoring benefits and issues for public health nurses. *Public Health Nursing, 18*(2), 101–107.

Stewart, B. M., & Krueger, L. E. (1996). An evolutionary concept analysis of mentoring in nursing. *Journal of Professional Nursing, 12*(5), 311–321.

Thorpe, K., & Kalischuk, R. G. (2003). A collegial mentoring model for nurse educators. *Nursing Forum, 38*(1), 5–15.

U.S. Department of Health and Human Services. (2002). *Projected supply, demand and shortages of registered nurses, 2000–2020.* Retrieved October 29, 2007, from ftp://ftp.hrsa.gov/bhpr/workforce/rnsupplyanddemand2002.pdf

Walsh, C. R., & Clements, C. A. (1995). Attributes of mentors as perceived by orthopaedic nurses. *Orthopedic Nursing, 14*(3), 49–56.

Washington, D., Erickson, J. I., & Ditomassi, M. (2004). Mentoring the minority nurse leader of tomorrow. *Nursing Administration Quarterly, 28*(3), 165–169.

Yoder, L. (1990). Mentoring: A concept analysis. *Nursing Administration Quarterly, 15,* 9–19.

Young, A. M., & Perrewe, P. L. (2000). The exchange relationship between mentors and protégés: The development of a framework. *Human Resource Management Review, 10*(2), 177–209.

Zachary, L. J. (2005). *Creating a mentoring culture: The organization's guide.* San Francisco: John Wiley & Sons, Inc.

17

THE NURSING ROLE IN THE NEXT DECADE

K. ALBERTA MCCALEB

DSN, RN, Administrative Director, UAB Center for Nursing Excellence, University of Alabama Health System, University Hospital Professor, University of Alabama School of Nursing University of Alabama at Birmingham

To know even one life has breathed easier because you have lived—that is to have succeeded.

–Ralph Waldo Emerson

LEARNING OBJECTIVES

At the completion of the chapter, the learner should be able to do the following:

1. Describe societal influences affecting the role of the nurse in the next decade.
2. Describe population trends for the next decade.
3. Discuss issues in the workforce today that will affect the work of the nurse tomorrow.
4. Discuss issues in health care that affect the role of the nurse.
5. Discuss trends and changes in the role of the nurse of the future.

KEY TERMS

Cultural Sensitivity
Ergonomics
Health Care System
Knowledge Workers

Nursing Role
Nursing Shortage
Professional Nursing Practice
Population Trends

Roles of the Professional Nurse
Workforce Diversity
Environment

INTRODUCTION

It's been almost a decade since the world was concerned about the predicted effects of moving electronic and computerized clocks and calendars from 1999 to the year 2000. Many predicted that our technology was not sophisticated enough to handle this change. Many citizens prepared for major catastrophe, including the destruction of our societal infrastructure and the loss of resources essential for daily living. Forecasters in almost every category of American life tried to direct our thinking as to what would happen in the next decade. The discipline of nursing was no different. For many decades, the profession of nursing has tried to predict issues that will be faced in the next decade, such as supply and demand, health care delivery, and the environment that will exist for the workforce of the future. Kerfoot (2001) wrote "nursing as we know it today will not exist in the future; to be a viable entity in the years ahead, nursing will need to reinvent itself several times over in order to survive" (p. 919). Certainly, the last 5–7 years have seen some change in the profession of nursing, but not catastropic change. Perhaps the greatest change has been in the increased seriousness of the **nursing shortage**, both in the practice and academic arenas. In addition, there has been continuing change in the work of the nurse as it relates to technology advancement, cultural diversity of the population, and health care delivery system mergers (Figure 17-1). Many of these

Figure 17-1
Change faced by nurses in the next decade will continue to involve advancements in technology, as well as the nursing shortage, the diversity of the population, and health care delivery system mergers, among others.

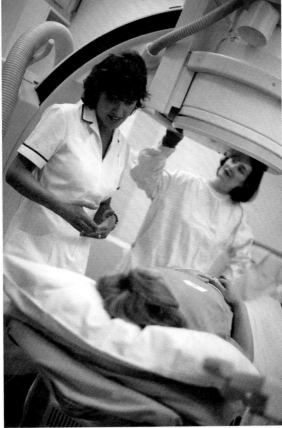

COURTESY OF GETTY IMAGES.

issues will continue to drive changes in health care delivery, professional **nursing roles**, and work-force alterations well into the next decade.

Currently, our society and the health care delivery system face a number of challenges. Nursing as a practice discipline has the opportunity to be a solution to many of the issues relative to health and health care delivery for the nation's public. These opportunities will be laden with challenges such as: population trends, **workforce diversity**, global economics, health care delivery shifts, and continuing advancements in technology and health care-related information systems. Without question, nurses must continue to plan now for the next decade and the challenges the discipline faces. In fact, the resolution of some of the re-occurring issues in nursing must be addressed in the next decade. These issues include differentiated practice, educational entry into **professional nursing practice**, re-engineering workforce delivery models, work environment improvement, and access to health care for America's citizens. To continue to be passive about these issues will pave the way for other disciplines to replace nurses in some sectors of the health care delivery system. What a travesty for the citizens that nurses serve! In 2020, will nursing look back and wonder why? Or, will nurses be working together with a unified vision of their legitimate roles in the health care delivery system of the future?

Writing Exercise 17-1	Explore the Internet for literature to support each question below. Discuss the latest information relative to future trends in nursing and the health care delivery system. Which one is the hardest to predict and why?

1. What U.S. trend will affect the practice of professional nursing most in the future?

2. What are the traditional roles of the professional nurse?

3. What role shifts have already occurred in nursing in the first decade of the 21st century?

4. Where will nursing practice be delivered in 2010, 2015, and 2020?

5. What level of education will the nurse need to implement the roles needed by society?

TRENDS FOR THE FUTURE

There are several societal issues that will affect nursing and the nursing workforce in the next decade. To better understand how these trends and issues will affect nursing, it is important to recognize the effect that these variables will have on society, health care delivery, and global economics in general. According to Snyder (2007), two of the most dramatic changes that will affect nursing are the aging population trends and the shift of patient care from a hospital-based-delivery to home-based-delivery care model. Likewise, the future will continue to hold advances in technology, new discoveries related to treatment modalities, and the globalization of society. These changes in health care delivery will be more complicated as the general patient population expands in life expectancy. In addition, the patient population will consist of a plethora of cultural differences and ethnic backgrounds.

Changing Population Trends

One of the most publicized changes occurring in American society is that of an aging population. According to the U.S. Department of Health and Human Services (2006), in 2006 just over 12% of the population was over age 65; however, by 2030 that number is expected to be around 20%, with almost 9% of the elderly aged 85 or over (see Figure 17-2). This aging of the American population will affect every aspect of society including challenges for families, businesses, and health care providers. The effect on America's workforce is yet to be realized; however, it is likely that the multigenerational market for employment of America's workforce will continue. Currently, larger businesses have faced the unprecedented challenge of three generations

Figure 17-2
Number of Persons 65+, 1900–2030 (numbers in millions). *(Courtesy of U.S. Department of Health and Human Services Administration of Aging, 2006.)*

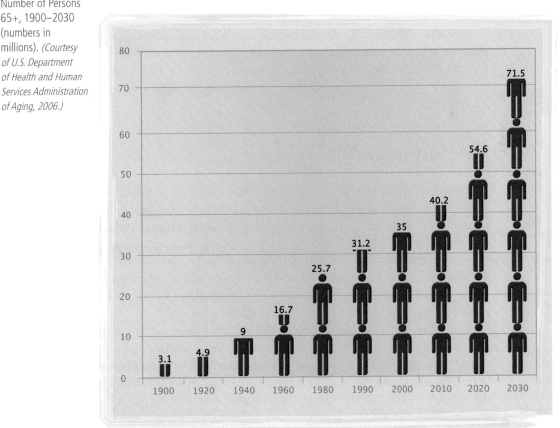

**Number of Persons 65+,
1900–2030** (numbers in millions)

Year (as of July 1)

working together in the workforce. In the baby-boomer generation alone, there are 78 million persons born between 1946 and 1964 all turning 65 or older in the decade between 2010 and 2030 (Bleich, Connolly, Davis, Hewlett, & Hill, 2006). With the changing life cycles of an aging population, and with life expectancy promising to increase above 77 years of age, the workforce will continue to experience four generations of workers. A workforce mix with multiple generations that exhibits differences in values and work ethics will likely cause role conflict and role transition to occur not only in the health care provider professions, but in many disciplines in the American industry.

Another **population trend** that is likely to affect many disciplines, nursing notwithstanding, is the declining number of precollege students available to enter the disciplines that require higher education and work/practice experiences. Byrne (2005) described the pipeline for high school students who will be matriculating into higher education by the middle of the next decade. Freshman who will enter college in 2015 were born in 1997. The number of entering freshman is expected to continue to rise slightly for the remainder of the 2000s. By 2010, high school graduates are estimated to be nearly 3.2 million, but begin to decrease after that. It is estimated that by 2015 there will be a more diverse student population entering higher education: approximately 1.58 million white, 367,000 black, and 546,885 Hispanic high school graduates. The challenge for disciplines like nursing is to attract these young students to a service-oriented profession in the midst of highly competitive offers from other professional disciplines. Certainly, nursing as a predominantly female discipline has seen great change in the number of males coming into the profession; however, numbers relative to racial diversity continue to lag behind population trends in society (AACN, 2007). There is opportunity in the future to increase the number of recruits into nursing with racially diverse backgrounds.

Health Care System Changes

Another observation seen already in this decade is the shift in health care services from an acute-care-focused model to a home-and-community-focused model of care. The aging population will continue to cause a strain on the costs of health care services. Patients and their families will seek nursing care services to assist them in making decisions about health care as well as serve as a health care coach who can teach, monitor, and promote health care behaviors. Nurses are educated to care for the holistic needs of the patient and their families. It is only logical that the nurse will be one of the first health care providers accessed by the patient and family in time of need for services, health education, coaching, and counseling.

Of particular concern to every American citizen is the rising cost of health care. This scenario will likely continue well into the future; as citizens age, new technologies are discovered to improved health care delivery, and new therapies are discovered to enhance the human condition. Who will pay for the health care services of tomorrow? Will third-party payers survive the increasing costs of health care services coupled with an aging population in need of those services? What role will the government and policymakers play in trying to decrease the overall rising cost of health care for the entire country?

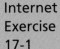

Internet Exercise 17-1

With regard to policy makers and governmental monitoring of health-care policy, the nurse can be a major influence on the passage of legislation that affects the nursing discipline. Nurses must be astute and knowledgeable about the policy process as well as current legislation at the local, state, and national levels that will inform future health policy. To increase your own knowledge, follow the steps below:

1. Go to the Web site http://thomas.loc.gov and enter the word "nursing" in the "search bill text" screen. This will send you to all current legislation, both House and Senate, that contains the word "nursing."

2. Choose one of the bills and read it.

3. Analyze the bill in terms of your own nursing knowledge. Is the bill one that promotes nursing? Are you supportive of it?

4. How would this bill inform and impact policies and your own practice?

Health Care Technology and Treatment Innovations

The demands of new technology and treatment innovations will call for the most knowledgeable health care provider seen in the health care arena. Not only will the sophistication of technology and treatment modalities increase, but the need for knowledge workers in the **health care system** will continue to escalate. Patients, who are more knowledgeable themselves due to improved health information access via the Internet, television, and news media, will continue to demand the most knowledgeable worker for guidance and assistance in planning care activities to promote health or recovery from illness. With improvements in technology and access to treatment options that are available independent of the health care provider, some patients and families have been able to regulate their own health care and access to services in a traditional primary care setting.

New innovations in technology and information systems will likely increase electronic access to health care information not only by health care providers, but also patients and their families (Figure 17-3). Electronic pathways and digital technology will continue to increase access to health care information by consumers as well as improve diagnostic processes for patients. Robotics and computerization will continue to increase across businesses, homes, and the health care system. Nurses must be knowledgeable in the use of such technology in order to promote the health of patients and families.

Globalization of Society

Advances in technology, communication, and international mobility have expanded the world view of society. Today, the term "distance" seems relative. World globalization of the economy, intercultural access, and increased knowledge of issues that face the people of any country have

Figure 17-3
Innovations in technology and information systems will increase health care providers' access to health care information.

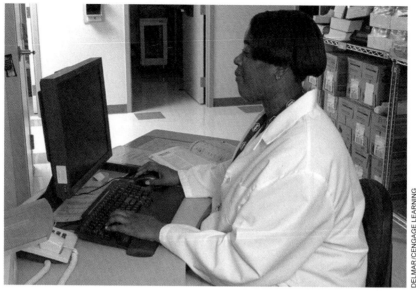

caused the perception of the world to be not so "distant" or to be "small." The societal mix of many cultures affects every citizen and the economy, especially the health care enterprise. **Cultural sensitivity** in the workplace will be a primary focus for ongoing education of health care providers. The need to understand and be sensitive to the needs of people from different cultures will continue to increase throughout the next decade.

Writing Exercise 17-2	Given the discussion about societal issues that will affect the people of our country in the next decade, write a short story about your neighborhood and how population trends and changes in culture have affected your community. Include examples from business, education, religion, and government. Include any issues obvious in your community that were not mentioned. Decide on the top two priorities for participating in the change process in your community.

TRADITIONAL ROLES OF THE PROFESSIONAL NURSE

Professional nurses assume a number of roles when providing nursing care to patients and families. Simply defined, a **role** is "a cluster of prescribed actions; the behaviors we expect of those who occupy a particular social position" (Myers, 2005, p. 90). Nurses are prepared to implement multiple roles depending on the needs of the patient, their family's situation, and the environment. Traditional roles of the professional nurse include caregiver, communicator, teacher, client advocate, counselor, change agent, leader, manager, case manager, and research consumer (Berman, Snyder, Kozier, & Erb, 2008). When describing the roles of the professional nurse today, Ellis and Hartley (2008) included the roles of therapist, role model, and coach. It should be noted that these roles are not utilized in isolation of each other, but rather, the nurse is knowledgeable and skilled in the use of multidimensional role sets to enhance the quality of patient-care outcomes. The future in health care delivery will require a knowledgeable, educated nurse who is able to work within multisystem structures to plan, implement, and evaluate the highest levels of quality-care outcomes for the patient and family.

While these traditional roles are often associated with clinical practice, it must be noted that the roles are also applicable to the advanced practice nurse, academician, researcher, and policy maker. Nurses must continue to advance their experiences, educational backgrounds, and leadership skills in order to affect change not only within the profession of nursing, but also at the systems level within health care delivery and academic educational settings.

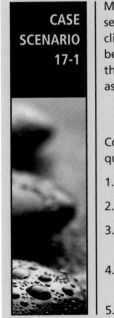

CASE SCENARIO 17-1

Mike is a master's-prepared nurse who has decided to leave the clinical practice setting and join the ranks of academic faculty. He has been working in his role as a clinical nurse specialist in oncology nursing for the last five years. In addition, he has been serving the local university nursing program as a clinical instructor for the last three years. In his new role, he will be engaged in teaching, scholarship, and service as it relates to his expertise in clinical practice.

CASE ANALYSIS

Considering Mike's history and new role as a faculty member, answer the following questions:

1. What are the specific roles for Mike in the academic setting?

2. Differentiate between role confusion and role conflict.

3. What role confusion is possible in the transition from practice to the academic setting?

4. Considering Mike's expertise in oncology, what are the roles that he will likely focus on with students at the undergraduate level? Master's level?

5. Describe any areas of role conflict that Mike might have in his new job.

FUTURE TRENDS AND THE NURSING ROLE

In the next decade, nursing will be affected by changes within the larger context of society. The population cannot get older, new technologies continue to go where no one has ever gone before, and the health care settings expand to meet the needs of the consumer without a tremendous re-evaluation of nursing and its role in society. Heller, Oros, and Durney-Crowley (2007) purport ten changes that will affect nursing as a discipline (Figure

Figure 17-4

Ten changes
that will affect
the nursing
discipline *(Heller,
Oros, and Durney-
Crowley, 2007.)*

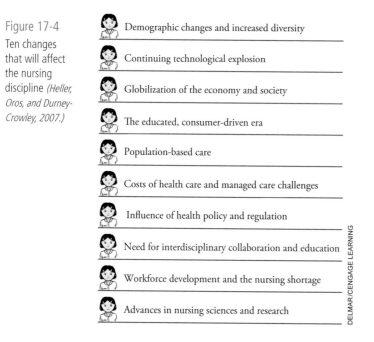

Demographic changes and increased diversity

Continuing technological explosion

Globilization of the economy and society

The educated, consumer-driven era

Population-based care

Costs of health care and managed care challenges

Influence of health policy and regulation

Need for interdisciplinary collaboration and education

Workforce development and the nursing shortage

Advances in nursing sciences and research

DELMAR/CENGAGE LEARNING

17-4). These include: demographic changes and increased diversity; continuing technologi-cal explosion; globalization of the economy and society; the educated, consumer-driven era; population-based care; costs of health care and managed-care challenges; influence of health policy and regulation; need for interdisciplinary collaboration and education; work-force development and the nursing shortage; and advances in nursing science and research. The beginning of the new millennium has been a time to analyze the roles that the nurse will need to assume for the future. There is still much to do as the profession continues to examine the traditional roles of the nurse and the potential need for new and expanded roles in the future.

Workforce Demographics

Population statistics provide a projection of the issues that nursing will face both in aca-demia as well as the practice setting. Simply stated, it can be predicted that many positions in both practice and educational settings will be left unfilled when the baby-boomers begin to retire over the course of the next decade. With the largest number of practicing nurses in their mid-forties, coupled with increasing vacancies left by retirements, it is expected that the nursing shortage will continue to increase in both practice and academic settings. The American Association of Colleges of Nursing Fact Sheet (2007) pointed out an often-quoted statistic from the U.S. Bureau of Labor Statistics, "the U.S. nursing shortage will grow to more than 800,000 registered nurses" by 2020. This statement coupled with the potential decline in number of possible high school graduates available to recruit into nursing yields quite a concern for the next decade and beyond. Likewise, Auerbach, Buerhaus, and Staiger (2007) provided workforce data that projected a shortfall of nurses by 2020 of approximately 800,000. Of interest in the projections is the need for entry-level nurses to meet the growing needs of high-acuity patients. Nothing in the data mentions the shortfall of nurses who will move from the high-acuity sector to home and community-based care as health care delivery shifts. In addition, it is likely that the shortfall of master's- and doctoral-prepared nurses needed to educate the entering nurses of the future will continue to exist. These two indicators alone will add to the nursing shortage complexity. Without question, as the shortage worsens, the roles of the nurse will need to expand to create mechanisms for meeting the needs of the consumer.

Workforce Redesign

The literature is compelling with regard to the need to further define the role of the nurse based on educational, experiential, and credentialing backgrounds. It is time to take a serious look at the knowledge and skill outcomes of educational programs and to modify practice models

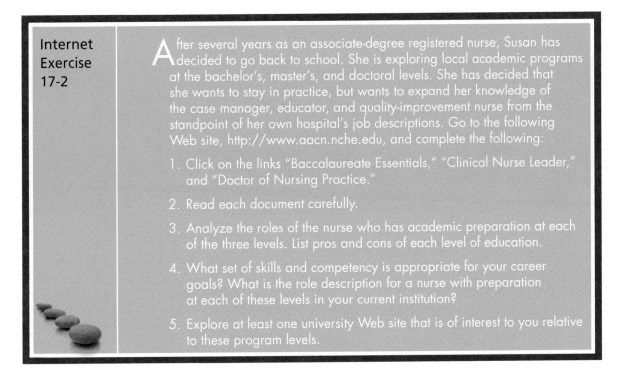

Internet Exercise 17-2

After several years as an associate-degree registered nurse, Susan has decided to go back to school. She is exploring local academic programs at the bachelor's, master's, and doctoral levels. She has decided that she wants to stay in practice, but wants to expand her knowledge of the case manager, educator, and quality-improvement nurse from the standpoint of her own hospital's job descriptions. Go to the following Web site, http://www.aacn.nche.edu, and complete the following:

1. Click on the links "Baccalaureate Essentials," "Clinical Nurse Leader," and "Doctor of Nursing Practice."

2. Read each document carefully.

3. Analyze the roles of the nurse who has academic preparation at each of the three levels. List pros and cons of each level of education.

4. What set of skills and competency is appropriate for your career goals? What is the role description for a nurse with preparation at each of these levels in your current institution?

5. Explore at least one university Web site that is of interest to you relative to these program levels.

accordingly. A total, comprehensive evaluation of the work environment with careful planning for a work model that encompasses safety design, **ergonomics**, efficiency in resource utilization, and cost/benefit financial indicators point to the need for overall work environment redesign as a major priority. The next decade will provide the opportunity to change work teams and design of patient care delivery to include new **knowledge workers** such as the Clinical Nurse Leader (CNL) and the Doctorate of Nursing Practice (DNP). While educational outcomes can assist in job redesign, patient outcomes and the expertise needed for patient care delivery must also be considered.

Another element of work redesign is the inclusion of nurses who are at retirement age but not ready to leave the work environment. These nurses add a dimension of experiential wisdom, knowledge, and skill that would cost several thousand dollars to replace through the orientation of an inexperienced, less-knowledgeable nurse. Work settings must examine the value added to the organization by assisting these nurses to stay in the workforce. Bleich, et al., (2007) gathered data from "seasoned" nurses to identify new, innovative positions that institutions could create for aging nurses. These new positions included: "Team Builder, Chief On-Boarding Officer, Best Practice Coach, Quality Coach, Technology Facilitator, Senior Consultant/Cost-Benefit Analyst, Preceptor/Mentor, Community Liaison, Research Assistant, Relief Nurse, Safety Officer, Communicator, Patient Educator, and Family Advocate" (p. 30). Without question, the loss of a "seasoned" registered nurse with sage wisdom is not only a knowledge drain on the nursing services department, but also a financial burden for the system. Visionary nurse leaders must engage in a careful analysis of the overall nursing staff and make hypothetical projects of retirement timelines, succession planning, and career development opportunities that provide incentives for the retention of the most qualified nurses in the institution.

| Writing Exercise 17-3 | Given the concepts of work redesign, identify the characteristics of the unit that you currently work on or last worked on. Identify the unit layout issues, material and human resource issues, patient population, and economic concerns. Plan a different, but efficient, work redesign model for the future. Include physical, human, and economic resources needed to implement the plan. If there are retirees on your unit that need to be reassigned, describe the institutional needs for their knowledge and expertise. |

Health Care Delivery System Shifts

Due to health care costs, population projections, and shifts in delivery-of-care settings, it is estimated that the future will hold a drastic shift from care delivered in acute-care settings to community and home environments. This shift in health care will cause some variation in the role of the nurse, with primary caregiver responsibilities shifting from the health care provider to the family members. Nurses will become facilitators of care, coaches, health educators and counselors. Not only will this shift in care affect the role of the practicing nurse, but also the educational programs that prepare entry-level nurses. Critical thinking and decision-making skills are essential in work environments that are unpredictable. The nurse will have to be knowledgeable and flexible in not only identifying priorities but changing them based on the situation encountered in the home.

As health care shifts to the community from hospital settings, the profession of nursing has the opportunity to be the answer to problems with health care access. Nursing is the answer to high-quality, lower-cost access to health care, and subsequent triage to higher acuity and specialty care, if needed. Advanced practice nurses and nurse faculty are in strategic positions to form a partnership link between consumers and the health care system. In the collaborator role within the health care team, the nurse functions in the role of primary care provider, health educator, health coach, and liaison for the entire health care system experience. For the patient, the nurse becomes the health care "concierge" in assisting the consumer to access quality health care services.

SUMMARY

Without question, the next decade will hold many opportunities for professional nursing to modify its roles, work design, and practice models. Population trends will not only affect society as a whole, but also workforce development trends in nursing. The nursing shortage will continue to be affected by such population and workforce trends. While the nursing practice shortage is a challenge, it is compounded by the same population statistics and workforce shortage issues in the academic institutions. In order to ease the challenges of the nursing shortage, institutions should strategically plan for retirements of the workforce, engage in succession planning and leadership development, and develop new models of care delivery that include workers from at least four generations.

Nurses and consumers will be faced with continuing escalation of health care costs coupled with fewer consumers who are adequately insured. As the population ages, there will be a rise in age-related illnesses, typically chronic in nature, that require longer periods of high-costs treatments. Health care cost will drive a shift from hospitalization and fewer days in the hospital to more home-care service needs. Patients will be forced to move home, into intermittent care facilities, and into long-term care facilities to receive assistance in meeting their health care needs. Professional nurses and advanced practice nurses can assist in bridging the gap between high-acuity stays in the hospital and a return to independent or interdependent living outside the hospital.

The ladder of success is best climbed by stepping on the rungs of opportunity....

–Ayn Rand

REFERENCES

AMERICAN ASSOCIATION OF COLLEGES OF NURSING. (2007). *Nursing Fact Sheet*. Retrieved November 19, 2007, from http://www.aacn.nche.edu/Media/FactSheets/nursefact.htm

AUERBACH, D. I., Buerhaus, P. I, & Staiger, D. O. (2007). Better late than never: Workforce supply implications of later entry into nursing. *Health Affairs, 26*(1), 178–185.

BLEICH, M. R., Connolly, C., Davis, K., Hewlett, P. O., & Hill, K. S. (2006). *Wisdom at work: The importance of the older and experienced nurse in the workplace*. Barbara J. Hatcher (Ed.). Princeton, NJ: Robert Wood Johnson Foundation.

BERMAN, A., Snyder, S. J., Kozier, B., & Erb, G. (2008). *Fundamentals of nursing: Concepts, process, and practice* (8th ed.). New Jersey: Pearson, Prentice Hall.

BYRNE, R. (2005). Higher education 2015: How will the future shake out? *The Chronicle of Higher Education,* vol. LII, no. 14, A10–A11.

ELLIS, J. R., & Hartley, C. L. (2008). *Nursing in today's world: Trends, issues and management* (9th ed.). Philadelphia: Lippincott. Williams & Wilkins.

HEALTH RESOURCES AND SERVICES ADMINISTRATION. (2007, February). *The registered nurse population: Findings from the March 2004 national sample survey of registered nurses*. Washington, DC: U.S. Department of Health and Human Services.

HELLER, B. R., Oros, M. T., & Durney-Crowley, J. (2007). The future of nursing education: Ten trends to Watch. In *NLN National League for Nursing newsletter*. Retrieved August 10, 2007, from http://www.nln.org/nlnjournal/infotrends.htm

KERFOOT, K. M. (2001). Nursing in the new world of health care: A vision or an illusion? In N. L. Chaska (Ed.), *The Nursing Profession: Tomorrow and Beyond*. Thousand Oaks: Sage Publications, Inc., 919–930.

MYERS, D. G. (2005). *Exploring psychology* (6th ed.). Holland, MI: Worth Publishers.

SNYDER, L. (2007). Fundamental shift in nursing's future. *Advance for Nurses, 9*(27), 21–22.

U.S. DEPARTMENT OF HEALTH AND HUMAN SERVICES ADMINISTRATION OF AGING. (2006). *A statistical profile of older Americans aged 65+*. Retrieved December, 2007, from http://aoa.gov/PRESS/fact/pdf/Attachment_1304.pdf

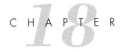

CHAPTER 18

TEST TAKING STRATEGIES, INCLUDING NCLEX, GRE, AND CERTIFICATION EXAMS

CATHLEEN M. SCHULZ

PhD, RN, CNE, FAAN, Dean and Professor, Harding University

The most important practical lesson that can be given to nurses is to teach them what to observe—how to observe—what symptoms indicate improvement—what the reverse—which are of importance—which are of none—which are the evidence of neglect—and of what kind of neglect. All this is what ought to make part, and an essential part, of the training of every nurse.

–Florence Nightingale

LEARNING OBJECTIVES

At the completion of the chapter, the learner should be able to do the following:

1. Determine the testing points of a nurse's career.
2. Discuss the relevance of predictors and personal characteristics to test-taking success.
3. Describe useful test preparation and test-taking strategies.
4. Use test anxiety reduction strategies to enhance testing success.
5. Locate personal resources for test preparation and remediation.
6. Prepare a study plan for passing a test such as the NCLEX-RN®.
7. Discuss personal surviving and thriving strategies following a test failure.

KEY TERMS

Computer Adaptive
    Examination
Diagnostic Test
First-Time Test Taker
Licensure Examination

NCLEX® Test Plan
NCLEX-RN®
Temporary Permit
Test Anxiety
Test Difficulty Levels

Test Preparation Plan
Test-Preparation Strategies
Test-Remediation Strategies
Test-Taking Skills

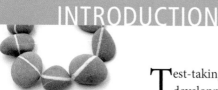

INTRODUCTION

Test-taking is a skill as critical to a nursing student's academic success as to a nurse's career development. Florence Nightingale gave "hints" for nurses to formalize their practice in her classic book, *Notes on Nursing* (1859). However, she never envisioned the testing expectations currently facing nursing students and nurses in practice. Tests will be encountered to meet program preadmission criteria, progress through a course or an entire program, graduation requirements from a program, prepare for the **licensure examination**, attain continuing education units or hours, achieve a job or promotion, enter and exit graduate school, and obtain national certification. Employers may test knowledge prior to employment such as requiring a new applicant to pass a pharmacology content test, to ensure competency such as before using a new procedure, or to demonstrate mastery of management content prior to granting a new title or position.

Nursing students have usually been tested in various ways prior to entering a nursing program. In the U.S., most of today's nursing students are very familiar with forms of computerized, oral, written, and standardized tests. Nontraditional students, such as those reentering academics after time away from studying and those with English as a second language, may find the testing environment, particularly computerized testing, more unfamiliar.

Few nursing students are prepared for the type, volume, and rigor of testing that they encounter in the nursing profession. Other health care professionals, such as pharmacists and physicians, have similar career-testing adventures; however, most health care professionals are educated and tested separate from nurses. Health care professionals are frequently prepared in educational "silos," with little opportunity for collaboration and interdisciplinary interaction. As a result, it is easy for nursing students to feel highly stressed when around colleagues who are not experiencing similar testing and program rigors.

Nursing education and nursing practice are regarded as demanding, and nurses will encounter tests throughout their careers, as displayed in Table 18-1. The important point is that nursing is a highly tested and legally regulated profession. Also, patient safety remains an ongoing national priority and testing of health care professionals is likely to be part of the public's effort to ensure that graduates have earned the privilege to care for them and to remain licensed nurses (see Figure 18.1). In preparation for the academic and practice environments, becoming the best possible test-taker precludes success in the profession of nursing.

An influential organization, the Carnegie Foundation, published a research report (Benner, Sutphen, Leonard, & Day, 2007) that said nursing education programs and nurse employers will face recommendations to meet the increasing demands of complex care environments and systems. Practice settings are not only complex because of the knowledge and skill required to practice, but also because practice takes place in complex bureaucratic settings with limited resources and economic constraints. Nurses will be asked to further form the capacity to develop a self-improving practice—one which demands habits of ongoing self-evaluation and self-improvement—and these habits involve testing skills. Preliminary recommendations include that, beginning in 2010, all entry level nurses who pass the NCLEX® after 2010 be required by

Table 18-1 Timeline of Testing Points of a Nurse's Career

	Testing Points					
Pre-College	**Pre-Admission to Nursing Program**	**During Nursing Program**	**Entry Into The Profession**	**Following Initial Licensure**	**Advanced Licensure**	**Graduate School**
ACT SAT (only taken while in high school)	Nursing pre-admission exam ATI HESI Kaplan NLN Pre RN Exam NET Pre-nursing course exams	Nursing Course Exams • Knowledge • Skills • Clinical • Simulation Benchmark Tests CPR or ACLS Tests Universal precautions test Certification test such as American Red Cross First Aid Test Outcomes • Critical Thinking • Communication • NCLEX® predictor test	Licensure Examination—NCLEX®	Pre-employment exam such as a pharmacology exam Employer competency exams such as those for critical care units Continuing education tests for CEs or CEUs (may be required for license renewal.) CPR or ACLS Testing Certification exam (may be state or employer required for a position)	Pre-employment exam Employer competency exams National certification exam (required for advanced licensure such as for nurse practitioners or nurse anesthetists) Continuing education tests for CEs or CEUs (may be required for license renewal)	Admission • GRE • MAT Progression Comprehensive exams Graduation Defense of dissertation or project may be required

Figure 18-1
Testing of health care professionals is likely to be used to help ensure that nursing graduates and licensed nurses are qualified to care for patients and ensure their safety. *(Photo by Jeff Montgomery. Used by permission.)*

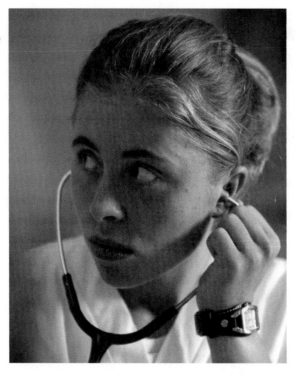

boards of registered nurses to complete a master's degree within five years of graduation (p. 21). Also recommended is that at least a one-year, planned, mandatory, post-graduation internship, focusing on one area of specialization in nursing, be offered (Benner, et al., 2007, p. 22). To prepare for this current environment and impending educational and practice changes, a nurse can little afford to not address test preparation and **test-taking skills**.

TYPES OF TESTS

The typical nursing student takes many tests, which evaluate the student's knowledge, skills, abilities, performance, and competencies. In most programs, the **test difficulty levels** increase as the students progress through the program. Essential to progression through and graduation from a nursing program is successful test taking. The wise student will spend time and energy to master test-taking skills that are as essential as writing and clinical practice are to ongoing professional success. Tests can be teacher-made or written as a professional product by a company or vendor that sells and administers tests. Table 18-2 contains common types of formal tests identified in the literature, their descriptions, and test examples likely to be encountered during a nurse's career.

Nurses are tested to determine knowledge, clinical experience abilities, critical thinking abilities, competency, promotions, course requirements, and progression towards and meeting program outcomes. Often, nursing programs require that a purchased diagnostic test be taken to assess the student's readiness for the licensure examination (NCLEX-RN®); more programs require a specific test score as a course or graduation requirement than ever before.

Table 18-2 Overview of Types of Tests Used in Nursing Education and Practice

Type of Test	Description	Examples
BENCHMARK	A test that measures a quality that faculty desire students to achieve. This may be during or at the conclusion of a course or program. A score may be used for remediation.	• ATI end-of-course test, which reports scores of variables such as communication and therapeutic nursing interventions. • NLN Physical Assessment, Community Health Nursing, Comprehensive Psychiatric and Health and Illness: Adult Care Tests
OUTCOME	A test completed at the end of a course or a program. Most often, it is an end product of a program.	• Critical Thinking Test • NLN Baccalaureate Achievement
PRENURSING	A test taken prior to admission to a nursing program. The test score may be an admission requirement or used for student remediation or placement.	• TEAS (from ATI) • NLN Preadmission Exam • NET • PreRN Examination
PRECOLLEGE	A test taken, usually in high school (or an equivalent), prior to entering college. The score may be used to determine financial funding or remediation.	• ACT (American College Test) • SAT (Scholastic Aptitude Test)
GRADUATE	A test taken prior to entering graduate school. Individual programs determine cut scores if the test is an admission criterion. The score may determine entrance status or remediation.	• GRE (Graduate Record Exam) • MAT (Miller Analogies Test)
LICENSURE	A test required by law (nurse practice act) to practice nursing in the U.S. and its territories. Note, the test is being offered abroad.	• NCLEX® • RN for registered nurses • PN for practical nurses
DIAGNOSTIC	A pretest similar in content and testing method to an actual test. Usually the test-taker receives an overall score with identified strengths and weaknesses useful for **test-preparation strategies.**	• ATI **Diagnostic Test** • HESI E^2 • NLN PreNCLEX® Readiness Tests
CERTIFICATION	A test that evaluates the test-taker's ability or knowledge about a nursing practice specialty. In nursing practice, the certification test is usually administered by a national organization and taken postlicensure. The certification may be a requirement for advanced licensure.	• Family Nurse Practitioner • Pediatric Nurse Practitioner
COMPETENCY	A test that measures or evaluates aspects of an employee's job performance.	• Drug calculation • Demonstration of a procedure • Observation while providing patient care

Success on the NCLEX-RN®; What Is at Stake?

Because all nurses take the licensure examination and nurses are unable to work unless the criteria of passing the NCLEX® is met, the NCLEX® **computer adaptive examination** is probably considered the single most important test by nurses. Even with graduation and preparatory materials, the graduate faces about an 85% chance of passing, based on national pass rates, as a **first-time test taker** or candidate; the latter term is used by regulatory bodies, such as a state board of nursing or the National Council of State Boards of Nursing, to describe a person taking the NCLEX® for the first time.

The stakes are high in many states, especially those in which graduates can work using a "**temporary permit,**" a temporary nursing license, until test results are received. Employers routinely grant a new graduate the same pay that a registered nurse receives, and the graduate often completes the same nursing practice activities permitted by state law, the nurse practice act, as a registered nurse. When a failing NCLEX® test result is received, the graduate may receive a pay decrease and no longer be able to work using the temporary permit; the state's nurse practice act and the employer's policies will determine the new graduate's work assignments or whether the graduate may remain employed. In states without "temporary permits," the graduate is unable to work until the NCLEX® is passed. Due to the nursing shortage and an attempt to speed the test retake process, graduates who are unsuccessful in taking the NCLEX® initially may retake the test within forty-five days of the previous test date. The time between testing has gradually been shortened from ninety days to forty-five days due to nursing shortage pressures in work settings. Between testing sessions, the graduate is encouraged to create a test preparation plan for success. (See Writing Exercise 18-2 presented later in this chapter.) See Table 18-3 for national pass

Table 18-3 National Pass Rates Based upon Frequency of Taking the NCLEX-RN®

Days*	Overall	U.S. Educated		Internationally Educated	
		First-time	Repeat	First-Time	Repeat
0–21	79.7%	90.1%	60.8%	70.7%	36.3%
22–33	80.9%	88.1%	54.9%	66.1%	33.7%
34–54	75.2%	85.0%	50.4%	63.6%	31.3%
55–365	49.6%	77.0%	39.2%	51.4%	21.8%

Adapted from: Eich & O'Neill, 2007, p. 1
* Days between obtaining eligibility and actually taking the NCLEX-RN®.

rates based upon the number of times test-takers take the NCLEX®. What is known about test pass rates is that the longer the candidate's time between eligibility for testing and actually taking the examination, the more passing rates tend to decrease (Eich & O'Neill, 2007).

Unsuccessful licensure testing, by law, removes a "temporary permit" or keeps new graduates from practicing nursing. Physicians, unsuccessful at licensure testing, are not kept from employment or practicing as a physician. Fair or not, the nurse faces a "no-practice situation" until the NCLEX® is passed.

The test result stakes are not only high for the graduate; the stakes are high for the nursing program and employer (Schwarz, 2005). Nursing differs from many professions, including law and medicine. No other discipline faces the publicity that a nursing program does regarding its graduates' success on a professional examination. High or low pass rates affect program funding, attraction of future students, employer desirability of graduates, donors who provide facilities and scholarships, faculty retention, and the general reputation of the nursing program. News casts, newspapers, blogs, radio and television announcements, and other forms of media are quick to publicize programs' NCLEX-RN® pass rates. Unfortunately, a negative pass rate or a 100% pass rate receives more attention than other program pass rates. The public needs reminding that the published NCLEX® pass rates indicate first-time test takers and that the total pass rate story, which includes all graduates who ultimately pass the examination, is rarely available to the public.

Employers that hire a new graduate using a "temporary permit" assume the graduate will shortly be fully functioning as a registered nurse. Employers invest time, staff, and money into orienting and preparing a new graduate for the specific organization; graduates frequently report that employers pay for them to attend an NCLEX® review course, such as HURST Review or KAPLAN Review courses, or offer a review course during orientation. Although no published quantifiers of employer resources used for NCLEX® preparation exists, it is reasonable to believe that the dollar amount is in the thousands. Hiring an employee unable to fully function, at a minimum of forty-five days between NCLEX® testing, is costly to the employer, the consumers, and industries, which pay the bill.

Regardless, graduates who do not prepare for the examination and are unsuccessful affect themselves as well as future students, employers, and health care consumers. It is in everyone's best interests, and the public's most of all, that the graduate succeed during the first test-taking opportunity.

CONCEPTS IMPORTANT TO TESTING

A few general concepts are important to understand the testing language used by nurse educators and nurse employers. The concepts are woven into nursing's education and practice fabrics. The more meaningful concepts to a student or new graduate facing tests are benchmarking, outcomes, competency, and remediation. These four concepts will drive the nurse's educational and employment expectations more than the requirements for other disciplines. In fact, these concepts permeate the rigorous demands experienced by nurses throughout their education and employment.

Benchmarking and Outcomes

Currently, benchmarking is best known by nurses as a method to identify and determine high-quality care by analyzing patient-outcome data such as patient satisfaction with care providers such as nurses, and days in the hospital. Collected by health care agencies, the data is published as hospital or agency report cards; these reports track the hospital's benchmark for quality care as compared within the industry. The cost effectiveness of the services offered, such as how many hours the patients remain in the outpatient department following surgery, is also reviewed (Rudy, Lucke, Whitman, & Davidson, 2001). The data are trended for management decisions and strategic planning.

Nursing's response to the benchmarking movement, which originated in business and industry (Rudy, et al., 2001), emerged from the American Nurses Association (ANA) as early as 1995 (ANA, 1995; 1996). Nursing-sensitive patient-outcome indicators captured the nursing role in delivering quality patient care. Both health care agencies and nurses identified "best practices" through the report cards, which compared performance to standards, also known as variables (Billings, Connors, & Skiba, 2001). Excellent results were used to describe best practice as a model for others to follow. Benchmarking is now an industry (benchmarking) within an industry (health care), and new graduates will find benchmarking an active component of employment settings.

Benchmarking in education is an emerging industry fueled mainly by political and public desires for accountability for program outcomes. Adoption has been slow and complicated due to lack of measurable standards unique to all programs. One success area has been in the student selection process because of standardized tests such as ACT and SAT. A well-known method of benchmarking in higher education involves the SAT. Annually, each U.S. state identifies a benchmark score to select National Merit Scholarship semifinalists (Hewitt, 2002). The scores vary among states depending upon the number of high school seniors residing in the state and their specific scores. All junior students who score at or above the PreSAT benchmark score are named National Merit Semifinalists.

Currently no "gold-standard" benchmarks exist for nursing education at the national level. The NCLEX® is not a gold standard, as the test addresses minimum competency to enter practice. However, the public most likely considers program NCLEX® pass rates as the gold standard

Writing Exercise 18-1	An entry-level program outcome is "critical thinking." In a final semester course, you are required, in an essay test, to analyze changes in your critical-thinking skills since the beginning of the program.

1. Identify your strengths and weaknesses in using critical thinking during practice.

2. Discuss in two typed, double-spaced pages your change in critical-thinking abilities from the beginning of the program to the present.

of a program's achievement. In addition, many state boards of nursing require continuing education to demonstrate meeting a competency for licensure renewal.

Nursing programs frequently use benchmarks such as a standardized test taken during a designated time, such as the first year, within the curriculum. These test scores are compared with scores from other programs' students taking the test at the same time. Basically, the scores are used for remediation. However, identifying and placing at-risk students in remediation programs remains the result of professional judgment based upon trends or experiences rather than empirical evidence of student or employee competence. A quickly growing trend is benchmarking competency, which involves identifying progression and graduation requirements, usually through commercially made test scores. The main purpose is to identify students in need of remediation prior to graduation and taking the NCLEX®. Although reports of successful use of progression and graduation policies appear in the literature (Morrison, Free, & Newman, 2002), the samples are too small to firmly generalize findings. This remains an area needing evidence-based nursing education research to further guide faculty who adopt benchmarking strategies and desire to create "best practice" exemplars in education.

Competency

The competency movement began in the early 1970s when the U.S. State Department wanted a new method of selecting junior foreign service information officers. Existing knowledge and aptitude tests did not accurately predict on-the-job success, plus the tests were discriminatory against minorities and people from less fluent backgrounds. McClelland (1993) and his associates sought to identify job-success-predicting factors known as competencies. By interviewing superior, average, and poor job performance officers, a set of behaviors combined with skills, knowledge, and personal attributes were identified, observed, and measured. Differences between the performance categories were used for officer selection, and these differences were placed in three categories:

1. Cross-cultural interpersonal sensitivity.
2. Positive expectations of others and the ability to maintain this outlook under stress.
3. Speed in learning political networks of influence and interests.

These same competencies would benefit nurses who work in complex, stressful, and political environments and are required to practice skills, collaborate, advocate, and think critically. Most competency evaluations in practice focus on clinical skills, a narrow focus that has a limited measurement of practice. The health care industry has been attracted to competency measures for almost three decades, primarily due to the belief that caregiver characteristics can predict or contribute to successful job performance and positive or desired patient outcomes.

Competency development in health care typically refers to improving employee job performance and care outcomes. The focus of a competency-based employee orientation or development program is the end result; that is, the ability of new employees to do their jobs. The actual driver for comptencies in nursing began in 1991 when the Joint Commission on Accreditation of Healthcare Organization (JCAHO) began requiring hospitals to prove that its workers had the ability to meet performance expectations stated in job descriptions. Hospitals have since been engaged in ever-evolving mandates on competency assessment while assuring these are relevant to the real work world of daily practice.

Competency assessment is not new to nursing and continues to evolve as a response to changes in practice patterns. Passing the NCLEX® assures the public and the law that a graduate has met a minimum competency to practice. The NCLEX® competency is based upon surveys of the practice of new graduates within six months of graduation. Numerous state boards of nursing require continuing education to demonstrate continuing competency for license renewal; generally this also meets a minimal competency requirement.

Employers rarely take a holistic approach to their competency programs due to time and costs involved in development and implementation. The outcome of a competency approach that complies with minimal standards is a competency program consisting of skills checklists outlining interventions that nurses usually provide. High employee performers are not developed and mediocre practice is accepted as satisfactory. Understanding the employers' competency approach prepares the nurse for job performance reviews, testing and evaluating competencies (see Figure 18-2), and the quality of expected nursing care. Competency assessment and

Figure 18-2
Understanding the employers' competency approach prepares the nurse for job performance reviews, testing, and evaluating competencies. *(Photo by Jeff Montgomery. Used by permission.)*

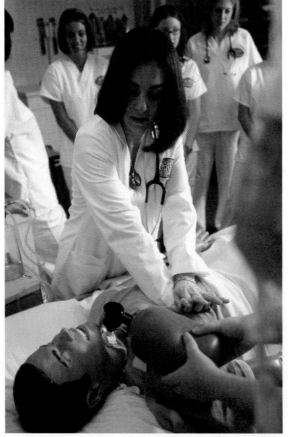

programs should emphasize what the nurse actually does and promote the development of new and experienced nurses; unfortunately, many nurse practice settings do not have a strong competency approach to employee development.

The nurse's education and practice arenas abound with competency assessments, which test knowledge, skills, and abilities (competent performance). The practice environment contains testing measures that vary by employer. Table 18-4 contains nursing competency examples expected in the three dimensions of competency (del Bueno, Griffin, Burke, & Foley, 1990).

Remediation

Students and employees may find themselves involved in test remediation activities. Trends, particularly in this time of nursing shortage, foster implementation of success strategies; many resources, including time, money, and people, were operationalized to enhance the nurse's

Table 18-4 Examples of Performance Competencies

Competency	Examples
CLINICAL AND TECHNICAL SKILLS	Knowledge Psychomotor Skills
CRITICAL-THINKING SKILLS	Planning Priority Setting Managing Change Time Management Resource Allocation Application of Ethical Principles
INTERPERSONAL SKILLS	Communication Conflict Management Delegating Collaboration Team Building Customer Service Understanding Diversity

Figure 18-3
Test Remediation
Strategies.

Informal and formal support programs can help with test remediation by:
- Increasing academic skills
- Addressing nursing knowledge deficits
- Promoting social support systems

Informal and formal support programs can offer:
- Review course
- Preparatory review books and software
- Simulated testing
- Faculty, peers and preceptors tutoring
- Test-taking skills training
- Master English language and medical language competencies

development. The capable person is too valuable to abandon to his or her own methods of test preparation. If you find yourself in a remediation situation, your attitude toward the process may affect the outcome. No person is the perfect student or employee. Shifting your attitude from one of a "victim perspective" with shame and doubts, to one of "this is part of my continuing self-development as a lifelong learner," contributes to the likelihood of a successful result.

Remediation, defined as any additional study or preparation activities, takes time. The time will be above current school or work demands. Remembering that success is in sight enables the nurse to alter present plans for the long-term goal. Engaging family and friends in a supportive way reduces the role-strain that is often felt during periods of intense test preparation. Examples of some of the more successful **test-remediation strategies** are listed in Figure 18-3. Many campuses and employers provide tutors free or for a nominal cost.

TEST-TAKER CHARACTERISTICS THAT AFFECT TESTING OUTCOMES

Predicting testing success is a complex endeavor. However, a test-taker needs to know that if more than one at-risk characteristic is present, then test preparation and test-taking skills will need increased attention for success. Knowing one's own test-taking strengths and weaknesses is critical to essential test-taking self development. For example, higher nursing GPAs from courses that lead to the diploma or degree, past positive performance on standardized or multiple-choice test items, work experience, passing an NCLEX®-PN exam, not repeating prerequisite or nursing courses, and higher preadmission test scores are all indicators of test-taking success. Licensed practical nurses, having passed an NCLEX® test, are more likely to pass the NCLEX®-RN than first-time test candidates.

There are other personal characteristics, often little known, that can be modified by the test-taker and his or her social support system to further the probability of testing success. These include family and personal stress levels, reading levels and comprehension, time management skills for test preparation, role strain due to personal and family responsibilities during school, health status, quality of sleep, and personal economic factors (Sayles, Shelton, & Powell, 2003). Each of these can contribute to a phenomenon known as test anxiety. The test-taker is provided an overview of test anxiety and strategies to prevent, minimize, and control anxiety, which impairs test-taking ability.

Test Anxiety

Anxiety, a normal human condition and a motivator in preparing for tests, can be detrimental when too much is experienced by a test-taker. In this section, test taking as a source of anxiety is a focus in the situational context of test anxiety. Test anxiety, a form of general anxiety, refers to physiological, behavioral, and personal responses that result from concern about possible failure. Too much test anxiety can interfere with the ability to prepare for and perform on tests. Most often, deficits in study habits and test-taking skills, not anxiety, are central to impaired test-taking performance. Successful strategies include targeting both test anxiety and test preparation and test-taking skills (Sheil & Meisenheimer, 1992).

The first step is to face the anxiety, then distinguish between the two types of anxiety. If the anxiety is due to lack of preparation, consider the reaction normal. If, however, you are adequately prepared but still overreact or panic, your reaction is not rational. Anyone can have these reactions, but it is helpful to know how to overcome their effects.

Preparation is the best way to minimize rational anxiety. Avoid cramming and master the main concepts of the course. Change your attitude by not overplaying the grade's importance; the grade is not a reflection of self-worth, nor does it predict future success. Consider the anxiety reduction recommendations in Figure 18-4.

If anxiety becomes unmanageable, most universities have counseling programs or support staff who work with students with a need to refine their test-taking skills. Discussing positive effects of anxiety with peers, recognizing physical responses and feelings related to test anxiety, and using biofeedback to promote relaxation are helpful anxiety-reduction strategies.

Figure 18-4
Strategies to reduce
test anxiety.

- Remind yourself that the test is only a test — you will have others.

- Reward yourself after the test (reward affirmation).

- Avoid thinking of yourself in a negative manner.

- Once you've adequately prepared for a test, do something relaxing.

- Avoid classmates who generate anxiety and tend to upset others; anxiety is "contagious."

- If waiting for a test causes anxiety, distract yourself by:
  - Thinking about the post-test reward
  - Going to the restroom, if permitted
  - Telling yourself "I can be anxious later, now is the time to take the exam" (positive self-talk)
  - Tensing and relaxing muscles; use progressive relaxation techniques
  - Using success imagery
  - Maintaining a positive attitude
  - Taking several deep, slow breaths

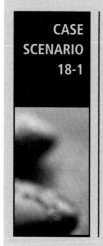

CASE SCENARIO 18-1

A registered nurse completed his master's nurse practitioner program ten months ago. He has now completed all clinical hours required for family nurse practitioner certification. The next step is to take the national certification examination so he can obtain his advanced practice licensure. He has considerable test-related anxiety but has never tried to reduce the anxiety before. He passed the NCLEX®-RN on the second testing attempt.

CASE ANALYSIS

1. What are the test-taker's strengths and at-risk testing-related behaviors?

2. Should he take a review course for the national certification test? Why?

3. What specific test-taking strategies would be helpful to him?

4. Describe techniques available to him to manage his test-taking anxiety.

TEST PREPARATION

Preparation is fundamental to successfully passing tests during a nurse's career. Considerable proven strategies are available to become the best possible test-taker.

General Preparation

The only time that an exam should be a problem is when test-takers are unprepared. One of the best indicators of being unprepared is "cramming" before an exam, which may lead to increased anxiety and decreased focus during testing.

Start preparing the first day of class by taking useful, legible notes and reviewing the syllabus to find test dates, number of tests, and the weight of tests toward the final grade. Plan reviews as part of a weekly study schedule and not just at testing time; budget your time. The brain needs time to process and retain information. Reviews are more than reading and rereading class notes and assigned readings. Outlining essential content transfers the knowledge from your head to a paper. In addition to reading (visual), use another learning style, such as reading notes out loud (auditory) to promote retention. Flash cards may seem outmoded, but they work, especially when learning new terms. Review for several short periods; if possible, right after class is the best time, while content is fresh. Use study groups to reinforce retention and turn main topics into questions the group answers for understanding. Go to instructor-held reviews. There is a correlation between class attendance or online presence and success in all aspects of passing a course.

Directly prior to a test, make sure you have eaten protein, which sustains and provides energy and focus during tests. Avoid foods that make you feel groggy. Get at least three hours, and preferably a total night's, sleep before the test. Arrive at the test site early so you will start on time to diminish anxiety. Set your alarm and a back-up alarm; being late may have severe consequences, especially if the test is timed. Think about what you will do to relax after you take the test.

Standardized Tests

Standardized tests like the Graduate Record Exam (GRE), Miller Analogies Test (MAT), American College Tests (ACT), and Scholastic Aptitude Test (SAT) are not only used for admission to various programs, but also to determine eligibility for scholarships, program placement, and remediation requirements. Many standardized test takers participate in review courses, use preparatory online software, or purchase books with sample test items that are specific to the standardized test. Some take the tests, if permitted, several times to obtain the best test score. Attaining the best score is important for future success. Consequently, this contributes to a highly competitive group of people taking the exams.

Unless test-takers are very confident of their testing abilities, preparation includes taking pretests and spending time with resource materials to familiarize the test-taker with the type of questions, details about the tests, and for experience with similar sample tests. All standardized tests have Web sites with resources for information, registration, and preparatory resources. Some companies, such as Sylvan Learning Centers, offer preparatory information for all the standardized tests. Consider the example in the next Internet exercise (18-1). To reduce expenditures related to testing, consider using campus or community libraries, which have test resources specific to the standardized tests. Software and online practice tests are available. It is okay to not know everything. These tests have some questions designed to challenge the limits of your knowledge above what you already know; perspective is helpful.

Familiarize yourself with what is being tested, the length and number of questions, the preparation resources, and the score or range of possible scores. Practice preventing hand and arm fatigue during testing. If your arm tires during standardized tests, which can be lengthy, it is probably due to the grip you have on your pen or pencil. Relax your grip, forearm, upper arm, and shoulder. Give those muscles a rest. Do NOT do elaborate arm exercises during the test, as these movements disturb others. Preparation can contribute to higher scores, which may be invaluable to obtaining increased scholarships or ensuring your successful entry into a desired school or program.

Internet Exercise 18-1	Locate the Web site http://www.Kaplan.com/testpreparation. Kaplan/Lippincott Williams & Wilkins is an example of a test preparation company that addresses testing for numerous standardized tests and some professional tests such as nursing. Separate preparations exist for the precollege tests of ACT and SAT, the graduate tests of GRE and MAT, and nursing's NCLEX®.
	1. Examine the introductory descriptions of the various tests.
	2. Take sample test items.
	3. Identify the resources available to prepare for the tests. Do these resources meet the studying, budget, and learning styles of the test-taker?
	4. What company guarantees, if any, are offered to the test-taker who fails the examination?
	5. What is the length and method of preparation?

NCLEX® Predictors for Success

Predictors for success on tests are worth knowing and using. Clearly, though, there is no magical, fool-proof formula that predicts a person will absolutely pass a test. Nothing, repeat nothing, substitutes for consistency in studying, attending to the test expectations and methods, investing time and energy in preparation, and learning test-taking skills.

Nurse educators have searched for test-success predictors for over fifty years. In nursing, most efforts have been expended on predictors of testing success particularly on the NCLEX-RN®. Numerous authors have published literature reviews that condense the findings (Carpenter & Bailey, 1999; Waterhouse & Beeman, 2003; Jacobs & Koehn, 2006). These findings span the licensure examination from when it was a two-day, paper-and-pencil test in the 1960s to the present computer-adaptive licensure test, adopted in 1994, which may be taken for a maximum of six hours. Student predictor variables included items such as SAT scores (Alexander & Brophy, 1997; Beeman & Waterhouse, 2001), GPA (Ashley & O'Neill, 1994), age at time of testing (Beeson & Kissling, 2001), and specific course grades (Campbell & Dickson, 1996; Jacobs & Koehn, 2006). The studies with the largest samples of students involved commercially prepared predictor tests such as the NLN Diagnostic Readiness Test (Schmidt, 2000, n = 5,698) and HESI Exit Exam E² (Nibert & Young, 2001, n = 6,277; Nibert, 2003, n = 6,300).

No one predictor has remained a stable predictor for testing success due to changes in testing and learners. The characteristics of the student applicants and the licensure examination continue to change; this causes the predictors to be unstable from a research perspective. Along with the studies, the NCLEX® examination difficulty level has increased frequently during the annual National Council of State Boards of Nursing meeting. Also, the type of NCLEX® test items have changed; items were once all multiple-choice tests written in a specific format. Among newer test items include computing drug calculations, filling in a blank, multiple answers to the same test item, and locating answers on a drawing. Nursing does not have a consistently stable predictor of success, but it is certainly closer than even fifteen years ago. Largely, this was made possible by computerized technology becoming embedded in most nursing curriculi and the national educational outcomes movement, which requires reporting of program outcomes, including NCLEX-RN® results, through the program's accreditation process.

The years of studies demonstrated limited success with a few predictors used to determine students at risk of failing the NCLEX®. Academic predictors such as science course grades, nursing course GPAs, admission criteria such as the Scholastic Aptitude Test (SAT) and American College Test (ACT) scores, and high school percentile rank are correlated with NCLEX® testing success. Nonacademic predictors that trend with NCLEX® testing success are parent's education level, age at time of testing, emotional state, ethnicity, self-esteem, time management, role strain, and test anxiety; however, these are generally less predictive than the academic factors. Factors associated with the highest predictability of NCLEX® success, such as the cumulative GPA, senior course grades, and predictor test results usually occur at the end of the nursing program; little time remains for remediation prior to graduation.

More nursing programs have resorted to using computerized NCLEX® predictor tests (Billings, Hodson-Carlton, Kirkpatrick, et al., 1996; Riner, Muller, Ihrke, Smoten, et al., 1997) early in the last half of the final semester. A growing trend is the implementation of a comprehensive student test-preparation plan that permeates the curriculum (Davenport, 2007; Jacobs & Koehn, 2006; Uyehara, Magnussen, Itano, et al., 2007) and includes the predictor test as one strategy. Programs and companies view the tests as diagnostic in that the results give test-takers a summary snap-shot view of their readiness to take the test; the relevance to the student is truly dependent upon how seriously the student answers test items. If answers are quickly or thoughtlessly chosen, then the predictability score has little relevance to the student. Diagnostic test results often include test-taker strengths and weaknesses, suggestions for study, resource suggestions, and rationale for wrong answers.

Programs generally use predictor test scores as the main indicator of need for remediation. Those students identified as at risk for NCLEX® failure can receive remediation as early as possible, while still in the supportive academic environment. These tests provide an overall predictor score as well as separate scores for strengths and weaknesses based upon the actual **NCLEX® test plan.** The diagnostic test is most beneficial when reviewed in detail relative to the student's placement in the program. The responsibility remains with the student and, later, as a graduate, to pass the NCLEX® per U.S. state and territory laws known as the nurse practice act.

How does this information assist the student or nurse being tested? The predictor tests are important to focus test preparation efforts (see Figure 18-5). But considered alone, without attending to other life factors, can lead one to falsely conclude that studying alone will lead to test-taking success. For example, the graduate who has obtained a high predictor test score completes no further study prior to the examination, delays taking the NCLEX® for four months following graduation, and plans a wedding two weeks before the scheduled NCLEX® test date will be at risk for being unsuccessful. Weddings, divorces, birth of a child, illnesses, death of a family member, and other major life events distract the learner from focused test preparation. The student or graduate can have the highest GPA and predictor test score, but without managing nonacademic predictors, such as life stressors, testing vulnerability increases. The test-taker is encouraged to plan the manageable life events separate from the scheduled test, if possible. Nonplanned events may warrant the test-taker delaying the scheduled test time to ensure increased testing success.

Figure 18-5
Predictor tests are useful in focusing test preparation efforts. *(Photo by Eric Swanson. Reprinted by permission.)*

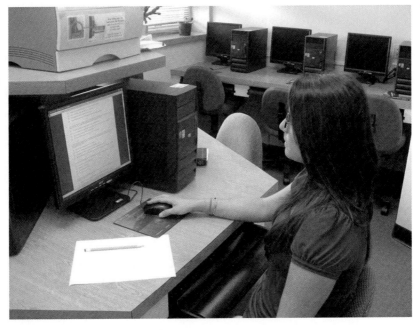

Test Preparation Specific to NCLEX®

Preparation for the NCLEX® begins the day a student enters a nursing program. Abundant resources exist to ensure students' academic successes in American nursing programs, colleges, and universities. A growing trend is that programs are embracing a holistic approach to preparing students for NCLEX® success (Mills, Wilson, & Bar, 2001). The approach teaches and encourages strategies of successful test-taking from admission to the program through graduation.

For the nursing student, mastering computerized tests, especially multiple-choice test items, is a key preparation for NCLEX®. The more computerized, multiple-choice nursing practice test items that a student takes, the more prepared, and therefore more likely to pass, the first-time test candidate will be. A useful NCLEX® study plan would include taking hundreds of computerized test items in various nursing categories such as adult nursing, psychiatric-mental health, women's health, and children's health, and from different companies using different venues. Exposure to different test writers broadens the students preparation for NCLEX®, which is written by many nurse faculty. After knowledge and clinical experiences are attained, nothing replaces the three Ps of practice, practice, practice as a strong test preparation strategy.

Test review books are helpful in providing test rationale, plus the books may be used where computer use is not accessible. Some learners prefer paper products that they can mark or tab for study purposes. Most review books also have access to electronic test banks, so the learner may take the tests in written and computerized formats.

For the NCLEX®, being on time to the testing center is essential. Most of the centers are located in metropolitan areas. Consider staying in a hotel near the testing center if weather is predicted to be problematic or you live hours away from the testing location. Take care of bodily needs before entering the exam room so to avoid being distracted or waste time during the exam.

Employers often offer or pay for a review course during an orientation program (Wray, Whitehead, Setter, et al., 2006). The approach is more cost effective to ensure first-time candidate test success than to remediate someone who has failed the test and is no longer eligible for an RN position. While interviewing for new positions, ask the employer as a new graduate if this is a benefit of the position.

Review or preparatory courses are prolific for most standardized and nursing licensure tests. Thoroughly read the company's description and claims about the course. Facts such as the length of the course, what the course includes, cost of the course, claims for success in passing the test, and services available if the test is failed are important items to explore before applying and paying for the course. Most companies have online or printed tests and other review resources available between the time of attending the course and successful test taking; this is typically included in the purchase price. Research indicates that graduates who take a review course are more likely to pass the licensure exam. Many review course companies will provide additional resources, such as DVDs, tutors, or books to use once the online or traditional course is completed.

Often unknown to students is the fact that the NCLEX® test plan changes every three years based upon a national survey of new graduate's work activities (Aucoin & Treas, 2005). The NCLEX® is a practice-driven exam and is required for entry into practice. Graduates are

Writing Exercise 18-2

Develop your test preparation plan to successfully pass the NCLEX-RN® as a first-time test candidate. Use the following sample format with examples to personalize your plan.

Goal	Activities	Target Dates
To successfully pass the NCLEX-RN® by <insert date>; review Table 18-3.	1. Review the important Web sites. • http://www.ncsbn.org • <state board of nursing Web site> • http://www.vue.com/NCLEX	Insert your own schedule. Do this early in the term of graduation or before.
	2. Obtain test review materials. • Test review book • School's test preparation software & resources • From http://www.ncsbn.org take NCLEX®-RN practice test • Obtain NCLEX® test item of the week • Download the NCLEX®-RN test plan	Do this early in the term of graduation.
	3. Take an NCLEX®-RN predictor test and use results to identify areas to study.	Allow time to study based on test results. If the school has a required score, consider need for test retakes.
	4. Take 2,000 computerized test items similar in format to the NCLEX®-RN; review the results for test plan areas to strengthen.	Pace yourself. These can be taken beginning two semesters prior to graduation.
	5. Prepare a list of weak areas based on various test results.	Make a timeline to take practice test questions per weak area.
	6. Take a traditional review course.	Allow time to study deficit areas identified during the review.

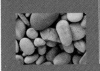

surveyed and asked to delineate the frequency and priority of more than 130 nursing care activities (Smith & Crawford, 2003). The test plan, developed from the survey, becomes the test blueprint for test item development (Poster, 2004). The exam is developed as a difficult test with most questions requiring analysis and application of cognitive skills. A graduate takes no less than seventy-five test items and has up to six hours to pass the exam. No pass score exists. When test-takers receive test results, they are told that they "passed" or "did not pass." Once passed, the licensed nurse may practice in any state or U.S. territory; the test will not be required again to remain licensed. Writing Exercise 18-2 is an outline that can be used to prepare a timeline for taking the licensure examination. All of the preparation strategies are known to enhance success on passing the NCLEX-RN®.

TEST-TAKING STRATEGIES

Tests made by commercial companies, especially the licensure and certification exams, have educated, experienced test writers. Test items are piloted and statistically scrutinized for validity and reliability. Test experts and statisticians are consulted throughout the test-making process. The NCLEX® tests are constantly reviewed for currency and relevance to practice. Considering the knowledge and experience of test writers to which students and nurses are exposed during a career, a developmental goal to become a prepared test-taker would serve a nurse well in the demanding, commercially-prepared testing market.

What Is Known About Test-Taking Strategies?

How do you learn? How do you process information? Do you learn best alone or in study groups? How do you retain and recall information for future testing use? These are samples of questions to assess your most effective learning and study methods. They are foundational to selecting test strategies that are customized to be most beneficial to the test-taker.

Tips and lists of test-taking strategies abound in the published literature and on Web resources (see Figure 18-6). Few are evidence-based; most are generated through educator and learner experiences. They are particularly helpful to novice test takers, those unaccustomed to difficult tests, and those who have seldom prepared for academic tests prior to entering a nursing program. Widely used test-taking tips for teacher-made tests are summarized in Figures 18-6 and 18-7. Tips in Table 18-8 generally do not apply to commercially prepared tests such as the NCLEX®.

There is a science behind test-making. Nursing faculty have taken courses, certification programs, and continuing education activities, and pursued self-development strategies to learn principles and techniques of testing and grading. Often nursing course tests address the application of information to a clinical situation, with test items becoming increasingly difficult as the student progresses through the course or program. Most nursing faculty are excellent test-makers as compared to faculty in other campus disciplines. When meeting the challenges of tests that are teacher made and standardized, the test-taker recognizes that mastering test

Figure 18-6

Multiple Choice
Test-Taking Tips for
Teacher-Made Tests.

- Read the question before you look at the answer.

- Answer in your head before looking at the possible answers, then search for your answers in the options.

- Eliminate answers you know aren't right; mark these on the test if allowed.

- Read all the choices before choosing your answer.

- A positive statement choice is more likely to be true than a negative one.

- Usually the correct answer is the choice with the most information or the one with the largest number of words.

- In a question with an "all of the above" choice, if you see that there are at least two correct statements, then "all of the above is probably the answer.

- In "all of the above" and "none of the above" choices, if you are certain one of the statements is true, don't choose "none of the above" or, if one of the statements is false, don't choose "all of the above."

- Don't keep changing your answer. Usually your first choice is the right one, unless you misread the question.

- If there is no guessing penalty, always take an educated guess and select an answer.

- Work toward spending no more than 1 minute per test item to be better prepared for timed tests.

DELMAR/CENGAGE LEARNING

Figure 18-7

Open Book
Test-Taking Tips
for Proctored Tests.

- Spend an equal or greater amount of time preparing as you would for a normal test; the open book test will most likely be harder than if it were a closed book exam.

- Familiarize yourself with the book and relevant course materials.

- Focus on learning the main ideas and get a feel for where they are located in the book, learn the details later if there is still time.

- Highlight important points, use post-it notes as bookmarks, and make notes in your book, if allowed.

- If it is allowed, write down all the important formulas and key information on a separate sheet so you don't have to search through your book for them.

- Bring all the resources that your teacher allows.

- Answer the easy questions that you know first, then go back and answer where you need to reference your book.

- Use quotations from the book to support your view, but don't over-quote; be sure to give your own insight and commentary. Be sure to know the plagiarism policy for the test and how quoted material is to be included.

DELMAR/CENGAGE LEARNING

preparation and test-taking strategies to obtain the best possible test scores is an imperative goal.

Test Strategies During Testing

First, read directions carefully, determine the type of questions and the point allotments to test items. Bring a watch and see how much time to plan for each section. Efficiently pace time and, if possible, mark the quarter and half points of the test as a reminder to check time. Work on the easiest items first and the items with the most point value. If your testing strength is essay items, do them first to gain maximum points. Organize time to address the difficult parts. Figure 18-7 summarizes tips for open-book tests.

When answering an essay question, make an outline in the margin before writing begins. Organization, clarity, and good writing are important and so is neatness; write legibly. Find out if penalties are given for incorrect answers; if not make educated guesses. If a penalty exists, avoid guessing.

Always read the whole question carefully. For multiple-choice items, consider covering the answers while reading the stem; try to answer the stem statement, then uncover the answers to see if your response is among them. If stuck on a question, continue to the next, and return to the unanswered question at the end of the test. The last sentence does not apply to the NCLEX®. Once you submit an answer choice in that test you will not be able to return to the previous question. Previous test item answers influence the choice of the next test item entered on the computer screen.

Nursing tests rarely require only memorization, except when essential facts are initially taught. For example, when first taught lab values, a test item may request the normal range of a lab test value or the safe range of a medication dosage. Later in the course or program, an application test item will require knowledge of lab values or medication dose ranges to test selection of an answer of safe nursing interventions. The earlier memorization and retention promotes more rapid problem solving, an important nursing skill.

Don't worry if others finish first; focus on the test in front of you. Keep your eyes on your own test; don't give others the opportunity to question your ability or integrity. Academic misconduct in nursing programs is considered a serious matter.

Maintain a positive attitude throughout the test. Stay relaxed and confident. Remind yourself that you are well prepared and are going to do well. Picture yourself answering questions easily and passing the test (known as positive imaging). If you find yourself getting anxious, take slow, deep breaths with your mouth open. The technique diminishes anxiety and promotes relaxation. If the test is lengthy or eye strain becomes evident, use the technique in Figure 18-8 to moisten your eyes.

Resist the urge to leave as soon as the test is completed. If there is time, make sure all items are answered, not mismarked, and other potential mistakes are corrected. Contrary to popular opinion that urges test-takers to always keep their first answer, evidence-based education research does not support that suggestion. However, if you have encountered information elsewhere on the test that indicates the first choice is wrong, change it. Proofread any essay or short-answer questions. Double check to be sure your name and other identifying information is on the test and any answer sheet.

Figure 18-8
Technique to reduce
eye strain and
increase moisture
during testing.
(Adapted from http://
learningext.com/
resources/rejuvenation.
asp, retrieved July 28,
2007.)

- Remove any glasses.
- Place the tip of the index finger between the eyebrows.
- Without blinking, slowly move the finger down to the nose tip.
- Follow the finger with your eyes.
- Tears are released naturally, blink several times.
- Repeat the technique.

TESTING RESOURCES FOR NURSES

Today's student and graduate have a plethora of testing resources available for successful test taking. Many resources are free and available through Web searches using key terms, textbooks, campus support services, and colleagues. Software companies have responded by offering a variety of computer products that are available through purchase. It is important to know which products are the best test predictors for the nursing program from which the student graduates. Most programs have predictor information available and share it with nursing students preparing for the NCLEX-RN®. For example, faculty may know the nursing GPA and predictor test score, when considered together, that predicts, with a high degree of accuracy, which graduates will succeed in passing the NCLEX-RN® as a first-time test candidate. The predictors that are most relevant to the students enrolled in the program will likely be the best predictors to consider for test preparation.

Testing Centers

Testing centers are professional companies that administer a variety of standardized and professional tests, such as the nursing licensure and certification exams. A campus may have its own testing center. When unfamiliar with the center's location, find it at least prior to the day of the test. The professional centers, such as the one in the next exercise, may have their own Web sites; the sites contain valuable preparation and testing information.

National Council of State Boards of Nursing (NCSBN)

The NCSBN has a Web site useful to NCLEX® test candidates. Through e-learning for the nursing community, NCSBN has a section labeled as a learning extension. The site has study tips specific for the NCLEX® exam, NCLEX® test information, online NCLEX® preparation tests, and a place

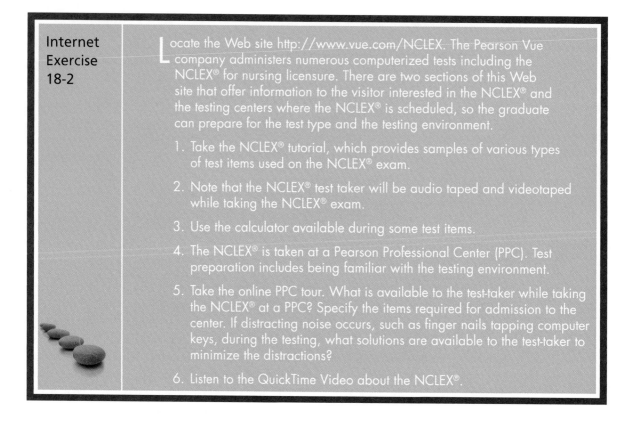

Internet Exercise 18-2

Locate the Web site http://www.vue.com/NCLEX. The Pearson Vue company administers numerous computerized tests including the NCLEX® for nursing licensure. There are two sections of this Web site that offer information to the visitor interested in the NCLEX® and the testing centers where the NCLEX® is scheduled, so the graduate can prepare for the test type and the testing environment.

1. Take the NCLEX® tutorial, which provides samples of various types of test items used on the NCLEX® exam.

2. Note that the NCLEX® test taker will be audio taped and videotaped while taking the NCLEX® exam.

3. Use the calculator available during some test items.

4. The NCLEX® is taken at a Pearson Professional Center (PPC). Test preparation includes being familiar with the testing environment.

5. Take the online PPC tour. What is available to the test-taker while taking the NCLEX® at a PPC? Specify the items required for admission to the center. If distracting noise occurs, such as finger nails tapping computer keys, during the testing, what solutions are available to the test-taker to minimize the distractions?

6. Listen to the QuickTime Video about the NCLEX®.

where the student may sign up to receive an NCLEX® question of the week. The study tips listed in Figure 18-9 are further discussed on the Web site. Once you review Internet exercises 18-1 and 18-2, write your own NCLEX-RN® test preparation plan as discussed in Writing Exercise 18-2; additional preparation is available there.

TESTING ENVIRONMENT

The test environment, ideally, is conducive to test-taker success. Keeping the room temperature comfortable, the environment free of distractions such as loud noises, and providing ergonomic seating promote the test-taker's focus on the test. When others in the room interrupt focus, such as by tapping the desk with a pen or the computer keyboard with finger nails, the test-taker can request the test proctor to keep the environment quiet. Most professional testing centers provide ear plugs during testing when requested. More universities are creating campus test centers to provide test security and the best testing environment.

Dressing in layers enables the test-taker to accommodate for the room being too hot or too cold. Frequently, test-takers are not permitted to have any personal belongings including a backpack, cell phone, personal pen, or ball cap with them. These steps go far to maintain test security and minimize cheating.

General Study Tips
- Build confidence through practice.
- Practice as if it is the "real thing."
- Create flashcards.
- Use mnemonic devices (memory triggers).
- Aim to understand instead of memorize.
- Make a study schedule.

Test Taking Hints
- Get a good night's sleep.
- Reach each question carefully.
- Try to answer the question before looking at the options.
- Go at your own pace.

Relaxation Techniques
- Be confident in what you know.
- Be prepared in advance.
- Use tension-reducing techniques.
- Try meditation.

Professional testing centers, such as those used for the NCLEX® and certification exams, will take a picture and fingerprint the test candidate. Picture IDs are checked to match test applications. Cameras are on throughout the testing session. Generally, no gum or food is permitted during testing.

Be assertive when the environment is problematic. Proctors and teachers are responsible to ensure that testing is conducted in a safe, secure, comfortable situation. If testing at home, the same environmental factors apply for successful testing. In preparing for the NCLEX®, take the practice exams in as close to a simulated test environment as possible. For example, time the test items, minimize distractions, and practice relaxation techniques during testing.

SURVIVING AND THRIVING AFTER FAILING A TEST

Tests vary in importance. Failing a pop quiz may hold little significance. Whereas failing a course final exam, the licensure exam, an employer's competency test, or a certification exam may have consequences considered devastating to the test-taker. How one reacts to failing such an important test affects one's ability to function personally and professionally.

Just as important as planning to pass a test is to think through an additional plan should the test results be negative. When test results have much at stake, like progressing in the nursing program, becoming a licensed nurse, obtaining employment or a promotion, entering graduate school, or meeting criteria for advanced practice licensure, disappointment

Internet Exercise 18-3

Locate the Web site http://www.ncsbn.org. The Web site is the home page of the National Council of State Boards of Nursing (NCSBN), headquartered in Chicago, Illinois. Every state board of nursing is accessible through links at this site. NCSBN authorizes, following job analysis research of new graduates, the test plan for the NCLEX® (PN and RN). The site also contains access to the NCSBN products produced for test preparation.

1. What test preparation resources does the bar labeled "NCLEX® Examinations" offer the visitor?

2. Compare the "candidate" and "educator" NCLEX-RN® test plans. Describe the essential features of each. Which is most helpful for NCLEX® preparation?

3. Print the NCLEX® test plan for testing preparation. The test plan is free.

4. Review the sample NCLEX® test items. These are located in at least two sections of this site.

5. Find the "Student" section to access a diagnostic test for the NLCEX and to access an online preparatory course for the NCLEX®.

6. Sign up to receive the NCLEX® Test Item of the Week.

may be quite intense. Being upset about the results is a normal reaction. If one's self-worth is linked to test results or if the test outcome is widely known, such as when classmates or coworkers are aware that testing occurred, there may be accompanying shame, self-doubt, withdrawal, and depression. Loss of status, income, opportunities, and plans may occur, and the person may experience stages of grieving. If family's or significant other's plans depend upon the test scores, they may encounter similar feelings and not be fully available as a support system.

Following the initial shock, it is important to encourage the test-taker to respond ultimately in a healthy manner. That response would eventually be proactive and a response that does not impair relationships, school, or work. If able and motivated to retake the test or repeat a course, focus on developing a plan of action that promotes successful test taking the next time. Should reactions lead to ongoing anxiety or depression, consider seeking a campus or private counselor. Friends and family are unable to effectively meet the need for counseling, especially if the emotional response creates impaired functioning.

Surviving and thriving, that is, optimal functioning, are the ultimate goals following a test failure. Spend time with those who encourage you toward your goals. Resist the urge to fall into the "blame game"; it takes away energy needed for constructive strategies to rebound. Case Scenario 18-2 helps you assist a colleague who failed the NCLEX-RN®. Regroup and gain perspective knowing that testing success, with effort, capability and planning, is possible.

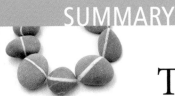

CASE SCENARIO 18-2

A recent nursing program graduate prepared for the NCLEX-RN® licensure examination by taking and scoring above the program's recommended score on a diagnostic test prior to graduation. In addition, she completed the program's online review course and her employer paid for a traditional, five-day review course; both companies are nationally known and reputable. The online company provided six months of access to test items following graduation. She used the online course, a test book, and the diagnostic test results to develop a study schedule, to which she adhered. She felt confident and prepared for the NCLEX-RN®. While taking the test she became anxious as she took more and more questions. She took 275 test questions over 5 hours, but still felt that she passed. Two days later, she found that she failed the NCLEX-RN®. Her father, per her request, called her at work when the results arrived early in the shift. As a coworker, you find her a few minutes later, crying in the lounge. She is inconsolable.

CASE ANALYSIS

1. Is your colleague's reaction typical? What will you do to assist her today and in the future?

2. What may this new graduate experience during the initial days after receiving the test results?

3. Is patient safety of concern in this situation? Why?

4. Discuss when and why the graduate must tell the employer about her test results.

5. Develop a preparation plan for retaking the test.

SUMMARY

Test preparation and test-taking skills are essential to a nurse's success as a student and employee. Because of the practice environment's complexity and the need to provide safe and competent care, nurses will face testing events throughout their careers. Nurses are expected to self-evaluate and self-develop; testing-success abilities are key to the framework a nurse creates for lifelong professional development. The nurse's habits of testing, self assessment, improving one's knowledge, skills, and attitudes, and being a proactive, successful test-taker begin in the nurse's first education program.

An overview of the types of tests encountered by nurses, including the nursing licensure exam, the NLCEX®, is provided along with test-taker characteristics; the NLCEX® is a focus of the chapter. Four concepts important to understanding tests that nurses may take during their careers are reviewed; these concepts are benchmarking, outcomes, competency, and remediation. Studies have identified test-taker characteristics that affect testing outcomes. One concept, testing anxiety, has been documented as influencing testing success. Strategies that relate to knowledge, skills, and attitudes are offered to give the test-taker options to prevent and minimize test anxiety.

Test-preparation strategies are divided into three categories of preparation—general test preparation, standardized test preparation, and NLCEX® preparation—and testing strategies are provided in detail. Current technology support and resources are identified for the adult learner and test-taker. Evidence-based test-taking strategies are presented specific to teacher-made multiple-choice tests, open-book proctored testing, NLCEX® testing, and general information applicable to all testing circumstances. Both personal habits such as eating, sleeping, and exercising, and testing habits such as reading test items and selecting the best multiple-choice answer are explained.

A review of testing resources leads the nurse test-taker to some of the best-known electronic test preparation sites. The testing environment, also important to testing outcomes, is reviewed and strategies presented for ensuring that the best possible testing environment is provided.

Finally, strategies for surviving and thriving following failing a test are discussed and personally related to the nurse, who is urged to be proactive to plan for a test retake, to determine whether post-test behavior affects personal and professional functioning, to assess knowledge, skills, and attitude changes needed for retesting, and to develop a plan for successful retesting. Methods to stay hopeful and motivated are discussed.

Considering all strategies, the test-taker is lacking nothing for testing success except the three Ps—practice, practice, practice. Use the best test preparation strategies to become the best test-taker possible. Career success depends upon knowing your testing strengths and weaknesses and proactively pursuing test-taking self-development as a life-long learner.

It is admirable to consider how many Millions of People come into, and go out of the World, Ignorant of themselves and of the World they have lived in.

–William Penn

REFERENCES

ALEXANDER, J., & Brophy, G. (1997). A five-year study of graduates' performance on NCLEX-RN®. *Journal of Nursing Education, 36*(9), 443–445.

AMERICAN NURSES ASSOCIATION. (1995). *Nursing report card for acute care.* Washington, DC: American Nurses Publishing.

AMERICAN NURSES ASSOCIATION. (1996). *Nursing quality indicators, definitions and implications.* Washington, DC: American Nurses Publishing.

ASHLEY, J., & O'Neil, J. (1994). Study groups: Are they effective in preparing students for NCLEX-RN®? *Journal of Nursing Education, 33*(8), 357–364.

AUCOIN, J. W., & Treas, L. (2005). Assumptions and realities of the NCLEX-RN®. *Nursing Education Perspectives, 26*(5), 268–271.

BEEMAN, P., & Waterhouse, J. (2001). NCLEX-RN® performance: Predicting success on the computerized examination. *Journal of Professional Nursing, 17*(4), 158–165.

BEESON, S., & Kissling, G. (2001). Predicting success for baccalaureate graduates on the

NCLEX-RN®. *Journal of Professional Nursing, 17*(3), 121–127.

BENNER, P., Sutphen, M., Leonard, V., & Day, L. (2007). *Educating nurses: Teaching and learning for a complex practice of care. Précis of chapters.* Stanford, CA: The Carnegie Foundation.

BILLINGS, D., Connors, H., & Skiba, D. (2001). Benchmarking best practices in web-based nursing courses. *Advances in Nursing Science, 23*(3), 41–52.

BILLINGS, D., Hodson-Carlton, K., Kirkpatrick, J., Aaltonen, P., Dillard, N., Richardson, V., et al. (1996). Computerized NCLEX-RN® preparation programs: A comparative review. *Computers in Nursing, 14*(5), 272–286.

CAMPBELL, A., & Dickson, C. (1996). Predicting student success: A ten-year review using integrative review and meta-analysis. *Journal of Professional Nursing, 12*(1), 47–59.

CARPENTER, D., & Bailey, P. (1999). Predicting success on the Registered Nurse Licensure Examination—1999 Update. In K. Stevens & V. Cassidy (Eds.), *Evidence-based teaching: Current research in nursing education* (pp. 135–170). Sudbury, MA: Jones and Bartlett Publishers and NLN Press.

DAVENPORT, N. C. (2007). A comprehensive approach to NCLEX-RN® success. *Nursing Education Perspectives, 28*(1), 30–33.

DEL BUENO, D. J., Griffin, L. R., Burke, S. M., & Foley, M. A. (1990). The clinical teacher: A critical link to competence development. *Journal of Nursing Staff Development, 6*(3), 135–138.

EICH, M., & O'Neill, T. (2007). *NCLEX® psychometric research brief.* Chicago, IL: National Council of State Board of Nursing.

HEWITT, P. (2002, October 30). Keeping score academically: National Merit semifinalists rate as cream of crop. *Houston Chronicle*, p. 22A.

JACOBS, P., & Koehn, M. L. (2006). Implementing a standardized testing program: Preparing students for the NCLEX-RN®. *Journal of Professional Nursing, 22*(6), 373–379.

McCLELLAND, D. C. (1993). Introduction. In L. M. Spencer & S. M. Spencer (Eds.), *Competence at work* (pp. 3–7). New York: John Wiley & Sons.

MILLS, L. W., Wilson, C. B., & Bar, B. B. (2001). A holistic approach to promoting success on NCLEX-RN®. *Journal of Holistic Nursing: Official Journal of the American Holistic Nurses' Association, 19*(4), 360–374.

MORRISON, S., Free, K., & Newman, M. (2002). Do progression and remediation policies improve NCLEX-RN® pass rates? *Nurse Educator, 27*(2), 94–96.

NIBERT, A., & Young, A. (2001). Predicting NCLEX® success with the HESI Exit Exam: A third study. *Computers in Nursing, 19*(4), 172–178.

NIBERT, A. T. (2003). *Predicting NCLEX® success with the HESI Exit Exam: Results from four years of study.* Denton, TX: Texas Women's University.

NIGHTINGALE, F. (1859). *Notes on nursing: What it is, and what it is not.* London: Harrison, Bookseller to the Queen.

PENN, W. (1903). *Some fruits of solitude.* New York: H. M. Caldwell Co.

POSTER, E. C. (2004). Psychiatric nursing at risk: The new NCLEX-RN® Test Plan. *Journal of Child and Adolescent Psychiatric Nursing, 17*(2), 47–48.

RINER, M., Muller, C., Ihrke, B., Smoten, R., Wilson, M., Richardson, V., et al. (1997). Computerized NCLEX-RN® and NCLEX-PN preparation programs: Comparative review, 1997. *Computers in Nursing, 15*(5), 255–267.

RUDY, E., Lucke, J., Whitman, G., & Davidson, L. (2001). Benchmarking patient outcomes. *Journal of Nursing Scholarship, 33*(2), 185–189.

SAYLES, S., Shelton, D., & Powell, H. (2003). Predictors of success in nursing education. *The ABNF Journal, 14*(6), 116–120.

SCHMIDT, A. (2000). An approximation of an hierarchical logistic regression model used to establish the predictive validity of scores on a nursing licensure exam. *Educational and Psychological Measurement, 60*(3), 463–478.

SCHWARZ, K. A. (2005). Making the grade: Help staff pass the NCLEX-RN®. *Nursing Management, 36*(3), 38–44.

SHEIL, E. P., & Meisenheimer, C. G. (1992). Helping new graduates succeed at the NCLEX-RN® experience: Evaluation of an anxiety-reducing workshop. *Journal of Nursing Staff Development, 8*(5), 213–217.

SMITH, J., & Crawford, L. (2003). *Report of the findings from the 2002 practice analysis: Linking the NCLEX-RN® examination for practice.* Chicago: National Council of State Boards of Nursing, Inc.

UYEHARA, J., Magnussen, L., Itano, J., et al. (2007). Facilitating program and NCLEX-RN® success in a generic BSN program. *Nursing Forum, 42*(1), 31–38.

WATERHOUSE, J. K., & Beeman, P. B. (2003). Predicting NCLEX-RN® success: Can it be simplified? *Nursing Education Perspectives, 24*(1), 35–39.

WRAY, K., Whitehead, T., Setter, R., et al. (2006). Use of NCLEX® preparation strategies in a hospital orientation program for graduate nurses. *Nursing Administration Quarterly, 30*(2), 162–177.

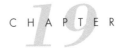

CHAPTER 19

TRANSITIONING FROM STUDENT TO PROFESSIONAL NURSE

PAMELA PATTERSON
MSN, RN, Nurse Manager, RN Intern Program and Coordinator, BSN Residency Program, University of Alabama Hospital

K. ALBERTA McCALEB
DSN, RN, Administrative Director, UAB Center for Nursing Excellence, University of Alabama Health System, University Hospital
Professor, University of Alabama School of Nursing, University of Alabama at Birmingham

Life, it seems, is nothing if not a series of initiations, transitions, and incorporations.

–Alan Dundes

LEARNING OBJECTIVES

At the completion of the chapter, the learner should be able to do the following:

1. Discuss issues related to transitioning from student to professional staff nurse.
2. Describe Benner's Model relative to new nurse competency.
3. Discuss issues in the workforce today that increase new graduate stress when entering the first professional nursing job.
4. Identify strategies important in seeking the first job as a staff nurse.
5. Describe strategies used in the workforce today to assist the new graduate nurse in role transition.
6. Describe work-related programs that assist new graduates to transition successfully.

KEY TERMS   Externships   Novice   Role Transition
                  Life Transition   Reality Shock

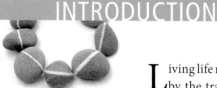

INTRODUCTION

Living life means preparing for new beginnings and experiencing endings. We are reminded by the transition of the seasons that time will change things—the color of dying leaves in the fall, the cold and barren trees of the winter, the new buds and flowers in the spring, and the green and flowering of nature in the summer. According to the Life Esteem Wellness Matters newsletter (2004), "**life transitions** are predictable changes in our lives associated with a discontinuity with the past" (p. 1). This phenomenon is a natural change from a protective, supportive comfort zone to one that is new, uncertain, and perhaps vulnerable. New graduates who leave the comfort of nursing school and accept their first job as a professional nurse experience one of life's most challenging transitions. The nursing school experience has been filled with many challenges of learning a new role, incorporating a whole new skill set into the daily routine, and growing developmentally both personally and professionally. It's important to recognize that the passage from student to practicing professional nurse is a stressful one (Quan, 2006). While the student nurse had many support mechanisms in place, transition to the new work environment will require the new nurse to develop additional coping and support strategies.

Learning to cope and successfully adapt to change are important developmental skills. In fact, coping and adaptation are two basic elements of human survival. Williams (2005) indicated that most transitions are "associated with significant life events," such as changes to a person's role in life, the environment in which they live, or the experience of a loss or traumatic change to life in general. His prediction was that it takes longer for a person to transition to changes in life events than we think; maybe six to twelve months or longer. Williams (2001) purported that a person may experience transitions up to ten to twenty times over the course of a lifetime. Not all changes in life require major life transitions. In fact, Williams indicated that small transitions can be achieved by learning new processes; however, major life-event transitions take time and may challenge our very identity of who we are, what we believe, and our life plans and goals. The transition process cannot be avoided; but rather, it can be looked upon as an opportunity for personal and professional development.

Without question the complex role of professional nursing practice in the health care delivery settings of today is stressful for any nurse, especially the new graduate nurse. In recent years, astute nursing service departments have recognized that changing work environments in health care settings has added to transition anxiety experienced by new graduates. Even the most successful nursing students have difficulty making the complex, challenging transition from the classroom to professional nursing staff (Quan, 2006). Partnerships between schools of nursing and nursing service departments are forming to better understand the demands placed on the new graduate nurse now and in the future. Positive outcomes for nursing practice, decrease in new graduate turnover, and a supportive workforce development plan can be a win-win situation for both the new employee and the health care organization.

PREPARING FOR TRANSITION

While the student is enrolled in the last year of the nursing program, it is a good strategy for the faculty advisor to discuss issues related to employment. Direction and guidance related to writing a résumé, conducting an interview, and professional dress for the interview should be discussed. In many cases, representatives from the local health care agencies begin to meet with potential new graduate hires by attending classes to discuss their organizational/nursing culture, hiring practices, and the process for employment. It is not too early to assist the student in planning for the senior capstone experience, in career planning strategies, and to provide important professional tips for seeking entry-level jobs in professional practice. Many nursing programs have decided to integrate these socialization concepts and issues throughout the entire curriculum pathway, with the understanding that these strategies are important to the healthy transition of the student to the world of professional nursing practice.

Keep Your Options Open: Where Will I Work?

As the new nurse begins to make the transition from student to staff nurse, the first major decision will be where to seek the first job. With the current nursing shortage there are more opportunities available in a variety of settings than ever before for the new graduate. As the graduate begins to look at different options, it is important to keep in mind that a job that provides the best support, educational opportunities, and benefit packages, not just at the beginning of employment but over the life of a career, is probably a better choice than the hospital with the most attractive sign-on bonus. If money drives the employment decision, look carefully at sign-on bonuses and the small print. Be sure to understand the terms of the agreement, the length of the commitment, and if there are penalties for terminating the agreement prior to completion. In addition, explore the potential earning power after the agreement is over. Is the agency offering larger dollars in the beginning—first six to twelve months—of the experience, but the opportunity to expand the salary base is minimal after that? An important question to ask would be, "What type of raise history does the organization offer the experienced nurses in the organization?" The lure of money at the beginning of a new career is very attractive; especially to new graduates with student loans. After all, remember that this is the business world and an excellent marketing strategy to entice the new graduate is to offer an extra "gift" at the beginning of the employment relationship. Keep in mind that while a high salary package is enticing, no amount of money can make up for an unpleasant and nonsupportive work environment.

Ideally, the job search will provide a number of work opportunities in several hospitals or other clinical agencies. This can help in further identifying and prioritizing the type of patient, health care setting, and work characteristics to pursue after graduation. For example, many hospitals offer their nursing assistant positions to nursing students as a recruitment tool for employment after graduation. In some of these nursing assistant positions, the nursing student has the opportunity to work in multiple areas, which helps to further define where one wants to work and what type of patient care is of interest. If an opportunity to work in a hospital presents itself prior to graduation, this is an excellent way to get not only valuable clinical experience, but also the chance to find out what its like to be an employee at this hospital. Networking with peers can also provide additional data about other hospitals and clinical agencies while determining places where employment applications will be sent. Part of the process of seeking employment upon graduation will be determined by the type and quality of learning experience and staff support received while the nursing student was in the clinical learning experience on a particular unit. The graduate nurse seeking a worksite will further refine the employment possibilities list by remembering experiences they had while in the clinical learning rotations in school.

Another option for getting into the hospital as a student for an extended time is through an **externship**. Externships are usually offered in the summer before the final year of nursing school. As an extern, the student nurse is assigned a preceptor and works with that nurse throughout the summer experience. This opportunity provides a small "reality check" related to patient workload and organization of care. Rather than taking care of one to two patients in a student role, as an extern the assignment is the same as that of the staff nurse preceptor. Depending on the unit and type of patient care, this will likely mean a workload of five to six patients on any shift. Obviously, an externship opportunity provides a mechanism to gain additional clinical experience, confidence in patient-care abilities, and information about the hospital work environment.

As the list of employment possibilities narrows to match your interest, it's important to remember the type of facility, mission, and characteristics of the agency. Do you want to work in a university teaching hospital or a private, for-profit hospital, or another type of agency in the community? There are positive and negatives to each type of work setting. In a hospital with a mission of service and teaching, work experiences are targeted toward more complex patients and cutting-edge experimental treatments; teaching is a primary focus of both patient care and professional development for all employees, and there is a focus on lifelong learning and implementation of cutting-edge "best practices" based on clinical evidence and research. While this type of work environment can offer excellent learning experiences and provide a quality foundation for graduate school, it can be intimidating for new graduates. The environment may be particularly stressful for the new graduate who had nursing student experiences in settings where acuity levels were lower, with less complex patient populations. If all the clinical learning experiences have been in community hospitals and primary-care agencies, with minimum to no experiences in a large teaching hospital, the acuity and treatment requirements of these very sick patients can be overwhelming. If adding this type of agency to your potential employment list, make sure that the hospital or agency provides a structured orientation plan, an organized work-transition development plan, support, and mentoring opportunities.

Now, what does that potential employment list look like (see Table 19-1)? Is there a list of pros and cons for each agency? Choose the top two or three as targets for the first job. Submit the

Table 19-1 Working List: "Places I Would Consider Working"

Agency	Contact Info	Pros	Cons	Comments
UNIVERSITY MEDICAL CENTER	Address Phone #	Close to apartment State-of-the-art women's health Friends already work there Tuition benefits after 6 months	Waiting list for OB unit No designated parking HR doesn't call me back	Working at a medical center may outweigh any of the negatives Very warm, supportive staff during school
TOUCHTONE HEALTH SYSTEM	Address Phone #	10 miles away Has moderate size women's and OB unit Good benefit package	Night shift a requirement at beginning Charge nurse role expected after 6 weeks Pay $5.00 less/hr	Good support when I met the nurses Can get the specialty I want Salary lower
TRI-COUNTY PUBLIC HEALTH	Address Phone #	Large agency with large client base Good chance of working in OB complications clinic Good retirement plan Good parking M–F day shift	Downtown area Pay $7.00 lower than hospitals No tuition reimbursement Not as flexible with schedule Not many psychomotor skills	Like the clients and the specialty Like M–F May not be flexible when returning to school Not sure about community right out of school?
LOVE BOAT CRUISE SHIP INCORPORATED	Address Phone #	Great work environment Great chance to travel Good salary for travel Nurse manager of ship clinic	Work 3 weeks/ off 1 week Poor benefit package No chance for upward growth No chance to return to school	Consider carefully for first 2 years Chance to travel and make good $$$/hr Think about time away from home and family
GOOD CAREGIVERS HOSPITAL	Address Phone #	300–400 beds OB small unit Salary competitive with local hospitals	No CEU opportunities No career ladder Parking is remote	Check out benefits and tuition reimbursement opportunities

application and résumé, arrange an appointment for the job interview, and do your homework—complete a comprehensive "knowledge" search about the employer via peers, human resources, and their Web site before the interview for the job. As more information is gathered about each place, add them to the "pros" and "cons" categories for your priority employer list.

Prepare a Professional Résumé

Most college students have a résumé that was prepared for entry into college, scholarship applications, or job interviews while at the university. It's time to make sure that this résumé is cleaned up and looks professional. A résumé is not a representation of all the awards, accomplishments, and activities since entering public schools. Rather, it is a two- to three-page account of education completed, work experiences, awards and other leadership accomplishments, community service, and volunteer activities over the past four to five years. Other additions could include: a short purpose or goal statement at the beginning; academic clinical experiences, especially if there is no work experience in a health care setting; future goal statement at the end; and a short summary of work expectations. A one-sentence listing of personal interests or hobbies is optional. Print the résumé on good-quality paper that is attractive and professional in appearance. Remember, it's better to have a short, concise résumé that accurately represents your experiences than to have a lengthy, highly embellished résumé that borders on misrepresentation of your past.

Writing Exercise 19-2	Visit the following Web sites: http://www.write-a-resume.org, http://www.how-to-write-a-resume.org, and http://www.monster.com

Prepare a cover letter, résumé, and job application for the top three agencies on your list of potential employers. It's important to send your information to the right person at the agency; so, do the homework necessary to find out names and addresses of those who will receive your materials. Often, it is more than one person in an organization. Today, materials may be asked for in electronic format; so, remember this as the cover letter, résumé, and application are prepared.

PLAN FOR THE INTERVIEW

The new graduate should never underestimate the professional interview process. This interview is a two-way pathway for information gathering by the potential employer, as well as the employee. Be prepared. It's human nature to think about the questions that may be asked by the employer and, naturally, there's anxiety attached to the fact that you are a new graduate with minimal experiences. Trust that everyone knows the issues related to transitioning from the student role to the staff nurse role. Be confident in the experiences that have been obtained from the educational process and convey an attitude of willingness to work hard to overcome deficits. Remember, every professional nurse has been a new graduate at some point in their career; you are not the first!

Figure 19-1
Important Questions
to Consider in
Interviewing.

1. What orientation and support programs are available for me? How long will I be actively involved in these programs?

2. What benefits do I receive after employment and when are they activated?

3. Does the agency have an educational assistance program? If so, what does it cover?

4. What are the opportunities for career advancement? If I transition well to work, when can I expect to work in a leadership role? When can I apply for the next level staff nurse position?

5. What were the retention rates for your new graduates last year? Over the past 3 years?

6. What is the average years of employment of the nurses in the hospital? On the unit I am considering for employment?

7. What is a reasonable projection for salary adjustments over the next year, 3 years, or if I stay for 5 or 10 years?

8. What is the philosophy of the institution regarding nurses who go back to further their education? Do you "grow your own" with regard to leadership?

DELMAR/CENGAGE LEARNING

One way to control your anxiety is to prepare your own questions for seeking employer information (see Figure 19-1). This is an opportunity to demonstrate to the new employer that you are a professional and this decision is an important one in your life. Decide what information is most important to learn in the interview process and write it down, if needed. In case time is an issue, decide the top three to five questions that are most important to know the answers to when making a decision about the first job experience. Depending on how the answers go, be prepared to use follow-up questions if an answer is not clear or you don't understand.

Another strategy for preparing for the interview is to search the Web sites of the hospitals that you are considering. At the Web sites, carefully explore the message that is being conveyed to the public, which means potential employees as well as patients and families. Review the benefits, types of units, and links to submit an application.

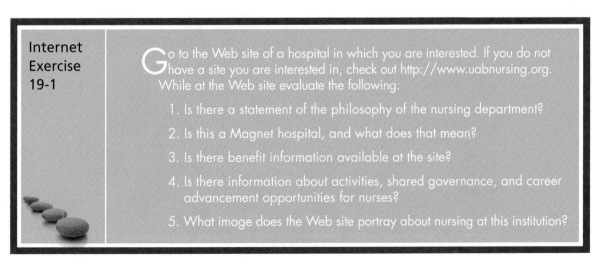

Internet
Exercise
19-1

Go to the Web site of a hospital in which you are interested. If you do not have a site you are interested in, check out http://www.uabnursing.org. While at the Web site evaluate the following:

1. Is there a statement of the philosophy of the nursing department?

2. Is this a Magnet hospital, and what does that mean?

3. Is there benefit information available at the site?

4. Is there information about activities, shared governance, and career advancement opportunities for nurses?

5. What image does the Web site portray about nursing at this institution?

The Interview Makes a Statement About You!

Once the application process is complete and an interview is scheduled, prepare for the interview. Plan for the interview by thinking about your answer to obvious questions that will be asked. The appointment process is the first step toward making an impression on the new potential employer. Don't schedule an appointment unless you know that the commitment will be kept and that there are no conflicts in your schedule before or after the meeting. Build in extra time to get to the appointment without being late, and then plan for the interview taking more time than expected. It could be that the institution will want for you to meet with multiple departments, which will take more time for the entire process.

Appearance is critical! First impressions are made quickly and are then hard to change. Whether you believe it is fair or not, that first impression can influence the decision of whether or not to extend a job offer. Don't make the mistake of believing that with the nursing shortage there are plenty of jobs out there waiting, and that appearance will be a low-priority issue. It's true that with the nursing shortage some institutions have high vacancy rates; however, all agencies are still looking for professional employees to represent the discipline and the organization. Professional appearance at the interview is important! (See Figure 19-2.) Regardless of gender, a business suit with minimal accessories is always best and makes a wonderful first impression. It's possible that male nurses will decide on a more casual business approach, with khakis and a sports jacket; however, a dress shirt and tie are still in order—and don't forget the socks. Female nurses may decide on a more casual business look with a pantsuit or blouse and skirt—don't forget accessories and proper shoes.

Remember to ask yourself what message/image you want the employer to receive from your appearance. Whatever decision is made about what is worn, make sure it fits appropriately. When selecting the outfit try sitting down in it and moving a little; make sure the fit of your outfit is

Figure 19-2
What kind of message does this nurse send by showing up to an interview wearing jeans?

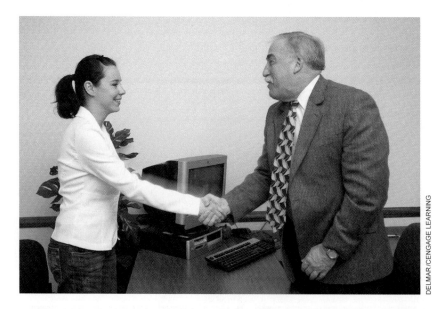

DELMAR/CENGAGE LEARNING

comfortable. Look in the mirror—are the seams and buttons bulging? It will be distracting for you and the interviewer if pulling and tugging is necessary to keep yourself covered. Regardless of your usual wardrobe, choose at least one outfit for the professional interview that is comfortable, stylish, and made just for you. It is never professional to show up for the interview in shorts, T-shirts, midriff tees, with visible belly buttons, or in revealing short or high-cut skirts. For males, it's best to avoid shorts, T-shirts, pants that sag, baseball caps, visible body piercing jewelry, tattoos, and sandals. When in doubt, decide to go professional and conservative.

Internet Exercise 19-2

Visit the following Web sites relative to strategies for the job search including how to dress for an interview: http://www.jobsearch.about.com, and http://careerplanning.about.com.

The first encounter with the interviewer should be relaxed and comfortable. Greet the interviewer with a handshake, a smile, and your name. A thank-you for sharing their time with you is always a professional courtesy. During the interview, maintain eye contact and use good verbal skills. Make sure to genuinely express interest in the hospital overall, but also be specific during the interview and let the interviewer know if you have an interest in a particular area. Progress through the interview in a calm, comfortable manner answering questions as openly and honestly as possible. When appropriate, use the list of questions that were prepared prior to the interview for gaining information. A prepared list of questions lets the interviewer know that you have taken the time to look at information about the institution and formulated your own questions of interest (see Figure 19-3). Target questions may include benefits, uniform requirements, and general nursing orientation. If the interview is with a representative from a particular area of the agency, it's time to ask more specific questions.

It is also a good idea to ask about malpractice insurance. What are the conditions of any coverage offered by the hiring institution? It could be in your own best interest to invest in malpractice insurance, even if your organization provides coverage for all nurses. Malpractice coverage is relatively inexpensive. Contact your state nurses association or specialty organizations for information on sources of coverage.

When the interview session is ending, make sure to cordially and genuinely thank the interviewer for the time and consideration for a new job opportunity. Clarify the process for making a hire decision after the interview is over. What is the length of time that can be expected before a decision is made, and will someone with the agency make contact to convey the outcome decision? Terminate interviews with a professional closing and a follow-up letter to the interviewer after the interview thanking them for the time and consideration.

Figure 19-3
Questions that
Clarify the Work
Environment.

1. What is the shift like that I will be working? What is the usual nurse/patient ratio?

2. Will I need to take call on this unit? Is there opportunity for over-time pay?

3. What is the orientation program like on this unit? How long does it last? Will I be assigned to staff nurses or is there a preceptor or educator who orients me?

4. What is the philosophy of the work schedule design on this unit? What do I do if I need to request a day off, vacation or holiday time?

5. If the census is not sufficient on a particular shift I have to work, what happens? Do I get called to take a vacation day? Do I come in and rotate to another unit?

6. What is the process for performance evaluation? While I am on orientation? At the end of a year? During the years to come?

7. What is the salary and raise history for new graduates on this unit?

MAKING A COMMITMENT

After all the interviews are finished, compare and contrast important information that was gathered during the interviews. Further identify pros and cons of each setting and information that is absolutely a "must" for consideration of employment. Consider the following: their orientation program and educational support services, such as unit educators and preceptors to serve as mentors and coaches; availability of relevant continuing education (CE) on the shift that you will be working; other CE paid or unpaid CE offerings; educational reimbursement plans; and the length of employment necessary to be eligible for these. Without question, salary is important and may be your bottom line for decision making, but try to keep it in perspective and weigh carefully whether other nonmonetary benefits offset the salary projections. In fact, benefit packages are also important and may become the most attractive element of the employment decision. Consider basic benefits like vacation, paid holidays, sick leave for individuals and family, and health insurance packages. Equally important are other benefits like tuition reimbursement, child care options, dependent care offerings, life insurance, and accidental injury coverage. While new graduates think little about retirement at this point in their career, it may be another attractive benefit for retention and long-term employment opportunities. Does the hospital offer any retirement matching dollars for the money contributed by the employee? What about retirement vesting; for example, how many years must you work before you are vested in the retirement system? Whether vested or not, what happens to the money contributed to the retirement plan if you leave the hospital? Many companies have multiple options for retirement plans.

What information was given at the interview about hiring practices? Were there particular rules about employment and unit assignments that affect only the new graduate nurse? After all, where your work will occur and with what type of patients is probably a high priority for new graduates seeking a first job experience. Many hospitals do not hire new graduates into intensive care units (ICUs). Think carefully as to whether this would be a real deciding factor for your employment decision. Even if high-acuity care is your top priority, it may be that a direct assignment into an ICU would not be the best option. Many new graduates want to work in an ICU setting, but it may be a good idea to get a good foundation in an acute-care unit. Think again about the career pathway you've selected for yourself; it could be that a logistical pathway based on patient acuity level is more appropriate and comfortable. When considering where to work within the agency, it is a good idea to listen to the experts who work in the facility every day. Demonstrating a desire to work in the facility first, and then progressing through different types of patient care experiences, may be the ticket to a long, successful career at one institution.

Once an offer has been made by the institution and accepted by the new graduate nurse, it's time to plan for the beginning of employment. Information should be received in writing from the agency that specifically outlines the official start date and specific nursing orientation schedules. Complete any required paperwork requested prior to the start date, if applicable. For the first day, arrive at the location for orientation prior to the time for the event to start—don't be late.

PREPARING FOR ORIENTATION

The entire orientation process is targeted toward a smooth and happy transition to the worksite. It's time to begin the first professional nursing experience at your new place of employment. You have probably already reviewed the nurse practice act for the places where you sent job applications, but just in case, it's a good idea to review your state's nurse practice act. This document is usually included with the professional nurse license packet received after you successfully complete the NCLEX-RN exam. You can also access a copy at your state board of nursing. Go to http://www.ncsbn.org. At this national site, select your state and the site will direct you to your state board of nursing. The document outlines what you can and cannot do as a registered nurse in your state of employment. It's essential to read and understand the legal regulations and limitations of the professional nurse before you begin work.

Internet Exercise 19-3	Locate the Web site http://www.ncsbn.org.
	1. Locate your state board of nursing site.
	2. Access your state's nurse practice act.
	3. What other resources are available at this site?

Another important document similar to the state rules and regulations for professional nurses is the clinical agency's job description for registered nurses. Many organizations provide a copy of this job description at the time of hire. If not, ask for a copy. Other important documents to review either before or during orientation include the organization's dress code,

CASE SCENARIO 19-1	Merry Nurse was contacted by human resources (HR) at the local medical center hospital to make an appointment for a job interview for a registered nurse position. While preparing for the interview, Merry decides to go ahead and send a résumé to the HR department and the nurse manager. Merry has thought carefully about what she wants in the first job; after all, this job will be a "stepping stone" for graduate school. Merry has a career goal to return to the Nurse Anesthesia program (CRNA) at the local university at the end of the first year of employment. On the day of the interview, Merry decided to wear one of the coolest outfits that she owns: a stylish, royal blue tank with her newest pair of designer jeans that are cropped at the ankles; four-inch, black, patent leather spiked heals; matching earrings and belly button ring; and her newest black, patent leather shoulder backpack. How lucky Merry feels that she just had a manicure with new nails applied and designer polish. She intended to get her hair trimmed and highlighted before the interview but ran out of time. At the interview, Merry conveys to the unit manager that she is very competent, earning only the highest marks in clinical courses in her nursing program. She is excited about the potential for this job, so she tells the unit manager that she is goal-directed and wishes to work only days so that she can get the most comprehensive experiences. She also hopes to enter the local CRNA School and wants to meet as many doctors as possible. When asked what type of patients/cases she likes to work with, Merry states that it really doesn't matter as long as she gets to meet some surgeons and anesthesiology doctors. While Merry acknowledges that she has a lot to learn, she tells the unit manager that she is very smart and can work extra if needed to learn the job and be successful.

CASE ANALYSIS

Based on this case, answer the following:

1. What transition issues would be expected for this new graduate?

2. Discuss potential problems with the job interview process.

3. Identify positive characteristics that you see in Merry.

4. List a minimum of five goals that Merry and her preceptor need to address to make transition easier and successful.

5. Identify professional and socialization issues that may be a problem for Merry.

policy, procedures, and standards-of-care guidelines. It's important to understand and review carefully the dress code for your particular job description. Some nurses think that appearance really doesn't matter; what's important and really matters is the kind of care they give. While the care delivered is important, others will judge you based on your appearance. Whether right or wrong, a sloppy or dirty appearance will cause people to question the quality of care you provide. A positive impression is made by wearing clean, wrinkle-free clothes and clean shoes that are in good repair. What about nails? Most agencies require short nails that are free of polish. If polish is worn, it must be in perfect condition, free of any cracks that can harbor bacteria. Artificial nails are always unacceptable because they harbor bacteria. Avoid hairstyles that interfere with patient care—whether long, dirty, oily, unwieldy, or uncontrolled. It's a good rule of thumb to read the policies yourself and develop your own interpretation of the dress code; don't look around at coworkers and model them until you know their appearance meets institutional rules.

Another important nurse hygiene issue that affects relationships with others is types of odors. Of course, it's always important to be clean and free of body odor, which includes mouth odor. It is likely that close contact with both patients and coworkers will happen on every shift. Remember to avoid strong scents of any kind. This includes cigarette smoke, perfumes, and other herbal scents. Many people are sensitive to perfumes, and this sensitivity can be made worse by illness. Strong odors can sometimes aggravate symptoms of nausea in patients who are ill, those who are experiencing nausea of pregnancy, and those who are allergic to odors in the atmosphere. Be sensitive to the needs of others in the work environment; just because you like the scent does not mean everyone else will.

UNDERSTANDING YOUR FIRST PROFESSIONAL ROLE

While nursing schools help prepare students with nursing knowledge, skill competency, and guidance for licensure to practice, there are many issues that new graduates will face as they enter the workforce. These issues, dilemmas, and challenges cannot be addressed in depth and scope by nursing schools due to time constraints and limited clinical practice opportunities. However, nursing schools can equip new graduates with a way of knowing, thinking, and problem solving that can enhance their decision-making abilities as situations are encountered in the clinical setting each day. Without question, new graduates sometimes leave the nursing program with a gap between the knowledge of their first professional role as a nurse and the reality of how to integrate the roles of the nurse in everyday practice. When faced with the complexities of the health care delivery system of today, new nurses may feel that successful transition is not attainable, and that the nursing program did not prepare them for the reality of today's practice environment. One reminder for the new nurse is that every nurse has walked in the same shoes of reality. Realistic self-assessment, patience, an openness to learn each day, and establishing relationships that are supportive and encouraging will help the new graduate to undergird daily stress and anxiety.

Concepts of Role Transition Theory

Every new graduate is faced with learning a new role, understanding the organizational culture in which this new role exists, and establishing new relationships and a new support system within the context of the health care delivery team. Learning to trust others and building integrity with new members of a support team are essential in the transition process. Myers (2005) defined a "role" as "a cluster of prescribed actions; the behaviors we expect of those who occupy a particular social position" (p. 90). Simply stated, this definition covers many of the role changes that the individual will experience throughout life, including new jobs, being a new nurse, marriage, parenthood, and taking care of elderly parents. More specifically, Hardy and Hardy (1988) described the concept of **role transition** that occurs when a person moves from one position to another and requires an individual to take on a new or modified set of role expectations.

The transition from an educational setting to a work environment is one example of role transition that can cause role conflict and uncertainty. The concept of role shock, sometimes referred to as **reality shock**, has been used by Kramer to describe the role strain, conflict, and incongruity experienced by the new graduate nurse while transitioning from the ideal role of student to reality of staff nurse (Hardy & Conway, 1988). The transition process has been described as similar to the change process, requiring an individual to experience a change from a comfort zone, through a readaptation phase, and finally to stability, or comfort in a new role position. Williams (2005) indicated that a practical approach to successful change or transition management is to have a greater understanding of transition awareness. According to Williams, issues in transition management are affected by an awareness of the following:

- Individuality is central to coping with transitions…no two people exhibit the same levels of vulnerability.
- Transitions can reach a crisis level at approximately six months (plus or minus one month).
- Transitions have different outcomes based on a difference in circumstances.
- Successful transitions and the effects are based on variables at work and at home.
- Transitions affect significant others: family, friends, peers, and coworkers.
- Change is based on situations and personal abilities.
- Transitions involve adaptive behaviors and cognitive restructuring (p. 5).

A goal of any transition plan is to avoid transition crisis. Conditions that support successful transitions include a feeling of security, both economic and emotional, a healthy lifestyle, prior experience leading to self-determined transition skills, a supportive work environment, and strategic transition support (Williams, 2005). It only makes sense that organizations that invest in successful transitions for its employees can create an organizational culture that promotes

---

Internet Exercise 19-4

Visit the Eos Career Services and Work resource center Web site at http://www.eoslifework.co.uk. Click on the Eos Lifeline Chart. The exercise will assist in self-assessment of previous work and life transitions and how one copes with change.

individual personal and professional growth, optimal morale, innovation, job satisfaction, and high-quality and productive outcomes.

TRANSITION TO THE ROLE OF THE PROFESSIONAL NURSE

New graduates who are making the transition from student to the first professional role are faced with many challenges and new responsibilities. While nursing programs do an admirable job in a short period of time in preparing new nurses for their first role, there is no replacement for the actual day-to-day experiences that require critical thinking, problem solving, prioritizing, and organizational skills. Benner (1984) described a socialization process that nurses go through as they transition into the professional work setting. According to Benner, the new registered nurse moves through five stages as the nurse gains experience in the patient-care setting. Stage I of Benner's model is called the **novice** stage and begins as the student nurse enters the nursing program. In the novice stage, skills are limited because of a lack of knowledge and the background necessary to make clinical judgments without concrete rules and practice expectations.

The new nurse graduate entering the workforce moves into stage II, which is "advanced beginner." The advanced beginner can base clinical decisions on theory and principles, realizing that there are standards of care and a particular order to practice situations in the clinical setting. Weaknesses generally center on the lack of actual clinical time and experience causing difficulty with organization and prioritizing. According to Benner, Tanner, and Chesla (1996), it takes approximately two to three years to move to Stage III, or the "competent practitioner." Competent practitioners feel confident and organized in most complex clinical situations.

The next stage (IV) is the "proficient practitioner" stage described as requiring three to five years of experience. The nurse in stage IV is able to think of each patient situation holistically and focus on both short- and long-term goals as well as desired outcomes. The "expert practitioner" of stage V is reached when the nurse is able to synthesize the entire patient-care situation, moving from interventions, to evaluation, to revision of plans based on intuitive thought. Stage V is achieved after extensive practice experience; nursing actions and decisions come naturally and automatically based on the depth and scope of expertise.

Benner's work has been highly publicized and utilized in describing the process that new graduate nurses encounter as they are socialized into the professional nursing role. Institutions that are interested in assisting the new employee to transition successfully will recognize that the first three to five years of employment require a steep learning curve, most drastic during the first year of professional nursing practice.

Strategies to Promote Successful Transition

The most astute institutions and nursing departments acknowledge that transition issues are real for the new graduate nurse. These agencies prepare for the new graduate hire with a transition management plan. The purpose of such a plan is not only to assist the new graduate nurse with the transition into professional nursing practice, but also to increase awareness of transition issues and potential crisis that may be experienced by the new graduate among the other staff and managers. Strategies such as flexible orientation plans, preceptors to support orientation at the unit level, and extended skill proficiency programs are excellent approaches to minimize the reality shock experienced by new graduates (Chitty, 2005).

In recent years, many institutions have implemented formal programs such as clinical preceptorships, internships, and nurse residency programs to improve transition outcomes, including retention (Goode & Williams, 2004; Herdrich & Lindsay, 2006; Schoessler & Waldo, 2006; Thrall, 2007). Some of the most successful nurse residency programs for new graduate nurses are found at hospitals that are implementing the standardized postbaccalaureate residency program under the auspices of the University Health-System Consortium (UHC) and the American Association of Colleges of Nursing (AACN) (Williams, et al., 2007). The year-long program is a partnership program implemented by the hospital and a local school-of-nursing coordinator and faculty, and includes elements such as monthly classes and small group discussions, evidence-based nursing practice activities, collaborative mentorship and support from experienced nurses, and the opportunity to participate in a national research database that further describes the perceptions and issues that new graduate nurses experience in the first year of employment. The UHC residency program has turnover outcomes (11–13%) well below the national average for turnover (35–60%) in the first year. In many institutions, the year-long residency provides the foundation for advancing to the next level of the career advancement program for the institution. Obviously, this type of strategy is an excellent incentive for assisting with successful transition, enhancing knowledge and professional development, and increasing the salary base after the first year of employment.

Regardless of strategies used by the employer to assist the new graduate with transition to the work setting, the new professional nurse must also self-assess strengths and weaknesses, be motivated to perform at a high level, and handle personal and professional issues that may arise. The following strategies can assist the new nurse with personal transition awareness and success:

1. Be patient and allow time for a smooth transition.
2. Identify ways that appeal to everyday living and offset the stress of transition.
3. Take care of yourself…always.
4. Find appropriate support from others in the workplace and at home.
5. Be willing to admit weaknesses and seek assistance to overcome them.
6. Be willing to tolerate some discomfort during the transition period; after all, "growing pains" can be uncomfortable for a while.
7. Despite uncertainty, find inner confidence and the motivation to succeed.

The first year of employment will pass by very quickly, allowing for new and challenging opportunities in the future. It will not be very long before the successful transition will pave the way for the once-new graduate to become the preceptor for new employees and nursing students.

SUMMARY

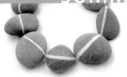

The next decade in nursing will hold many new and exciting challenges for all nurses. As health care systems survive and become more complex, new graduates will continue to experience transition issues as they leave the nursing student role and become a practicing professional nurse. Understanding transition issues, employment strategies, and institutional expectations will assist the new graduate in successfully transitioning to the new role of professional nurse. Cutting-edge health care facilities are those that understand and establish realistic expectations for the new graduate. In addition, these facilities plan, implement, and conduct ongoing evaluation of strategies that assist the new nurse in transitioning successfully. Isn't it comforting to know that all nurses were new at one time in their career? It is further comforting to realize that all nurses will experience transition anxiety as they progress through new career opportunities. In other words, transition is not just for the new graduate nurse, it's for everyone who continues to grow and develop throughout their career.

The quality of a person's life is in direct proportion to their commitment to excellence, regardless of their chosen field of endeavor.

–Vince Lombardi

REFERENCES

Benner, P. (1984). *From novice to expert: Excellence and power in clinical nursing practice*. Menlo Park, CA: Addison-Wesley.

Benner, P., Tanner, C. A., & Chesla, C. A. (1996). *Expertise in nursing practice: Caring, clinical judgment, and ethics*. New York: Springer.

Cardillo, D. W. (2001). *Your first year as a nurse: Making the transition from total novice to successful professional*. New York: Three Rivers Press.

Chitty, K. K. (2005). *Professional nursing: Concepts and challenges* (4h ed). St. Louis, MI: Elsevier Saunders.

Goode, C. J., & Williams, C. A. (2004). Postbaccalaureate nurse residency program. *Journal of Nursing Administration, 34*(2), 71–77.

Hardy, M. E., & Conway, M. E. (1988). *Role theory: Perspectives for health professions* (2nd ed). Norwalk: Appleton & Lange.

Hardy, M. E., & Hardy, W. L. (1988). Role theory: Role stress and role strain. In M. E. Hardy & M. E. Conway, *Role theory: Perspectives for health professionals* (2nd ed.). Norwalk: Appleton & Lange.

Herdrich, B., & Lindsay, A. (2006). Nurse residency programs: Redesigning the transition into practice. *Journal for Nurses in Staff Development, 22*(2), 55–62.

Kelly, P. (2008). Leadership and Management of Patient-Centered Care-Unit III, table 17-2. In P. Kelly (2nd ed.), *Nursing leadership and management* (2nd ed.). Clifton Park, NY: Delmar, Cengage Learning.

Life Esteem—Wellness Matters Newsletter. (2004). Life's Transitions: Self renewal involves letting go of the old and embracing the new. Simmonds Publications. http://lifeesteem.org/wellness/wellness LF.html

MYERS, D. G. (2005). *Exploring psychology* (6ᵗʰ ed.). Holland, MI: Worth Publishers.

QUAN, K. (2006). *The everything new nurse book.* Avon, MA: Adams Media.

SCHOESSLER, M., & Waldo, M. (2006). The first 18 months in practice: A developmental transition model for the newly graduated nurse. *Journal for Nurses in Staff Development, 22*(2), 47–52.

THRALL, T. H. (2007). Shock absorbers: Hospital residency programs smooth the bumps for new nurses. *Hospitals and Health Networks,* June, 60–64. Retrieved May 20, 2009, from http://www. hhnmag.com

WILLIAMS, D. (2005). *Life events and career change: Transition psychology in practice.* British Psychology Society Symposium.

WILLIAMS, D. (2001). *Transitions: Managing personal and organizational change.* Eos Career Services.

WILLIAMS, C. A., Goode, C. J., Kresek, C., Bednash, G. D., & Lynn, M. R. (2007). Postbaccalaureate nurse residency 1-year outcomes. *Journal of Nursing Administration, 37*(7/8), 357–365.

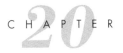

ACHIEVING LIFE–WORK BALANCE

KARIN A. POLIFKO
PhD, RN, NEA-BC, Vice President, Operations and Academic Affairs, Remington Colleges

Happiness is not a matter of intensity but of balance and order and rhythm and harmony.

–*Thomas Merton*

LEARNING OBJECTIVES

At the completion of the chapter, the learner should be able to do the following:

1. Discuss predominate issues of the working professional as the issues pertain to work and life balance.
2. Analyze the current work environment for registered nurses.
3. Differentiate among professional, family, and personal life goals.
4. Describe several recent theories relating to work–life balance.
5. Review work and gender issues several decades ago as compared to today.
6. Discuss at least five options or strategies for developing a healthier work–life balance.

KEY TERMS

Care Networks
The Fair Labor Standards Act
Family Medical Leave Act
Fast Track
Harmony
Imbalance

Macho Maternity
Mommy Track
Right to Work States
Role
Role Conflict
Role Overload

Role Stress
The Sandwich Generation
Spillover
Work–Family Conflict
Work/Family Border Theory
Workweek

INTRODUCTION

Our lives are becoming increasingly complex. We are busy. As Bunting (2004) discusses in her recent book, *Willing Slaves—How the Overwork Culture is Ruling our Lives*, work is consuming us, regardless of culture, location, or specialty. Workload is ever increasing, especially as technological advances such as cell phones, instant messaging, and virtual conferencing go beyond the physical boundaries of time and location (Figure 20-1). No longer does one leave the office—and its subsequent work—behind for the next day; it follows you as you drive home and continues late into the evening, unless one willingly disengages from all connectedness. Further complicating the intensification of work is the increased competitiveness among companies and sectors, as work becomes more global in scope. Production continues to migrate from the United States to countries that provide cheaper sources of labor, stressing American companies and their employees to continually churn out higher levels of productivity while discounting costs.

The environment and culture of the workplace is changing, in that company, and employee, loyalty is declining, resulting in a higher level of turnover and less of a sense of community among workers and those who supervise. No longer do you start a new job with the thoughts of retiring in the same organization. In fact, the average number of jobs that the average American holds in a lifetime is quite high. According to the U.S. Department of Labor, Bureau of Labor Statistics (2006), Americans between the ages of 18 and 40 hold an average of 10.5 jobs, with women holding 10.3 different jobs and men with 10.7 jobs (p. 1). As can be expected, both genders hold more positions during their late teens to early twenties as compared to later in life. In addition, men average being employed about 85% of the time during the years of 18–40, as

Figure 20-1
Technology has made it increasingly more difficult to keep work separate from other areas of all people's, including nurses', lives. *(Image copyright Monkey Business Images, 2009. Used under license from Shutterstock.com.)*

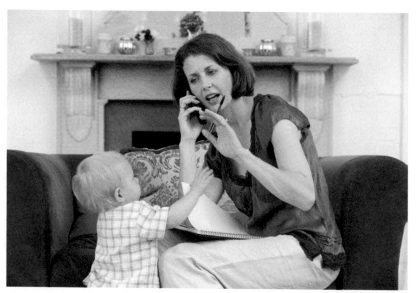

compared to women's average of 70% of all total weeks (p. 1). Women were predictably out of the workforce for up to 26% of the total weeks employed per year as compared to men's 10% of the total weeks employed (p. 1). Primarily due to taking time out for family obligations. Further, women who earned college degrees held more jobs than their male counterparts (11.2% as compared to 10.4%) who earned college degrees (p. 2).

The American Workweek

How is the **workweek** defined? The boundaries between work, and social and home life continue to blur, as employees are "on" much of the time thanks to computerization and instant access. Atack and Bateman (1992) estimated from early census worksheets that the average worker put in 60.1 hours per week in 1880. Daily hours declined during World War I; by 1919 the six-day workweek and eight-hour workday were the norm. There were some who advocated a shorter workday, arguing that workers were more productive working shorter hours. Scientists began providing evidence that long work hours resulted in "health-threatening, productivity-reducing fatigue" (Whapple, 2001), yet businessmen remained steadfast in their mindset to decrease hours for economic reasons. Weekly hours began to fall at the beginning of the Depression, when many workers were laid off. Certain segments of the population had been advocating for a shorter workweek as the country came out of the Depression, with thirty hours a week the preferred choice for workers, and industry and businessmen again arguing against this shortened workweek. The most common workweek was a forty-hour week.

Several key pieces of legislation were passed by President Franklin Roosevelt, including the Wagner Act, the Social Security Act, and the Fair Labor Standards Act of 1938. **The Fair Labor Standards Act** established a national minimum wage, child labor standards, and overtime rules for both full-time and part-time workers. The act designated that work beyond forty hours per week would be paid at one-and-a-half times the base rate in specific industries and later established equal pay parameters (http://www.opm.gov/flsa). The forty-hour, Monday-through-Friday workweek has been the norm ever since.

Americans who are employed full time continue to increase their weekly hours of work. According to Bunting (2004), between the years 1977 and 1997, the weekly average increased by 3.5 hours, taking it to 47.1 hours worked per week. While it may seem like work is never ending, work was significantly longer when people worked in a more agricultural setting; at that point, Americans were working almost 80 hours per week, most certainly without benefits including sick and vacation pay.

Right to Work States

With the advent of total quality management and continuous quality improvement that began in the 1970s, more and more output is expected from employees, yet the corporate world offers less and less employment security. There are laws that govern the employee under "At Will" doctrines that define the relationship between the employer and the employee as such that either

Figure 20-2
Right to Work
States in 2009.

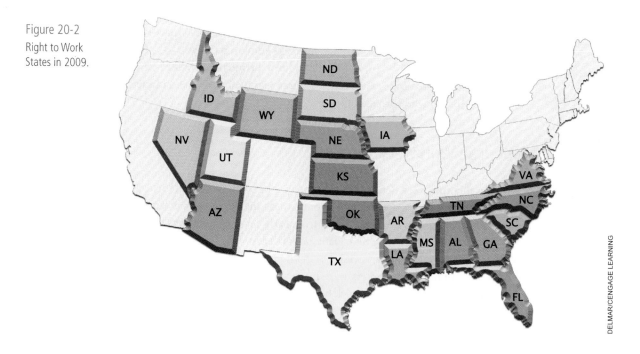

DELMAR/CENGAGE LEARNING

one can terminate the relationship without liability. This has generally meant that an employer can legally terminate an employee for no reason and without cause. Another interesting piece of legislation is the Right to Work, which governs employment in twenty-two states functioning as **Right to Work States** (http://www.nrtw.org). If you are employed in one of the states with these laws, most likely you are protected and cannot be required to join a union or pay dues to a union as a condition of employment or continued employment. There are a few exceptions to this ruling, such as if you are employed by the airline or railroad industries. Figure 20-2 illustrates the current Right to Work states where union membership cannot be forced upon an employee, nor can union fees be required of nonunion members in order to remain employed.

Internet Exercise 20-1

Locate the National Right to Work Foundation site http://www.nrtw.org.

1. What type of information does this site provide? Who is the audience?

2. Identify both the pros and cons of being employed in a Right to Work State. Is your state a Right to Work State?

3. Discuss some of the legal parameters surrounding the employee's rights in a Right to Work State. Discuss the employer's rights. Who is favored and why?

AMERICAN EMPLOYMENT STATISTICS

No longer does the American employment profile of "family" consistently present a working father and a stay-at-home mother. Due to ever-greater financial demands on the vast majority of families, two incomes are increasingly *required* just to provide basic life necessities. According to the U.S. Census Bureau 2004–2005, more women work outside the home than ever before. The number of working women has more than doubled over the last two decades, with almost 60% of able women employed, as compared to 44% four decades ago. The largest increase has occurred with women who are married, 41% in 1970 as compared to 62% in 2003 (U.S. Census Bureau, 2005, p. 377).

One of the professions in the United States with the highest percentage of females is that of registered nurse; of the almost 2.9 million holding licenses, over 92% of nurses are women, followed by elementary and middle school teachers who are 82% female (U.S. Census Bureau, 2005, p. 386). Eighty-three percent (an estimated 2.4 million) of the registered nurse workforce are actively employed in the field of nursing, with 58.3% (or 1.6 million) working full time, almost 25% (0.74 million) working part time, and 16.8% not employed in nursing at all (NSSRN, 2005). Figure 20-3 illustrates the employment status of American RNs.

According to the Health Resources and Services Administration (HRSA, 2005), the number of actively working RNs varies from state to state; however, there is consensus that there is a moderate shortage on the national level. By 2020, the moderate shortage turns to critical,

Figure 20-3
Employment status of American registered nurses.

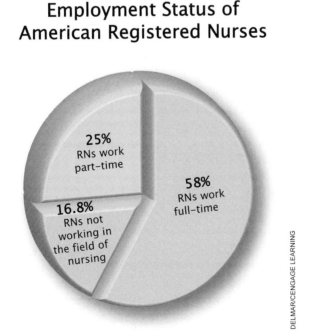

Employment Status of American Registered Nurses

25% RNs work part-time

58% RNs work full-time

16.8% RNs not working in the field of nursing

DELMAR/CENGAGE LEARNING

primarily due to many baby boomers retiring, nursing faculty retiring, and nurses in general leaving the profession. The nursing shortage will escalate tremendously; it is predicted that by 2020 there will be a shortage of more than *one million nurses throughout the United States*. By 2020, California will have the highest shortage of 116,600 nurses, followed by Texas with a shortage of 83,600 RNs, and then Florida with a shortage of 81,200 RNs (a 148% increase from the 2010 estimated 32,700 shortages). It is projected that all states will experience some level of the RN shortage (HRSA, 2005).

Logically, as the population continues to age, so does the RN workforce. One of the greatest concerns in health care today is that as the demand for services increases due to an aging population, the actual number of registered nurses able to provide care will continue to decline. Direct patient care is physically challenging, and a person may not have the stamina or the physical strength to perform many of the functions consistently during a twelve-hour shift, such as lifting patients or pulling patients in their beds, or dealing with ten simultaneous emergencies. Without a continuous influx of new, younger nurses, the profession may not be able to meet America's future health care needs.

One key area of employment growth is in women with children, especially those with young children under the age of six. In the 1950s, only 12.6% of married mothers with children under seventeen worked outside the home; by 1994 that figure rose to 69% (Hochschild, 2001, p. 6). Remarkably, the number of working mothers with children under one in that same year was almost 59% (Hochschild, 2001, p. 6). The largest increase in married working people has been in the category of women with children fourteen to seventeen years of age, growing from 54% to 81% from 1975 to 2003; however, almost 60% of married women with children under six are working (U.S. Census Bureau, 2005, p. 377). For single mothers, the numbers increase to 77% who work, and over 82% of single fathers work (U.S. Census Bureau, 2005, p. 378). Families, in order to remain financially solvent, will continue to have stressors and expectations placed not only on the wage earners, but on the children as well, as family time increasingly becomes compressed.

Unfortunately, while there has been an increase in the overall number of work hours for American employees, many days are missed due to "illness" and/or family obligations. The average employee misses nine days a year of work, excluding vacations and holidays (Hochschild, 2001). That number increases to fourteen days a year missed if that worker has children (p. 27). Having children does not dramatically expand days missed of work; working parents cannot afford to take additional time off in order to meet other demands on their time. How many times has a child been sent to preschool or school that has not felt well because there wasn't any available child care or because the parent could not use sick time (or didn't even have that particular benefit)? However, there are some forward-thinking organizations that have care for sick children on site at a workplace, so that if a child is sick with a minor illness, parents can still come to work, yet be assured that their child is being watched. This type of situation benefits the working parent, the child, and the employer, yet companies are reluctant to institute these family-friendly centers. Care centers for children with minor illnesses is just one example of what makes a family-friendly workplace; the Working Mother Web site (http://www.workingmother.com) lists annually the top one hundred family-friendly American corporations.

Men who take time off to parent full time also run into prejudices and bias. Many in corporate America cannot understand how a man can take time off to be with his family, since it is usually not as acceptable for a man to be the nurturer rather than the provider. Almost 160,000 American men stay home as the primary caretaker of their children, almost three times the number that were staying home just a decade ago (Tahmincioglu, 2007). So much of the popular definition of success is focused on achievement, salary, and professional accomplishments, particularly for men. The Web site http://mrdad.com, written by a stay-at-home dad, has unique perspectives that are encouraging and enlightening at the same time.

Internet Exercise 20-2	Locate the Working Mother Web site (http://www.workingmother.com).
	1. Who are the top one hundred family-friendly companies for the latest year?
	2. What are some of the common elements that make them family friendly?
	3. Are there any health care companies? Any health care systems? Why do you think there are not more health care systems listed in the top one hundred?
	4. Can you identify the essential requirements that are important to you as a potential employee?
	5. Does this information have any implications for men? Working fathers?

DEFINING BALANCE

Ask just about anyone who works if they have enough time to accomplish everything they want to do, and the answer would almost always be a predictable "no." As work becomes more intertwined with life, keeping the two separate may be impossible. There is an underlying perception in American culture that there are several particular components to being successful; what accomplishments do you have at work, what are you doing for your community, are your children excelling in school, and what does your personal social calendar look like? Many are struggling to attain simultaneous success in these areas, regardless of the type of work and a family's needs (Kossek & Lambert, 2005).

Work and family at-home time have been considered separate entities until the last few decades. In today's economy, two incomes are almost a necessity to maintain a household. Work influences home life, and home life invariably influences the work situation, with both scenarios having a direct effect on personal well-being. When one thinks of balancing work and family, it conjures up a perception of a scale, where one scale tips downward when one scale is tipping upward (see Figure 20-4). When one area is in conflict, then the balance is askew, resulting in an imbalance between the two domains. Is there always balance between work and family life? For most, the answer is no, with oftentimes an expression of dissatisfaction for both areas since neither is feeling complete, guided by the individual's perception of satisfaction and his or her ability to meet both domains' demands.

Figure 20-4
Work–Life Balance.
When one area
of a person's life
is stressed, the
work–life balance,
represented here
as a scale, is
tipped, causing
imbalance between
the two domains,
often leading to
dissatisfaction
with both area's
of a person's life.

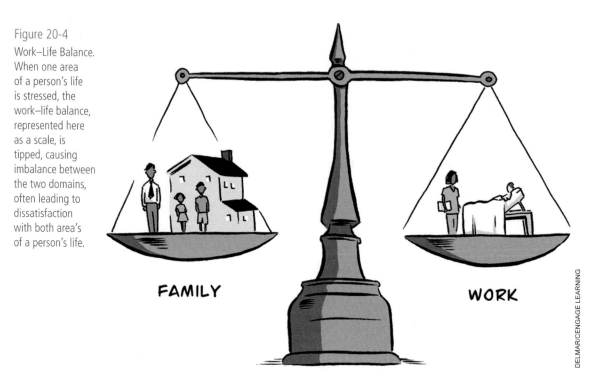

FAMILY   WORK

Greenblatt (2002) and Clark (2000) propose that work–family balance occurs when there is functioning both at home and at work, providing an *acceptable* level of conflict does not disrupt the system. If work is to be satisfying, there should be sufficient resources available so that work can be accomplished on work time, rather than being brought home. Likewise, there needs to be an adequate support system in place for home and family life, such as babysitters who can pick up the kids at the last minute if a critical meeting runs over, or a pediatric practice with alternative hours so that minor health care issues can be taken care of immediately. Within the definition of balance, one has to consider the demands of both work and home life. There are numerous issues to keep in mind when determining if there is sufficient balance, such as ample flexibility within the work environment when there is a need at home, the ability to actually take a planned vacation, having adequate rest to work a full day without being tired, and realizing both personal and professional successes.

Greenblatt (2002) suggests that there are real and perceived work and life obligations that have to be in place for conflict to be minimal. She suggests that there are four categories of resources to consider: financial, temporal, control, and personal, with the latter encompassing psychosocial, physical, and emotional areas. It appears that when one area is discordant, then the others compensate in order to keep the balance between work and family life—never an easy task. It is generally easy to feel accomplished in one or two categories, but to achieve fulfillment in all is quite challenging and, one would argue, not often done, even with numerous support systems. In keeping with the visual of a balance, when one area such as personal finances is in deficit, it can wreak havoc on one's professional life as the need for employment becomes essential and takes priority. Likewise, if a family member has a health crisis requiring constant care, work flexibility and benefits such as the Family Medical Leave Act come into focus.

Writing
Exercise
20-1

In thinking about the above writing about work–life balance, what is your personal belief set regarding this topic? Are these areas distinct? Are they interdependent? For this exercise, define the areas critical to your model of understanding, and illustrate accordingly.

Work and family issues cannot be so easily divided, with overflow from one domain encroaching on the corresponding domain (Polifko, 2007). Instead of the term integration, the term harmony is introduced in the context of work–family-life harmony. **Harmony** is defined by the author as a complementary balance of the physical, psychosocial, and emotional elements of a person's life. Harmony illustrates the concept of being in synchrony, being in accordance and agreement with all facets of work and family life. How often does one consider giving up something in the work (or family, or life) domain to "fit in" the other domains' demands and requirements? For example, whose turn is it to stay home with a sick child? Is it the spouse with the less hectic meeting schedule? Is it always the mom? Or the dad? Or is it the one with the most generous sick leave? Life can often feel like a constant tug and pull between competing forces.

Harmony also connotes satisfaction with one's life situation, without pitting one domain against another. Unlike balance, which can be perceived as give and take, in a harmonious situation, everything can coexist without struggle, and with acceptance. Like integration, harmony speaks to achieving inner peace, having resilience, and going about life with grace, humor, and enthusiasm. Harmony is working together, rather than competing against; having reached equilibrium that is comforting. Both work and home life can be accommodated.

Early on, the review of literature on work–family interactions began with a discussion of how the two areas developed into conflict; much of the literature even today focuses on work–family conflict (Lewis, 2002). After it was identified that there was conflict between these two domains, the research developed to focus more on work–family balance; how to achieve and master it. Do these two domains work independently and distinctly from each other? Or are these two domains somehow intertwined in an open-systems format, where there is fluidity between the parameters, with each affecting the other?

Spillover

One current theory that utilizes an "open-systems" approach is spillover theory (Staines, 1980), proposing that work and home life do interact and affect one another, regardless of the real or imaginary boundaries imposed. **Spillover** is the extent to which family life interferes with work or vice versa. When there is spillover, a situation that Greenhaus and Parasuraman (1987) identify as "carryover stress" occurs. Carryover stress becomes significant when one area interferes and places demands on the other area, which may not be able to accommodate the added strain. These

Figure 20-5
Factors that Affect
Work–Life Balance.

• Work Environment	• Flexibility at home and work
• Home Environment	• Physical stamina
• Support mechanisms at work	• Emotional stability
• Supervisor	• Social networks
• Supportive family relationships	• Financial security
• Role identification	• Physiological status
• Values	• Psychological status

DELMAR/CENGAGE LEARNING

negative stressors can be emotional, physical, and/or social, resulting in a variety of outcomes and consequences. For example, a hospital is faced with a severe nursing shortage, requiring RNs to work mandatory overtime. For most people, this would prove to be a hardship, even more so for those who are single parents with young children, and without familial support and backup. The work domain significantly affects the family/home domain so that both are overextended and stressed. The consequences of the family–work spillover may include bad decision-making due to lack of sleep, poor quality of work, decreased productivity, inferior people-management skills, physiological symptoms, missed deadlines, and fewer hours spent on the job. Likewise, if there are stressors at work, the spillover stress could potentially result in anxiety and short tempers at home, poor sleep patterns, longer hours at the office, and general house maintenance responsibilities placed on hold. Carryover stress can equally upset and negatively impact the individual and his or her family, and depending on the situation, can negatively impact the employee's organization as well. Figure 20-5 illustrates those factors that affect work–life balance.

Work–Family Conflict

The two primary areas of research for many years have separated the focus into two distinct categories: the work domain and the family domain. Lately, there has been additional research of **work–family conflict** discussion that also includes the life domain and the social domain. Issues are not distinctly isolated neatly into work and family; not everything occurs at work, nor are issues found distinctly within the family domain. In addition, there are personal needs, emotional needs, and social needs that focus on the person's place within his or her community or society.

Conflict between work and family occurs when there are pressures in one role due to interference from another role. Greenhaus and Beutell (1985) define work–family conflict as "a form of inter-role conflict in which the role pressures from the work and family domains are incompatible in some respect" (p. 77). More often than not, this conflict is due to the overlapping of roles and the "juggling" that creates the stress and internal strife. The conflict can initiate in the work domain or in the family domain; regardless of the starting point, it can quickly deteriorate (Figure 20-6).

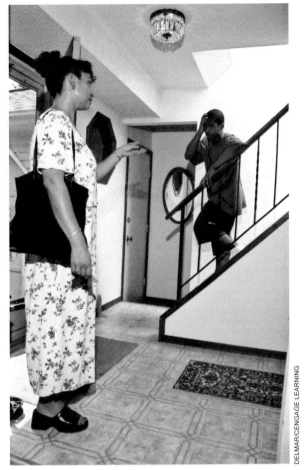

Figure 20-6
Work–family conflict can initiate in either the work domain or the family domain, when pressures on one role affect the other, for example when the role of being a nurse and working long hours interferes with the role of being a mother or father.

DELMAR/CENGAGE LEARNING

THEORETICAL EXPLANATIONS IN WORK–FAMILY BALANCE

Earlier in the chapter, spillover theory was discussed as the level to which work interferes with family life and vice versa as a possible explanation for emotions that "spillover" from one domain into the other. Having a deadline at work that necessitates long hours spills over into family and home time, as does a sick child requiring that a parent stay home, missing work. Staines's (1980) work in compensation theory postulates that people try to make up for the domain they feel lacking in; in other words, if people are unhappy with their marriage, they may put extra energy into a work assignment so that they do not have to go home at a regular time, achieving satisfaction and recognition. Both spillover and compensation theory connote that work and home life spheres are intertwined and codependent, influencing each outcome so that they cannot be ignored.

In one of nursing's most widely used models, Roy's Adaptation Model, **role** is defined as predetermined expectations that others have toward one another (Roy & Andrews, 1999). A role set consists of those multiple roles that someone holds simultaneously, such as father, husband, student, and professional. Common among adult learners is the concept identified as **role stress**, which is the pressure or strain resulting from a variety of expectations that the multiple roles require, and exhibited as physical and psychosomatic symptoms, such as headaches, anxiety, stomach aches, and shortness of breath. **Role conflict** occurs when a person is expected to play the part of two different and incompatible roles simultaneously.

Roles identify patterns of behavior that correspond to expected reactions by others. Regardless, **role overload**, particularly in women, is found to be detrimental, and is caused by "multiple and conflicting expectations from others" (Nelson & Burke, 2002, p. 5). Role overload occurs when there are multiple expectations, and people may feel as if they are unable to devote enough time to any one role, only fulfilling several halfway. Historically, women have had a higher overall workload, with the primary responsibility of dependent care, elder care, housework, plus vocational career work. According to Frankenhaueser (1991), women averaged 78 hours a week of workload as compared to men's 68 hours per week. While men may be increasing their contribution to the running of the household and time spent with children, Bond, Galinsky, and Swanberg (1998) found that the gaps over a twenty-year study still are significant and only mildly improving.

Clark (2000) proposes a relatively new theory entitled **Work/Family Border Theory**. This theory clearly delineates the spheres of "work" and "family" and states that while they both influence one another, there are significant differences. Borders are the "…lines of demarcation between domains, defining the point at which domain-relevant behavior begins or ends" (p. 756). Borders can be physical (the walls of your ICU), temporal (work hours), or psychological (emotions used in one domain but not the other). Some borders are more permeable than others, allowing physical movement from one domain to another, or they can be psychological in nature. Two other characteristics of borders is flexibility (can one domain stretch to meet the unplanned needs of the other domain) and blending (working at home can create seamless borders at times), with a resultant strength of the border wall.

People become "border-crossers" who "…make daily transitions between these two settings, often tailoring their focus, their goals and their interpersonal style to fit the unique demands of each" (Clark, 2000, p. 751). In Work/Family Border Theory, balance is defined as "…satisfaction and good functioning at work and at home, with a minimum of role conflict" (p. 751). What is interesting about this particular theory is its realization that work and home life really do have differing expectations, rules, responsibilities, and cultures. Both domains satisfy different goals, whether they are measured in accomplishments, friendships, or personal happiness. Total integration of both domains is not required for true balance, nor is the total separation of both domains necessary.

Border-crossers travel both domains repeatedly, and can be either peripheral or central participants to either domain. Characteristics of border-crossers include their ability to influence the domain and to identify with a specific domain. Border-keepers facilitate the frequent transitions for border-crossers, exhibiting commitment or antagonism.

Everyone is busy, especially nursing students. Develop a diagram of your life that resembles Clark's theoretical representation of the border-keepers, the border-keepers/domain members, and the border-crossers. Be sure to identify everyone and describe his or her relationship to others.

GENDER AND WORK–FAMILY BALANCE

According to Higgins, Duxbury, and Lee (1994), one of the most significant alterations in the labor market landscape over the last decade or so has been the increased participation of women with children in the workforce. Gendered differences, or the division of labor based upon gender, have been narrowing, as the male is no longer the primary wage earner in the vast majority of American households.

As nursing is a predominately female profession, with the majority of workers also mothers, it can be concluded that there may be significant role stress, overload, and conflict within their multiple roles, all requiring various levels of energy, time, and dedication. Multiple roles can negatively affect women's health and psychological well-being (Frone, 2000), as they are constantly under stress. Even though it may appear that society is increasingly more accepting of a change in gender roles, such as stay-at-home dads, a disproportionate amount of household and child-care responsibilities still fall to women, even when they are employed full time outside the home (Yoder, 2003). Some may postulate that many women who work may feel ambivalent about their desires to achieve professional success, others say that there really are limited options since so much of the childrearing and home maintenance responsibilities—such as grocery shopping, laundry, and meal preparation—are still completed by women (Smithson & Stoke, 2005). Real or imagined, many promotional opportunities may be lost when a woman cannot take on the same workload as a man because of familial and outside obligations.

Barnett (2004) discusses the need for understanding why many believe that marriage and motherhood are "natural" roles for most women, and that when employment is added to the mix, it may result in terrible discontent and role conflict. Are these roles really "natural" and expected? Can one handle multiple roles simultaneously and successfully? The overlapping and complexity of roles potentially leads to conflict whether they are intrapersonal or interpersonal strains. So much of the literature has illustrated the negative consequences for working parents, yet there are as many positives as there are challenges.

Diversity management, popularized in the 1990s as an effective method to sensitize the workforce to gender, racial, and ethnic differences (Polifko, 2007), continues to assist with highlighting women's needs in the workforce, particularly with maternity rights. As workforce policies continue to evolve, the focus turns from just women's needs to a more gender-neutral approach as work–life issues become popularized for men and women alike (Smithson & Stoke, 2005). Terminology such as flexible working has become a more politically correct phrase to better accommodate circumstances beyond the maternity leave to instead promote an enhanced work and family life. Both men and women can take full advantage of a flexible work schedule, whether it involves parenting a newborn or newly adopted child, or caring for a sick relative. Gender-neutral terms are much more acceptable than strictly feminine terms as companies attempt to achieve diversity awareness. The goal, after all, is supposedly to have equal choices and opportunities in salary and the ability to meet commitments outside of work. The thought is that if a work environment is nonsexist, and both males and females have the same and equal opportunities, then there should not be any need to address specifically gendered topics and concerns. Or is there? Are organizations able to provide gender-blind decisions and services without regard to the person being male or female?

Gender-Specific Issues

While many administrators may espouse that their organizations are gender blind and equal opportunists, is it more difficult to be a female, especially with young children? Hospital schedules can be notoriously challenging; after all, needing to be on-shift at 6:45 a.m. or 2:45 p.m. is not exactly conducive to school hours for small children. Likewise, men may be in a similar position if they have child-care responsibilities, or if they are single parents. A female, equally as qualified as a male, or maybe even more so, may perhaps not be considered for a promotion because she is not able to put in the "extra" hours after work, or she needs to alter her schedule to adjust to the after-school program's hours. Smithson & Stoke (2005) state that many management-level women, in order to be successful and continue to climb the corporate ladder, need to work "just like a man," including taking a "macho maternity." **Macho maternity** leave occurs when a woman only takes the absolute minimum time off to recover from childbirth in order to return to work earlier than scheduled in order to show others that having a baby doesn't interfere with work. It is not unusual for women in academe to attempt to schedule childbirth during the summer, when many are not in class teaching, or for others to attempt to time delivery for a slower season at work. Many women do not want to be relegated to the "mommy track," knowing that choice assignments and promotion opportunities may go to someone else without time and child-care restrictions.

Regardless of seniority, many women feel compelled to work the same hours as their male counterparts, lest they be looked upon as not being able to maintain the same outputs and achievements. Is it appropriate to measure time at work as the desired result, or are the outcomes really the true gauge of performance? Is it necessary to insist that someone put in an eight-to-five day when flex time may result in more productivity? The other side of the argument can be had from those without children who may feel penalized. Childless workers may have to take vacations after those employees with children have chosen their time, they may need to stay after work since they don't have any pressing "obligations," and they may be called upon at the last minute for an assignment rather than someone else who has children at home. Sometimes childless female bosses are even more demanding of their female subordinates who have children, producing a frustrating—and unexpected—work environment.

The Family Medical Leave Act of 1993

While balancing home and work life continues to be a challenge in the United States, numerous countries throughout the world place different expectations on working parents, especially new parents. How have companies in Europe been so successful with retaining working mothers and fathers? Nyberg (2003) suggests it is a change in perception from parenthood as an *individual* issue to parenthood as a *social* issue. While some American companies allow maternity, and some paternity, leave, in Europe it is called parental leave. In fact, in Sweden, parents are entitled to two months *paid* time off, or they lose the time (Nyberg, 2003). In the United States, the **Family Medical Leave Act** of 1993 allows up to twelve weeks of unpaid leave during any twelve-month period for:

- The birth of a son or daughter of the employee and the care of such son or daughter.
- The placement of a son or daughter with the employee for adoption or foster care.
- The care of spouse, son, daughter, or parent of the employee who has a serious health condition.
- A serious health condition of the employee that makes the employee unable to perform the essential functions of his or her position (http://www.dol.gov).

With FMLA, specific parameters must be met. It is important to note that this is time off without pay, and only certain employees and organizations are eligible. For example, the organization needs to employ more than 50 employees, and the employees themselves have to have worked in the organization for 12 months preceding the request for a minimum of 1,250 hours in that year, and the request has to be made at least 30 days in advance of the requested leave. It is estimated, however, that one in three employees are not eligible for FMLA benefits (U.S. Department of Labor, Monthly Labor Review, 2001). Some argue that while FMLA is a great benefit if you have enough vacation and sick time to be paid, others are critical that unpaid leave may produce a financial hardship for those who need it the most.

What Is Women's Work?

Some hold the belief that it is the social responsibility of the female to focus on her children rather than focusing on career development, and that regardless of the situation, all females should want to become mothers, with the primary identity of a woman being that of mother. Along the lines of this thinking is the notion that one must accept that a career is "sacrificed" for the good of the children, and that a mother should always be available for her family, regardless of the situation. Russo (1976) labels this the "motherhood mandate."

Given a choice, probably most of us would prefer to work part time and receive full-time pay and benefits; however, that situation most likely will not happen in our lifetime. Compared to men, many more women choose to work part time as opposed to full time. Do women "choose" part-time work when they could be working full time, which in most situations is looked upon more favorably in terms of current and future employment? Does part-time work mean less commitment to work and more to family?

Feminist scholars tend to see that women's choices of full-time or part-time work fluctuate during their careers. Tomlison (2006) sees career transition as a primary activity, with women fluctuating between work and domestic and family responsibilities depending on the point in time. There are significant implications for transitioning in and out of full-time work, including fewer promotional opportunities, fewer responsibilities, and perhaps a decrease in the social-circle standing at work. Several occupational fields are more conducive than others to flexible time, including nursing, allied health care, teaching, and service occupations such as restaurants, cleaning, and sales. Many women, after maternity leave, return to work on a part-time basis (Tomlison, 2006), possibly to negative consequences to upward career mobility. Further, many women, as compared to men, have a fluid career path that accommodates additional situations and concerns, such as family issues, self-growth, financial need, or a crisis. While various situations may be difficult and compromising, they may also be enabling and encouraging of a new path or trajectory.

Tomlison (2006) proposes that one's career trajectory is assisted or hindered by several situations, including care networks, work status, policy status, and work–life balance preferences. **Care networks** are those formal or informal structures that enable one to work. Care networks can be family members who watch children, friends, day care, and school programs. The richer and more extensive the care network is, the more the employee can explore options that are full time, or that are on off-shift. However, if there is a breakdown in the care network, a person's career options become severely limited, especially if there are children who require care or an elderly parent who needs watchful vigilance. When these networks collapse, many face constraints as they attempt to resolve issues of work and family needs.

Work status is often defined by what role people have at their place of employment, with those employed full time usually having more power and advantages than those who work part time. Further, those in more senior positions, or higher in the management chain, may have slightly more leeway than those with lower status if family issues arise, being able to adjust their work schedules accordingly, whether temporarily to take a sick child to the physician's office, or with flex time after a maternity leave.

In consideration of policy status, many who receive state-aided funding have limited work choices that directly influence family life choices. Many states have welfare-to-work policies in an attempt to break generational welfare dependence; however, not all communities have the support mechanisms in place to see these policies fully enabled. If a parent does not have sufficient resources, or an effective care network established, then it is almost futile to expect a fully successful transition back into the workplace. Parents cannot work when there isn't affordable day care, nor can people be into work on time if they do not have reliable transportation. There are many variables to consider when wondering why someone does not work.

VALUES, WORK, FAMILY, AND BALANCE

Work–family balance preferences are determined by the values one holds; given options, is it more preferable to work full time, stay at home, or work part time and juggle schedules? Given the availability of choices, some may believe it is critical that a mother stay home with young children. For others, this is not a financial or even personal option. Some would prefer to adjust spending habits, resulting in a lower income, than to place their children in day care. It is all a personal choice. **Mommy track** is a term that has been popularized in recent years, used to describe a woman who, usually in a white-collar career, willingly leaves the workforce in order to spend time with her children. The opposite viewpoint is being on the **fast track**, which connotes career progression and achievement in an accelerated fashion. There is considerable debate between the camps of mothers who work and mothers who choose to stay at home to raise their children, with both sides furiously believing they are doing the best for their children and their families. Numerous articles, Web sites, and even books have been developed that discuss this topic, all presenting their personal viewpoints, often in controversial terms.

Internet Exercise 20-3	Review a Web site that discusses the mommy track, such as http://www.mommytrackd.com.
	1. What is the focus of this Web site?
	2. Does it fairly portray the opposite perspective of the woman (or parent) who wishes/needs to work and raise children?
	3. Are there positive and negative angles to both views?
	4. Can you locate several current articles online that discuss the mommy track?

The Sandwich Generation

The Sandwich Generation is a relatively new term that defines those who are "sandwiched" between taking care of their children, and at the same time caring for their aging parents (see http://www.thesandwichgeneration.com). A new phenomenon is occurring in the United States: people are waiting longer to begin their families, while those who age are living much longer lives, with both groups needing protection, attention, and sometimes financial assistance. Adult children become parents to their parents. This dual parenting often occurs when one's career begins to peak, and retirement looks like a very real possibility. The sandwich generation often gets squeezed helping children pay college expenses, while perhaps beginning to pay for elderly parents' medical needs, all while one is attempting to save toward retirement.

In 2006, nearly 22 million workers in the U.S. were caring for their elderly parents or other relatives (Pitsenberger, 2006). According to the National Alliance for Caregiving & AARP (2004), almost 25% of all American households have cared for an elderly person within the last year, with care giving lasting an average of 4.3 years. Mothers are the ones who are most often cared for, typically widowed and approximately sixty-six years old. Their primary reasons for needing care are most often aging, or a medical condition such as cancer, diabetes, or stroke (National Alliance for Caregiving & AARP, 2004), needing on average eight hours per week of assistance. For those under fifty requiring care, emotional or mental illness is often the primary reason.

What impact does caring for an elderly parent or relative have on the caregiver? Emotional stress, financial stress, and physical stress are all reported, along with a direct and indirect impact on work. Schedules may need to be adjusted when taking time off to transport a parent to a medical appointment, or assuring that a home health aide arrives to help with activities of daily living, or managing dwindling finances. In caring for an elderly parent, 25–30% of caregivers state that they need to take time off work without pay; almost 15% of female caregivers actually quit their jobs due to the hardships and increasing physical and emotional needs of their parents (AARP, 2004). Regardless, many caregivers find themselves with limited promotional opportunities, income reduction, or missed assignments due to their home requirements. Coupled with assisting their parents with food, medicine, and transportation expenses, caregivers' personal incomes can be quickly depleted, often when they need to be bolstered and readied for pending retirements.

While child care is probably the first thing that comes to people's minds when care giving is mentioned, elder care places a significant impression on the worker's organization. There are estimates that up to 15% of all workers have elderly care-giving responsibilities at any one time. The most common effect that organizations see from their care-giving employees is absenteeism, costing national productivity losses up to $29 *billion annually*. Interestingly, only about 25% of all American companies offer any elder-care benefits, clearly a gap in services (National Alliance for Caregiving & AARP, 2004).

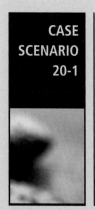

CASE SCENARIO 20-1

You currently are the assistant manager of a labor and delivery unit, interviewing for a new position. You just received the good news—you were selected to be the manager of a new labor and delivery unit in a hospital about six hours away. Unfortunately, your mother, who lives with you, has Alzheimer's and recently suffered a stroke. She is ever so slowly progressing. There are no rehabilitation facilities near the new job.

CASE ANALYSIS

1. There are several issues at hand besides the obvious one. What are they?

2. Can you come up with several options? How would you determine which one(s) has the greatest potential for you? For your mother?

3. How do you determine your decision?

THE CONCEPT OF IMBALANCE

Achieving work–family balance is much more than having a flexible schedule, working from home, or even working part time; it is about having satisfaction in all domains in which you are involved. For the past few decades, the concept of imbalance has prevailed in the literature as the primary consequence of work–family and family-work conflicts. Hall and Callery (2003) define imbalance occurring when "goals were in jeopardy and processes were unacceptable over the longer term" (p. 409). **Imbalance** occurs when either the work or family life area becomes controlling, resulting in problems exhibiting as stress, absence from work, physical symptoms, anxiety, and eventually lower work productivity and generalized unhappiness both at home and at work. Having multiple priorities only intensifies the feeling of imbalance.

People progress on trajectories that lead to the achievement of goals and desires, both in their family lives and in their professional careers. Trajectories are often determined by values and goals, and may change depending upon circumstances. As long as goals are being met, either personally or professionally, the situations are viewed as being in "balance," and become imbalanced when current goals are not achieved (Hall & Callery, 2003). When one works toward predetermined objectives, and is successful in achieving these objectives, there is a feeling of accomplishment, success, and personal fulfillment. It is when personal and professional goals appear to be in conflict with one another that we experience imbalance, struggling to rectify those conflicting situations or expectations by elimination of the causative factor or by overcompensating. A disruption can force us to reevaluate priorities, negotiate, compromise, and reassess goals.

What are the symptoms of imbalance? When forced to set priorities, there may be guilt over one area demanding so much, and taking so much time from the other, as well as disappointment, anger, isolation, and fatigue. Mental as well as physical exhaustion may also be apparent, with depression and feelings of helplessness and lack of control. When work is involved, there may be a decrease in productivity, an increase in mistakes, and resentment that one cannot be as equally devoted to work obligations as to family responsibilities. Real issues of financial concern may also be present when there is a significant and longer-term imbalance between work and family. Lastly, moving off a predetermined career trajectory for family needs, however temporary, may result in issues of personal failure, career viability, and professional aspirations.

WORK QUALITY AND FAMILY INTERDEPENDENCE

Work environments have multiple variables that influence people and their level of stress. These influential variables include the presence of children and their ages, the professional status of spouses, marital status, racial and cultural markers, work roles, and family responsibilities, including dependent relationships outside of children. When family variables mix with work variables, numerous results are possible, with many potential situations that can arise in conflict. For example, work–family conflict can be manifested when there are issues of job satisfaction, life satisfaction, family satisfaction, role overload, or role ambiguity. An inadequate work environment can result in tremendous anxiety and stress, both mental and physical, eroding confidence resulting in self-doubt, feelings of powerlessness, and poor self-esteem, not to mention decreased productivity, higher levels of mistakes, and inferior work quality.

What are some of the work stressors that may not be so obvious? Job monotony, nonautonomous decision making, and unpleasant environments lead to innocuous stress. Sometimes the accumulation of little annoyances can be even more stressful than an emergency situation, where at least there is an endpoint. Examples such as being closely watched for time at work, rather than being evaluated for quality of results, or being asked to explain the minute details of a process rather than focusing on the desired outcomes, can be incredibly demoralizing and stressful. Likewise, Frye & Breaugh (2004) found that a supportive supervisor could greatly decrease stress for a working parent, particularly among those of preschoolers. Parents who found their supervisors to be supportive, sympathetic, and flexible when there was a family emergency were less likely to feel work–family or family-work conflicts. What happens at work can greatly affect home life and vice versa.

WORK–FAMILY BALANCE AS SATISFACTION

As previously discussed, there are numerous variables that contribute to work, family, social, and life satisfaction. Listed among these variables are gender, age, educational attainment, marital status, having children, and a desirable occupation. Satisfaction occurs when one is content over a decision that was made or done correctly, or if gratification is present. When viewed in light of work or life satisfaction, another consideration is how closely the results concur with the values to which one is emotionally tied.

Hochschild (2001) states there are several issues that may make work seem like a refuge from the stressors at home, such as when one is experiencing a divorce; has preschool children, especially if both spouses are working full time; or has additional job responsibilities or is learning a new skill. Another key satisfaction aspect is that of financial stability; it probably goes without saying that the more financially secure a family is, the less work–family stressors that arise from financial worry occur. However, it is curious that perhaps many family incomes are rising due to the increasing number of dual-income earners, rather than one spouse earning significantly more than in previous years.

Another major satisfaction variable is the number of hours worked versus being at home. It can be assumed that many professionals and managers work longer than the expected forty hours per week, sometimes bringing work home and working weekends. It is not uncommon that in higher- and dual-income families, one of the spouses—and not necessarily the wife—may decrease the hours worked, or choose to stay home as a way to ease family, social, and life stressors. Work can also become less rewarding and less satisfying, resulting in resentment and a desire to shift priorities to home. Part of the difficulty, at least with some of the professions that attract a high number of females, such as nursing, librarianship, social work, elementary school teaching, and restaurant work, is that they are lower-paying jobs, with less autonomy and more restrictive schedules that often conflict with child-care options. Coupled with less opportunity for advancement, some of these variables inextricably add to spillover stress between work and home life, and may also decrease satisfaction significantly.

AGE AND WORK–LIFE NEEDS

One challenge that many nurses encounter is the issue of balancing work and family needs and responsibilities. Some of the obstacles are well known: difficult schedules, long shifts, mandatory overtime, not to mention the hard physical work and the emotional toll that it takes daily. Schedules are altered, often without regard to personal and family needs, focusing on the needs of the organization instead. The nursing shortage affects everyone, including nurses themselves. How can one balance work and home life when three twelve-hour shifts are required in a row, and a parent has not seen his or her children off to school in the morning or tucked them into bed at night for the majority of the school week? Who picks up the slack for this challenging schedule and home life, especially if there is a single parent without a support network. Even day care and school programs are limited.

CASE SCENARIO 20-2

Robert has been licensed for almost a year, returning to school in a second-degree nursing program after a successful career as a stockbroker for fifteen years. He chose the nursing field because he wanted to be more fulfilled and be directly involved with people's lives, making a difference. He said he thoroughly enjoys his new line of work, believing his life has more meaning now that he is out of the stockbroker business, even when working the evening shift, the only shift with openings. He is married, with three boys, ages ten, thirteen, and fifteen. His wife Lisa works during the day as a secretary for a CPA firm, earning minimum wage.

Not all is well at home, however, since Robert began his new job. The boys are getting into trouble at school, and often don't come right home. Homework is a battle, and because Lisa is so tired at the end of the day, the kids often run the house instead of the other way around. Robert's strong presence is somehow needed at home, and Lisa has been dropping hints that perhaps Robert should return to his old job where he made more money and was home in the evening.

CASE ANALYSIS

1. What are the boundary issues? Who are the border-crossers and the border-keepers? Are the domains clear-cut?

2. List some of the issues that pertain to each of the participants. Which is (are) the priority and why?

3. Should Robert return to his old career temporarily? Does he have any options?

4. What are the options and how would you weigh the consequences of each?

5. Determine the best solution for the situation.

The Aging Nurse Workforce and Demands for Work–Life Balance

With the advent of the baby boomers (born between 1946 and 1964), the entire workforce in the United States is aging, and the nursing profession is no exception. An aging population carries numerous implications for those needing health care services, including increasingly complicated chronic disease processes with a subsequent rise in comorbidities, dwindling financial resources, loss of family members and, many times, social isolation. Over 12.4% of the U.S. population is over 65 (U.S. Census, 2000). The fastest growing group of elders is also the oldest; in the year 2000, almost 12.1% of older Americans were at least 85 years of age, raising some interesting points for future care needs of these frailest seniors (U.S. Census, 2000).

Interestingly, as the population ages, it becomes more imbalanced in terms of gender. For the age group 55–64, there were almost 92 men for every 100 women, but that number becomes more skewed as the age increases. For those over 65, there were 70 men for every 100 women, and by 85 and older, only 41 men were available for every 100 women. Further, the majority of elderly live either in the western United States (20%) or the southern United States (16%) according to the 2000 census (see Figure 20-7).

Consistent with the aging demographics of the United States, the registered nurse population is also aging, coming closer to retirement age and not being replaced as readily. The largest decline in the last two decades occurred among the under-thirty group of registered nurses, with the total numbers dropping from a level of 25.1% (1980) to only 9.1% (2000) to 8.1% in 2004. In fact, the General Accounting Office (2001) predicts that by 2010, the percentage of nurses over age fifty will be approximately 40% of the total nursing workforce.

The aging of the registered nurse workforce can be directly attributed to the declining numbers of new students into nursing, coupled with the higher age in which they enter their nursing program. Enrollment in baccalaureate nursing programs declined for the latter part

Figure 20-7

As the population ages, there are more women than men.

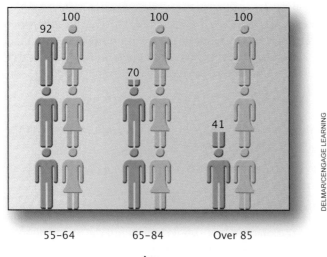

of the 1990s, with it only recently showing improvement in the last eight years (American Association of Colleges of Nursing, 2008). In 2008, the vast majority of nursing programs turned away numerous, well-qualified applicants who met the admission requirements; in fact, over 49,948 potential nursing students were not admitted—*and those numbers reflect BSN applicants only*. There are numerous justifications for turning away prospective nursing students, but the most frequently cited reason is the lack of qualified faculty, followed by clinical site availability.

The primary concern of employers and consumers alike is that a large group of registered nurses will be retiring from the nation's health care systems at about the same time as health care services are expected to dramatically increase for those sixty-five and older. Technological, pharmacological, and biomedical advances continue to improve life expectancy. Coupled with the significant decrease in younger nurses entering the workforce, a huge gap exists in the health care profession's ability to offer quality-nursing services to those who need them the most. We would be losing not only a significant human resource with these aging nurses' retirements, but many years of wisdom and knowledge in a variety of clinical areas and settings.

Nursing is a physically demanding profession, and as one ages, it gets more and more difficult to run up and down the long hallways (nurses surely did not design most hospital wards), to move and lift patients, and to multi-task ad nauseam while managing a team of nurses and para-professionals. It can be exhausting work filled with many stressors. It would seem logical that employers would rush to develop flexible and employee-friendly policies to help stem the nursing shortage on one hand and to attract more people to the profession on the other. However, many health care organizations appear oblivious to the real and pending issues.

Dissatisfaction and burnout, in addition to simply aging out of the employment arena, are additional causative factors for nurses leaving the profession. Buerhaus (2005) wrote that the nursing shortage does in fact influence work quality; more than 75% of RNs surveyed believe that the quality of patient care and the amount of time they spend with patients has declined directly because of the shortage. In projecting the future impact of the shortage, almost all the surveyed nurses predict that there will be increased stress on nurses (98%) and lowered patient care quality (93%), resulting in nurses leaving the profession (93%). Work that does not provide satisfaction eventually seeps into family life, causing a disruption in the fragile balance that one needs to maintain for a satisfying existence.

ACHIEVING WORK–LIFE BALANCE: IS IT POSSIBLE IN TODAY'S HURRIED WORLD?

For those who struggle with the daily balancing act, there are methods that can be used to regain a sense of work–life balance, establishing and maintaining harmony within the factions in everyday lives. Clark (2000) states that communication and central participation are key tools that can help achieve a more balanced life and work situation. In going back to her model of Work/Family Border Theory, she believes that "border-crossers" can increase their own support systems by talking about some of the challenges they face in both spheres of life; not whining, but fruitful discussions that can lead to mutual problem solving. Clark's stance is that balance is more likely to occur between work and home life when others understand and are up to date about the issues that arise from both areas. She goes on to say that relationship building is critical, as is increasing participation at both home and work, so that decisions that need to be made are done so with as many facts as possible. When people are informed about choices that are integral to decision-making both at home and at work, better decisions are made because of not being left out of the information loop. By taking a more active role in decision-making, more responsibility is taken, and ultimately, everyone will have a more balanced viewpoint of all areas needing attention.

How do we ensure that our lives are in check? How do we make sure that one area does not overtake the other area? What are some of the strategies that can be undertaken to create harmony

Figure 20-8
Strategies and Coping Mechanisms to Achieve Balance in the Work Domain.

1. Be realistic in what you can accomplish at work and what you cannot.

2. Is there any flexibility in work hours or scheduling? For example, is working four ten-hour days a possibility rather than a traditional five eight-hour days?

3. Is telecommuting—for a portion of the week—a possibility?

4. Is part-time work a temporary possibility rather than full-time work?

5. Does the employer offer on-site childcare that is affordable, and in the case of workers with unusual scheduling, offer expanded hours? Is there sick day care for children of employees too sick to go back to school, but not necessarily sick enough to be at home by themselves?

6. Managers and supervisors need to be supportive, understanding and flexible with employees with sick children, especially those with preschool children and without close family support mechanisms.

7. Employing organizations can actively encourage the values of work family balance by developing and implementing family-friendly policies. More than lip service needs to be paid, and in some organizations, there may need to be a major attitude shift as well as behavioral changes implemented.

8. Take breaks daily. Instead of eating lunch at your desk, get up and take a walk, enjoy conversations with someone else, or read the newspaper. If you do not normally sit at a desk, find somewhere to sit down. Don't eat on the run, don't skip lunch, or you won't have energy or patience to deal with issues as they arise.

9. Try not to take work home on a regular basis; everyone has occasional needs to work on a special project, or to complete an assignment that is due, but again, this is blurring the borders between work and home life.

10. Set priorities and work toward them, reviewing frequently.

between two competing forces? As work and home life continue to become intermingled due to the twenty-four-hour availability of computers, personal digital assistants, fax machines, text messaging, and cellular phones, it is increasingly more difficult to "turn off" the outside world. The boundaries of both domains can be controlled, but it is challenging in this information age when data is instantly available, and with everyone conditioned to have ready access to one another. Figure 20-8 illustrates strategies and coping mechanisms to achieve balance in the work domain, Figure 20-9 in the home/family/life domain, and Figure 20-10 in the personal domain.

Time-management is a challenge, regardless of one's profession or the size or composition of our family. As Robert Fulghum said in his influential book, *All I Really Need to Know I Learned in Kindergarten*, "Be aware of wonder. Live a balanced life—learn some and think some and draw and paint and sing and dance and play and work everyday some."

Figure 20-9
Strategies and Coping Mechanisms to Achieve Balance in the Home/Family/Life Domain.

1. Promote an equal (or as equal as one can) division of household family work, such as laundry, grocery shopping, cleaning, childcare tasks, eldercare tasks.

2. Encourage non-traditional roles for the wife and husband; perhaps it makes good sense that the father stay home with the young children if daycare services are not optimal and the mother can be the primary breadwinner.

3. Promote the authenticity of being childless and single by choice.

4. Acknowledge that perfection is not the goal, especially when it comes to household tasks and childrearing. A clean house only gets messy.

5. Acknowledge that parenting is difficult and a challenge—and yes, it can also be tremendously rewarding and fulfilling.

6. Appreciate that taking care of an elderly parent or relative can be incredibly challenging as well as exhausting. Know when you need help, and don't be afraid to ask. Also know when you need a break from care giving duties; there are resources.

7. Understand that when one spouse is having a particularly arduous time at work, then the other spouse can take on extra home chores, like meal preparation, taking children to and from activities and other cooperative tasks.

8. Better time management goes without saying: do you really need to go to the grocery store every night after work, or can you prepare several meals in advance and freeze them to streamline dinner after work?

9. Realize that having a family should not be a career liability for women—the logistics just need to be figured out.

10. Priority setting becomes paramount. Reassess often and regularly your priorities at work, at home, in your social circles. What are the obligations that are essential and which can be eliminated?

Figure 20-10
Strategies and
Coping Mechanisms
to Achieve Balance
in the Personal
Domain.

1. Regarding priorities, who comes first? Is it your children? Your spouse? Your work? Where do you fit in?

2. Realize that life is not perfect and certain amount of chaos and imperfections are to be expected.

3. Understand that you cannot be in two places at the same time—and give yourself enough time to go from point A to point B. Being early does take off some of the stress—really!

4. You cannot meet anyone else's needs successfully if your needs are not met first.

5. If possible, choose to live in an area that is geographically close to work, school, home and basic shopping needs. With the average commute to work time increasing, the less time in the car is better for everyone.

6. Can someone else be hired to do the housework? The gardening? Repair minor household problems? The more things that can be delegated, the more time you have to do those things that are most pleasurable.

7. Is there some way to carve out some personal time? As crazy as it may be, a little down time can make a world of difference in de-stressing and becoming refocused.

DELMAR/CENGAGE LEARNING

SUMMARY

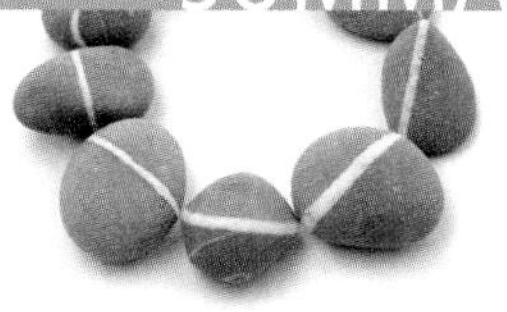

It appears that Americans are experiencing more stressful lives than previous generations due to shifting demographics, changes in the family structure, increased single parenting, and caring for elderly parents. As work boundaries become increasingly porous to outside influences such as societal expectations and home life requirements, it is no wonder that more people are becoming increasingly stressed about their life situations, often believing their world is unbalanced. To bring the issue home with regard to the registered nurse workforce, this chapter discussed how stress appears to be building in this arena as well; as the baby boomers age, so does the average age of an RN, concurrently with fewer young people entering the field. What the health-care systems are dealing with is a current shortage that, unfortunately, has not had its potential realized yet; the larger challenges lie ahead unless job satisfaction can be realized along with family life satisfaction. Gender and work–family balance issues are also discussed in this chapter, including timely topics such as "macho maternity," "the mommy track," and "the sandwich generation." While there are numerous discussions about the stress in everyday life, and the inability sometimes to feel fulfilled either at home or at work, there are various suggestions offered to assist in promoting balance and satisfaction in our multiple roles.

But what is happiness except the simple harmony between a man and the life he leads.

–Albert Camus

REFERENCES

AMERICAN ASSOCIATION OF COLLEGES OF NURSING. (2006). *2008–2009 Enrollment and graduations in baccalaureate and graduate nursing programs in nursing.* Washington, DC: Author.

AMERICAN ASSOCIATION OF RETIRED PERSONS. (2004). *Balancing work and caregiving.* Washington, DC: Author.

AMERICAN HOSPITAL ASSOCIATION. (2007). *The state of America's hospitals—Taking the pulse.* Retrieved June 28, 2007, from http://www.aha.org/aha/content/2007/PowerPoint/StateofHospitalsChartPack2007.ppt

ATACK, J., & Bateman, F. (1992). How long was the workday in 1880? *Journal of Economic History, 52*(1), 129–160.

BARNETT, R. C. (2004). Women and multiple roles: Myths and reality. *Harvard Review of Psychiatry, 12*(3), 158–164.

BOND, J. T., Galinsky, E., & Swanberg, J. E. (1998). *The 1997 national study of the changing workforce.* New York: Families and Work Institute.

BUERHAUS, P. I. (2005). Six-part series of the state of the RN workforce in the United States. *Nursing Economics, 23*(2), 58–61.

BUNTING, M. (2004). *Willing slaves: How the overwork culture is ruining our lives.* London: Harper Collins.

CLARK, S. C. (2000). Work/family border theory: A new theory of work family balance. *Human Relations, 53,* 747–770.

FRANKENHAEUSER, M. (1991). The psychology of workload, stress and health: Comparisons between the sexes. *Annals of Behavioral Medicine, 13,* 197–204.

FRONE, M. R. (2000). Work–family conflict and employee psychiatric disorders: The national comorbidity survey. *Journal of Applied Psychology, 85,* 89–99.

FRYE, N. K., & Breaugh, J. A. (2004). Family-friendly policies, supervisor support, work–family conflict, family–work conflict, and satisfaction: A test of a conceptual model. *Journal of Business and Psychology, 19*(2), 197–220.

FULGHUM, R. (2004). *All I really need to know I learned in kindergarten.* New York: Random House.

GREENBLATT, E. (2002). Work/life balance: Wisdom or whining. *Organizational Dynamics, 331,* 177–194.

GREENHAUS, J. H., & Parasuraman, S. (1987). A work-nonwork interactive perspective of stress and its consequences. *Journal of Health and Social Behavior, 24,* 300–312.

GREENHAUS, J. H., & Beutell, N. J. (1985). Sources of conflict between work and family roles. *Academy of Management Review, 10*(1), 76–88.

HALL, W. A., & Callery, P. (2003). Balancing personal and family trajectories: An international study of dual-earner couples with pre-school children. *International Journal of Nursing Studies, 40,* 401–412.

HIGGINS, C., Duxbury, L. D., & Lee, C. (1994). Impact of the life cycle stage, gender and the ability to balance work and family responsibilities. *Family Relations, 43*(2), 144–150.

HOCHSCHILD, A. R. (2001). *The time bind: When work becomes home and home becomes work.* London: Owl Books.

KOSSEK, E. E., & Lambert, S. J. (Eds). (2005). *Work and life integration: Organizational, cultural and individual perspectives.* Mahwah, NJ: Lawrence Erlbaum Associates.

LEWIS, S. (2002). Work and family issues: Old and new. In R. J. Burke & D. L. Nelson (Eds.), *Advancing women's careers* (pp. 67–82). Oxford: Blackwell Publishing.

MARKS, G., & Houston, D. M. (2002). Attitudes toward work and motherhood held by working and non-working mothers. *Work, Employment and Society, 16*(3), 523–536.

NATIONAL ALLIANCE FOR CAREGIVING AND THE AMERICAN ASSOCIATION OF RETIRED PERSONS. (2004). *Caregiving in the United States.* Washington, DC: Author.

NELSON, D. L., & Burke, R. J. (2002). *Gender, work stress and health.* Washington, DC: American Psychological Association.

NYBERG, A. (2003). *Economic crisis and the sustainability of the dual earner dual career model.* Paper presented at ESRC Seminar, "Work, Life and Time in the New Economy." Manchester, England, October 2003.

PITSENBERGER, D. J. (2006). Juggling work and elder-caregiving. *AAOHN Journal, 54*(4), 181–185.

POLIFKO, K. A. (2007). *Concepts of the nursing profession.* Clifton Park, NY: Delmar, Cengage Learning.

RUSSO, N. F. (1976). The motherhood mandate. *Journal of Social Issues, 5,* 143–153.

SMITHSON, J., & Stoke, E. H. (2005). Discourse of work–life balance: Negotiating "genderblind" terms in organizations. *Gender, Work and Organization, 12,* 147–168.

STAINES, G. L. (1980). Spillover versus compensation: A review of the literature on the relationship between work and non-work. *Human Relations, 33,* 111–129.

THE REGISTERED NURSE POPULATION: FINDINGS FROM THE 2004 NATIONAL SAMPLE SURVEY OF REGISTERED NURSES. (2005). Rockville, MD: Health Resources and Services Administration, Bureau of Health Professions, U.S. Department of Health and Human Services.

TAHMINCIOGLU, E. (2007). *Return to work not easy for stay-at-home dads.* Retrieved July 30, 2007, from http://www.msnbc.msn.com/id/19977348/

TOWNSEND, L. (2005). *Top work/family challenges and solutions.* Retrieved June 26, 2007, from http://www.bluesuit,om.com/career/balance/challenges.html

U.S. CENSUS BUREAU. (2000). *Quick tables DP-1 profile of general demographic characteristics: 2000.* Washington, DC: Author. Retrieved July 8, 2007, from http://factfinder.census.gov/servlet/QTTable?_bm = n&_lang = en&qr_name = DEC_2000_SF1_U_DP1&ds_name=DEC_2000_SF1_U&geo_id = 04000US12

U.S. CENSUS BUREAU, Statistical Abstract of the United States, 2004–2005, pp. 377–378, 386. Retrieved June 26, 2007, from http://www.census.gov/prod/2004pubs/04statab/labor.pdf

U.S. DEPARTMENT OF LABOR, Bureau of Labor Statistics. (2007). *Family Medical Leave Act of 1993.* Retrieved July 4, 2007, from http://www.dol.gov/esa/whd/fmla/

U.S. DEPARTMENT OF LABOR, Bureau of Labor Statistics. (2006). *National Longitudinal Surveys, NLSY97,* p. 1. Retrieved June 24, 2007, from www.bls.gov/news.release/pdf/nlsoy.pdf

U.S. DEPARTMENT OF LABOR, Monthly Labor Review. (2001). *Family and medical leave: Evidence from the 2000 survey.* Washington, DC: Author.

U.S. GOVERNMENT ACCOUNTING OFFICE. (2007). *Nursing Workforce: HHS Needs Methodology to Identify Facilities with a Critical Shortage of Nurses.* Retrieved July 8, 2007, from http://www.gao.gov/docdblite/summary.php?rptno = GAO-07-492R&accno = A68910

WHAPPLES, R. (2001). *Hours of work in U.S. history.* Retrieved June 24, 2007, from EH.Net Encyclopedia: http://eh.net/encyclopedia/article/whaples.work.hours.us

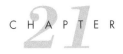

CHAPTER

21

HEALTH LITERACY

PAMELA SHERWILL-NAVARRO

MLS, AHIP, Librarian, Remington College of Nursing

Literacy is not a luxury; it is a right and a responsibility.

–President Bill Clinton

LEARNING OBJECTIVES

At the completion of the chapter the learner should be able to do the following:

1. Define health literacy.
2. Describe why health literacy is relevant to health care professionals, especially nurses.
3. Demonstrate the "Ask Me 3" or Teach Back techniques.
4. Describe how literacy can be a factor in patient noncompliance.
5. Formulate an action plan for assessing the readability of patient education materials.
6. Discuss tools to determine the reading level of patient education materials.

KEY TERMS

Communication
Health Literacy
Healthy People 2010

Informed Consent
Literacy
Medication Errors

Patient Compliance
Patient Education
Readability

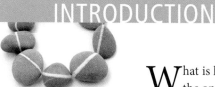

What is **health literacy?** The most popular and widely used definition of health literacy is the one used in **Healthy People 2010,** a set of health objectives for the nation to achieve over the first decade of the new century. Healthy People 2010 defines health literacy as "the degree to which individuals have the capacity to obtain, process, and understand basic health information and services needed to make appropriate health decisions" (JAMA, 1999). Why should health care professionals be concerned with health literacy? **Communication** is synonymous with safety. If health care providers and patients are not communicating, then patient safety may be at risk.

Literacy is a matter of degree, not an all-or-none situation. Unfortunately, according to the most recent study of national literacy, 29% of Americans have below basic ability and 14% have basic ability to read prose (Institute of Educational Sciences, U.S. Department of Education, 2007). That translates to 90 million people who do not possess the skills to read, understand, and act upon health information. The National Assessment of Adult Literacy (NAAL) conducted by the U.S. Department of Education evaluated more than 19,000 adults age 16 and older, representing the population demographics of the U.S. The latest NAAL survey, done in 2003, included an assessment of the nation's health literacy for the first time. Investigators measured more than 19,000 individuals' ability to read and comprehend health-related materials and forms. The results showed that the majority of Americans have intermediate health literacy. On average, women scored six points higher than men. The respondents were divided by highest educational level achieved. Many respondents with associate, bachelor, or graduate degrees were still among those that have low health literacy. Four percent of those with associate degrees and 3% of those who have earned bachelor or graduate degrees have health literacy levels that are below the basic level. When the percentage of health-literate college graduates is examined, 15% are associate degree recipients, 27% are bachelor's degree recipients, and 33% are graduate degree recipients (Institute of Educational Sciences, U.S. Department of Education, 2007).

A recent report on health literacy from The Joint Commission, the organization that accredits and evaluates hospitals and health care organizations, stated that 52% of hospitals report that they collect information from patients about their primary language; however, only 20% report that they collect information about patient literacy levels. The Joint Commission has recently required that the hospitals they accredit document a patient's preferred language and communication needs (The Joint Commission, 2007). Poor literacy can have a major effect upon a patient's communication needs.

Low health literacy can effect an individual's lifestyle choices; for instance, the likelihood of obtaining preventative health care such as annual mammograms, prostate exams, or regular physicals. It can also affect how individuals follow instructions on how to take prescription medicine and monitor their blood pressure or blood glucose levels, for example. Low literacy can also affect whether people can locate clinics and keep appointments. Research is showing that poor **patient compliance** is often a result of inadequate health literacy. If a patient does not understand what the test is or why it was ordered, they are less likely to take the time or spend the money to have it done.

Health literacy is necessary to read and comprehend the instructions and precautions on a pill bottle and take the medication properly (Keller, Wright, & Pace, 2008). These skills are also needed to discuss and understand what one is agreeing to on an informed consent form. Reading and complying with discharge instruction requires these skills. Failure to comprehend and follow discharge instruction may have serious consequences. Negotiating the complex health care system requires informed consumers who are able to advocate for themselves, their families, and their health.

Medicine and health care have languages of their own that are sometimes foreign to the general public's understanding. Frequently, health care professionals use this specialized language when communicating with patients and family members. Patients may believe that they understand the language used, or they may be too embarrassed to admit that they do not comprehend, so they do not ask for clarification. Patients, family members, and consumers are being encouraged to become more involved in managing their own health and to become active participants with their health care team, yet many lack the skills to do so (Davis, et al., 1991).

Major health care regulation and safety organizations such as the Institute of Medicine, the Joint Commission, Agency for Healthcare Research and Quality, the National Institute on Deafness and Other Communication Disorders and other health related groups are trying to raise awareness of the problem among health care professionals and determine the prevalence of low health literacy among the public.

DETERMINANTS OF HEALTH LITERACY

Health literacy is the result of many factors and is not just a problem for those for whom English is not their primary language, or individuals with low education levels. High school graduates or even college graduates may not possess the health literacy skills necessary to navigate the health care system and be active participants in their care. While adequate reading, mathematical, and writing skills are necessary, health literacy involves other competencies. People with inadequate health literacy come in all shapes and sizes. They come from all educational and economic levels. They may have been born in the United States or be immigrants to this country.

Literacy and the subset of health literacy are not constant through an individual's life span or across all subject areas. One can be a noted expert in British literature and know little about world history or medicine. Grade level completion does not correlate highly with reading level either. Some studies have shown that an individual's reading level may be as much as five grade levels below the last grade he or she completed (Davis, et al., 1991). Low health literacy levels are found more frequently in older individuals from lower income levels and among those with less formal education. Minority group members and sicker individuals are also more likely to have inadequate health literacy to comprehend health information. Health literacy is also likely to decline as one becomes older or sicker (Davis, et al., 1991).

Figure 21-1
A patient with inadequate health literacy may want a family member present while the medical history is being taken.

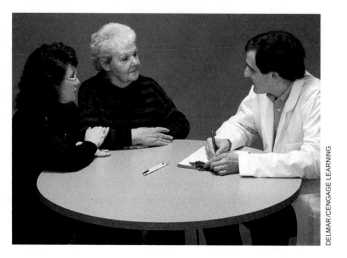

INADEQUATE HEALTH LITERACY AND THE IMPACT

In the initial encounter between a health care provider and patient or patient's family, medical history is taken (Figure 21-1). This process begins with the health care professional asking specific questions to obtain important background information and information about current symptoms. The accuracy and completeness of the information along with a clinical examination and any test results is used as the basis of the diagnosis and treatment of the patient. Health care personnel can determine some things by observation and test results, but when they are given incomplete or inaccurate information they might prescribe medication or treatments that are contraindicated or even inappropriate.

Patients with low health literacy may have a poor record of keeping clinic or doctor's appointments. Reading appointment cards may not be something that they can successfully perform. They may not be able to locate the clinic because they are not able to read a bus schedule or a map. When the health care professional sends patients to a laboratory or imaging center, they might not be able to find the location. They may not understand the reason for an appointment or the importance of a test or procedure, so they might not have them done. If a test or procedure requires fasting or preparation they may be unable to comply. Not understanding the reason for treatment can also be a factor in compliance. If you don't know the reason or importance of an appointment, test, or treatment, you are less likely to be compliant.

MEDICATION ERRORS

Recently there has been increased attention on **medication errors,** including the Institute of Medicine's report "Preventing Medication Errors" (Cohen, 2007). Numerous studies have investigated various aspects of the process, from the physician writing the prescription, to the pharmacy that processes and fills the prescription, to the nurses preparing and administering the medication, and finally the patients and how they fill, take, and follow the instructions (Beyea,

2007; Cohen, 2007; Dennison, 2005; A. L. Friedman, Geoghegan, Sowers, Kulkarni, & Formica, 2007). Patients are the final check point in preventing medication errors. However, to be effective in this role they must be knowledgeable, alert, and educated about various forms of the drugs that they have been prescribed, name brand or generic, dosages, adverse effects, drug and food interactions, and how to prevent errors. Until recently patient administration practices and errors were not a focus of study (Davis, et al., 1991). Some studies revealed that frequently pharmacists and physicians are failing to provide oral or written instructions to patients on managing their medications (Davis, 2006). The lack of oral instructions makes the written material more important. However, if patients cannot comprehend written instructions, the results may cause complications or even death. Mistakes were more common when the instructions were complex and contained several parts in the same sentence (Davis, et al., 1991). Research has shown that patients often ignore the warning labels on the container (Schiodt, 1997; Schrank, 2007). Confusing instructions are only one cause of patient medication errors. They may quickly read the instructions, trying to multi-task, or their literacy may not be adequate to read or understand the directions.

Medication administration can be difficult and confusing. Does "take two tablets four times a day" mean to take two tablets every six hours, even if you must wake up during the night, or does it mean to take two tablets at breakfast, lunch, dinner, and at bedtime? If you miss a dosage should you take it immediately as soon as you remember, or wait until the next dosage? If the instructions say avoid sunlight, can you go outside to get the mail or must you wait until it is dark? What does it mean when it says to take the medication on an empty stomach? When is your stomach empty?

Medications often have two names, the brand name and the generic. Patients may not know that fact. There have been cases of patients having both the generic and the brand name of the same medication and taking both since they did not realize that the bottles contained the same drug. If the medication is heparin or warfarin, blood thinning medications, the results can be serious or even deadly (Estrada, Hryniewicz, Higgs, Collins, & Byrd, 2000).

If a patient does not understand the oral instructions given by a physician or nurse, or cannot read the written instructions or medication container label, how can they follow those instructions? Research is showing that low literacy is often the cause of noncompliance with medication, testing glucose levels, missing appointments, and obtaining preventive screenings and care (Keller, et al., 2008).

A recent cohort study published in Archives of Internal Medicine of 3,260 Medicare patients age 65 or older examined the relationship between low health illiteracy and the ability to predict mortality (Baker, et al., 2007). Their degree of literacy was determined by their ability to perform such common medical information tasks as reading prescription labels, appointment slips, or instructions on how to prepare for common procedures. Results of these tasks determined that 25% were medically illiterate. Of the patients who were medically illiterate, 40% of them died during the study as compared to the medically literate group. When the researchers factored in the subject's health at the beginning of the study, the medically illiterate were 50% more likely to die than the literate group. These findings are very important due to the high incidence of chronic illness and the large number of prescriptions many elderly take. It seems that low health literacy is not only dangerous, it can be deadly (Baker, et al., 2007).

INFORMED CONSENT AND COMPREHENSION

The process of obtaining **informed consent** from a patient involves the preparation of a written document that lists the procedure, which is signed by the patient or guardian (Figure 21-2). This is a legal document that gives health care providers the legal right to do a procedure or perform treatment. It should be mandatory that the patient understands what is going to occur, why it is being done, and possible side effects that might occur. The National Quality Forum (NQF) reports that 44% of patients signing informed consent forms do not understand the type of operation that is going to be performed and the majority of patients (60–70%) did not read or did not understand the information contained on the informed consent form (Institute of Educational Sciences, U.S. Department of Education, 2007). To ensure patients comprehend what is about to happen and why, obtaining informed consent should be a dialog between the patient and provider. The patient should know and understand their diagnosis, the purpose of the test or procedure, the risks and benefits, alternative options and their risk and benefits, and finally the risks and benefits of not having the test or treatment. To insure this level of understanding the procedure of obtaining informed consent should be a two-way conversation with

Figure 21-2
Informed consent is a legal document signed by a patient or the patient's guardian that gives health care providers the legal right to do a procedure or perform treatment. However, the nurse should make sure a dialog occurs with the patient so the patient fully understands the procedure or treatment to be performed.

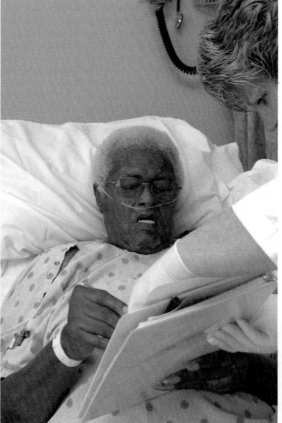

DELMAR/CENGAGE LEARNING

the patient. Talking with patients rather than at them takes time, patience, and commitment to their well being and what is best for them.

<table>
<tr>
<td>

Writing
Exercise
21-1

</td>
<td>

Practice explaining procedures to patients. Choose one of the following and write out a plan to discuss the procedure with these patients so that they understand why it is being done and what will occur.

1. The patient is a sixty-seven-year-old female retired factory worker who is hard of hearing. She is having a physical exam. The physician has asked you to explain to her how to do an occult blood fecal test, what it is, why it is being done, and what to do with it after collecting it.

2. The patient is a mildly retarded thirty-eight-year-old male who is scheduled to have blood drawn for a CBC. How would you describe the procedure and explain why it is being done?

</td>
</tr>
</table>

EMERGENCY DEPARTMENT CARE: THE MOST EXPENSIVE CARE

Individuals with high levels of health literacy are usually healthier. They do not smoke, limit alcohol intake, minimize their intake of fatty fried foods, drink more water than soda, attempt to eat the recommended servings of fruits and vegetables, and make other choices to promote good health. They also make time in their busy schedules for exercise. These individuals often have a primary care provider and have recommended screenings and health care. If their health care provider finds that it is necessary to put them on medication, either short term or long, health-literate patients understand the purpose of the medication, fill the prescription, and follow the administration instructions. When they notice a change in their own health status they schedule an appointment with their health provider. The majority of this group also has health insurance. Obtaining regular health care screening for conditions such as diabetes, hypercholesterolemia, or hypertension means they are often diagnosed in the early stages before a stroke, myocardial infraction, or other complication occurs. When they have such chronic conditions as asthma or diabetes, they do a better job of controlling them and make fewer trips to the emergency room for control (Schillinger, et al., 2003; Williams, Baker, Honig, Lee, & Nowlan, 1998).

People with low health literacy more frequently report their health status as poor. They may not completely understand their health problems, and are hospitalized more often than the health literate (Pawlak, 2005). When people have poor health literacy they may not make the same choices that health literate people do. They are more likely to smoke, consume diets high in fats, sugars, and sodium, and unwittingly make choices that impact their present and future health. When they are diagnosed with chronic conditions such as asthma (Williams, et al., 1998) or diabetes (Schillinger, et al., 2002), they do not control or manage their disease as well as the health literate. They may also practice risky behaviors such as unprotected sex, or fail to fill and take medications as they were prescribed. Those with low health literacy may be motivated to maintain their health but lack the knowledge and skills needed to do so. When health care providers take the time and effort to explain, and use the opportunity to teach these patients, compliance may increase. However, if patients do not understand what the provider is telling them, why it is important, and what they should do, then the chance of compliance is reduced.

Emergency departments are designed to deal with accidents and health emergencies. They are not designed to function as primary care providers. Individuals and families with low health literacy may lack health insurance or not understand their benefits. Without health insurance or a relationship with a primary care provider, regular screenings and care may not occur. They then seek care in hospital emergency departments (Felland, Hurley, & Kemper, 2008; Greene, 2007). Patients often use more than one hospital's emergency departments. Each hospital maintains their own medical records and typically they do not share or communicate those records with each other. Patients diagnosed with chronic conditions such as hypertension, diabetes, or hypercholesterolemia may be seen in the emergency department and given a thirty-day prescription for medication to treat the conditions diagnosed. If they mistakenly believe that the thirty-day prescription cured the condition, the patient may suffer serious complications as a result (Greene, 2007). When health care is obtained in this patchwork fashion, chronic conditions may not be properly managed and diagnosis of acute conditions may be delayed.

Universal medial records or personal health records are not common at this time. Patients using emergency departments for their main source of health care lack continuity of care, and do not frequently have routine screenings or monitoring. If they should be on medication to treat a chronic condition such as diabetes or hypertension, compliance to a regular administration schedule may not occur. A health care provider at one emergency department may prescribe a medication, and then if the patient arrives at another emergency department days or weeks later while still taking that medication, they might fail to inform the second emergency department what they are taking. This situation may result in the patient taking medications that are contraindicated to be taken concurrently, such as aspirin and warfarin. Patients with low health literacy may not follow dosing instructions for prednisone and abruptly cease taking it without reducing the dosage. This practice can be dangerous and even deadly.

TOO LITTLE TOO LATE

Many disease processes begin asymptomatically and can be detected early with testing, but by the time symptoms occur damage has often already begun. This is especially true with cancer, tuberculosis, diabetes, and hypertension or cardiovascular disease. All of these conditions can have better outcomes if they are diagnosed and treated earlier in the process. Treating the complications of cardiovascular disease, diabetes, and other conditions is often more expensive and invasive than early treatment and prevention. Diabetes is a disease process that can cause blindness, kidney failure, and other conditions when patients fail to exercise tight gylcemic control. The cost of dialysis and the effect that it has upon one's lifestyle is tremendous. Occasionally patients will arrive at either a physician's office or emergency department with difficulty breathing and coughing and be diagnosed with stage 4 lung cancer. For health care professionals there is nothing more devastating than diagnosing a patient with a terminal condition that could have been managed by medication, surgery, lifestyle changes, or treatment if that patient had access to regular health care.

Contagious Diseases

Tuberculosis, a disease that seemed to be almost eradicated a few years ago, has returned with a vengeance. Tuberculosis has developed resistance to many of the antibiotics that used to successfully treat it (Munsiff, et al., 2006). The current treatment now requires several medications and compliance by the patient in following the medication regime for almost a year. Compliance with the dosage and ongoing testing and monitoring is complex, but failure to comply may result in developing a strain that is even more drug resistant and difficult to treat. Hepatitis is an infectious disease that requires precautions and lifestyle changes to promote the patient's health and to prevent transmission to family and friends. HIV/AIDS is another catastrophic disease that can be spread by people who do not practice safe sex and other precautions to minimize transmission. Hepatitis, tuberculosis, and HIV/AIDS require complex therapies and patient compliance. However, if you do not understand or remember what the precautions are or why they are important, how likely is it that you will follow them? Failure to comprehend and follow the precautions and therapies could endanger a patient's health.

IMPROVING HEALTH LITERACY

Many health care professionals are frustrated by their patients' use of the Internet and the large amounts of material they find and bring with them to appointments. While almost anything can be found on the Internet, it is not evaluated or validated unless you restrict your searching to reliable sources such as government sites, university sites, or national organizations that support research and information dissemination on particular diseases.

There are also numerous books directed at consumers that do not confuse the reader with technical medical jargon, but contain just enough medical sounding words to convince the reader that the information is legitimate. While not recommending or criticizing these books, one must wonder how much research there is to support claims that taking supplements will improve your immune system to fight cancer, taking shark cartilage will prevent cancer, or killing parasites and removing benzene from the body cures HIV/AIDS. Unfortunately these books do an excellent job of being able to communicate with patients, making them believe they are being educated about their illness and learning how to treat it in a way that makes sense to them. If you are interested in learning more about Internet health hoaxes go to http://www.quackwatch.com. This site evaluates books, Web sites, and the backgrounds of the people promoting books, Web sites, and products that are not mainstream medicine.

The Internet has made a great deal of health information available to people who previously had few resources. A recent study of health-related Web sites revealed that 100% of the English-language sties evaluated were written at the twelfth-grade reading level and 86% of those written in Spanish were also (Schillinger, 2002). However, studies are showing the readability level of

Figure 21-3
Sample of Patient
Information
Written at the
Fifth-Grade Level.

Diabetes is a serious illness. Patients with diabetes have too much sugar in their blood and urine. They can control it with drugs, diet, and exercise. If they do not control it their heart, eyes, kidneys, nerves, and feet will be damaged.

DELMAR/CENGAGE LEARNING

Figure 21-4
Sample of Patient
Information Written
at the Twelfth-
Grade Level.

Diabetes mellitus occurs when glucose levels become high due to the body's inability to produce sufficient insulin. Insulin is a hormone produced in the pancreas which controls the amount of glucose in the blood stream. The absorption of glucose in the bloodstream stimulates the pancreas to produce and release additional insulin. Insulin facilitates the movement of glucose from the bloodstream into the individual cells where it is converted into energy. Diabetes Mellitus is an endocrine disease. Diabetes mellitus is a different disease than diabetes insipdus.

DELMAR/CENGAGE LEARNING

many published patient education materials and Internet sites are written at the tenth-grade reading level or higher (Friedman, Hoffman-Goetz, & Arocha, 2006). Functional literacy, however, is fifth-grade reading level. Much of the material that is written is just too complex for many patients to read. Since health education is one method that can be used to reach the goal of health literacy, material should be written such that patients can read and understand it. Figures 21-3 and 21-4 demonstrate the difference in information written at a fifth-grade level and twelfth-grade level.

People with low reading levels are often ashamed or embarrassed about their lack of reading skills, and many are very adept at concealing it. Frequently it is a secret that their spouse, children, friends, and relatives are not aware of. When given paperwork to fill out they may ask to take it home to fill out since they forgot their glasses or may ask you to read it to them for the same reason. The amount of energy that they expend to hide their secret is amazing. Many are so uncomfortable that they will not admit it when asked directly (Mayer & Villaire, 2004). Figure 21-5 lists tips for creating effective patient information.

DETERMINING PATIENT READING LEVELS

Literacy comes in degrees; it is not a black-and-white or yes-vs.-no situation. One's literacy is also not a constant during his or her lifetime. Individuals who were educated and very literate as young adults may find that as they age and lose acuity in eyesight, hearing, and short-term memory, their literacy decreases. When patients are ill, in pain, or taking multiple medications, their ability to focus, read, reason, and comprehend suffers. Nurses, physicians, pharmacists, and other health care providers suffer these same effects of time and illness and may not have the same level of health literacy later in life either. Therefore, health care providers cannot have just two sets of information, one for those who are literate and another for those who are not. Patients and situations must be evaluated individually.

Knowing a patient's educational level provides some information about literacy level, but it is not a fool-proof method to determining literacy level, as shown in the National Assessment of

Figure 21-5
Tips for Writing
Effective
Educational
Materials.

Tips for Creating Effective Patient Information Materials
• Begin with clear objectives of what you want to accomplish.
• Use everyday language — not medical jargon.
• Think of the audience and make it race, age, cultural or gender suitable.
• Provide clear steps that the reader can comprehend.
• Keep it positive — avoid negatives.
• A picture is worth many words and may be clearer.
• Use short sentences.
• Make it look easy — leave white space, use large print, bullet important points.

DELMAR/CENGAGE LEARNING

Adult Literacy (NAAL) results (Institute of Educational Sciences, U.S. Department of Education, 2007). Nursing programs do not typically teach skills that enable nurses to measure literacy or develop patient materials at appropriate literacy levels. There are resources available to assist health care professionals in writing materials at specific grade levels.

There are some subtle signs of low literacy that can become automatic in patient encounters. You and fellow health care professionals are perceived by your patients as confident, competent, intelligent, and educated. Patients with low literacy are often fearful that if you knew they could not read or understand what you have told them, you would have a poor opinion of them. Hiding this secret has become an automatic compensation for them. Patients who frequently say they have forgotten their glasses, want to take material home to read or to show and discuss with a family member, or regularly bring a "reader," "friend," or family member to routine visits might be patients demonstrating signs of low literacy (Mayer & Villaire, 2004). Patients who are consistently noncompliant may actually have low literacy. They may not be able to read or follow instructions. Some patients may truly have vision or hearing problems requiring evaluation. As you become more aware, observing these behaviors will become second nature and encourage you to investigate further.

While at the current time measuring a patient's literacy level is not standard practice, literacy has been identified as a vital sign (Committee on Health Literacy, Board on Neuroscience and Behavioral Health, Institute of Medicine, 2004; The Joint Commission, 2007). It may be only a matter of time until literacy is included in patient assessment. Sometimes an actual measure of a patient's reading grade level is required, and other times an approximation is sufficient. While testing patients' reading and literacy levels provides useful information, to tailor information to the proper level, it is a sensitive and emotionally charged area. Patients, regardless of their literacy level, may become hostile and upset. Patients with high literacy may be insulted that you are testing them. Patients with low literacy may be upset that you are testing them because low literacy is a very private situation. More than 67% of people with low literacy have not told their spouses about it, and 53% have not revealed their reading difficulties to their children (Parikh, Parker, Nurss, Baker, & Williams, 1996). Carefully determine if formal testing is necessary and then plan how best to initiate this conversation with patients.

The following information about literacy testing will not make you an expert in this area, but it will serve as an introduction and provide some basic knowledge on the subject. Some of the most popular instruments used for measuring literacy are the Wide Range Achievement Test (WRAT), the Test of Functional Health Literacy in Adults (TOFHLA), and the Rapid Estimate of Adult Literacy in Medicine (REALM). All of these tests are easy to administer and score; they do not require certification or training in order to administer. There is a high degree of correlation between the three tests.

The WRAT-4 measures word reading, sentence comprehension, spelling, and computational skills. This test can be used for individuals age five through ninety-four. It is widely used to obtain a rapid screening assessment and grade-level equivalent or percentile rank. It is a paper-and-pencil test that may be administered individually or in small group situations. Each question is worth one point. This test is not available free of charge. An introductory kit containing the manual, fifty response sheets, and other needed materials costs about $250.

The TOFHLA is another test that is commonly used in medical settings to assess literacy. One unique feature is that the test material is actually designed to measure patient health literacy, rather than general literacy. The test material uses actual health-related materials such as pill bottles or appointment slips. To view a sample selection of this test and to obtain ordering information go to: http://www.peppercornbooks.com/catalog/pdf/tofhla_eng_12pt_websmpl.pdf.

There are two versions of the test, a regular and a short version. The full version takes about twenty-two minutes to administer and has fifty items in the reading comprehension section and seventeen in the numeracy section. The short version takes approximately seven minutes and has only two reading comprehension sections. A Spanish version named the TOFHLA-S exists in both long and short format. The scores range from 0–100 on the long English and Spanish version and 0–36 on both short versions.

The purpose of the numeracy section is to measure how well a patient is able to understand and act upon that type of information. In one of the sample questions, the patient is handed a pill bottle with a label listing the name of the person to whom the medication was prescribed with a date, physician's name, medication name, and strength and dosing instructions (see Figure 21-6).

A typical question in the numeracy section would be, "If you took your first capsule at 7:30 a.m., when should you take your next one? When would you take the one after that? At what time would you take the last dose of the day? Another task in the numeracy section might be

Figure 21-6
Sample prescription label similar to those used in TOFHLA.

Miller, PJ   5/15/2009
RX: 237890   Dr. Chad Williams

Tetracycline
500 mg.
Take one capsule, by mouth 4
times a day
Qty: 40   MFG: TEVA
No Refills – Dr Authorization Required
              Use before 5/14/2018

to read a chart of family size and income limits after deductions from Medicaid or other free health care programs. The patient is asked questions, such as, if there are five people in your family and your monthly income is $1,950, would you qualify for this program?

The reading comprehension section uses a procedure known as CLOZE. A paragraph is written with certain words (the 5th word in every sentence, for instance) missing, and word choices listed below it. The materials used in this section are actual patient instructions for procedures such as an upper GI series, the patient rights and responsibilities of a Medicaid application, and standard language used on hospital informed consent forms (Committee on Health Literacy, Board on Neuroscience and Behavioral Health, Institute of Medicine, 2004).

The most commonly used tool is the REAHL, which takes less than five minutes to administer and score (see Table 21-1). This is the easiest test for health care professionals to administer and requires little training or preparation. The patient is given a laminated sheet with a list of sixty-six common medical terms divided into three lists. The first list begins with single-syllable words such as pill, eye, or fat. As you go down the lists, the complexity of pronunciation and number of syllables increases. Some of the words near the end of the third list include potassium, impetigo, and inflammatory. Patients are instructed to read as many aloud as they are able. The examiner has an unlaminated copy of the work lists on a clipboard turned away from the patient. The administrator marks a "+" by any word pronounced correctly, a "√" by mispronounced words, and a "−" by any words that were not attempted. To score, the number of + marks in each column is tallied, and the score is compared to those in the table of levels (Davis, et al., 1991). The actual grade level or raw score may be beyond your level of interest; the **patient education** implications are very relevant and should be considered when providing patient instructions or educational information. The following Web site provides a sample view of the REAHL test and ordering information: http://www.nursing.columbia.edu/informatics/HealthLitRes/pdf/REALM_1.pdf.

Table 21-1 REAHL Scores and Grade Equivalents

Raw Scores	Grade Level	Patient Education Implications
0–18	3rd grade or below	Not able to read most low-literacy materials; will need repeated oral instructions and materials composed primarily of illustrations, or audio or video
19–44	4th–6th grade	Need low-literacy materials; may not be able to read prescription label
45–60	7th–8th grade	Struggle with most patient education materials; will not be offended by low-literacy materials
60–66	High School	Able to read most patient education materials

Due to the fact that Spanish is much more consistent phonologically than English, simply translating the REAHL into Spanish would not measure reading ability as accurately as the English version. The inflated scores would not provide useful information. The SAHLSA or Short Assessment of Health Literacy for Spanish-speaking Adults was developed to be an easy-to-administer test for Spanish patients. In this test patients read aloud a list of medically related words, similar to the REAHL, but they are also required to associate each word with another word that has a similar meaning (Lee, Bender, Ruiz, & Cho, 2006).

There is a high level of correlation among these three, so the decision of which test to use depends upon which one the practitioner is most comfortable with and what they think will work best with their patients. Regardless of which test is selected, it is very important that you are direct with patients and explain why they are being tested and what you hope to accomplish with the results. If patients are hesitant or reluctant to be tested, it is usually best to not force the issue. You can always proceed with the indirect approach and observe their behaviors and employ some other techniques to check that the patient understands. When formal testing is used, it is important not to focus too much upon a specific grade-level equivalent. Reading and reading comprehension is a very complex process involving many skills. These tests are not comprehensive diagnostic tests. The value of these rapid screening tests is to identify those patients with low literacy, moderate literacy, or high literacy levels so that they receive information at the level and in the format that is most effective for them. Look to see if the score is high, average, or low. The purpose is to be more patient centered, not to embarrass or label patients.

The tests described above can be costly in terms of time and purchasing testing materials. Many health care professionals may not be comfortable testing the reading levels of patients in a formal method. Dr. Barry Weiss, an early researcher in the area of health status and literacy, developed an English or Spanish screening test that can be administered in approximately three minutes (Weiss, Hart, McGee, & D'Estelle, 1992). The instrument is named the Newest Vital Sign. This test consists of one scenario and six questions, which are scored either right or wrong. Patients are presented with a simulated label from a container of ice cream. Questions are based upon information on the label. The results of the Newest Vital Sign were tested against the TOFHLA, with a 95% confidence level that subjects testing greater than seventy-four on the TOFHLA would score between 71.5% and 78.5% on the Newest Vital Sign. During the development of the instrument, more than one thousand individuals were tested. The final version consists of one single scenario that measures both numeracy and literacy with six questions. The label and questions used in this test are found in the article, which is available on the Internet as open access (Weiss, et al., 2005).

VERBAL COMMUNICATIONS

The majority of communications between health care providers and patients is verbal. To speak effectively with patients on a level that they understand takes practice. There are a few tools available to assist you. One way to check that the patients comprehend what you are telling or teaching them is to ask them questions about what you told them. For example, if you are instructing the patient to reduce soda intake, ask them what they could drink that would be a better or healthier choice, or ask them to tell you strategies to cut sugar from their diet. Questions are very powerful, use them.

Ask Me 3

The Partnership for Clear Health Care Communication has a campaign to promote communication between health care providers and patients, because good communication equals healthy patients. The basis of this campaign is to educate patients to ask three pertinent questions when they visit a health care provider. These questions are: What is my main problem? What do I need to do? And why is it important for me to do this? There are posters, brochures, and other materials on the Ask Me 3 Web site (see Figure 21-7) that can be either downloaded or ordered for a fee. If you do not believe that this method would be effective with your patient population, an alternative would be to ask patients those three questions at the end of their visit. That will provide an opportunity to assess how much information they absorbed. To view the materials and to learn more about this campaign go to http://askme3.org.

Teach Back

Patient education is needed anytime a patient is newly diagnosed with a condition such as diabetes or asthma that requires self-monitoring or self-care performance. Performing these tasks properly requires the patient to learn detailed, multi-step processes. Listening to a description of performing the procedure or watching the procedure performed is usually not sufficient for a patient to be able to perform the task independently.

To insure that patients possess the necessary skills, have the patient demonstrate the procedure. Humans are multi-sensory beings, and the more senses involved in teaching, the better the learning outcomes. One method developed to assess patient comprehension and learning is Teach Back. When using Teach Back, health care providers ask patients to repeat the information or demonstrate the skill that they are being taught to assess their comprehension. This allows the health care provider to assess the learning and provide additional information or clarification to the patient. The situation should be as realistic as possible. Models or actual devices should be employed. Care should be taken to focus on two to three main ideas or skills per session. On subsequent visits, prior skills and information should be reviewed and repeated as needed. This method is endorsed by the American Medical Association (AMA) and the National Quality Forum's Safe Practices.

Closing the Loop

"Closing the Loop" is another tool developed to assist health care professionals to teach and assess patient learning. According to Dr. Dean Schillinger, a well-known speaker and writer on health literacy, patients recall only about one half of what they are told or taught. He advocates an

Figure 21-7
Ask Me 3: Good
Questions for
Your Good
Health. *(Courtesy
of Partnership
for Clear Health
Communication at
National Patient
Safety Foundation.)*

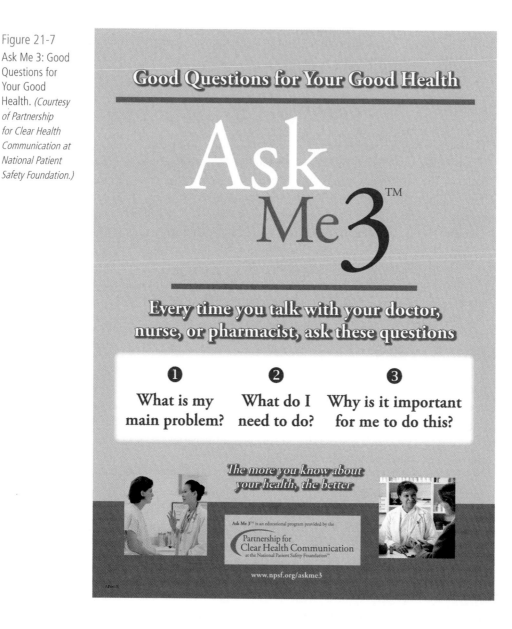

interactive strategy to increase patient comprehension and recall. He calls his method "Closing the Loop," which is based upon the "teach-back method." Dr. Schillinger used this method to evaluate the amount of information and skills patients with diabetes mellitus and low health literacy recalled, and how effective they were in maintaining gylcemic control. The basis of this approach is to ask the patient to explain what he or she is going to do by asking simple questions. When the patient cannot answer the question correctly, further teaching is performed (Schillinger, et al., 2003).

Using these two patient teaching opportunities, write out how you would teach them material, and then write how you would evaluate their learning utilizing either the Teach Back or Ask Me 3 techniques. After you have developed and written your teaching plan, it may be demonstrated through role play with classmates.

1. The patient is a forty-eight-year-old male who was born and educated in Mexico, but speaks English. He is hypertensive and is obese. The physician suspects that he is diabetic and has asked you to draw blood to obtain a blood glucose level. Plan how you would explain what you are going to do to the patient and why.

2. The patient is a sixteen-year-old female high school dropout who has recently delivered her second child. The physician has asked you to discuss birth control options with her. Describe how you would initiate the conversation and explain to her the available options.

MEASURING THE READABILITY OF TEXT

Assessing the **readability** of patient material first began in the 1920s. The recent NAALS survey provided a great deal of information about the state of patient literacy, but few answers about how to determine if material is at an appropriate level (Institute of Educational Sciences, U.S. Department of Education, 2007). Some of the scales and measurement instruments involve counting the number of syllables in the words and the number of words per sentence. There are tools available to measure the readability of material. Readability measured by the scales refers to the ease or difficulty of reading, and recognizing or being able to sound out the words; it does not measure the reader's comprehension of the material. Determining the readability level of material is much easier now with automatic calculators and Web-based tools. These tools, which are algorithms, provide only a rough guide and not an absolute level. They can be useful in determining if the content level is right for your intended readers. Sentence length and the number of syllables in the words are elements evaluated in most readability tests. Some of the tools are: the SMOG, Flesch-Kincaid, Automated Readability Index, Coleman-Liau Index, and Gunning Fog Index. The SMOG and the Flesch-Kincade are probably the most widely used tests of readability, so only those will be discussed here.

The SMOG, which stands for Simple Measure of Gobbledygook, was developed in 1969 to be an easier-to-calculate replacement for the Gunning-Fog Index. This index was developed in a world that did not have widespread availability of personal computers and the resources available on the Internet. There is a standard error in grade level calculation of 1.5159. Since its development, it has been widely used in the health care setting to estimate readability, especially in the Veterans Administration System.

The formula to calculate readability using the SMOG is to count the words containing three or more syllables in three ten-sentence samples, estimate the count's square root, and then add three.

$$\sqrt{\text{number of polysyllables} \times \left(\dfrac{30}{\text{number of sentences}}\right)} + 3$$

Computers and the Internet have simplified this process with the development of automatic calculators. To access a SMOG calculator go to: http://www.wordscount.info.

The second readability calculator is actually two tests; the Flesch-Kincaid Reading Ease and the Flesch-Kincaid Grade Level tests were developed by Rudolf Flesch. These two instruments use the same measures, but then use different scales. The two tests do not always correlate. The Flesch-Kincaid Reading Ease test results in a number that rates the text on a one-hundred-point scale. High scores indicate text that is easier to understand. For example, the sentence, "Nat is a cat," has a score of ninety-six with a grade equivalent of one, and the sentence, "Understanding written passages involves time-consuming concentration," was given a score of –thirty-four with a grade level of twenty.

The Flesch-Kincaid method is very widely used and has even been incorporated into several word processing programs, including Microsoft Word. To enable this tool in Microsoft Word, select "Tools" and then "Options," then click on the tab labeled "Spelling and Grammar." In the second section titled "Grammar," place a check in the box "Show Readability Statistics." When you complete a spell check of a document a box will open with the readability information. The results are divided into three sections: Counts, Averages, and Readability. The Counts section lists the number of words, characters, paragraphs, and sentences in the selection measured. The Averages section lists the average number of sentences per paragraph, number of words per sentence, and number of characters per word. The last section provides the readability measures. It lists the percentage of passive sentences, the Flesch Reading Ease score, and the Flesch-Kincade Grade Level.

Flesch Reading Ease Formula:

$$206.835 - 1.015 \left(\dfrac{\text{total words}}{\text{total sentences}}\right) - 84.6 \left(\dfrac{\text{total syllables}}{\text{total words}}\right)$$

Flesch-Kincaid Grade Level Formula:

$$0.39 \left(\dfrac{\text{total words}}{\text{total sentences}}\right) + 11.8 \left(\dfrac{\text{total syllables}}{\text{total words}}\right) - 15.59$$

In addition to the free readability tools and calculators, there are commercial computer programs available. Unless writing and measuring the readability of material is your full-time position or a major responsibility of your position, the free calculators are probably sufficient. Determining readability is not an exact science. These calculators are not a guarantee that the material will be understood; they are just tools. When writing patient education material, it is

Internet Exercise 21-2	Go to http://medlineplus.gov, http://www.noah-health.org, or http://www.webmd.com.

Select a disease or condition and copy a section of the text and paste it into the readability calculators at one of the following sites:

http://simbon.madpage.com (select FOG)

http://www.harrymclaughlin.com (select SMOG)

http://www.online-utility.org (select English and readability tests)

1. What did you estimate as the reading level of the material?

2. What is the SMOG rating of the material?

3. What is the Flesch Reading Ease score?

4. What is the range of grade levels assigned to the material?

5. How well do you think someone with low literacy would be able to read and comprehend the material?

6. How close were the grade levels assigned by the different calculators?

important to begin with a clearly identified purpose or objective and to focus the material on that purpose. Remember that less is more effective and less overwhelming, so preserve white space. Text size and font should be considered. Select a text font size of at least twelve points. San serif fonts, the ones that do not have bars on the bottoms or tops of the letters, are easier to read. Two common examples of san serif fonts are Arial and Tacoma. Times New Roman and Courier are two examples of serif fonts that should be avoided. Avoid writing the entire document in capital letters. However, use bolding, underlining, or capitalization to emphasize important points. Keep your writing in the active voice. It is more direct and less confusing. Carefully select words for the intended audience, e.g., use chicken not poultry for easier understanding. If you must use technical words, use examples to explain them. Using a question-and-answer format with short, direct answers can be very effective. Think bullet points rather than long, loose prose.

A PICTURE IS WORTH HOW MANY WORDS?

Pictures add interest and assist with comprehension for all of us, but are more important for people with low literacy; it gives them something upon which to focus that they can understand. We use multiple senses to learn, so involving multiple senses when teaching assists learning. Individuals tend to have a predominate style, and using multiple inputs increases learning, since

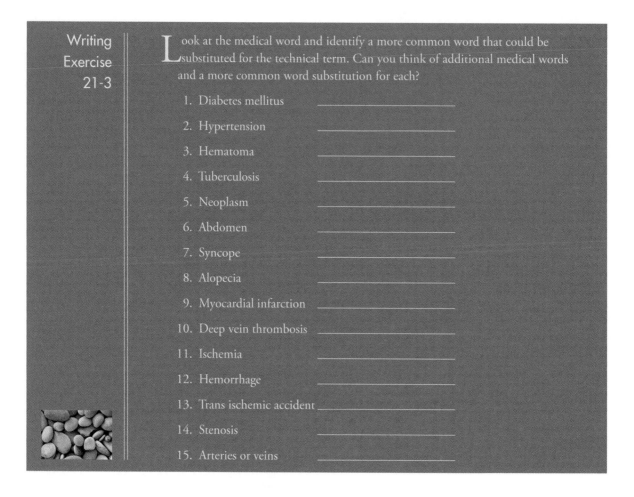

Writing Exercise 21-3

Look at the medical word and identify a more common word that could be substituted for the technical term. Can you think of additional medical words and a more common word substitution for each?

1. Diabetes mellitus _____
2. Hypertension _____
3. Hematoma _____
4. Tuberculosis _____
5. Neoplasm _____
6. Abdomen _____
7. Syncope _____
8. Alopecia _____
9. Myocardial infarction _____
10. Deep vein thrombosis _____
11. Ischemia _____
12. Hemorrhage _____
13. Trans ischemic accident _____
14. Stenosis _____
15. Arteries or veins _____

everyone utilizes more than one sense in a learning situation. When selecting graphics, keep them clean and focused on what you are teaching. Avoid busy and very detailed ones. Patients with very low literacy can be instructed with diagrams or pictures. Consider your audience—if it is predominately African American, do not use pictures of blond-haired, blue-eyed children. Golfing or skiing are not common exercises for low-income patients. Tattoos and multiple body piercings are not always acceptable to older patients. The selection of inappropriate graphics may disinterest your audience.

When patients are newly diagnosed with chronic health conditions such as diabetes, hypertension, asthma, or cardiovascular disease, typically the physician or nurse provides educational material and speaks to the patient about lifestyle changes that are beneficial. Often times the health care provider is frustrated due to the low amount of compliance to diet, exercise, or other lifestyle changes. When patients are newly diagnosed they are often given an overwhelming amount of information. They may not be in the best frame of mind to comprehend or absorb it, either.

Here is an example of how a simple but very clear patient education encounter impacted that patient and changed his life. Herb, a white male who was sixty-six years old and was employed as a general contractor, suffered a major myocardial infarction. Herb was a high school graduate and, while he was a good contractor, he had little knowledge of medicine. During his hospitalization a coronary angiography was performed to determine the state of his heart and blood vessels. The test showed substantial blockages, which were treated. After completing the procedure, the doctor came in to discuss the tests and necessary life-style changes. Instead of just talking to Herb, the doctor took out a pad of paper and drew a very simple line drawing of his heart and arteries. She then colored in the sections where the blockage was and wrote down the percentage of blockage. Herb was the "typical" construction worker type, and might have left the hospital wanting a cigarette, a burger, and a beer. The time and effort that his doctor spent with him on the drawing and explanation convinced him that he needed to make some changes if he wanted to maintain his health and enjoy the future. He agreed to participate in a cardiac rehabilitation program and made changes in his diet and exercise habits. He did so well in making lifestyle changes, that he began to be asked to speak to other patients recently diagnosed with cardiovascular disease. Over the course of time, he has spoken to more than one hundred people, and not one of them had been shown a drawing as Herb had been (Osborne, 2006).

Whenever Herb thought about going to a fast-food restaurant for a burger and fries, the picture of his occluded arteries flashed in front of his eyes. With a little thought, planning, and a bit of drawing skill, you too can be a health care professional who makes an impression and changes lives (Osborne, 2006).

ALTERNATIVE FORMATS

If this chapter was written a couple of years ago, you would have been encouraged to create cassette tapes, CD-Roms, or VHS tapes to provide alternatives to print materials for patients with low literacy. At this time we are in a state of flux on formats. The future seems to be embracing digital formats for audio that can be played on computers or MP3 players. However, you must first determine how widespread the access is to computers and MP3 players among the patients that you care for. While many people still have video recorders, they are also becoming obsolete. If you are going to produce any materials, it is probably best to ask your patients what format they would be able to use.

Before creating original materials, determine if free materials are available from national organizations or government agencies. There are some points to consider if you decide to produce multimedia materials (Figure 21-8). Carefully select the vocabulary in order to use words understood by the audience. Make sentences short and in the active voice. While the dialogue should sound natural, it is often helpful to write out a script. The use of a script insures that the main objective is addressed, that specific information is included, and that the vocabulary and sentence length are appropriate for the intended audience. If large or technical words must be used, give examples, define them, or show a picture if applicable. Keep the material short. It is suggested that eight minutes is about the maximum. If the necessary material cannot be covered

Figure 21-8
Tips for Producing
Multimedia
Patient Materials.

Do	Don't
Choose words comfortable to audience	Use jargon or medicalise
Use short sentences in an active voice	Use long sentences in a passive voice
Use natural sounding dialogue	Sound stilted and unnatural
Write a script and practice	Speak without a script that is practiced
Keep material short — 8 minutes max	Try to tell them everything at once
Use graphics, diagrams, or models	Be a talking head

in eight minutes or less, divide it into sections so that patients can view the next section at another time. Add interactive activities if possible. Talking heads are not interesting and do not encourage one to pay attention.

There are a variety of videos available for purchase. Some of the commercial videos are very good, while others may be too highly technical or dated for your patients. Videos can be expensive, so it is helpful if you can preview them prior to purchasing. If you have access to a medical library, either through a university or hospital, investigate to see if they have a video collection. It may be possible to borrow them or, if you cannot borrow them, it might be possible to preview them to determine if they are appropriate for purchase. More and more frequently, free, short health videos are becoming available on the Internet. If you screen them and determine that they are useful for your patients. sharing access information with patients with computers may be appropriate. For patients without computers or computer skills, an unused corner or small room might make a useful patient education center where a computer could be located, so that the videos could be cued up and viewed. A couple of resources for free online videos to investigate are http://healthlibrary.stanford.edu/index.html and http://www.medlineplus.gov.

IT'S ALL ON THE INTERNET, ISN'T IT?

The Internet has made a great deal of information available that was not available previously. However, not all of the information on health or other topics is reliable or reputable. Some physicians are not pleased when their patients decide to "research" their ailments and then bring the material to the office for their next appointment. Frequently the material that they bring is of poor quality or is not about the precise diagnosis that the patient has. Patients given a diagnosis of breast cancer have been known to go to a medical library and request everything that they have on breast cancer. They may not have been told the exact type or stage, and sometimes they did not hear, remember, or understand what was said, and they focused on what they knew. Patients have also arrived at the reference desk of a medical library wanting information about a condition that they have just been diagnosed with. Sometimes that condition is terminal, and the librarian does not want to be the one to tell them, especially since what they are saying they were diagnosed with may not be accurate. If you know that you have patients who will do research on their own, writing down the diagnosis, therapy, and other important facts will assist patients to locate information that is actually about their condition.

What about a situation where you have spoken to patients about their diagnosis, given them information at the appropriate level, and written down their diagnosis, but they still bring in material from Dr. Quack's miracle cure for foot and mouth disease? For health information for computer-literate patients who enjoy doing online research, develop a list of reputable Web sites for them to use. Many national organizations for diseases have Web sites with reliable patient information, and sometimes information about support groups. Universities and government agencies are additional sources to recommend. Prior to recommending ".coms" (commercial sites), examine the sites to determine who developed them and if the information is current and reliable. Commercial (.com) sites may be developed by drug companies or other companies to promote the use of their product. Do not automatically reject these sites, but investigate them prior to recommending them. A couple of general sites to recommend are;

Medline Plus	http://www/medlineplus.gov
	Produced by the National Library of Medicine
NOAH	http://noah-health.org
	Produced by New York Access to Health—Public & academic libraries in New York State
Merck	http://www.merck.com/mmhe
	Free online access to the Merck Manual, Home Edition

SUMMARY

Nursing is ranked as the most trusted profession in the country. Advocacy for patients is important at all levels of health care. Nurses are leaders in providing health education and information to patients, and are often better able to relate and communicate with patients than physicians. Being patient centered is how nurses function. Being aware of a patient's literacy levels, and adapting information and teaching accordingly, will improve the effectiveness of your interactions and potentially improve your patient's health. Patients expect nurses to listen to them because experience has shown that they do. They believe that nurses are more approachable than physicians. Often patients are reluctant to ask physicians questions because they are afraid of wasting the doctor's time or appearing ignorant or otherwise uneducated.

Since nurses are usually more accessible to patients than physicians, patients often approach nurses for information. Nurse advocates exemplify caring by functioning in the patient's best interest. Advocacy is such a key component that it is implied in the American Nurses' Association code. Characteristics of nurse advocates include leadership skills, excellent interpersonal skills, knowledge, passion and, most of all, commitment. Taking the role of advocacy to the next level and focusing efforts on providing appropriate education and information for each patient should be the standard.

Now that the concept of health literacy has been introduced, along with the effect that low health literacy has on patient compliance and an individual's health, how will you use this information in your professional practice? Which of the methods described will you utilize in patient education sessions? Health literacy is a relatively new area of interest and research. The interests of major groups such as the Institute of Medicine, the Joint Commission, the Agency for Healthcare Research and Quality, and the American Medical Association, along with other government agencies and national organizations, insure that health literacy will continue to be researched and promoted.

Additional Resources on Health Care Literacy

Agency for HealthCare Research and Quality
http://www.ahrq.gov
Go to the "Clinical Information" section, select "Evidence Based Practice," then select "Health Literacy" from the A–Z Quick Menu.

The Joint Commission on Health Care: What did the doctor say?
http://www.jointcommission.org
Use the site search feature to locate "What did the doctor say?"

Rhode Island Health Literacy Project
http://www.rihlp.org

National Network of Libraries of Medicine—Mid Atlantic Region
http://nnlm.gov/mar
Search the site for health literacy.

Ask Me 3
http://www.npsf.org/askme3/index.php

Institute of Medicine
http://www.iom.edu
Search the site for health literacy resources.

REFERENCES

BAKER, D. W., Wolf, M. S., Feinglass, J., Thompson, J. A., Gazmararian, J. A., & Huang, J. (2007). Health literacy and mortality among elderly persons. [Electronic version]. *Archives of Internal Medicine, 167*(14), 1503–1509.

COMMITTEE ON HEALTH LITERACY, BOARD ON NEUROSCIENCE AND BEHAVIORAL HEALTH, [INSTITUTE OF MEDICINE]. (2004). In Lynn Nielsen-Bohlman, Alison M. Panzer, & David A. Kindig (Eds.), *Health literacy: A prescription to end confusion*. Washington, DC: National Academies Press.

DAVIS, T. C., Crouch, M. A., Long, S. W., Jackson, R. H., Bates, P., George, R. B., et al. (1991). Rapid assessment of literacy levels of adult primary care patients. [Electronic version]. *Family Medicine, 23*(6), 433–435.

ESTRADA, C. A., Hryniewicz, M. M., Higgs, V. B., Collins, C., & Byrd, J. C. (2000). Anticoagulant patient information material is written at high readability levels. *Stroke; a Journal of Cerebral Circulation, 31*(12), 2966–2970.

FELLAND, L. E., Hurley, R. E., & Kemper, N. M. (2008). Safety net hospital emergency departments: Creating safety valves for non-urgent care. *Issue Brief (Center for Studying Health System Change), 120*(120), 1–7.

GREENE, J. (2007). Sending low-acuity patients away from the ED: Closing the door or stemming the tide? *Annals of Emergency Medicine, 49*(3), 317–319.

INSTITUTE OF EDUCATIONAL SCIENCES, U.S. Department of Education. (2007). *National assessment of adult literacy (NAAL)*. Retrieved August 1, 2008, from http://nces.ed.gov/naal/

KELLER, D. L., Wright, J., & Pace, H. A. (2008). Impact of health literacy on health outcomes in ambulatory care patients: A systematic review (October). *The Annals of Pharmacotherapy*, doi:10.1345/aph.1L093.

LEE, S. Y., Bender, D. E., Ruiz, R. E., & Cho, Y. I. (2006). Development of an easy-to-use Spanish health literacy test. [Electronic version]. *Health Services Research, 41*(4, Part 1), 1392–1412.

MAYER, G. G., & Villaire, M. (2004). Patient education: Low health literacy and its effects on patient care. [Electronic version]. *Journal of Nursing Administration, 34*(10), 440–442.

OSBORNE, H. (2006). Health literacy: How visuals can help tell the healthcare story. [Electronic version]. *Journal of Visual Communication in Medicine, 29*(1), 28–32.

PARIKH, N. S., Parker, R. M., Nurss, J. R., Baker, D. W., & Williams, M. V. (1996). Shame and health literacy: The unspoken connection. [Electronic version]. *Patient Education & Counseling, 27*(1), 33–39.

PAWLAK, R. (2005). Economic considerations of health literacy. [Electronic version]. *Nursing Economic$, 23*(4), 173–180.

SCHILLINGER, D. (2002). Researcher strengthens health literacy link. Retrieved August 1, 2008, from http://www.nidcd.nih.gov/news/releases/02/12_10_02.htm

SCHILLINGER, D., Grumbach, K., Piette, J., Wang, F., Osmond, D., Daher, C., et al. (2002). Association of health literacy with diabetes outcomes. [Electronic version]. *JAMA: The Journal of the American Medical Association, 288*(4), 475–482.

SCHILLINGER, D., Piette, J., Grumbach, K., Wang, F., Wilson, C., Daher, C., et al. (2003). Closing the loop: Physician communication with diabetic patients who have low health literacy. [Electronic version]. *Archives of Internal Medicine, 163*(1), 83–90.

UNITED STATES DEPARTMENT OF HEALTH & HUMAN SERVICES. (2000). *Healthy people 2010*. Washington, DC: U.S. Department of Health and Human Services.

WILLIAMS, M. V., Baker, D. W., Honig, E. G., Lee, T. M., & Nowlan, A. (1998). Inadequate literacy is a barrier to asthma knowledge and self-care. [Electronic version]. *Chest, 114*(4), 1008–1015.

WEISS, B. D., Hart, G., McGee, D. L., & D'Estelle, S. (1992). Health status of illiterate adults: Relation between literacy and health status among persons with low literacy skills. *The Journal of the American Board of Family Practice/American Board of Family Practice, 5*(3), 257–264.

WEISS, B. D., Mays, M. Z., Martz, W., Castro, K. M., DeWalt, D. A., Pignone, M. P., et al. (2005). Quick assessment of literacy in primary care: The newest vital sign. *Annals of Family Medicine, 3*(6), 514–522. doi:10.1370/afm.405.

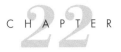

ADVOCACY IN THE PUBLIC ARENA

REBECCA BOWERS-LANIER

EdD, RN, Legislative Consultant, Macaulay & Burtch, PC

What do we live for if it is not to make life less difficult for each other?

–George Eliot

LEARNING OBJECTIVES

At the completion of the chapter, the learner should be able to do the following:

1. Discuss and compare the following: self-advocacy, patient advocacy, nurse advocacy, workforce advocacy, and public advocacy.
2. Describe advocacy in the public arena and compare public advocacy with patient advocacy.
3. Discuss the ethical basis for advocacy and the nurse's duty to advocate.
4. Identify the skills needed for effective advocacy.
5. Describe the process by which nurses become advocates for the profession in the public arena.

KEY TERMS

Coalition
Coercive Power
Compromise
Connection Power
Critical Thinking
Crucial Conversations
Electronic or
    e-Advocacy
Empowerment

Evidence-Based
    Nursing Practice
Expert Power
Information Power
Informed Consent
Legitimate Power
Nurse Advocacy
Patient Advocacy
Politics

Power
Public Advocacy
Referent Power
Reward Power
Risk-Taking
Self-Advocacy
Self-Knowledge
Workforce Advocacy
Workplace Advocacy

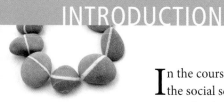

INTRODUCTION

In the course of their curriculum, nursing students learn how the biological sciences relate to the social sciences in the study of how to care for patients. They learn technical skills needed to care for their patients across the age and illness continuum. They also learn that nurses play a unique role in the care of their patients, as patients struggle to accommodate to changes in body and/or mind conditions, chronic or acute illness, and ways to prevent future illness or complications of their current illnesses. At some point in their work with patients, nursing students also learn that patients sometimes need help beyond the work they are already doing in their illness journeys. Patients may need a better explanation about treatment plans than they currently possess. They may need assistance from social services to return home after their hospitalization. Sometimes patients do not know they need help, such as when they receive an incorrect medication dosage. In these cases and many more, nurses provide help through advocating for their patients. Advocacy is a skill that is learned.

This chapter explores the various types of advocacy and the skills needed for effective advocacy, including self-advocacy, patient advocacy, nurse advocacy, e-advocacy, workplace or workforce advocacy, and public advocacy. Readers will review the ethical basis for advocacy, including the advocate's role in working through ethical dilemmas. The role of power and its relationship to advocacy are discussed. Finally, readers will learn how advocacy can be learned through incremental steps.

TYPES OF ADVOCACY

Advocacy ranges from the ability to speak up for oneself (self-advocacy), to speaking out for patients, nurses, and the public. The next section describes each of these types of advocacy and includes examples, case scenarios, and Internet exercises that further describe the concept of advocacy and its different types.

Self-Advocacy

Self-advocacy presupposes that one cannot be an effective patient or nurse advocate without possessing the ability to speak for oneself. That assumption is untested, but it probably helps if one understands the skills required of an effective self-advocate. Self-advocacy is the ability to speak up for oneself. Self-advocacy means one is able to ask for what one needs and wants, and to communicate this to others (Figure 22-1).

Inherent in successful self-advocacy are effective communication and problem-solving skills. Texts are written about effective communication skills, and nursing students learn therapeutic techniques designed to elicit from others their feelings, needs, and thoughts. With self-advocacy, one must know one's current state, one's desired state, how to achieve it, and how other persons can assist. The self-advocate also needs adequate problem-solving skills that can assess the

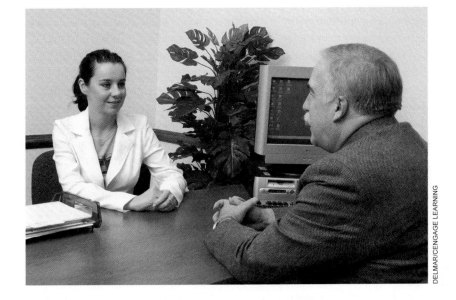

current situation, visualize the desired state, conduct a gap analysis, propose solutions to achieving the goal, and select a strategy to achieve the desired state.

Meecham describes the following characteristics of self-advocates: They are saying what they think and believe, taking responsibility for themselves, trying to change the way things are done, and willing to take risks (2003).

Patient Advocacy

Being an effective patient advocate requires skills similar to self-advocacy, except that to advocate for patients puts the primacy of the patients' needs before others' needs. Proponents of patient advocacy suggest that health care has become so complex that patients need someone to help them negotiate their way through the maze of health care options and systems (Oncology Nursing Society, 2007). There is an unequal relationship between the health care system and the patients it serves. The goal of advocacy, then, is to equalize that relationship by assessing patient/ family needs and understanding their circumstances, providing culturally sensitive information and education, ensuring equal access to appropriate care, and supporting the patient and family's decisions within the context of a multidisciplinary team (Oncology Nursing Society, 2007).

Patient advocacy, or the ability to speak up for one's patients, requires critical-thinking skills, appropriate assessment and intervention, speaking for the patient within the context of the multidisciplinary team approach, and ensuring that patient's wishes are honored and care is respectfully delivered (Oncology Nursing Society, 2007). For many nurses, serving as advocates for patients and families is the essence of their professional practice, but it is usually the least visible aspect (Foley, 2004).

When advocating for patients, nurses should employ **evidence-based nursing practice** or the use of research-based evidence to produce the best patient outcomes. To carry out evidence-based nursing, nurses should consider the following two factors: (1) sufficient research must have been published on the specific topic, and (2) nurses' practice must allow them to implement changes based on evidence-based nursing (University of Minnesota, 2007).

When nurses advocate for patients using decisions dependent on evidence-based practice, they bring not only their relationship skills to the effort, but also their ability to state the research base for the advocacy decisions they make. For example, the Oncology Nursing Society has developed a significant body of work defining evidence-based practice in oncology nursing. The society has compiled an analysis of evidence-based practice in oncology nursing care. Topics include management of symptoms such as fatigue, nausea and vomiting, and depression, as well as other physical and psychosocial symptomatology. This compilation supports best practice for oncology nurses and improved outcomes for patients (Oncology Nursing Society, 2007).

How do nurses become patient advocates? First, they need to have experience with the types of diseases/conditions, settings, and situations in which patients find themselves. Experience helps nurses build on their repertoire of examples of patient needs that may require advocacy. Second, they need a self-understanding of their own convictions, values, and beliefs (see section on ethics). This is important so that they can separate their own beliefs and needs from those of the patient. Third, nurses should have effective critical-thinking skills that enable them to assess the situation in which advocacy might serve as a useful tool, explore alternative solutions and, when possible, talk directly with their patients about these alternatives. Fourth, nurses need to know when patients are unable to participate in the decision-making and nurses themselves need to take action. Finally, nurses serving as patient advocates in some cases may be taking risks.

For example, a young nurse found herself in an untenable situation when the physician of her critically ill, ventilator-dependent patient ordered that the breathing tube be removed. Without the ventilator, the patient would expire. The nurse's moral beliefs precluded her from participating in what she considered to be murder. The more experienced nursing supervisor was called in to assess the situation. In doing so, the supervisor explored with the young nurse her refusal to participate in the tube withdrawal, supported her decision, but sought additional information. The supervisor discovered that the patient had a signed advance directive, indicating that no life-prolonging measures were to be used; however, the directives were not on file. The supervisor talked with the physician, who had failed to discuss with the nurse the family's and patient's wishes. She then engaged the patient and her family in a conversation about the patient's wishes. When she was assured that this was a decision that was made mutually by the family and the patient, the supervisor removed the tube and stayed with the patient, family member, and young nurse. After the patient's death, the supervisor debriefed the young nurse about her feelings and beliefs and those of her patient. She assisted the nurse in understanding that the patient's desires took precedence over others.

Not all situations are life-and-death situations like the previous example. Sometimes patients need as little as a call to the dietary department to ask for a visit by the dietitian. Others need nurses to draw attention to an overlooked reddened area on an elbow. Some need nurses to question the efficacy of a medication. And the list goes on. Patient advocacy involves placing oneself in the patient's place without taking over for the patient.

As in the example above with the breathing tube, new nurses need support to develop themselves into advocates. Nursing administrators must nurture advocacy. If nurses don't feel supported by nursing administration when they advocate, they are unlikely to fully develop that area of their practice. And yet, nurses often describe advocating for patients and families as what drew them to nursing. Nurses also describe advocacy as what keeps them in nursing (Foley, 2004).

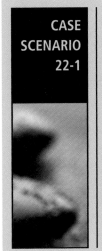

CASE SCENARIO 22-1

You are enrolled in the first of two medical-surgical nursing courses, and you are studying type 1 diabetes, a subject you know firsthand, having had diabetes since you were twelve. You consider yourself to be an advocate for yourself as a person with diabetes. In a lecture, the instructor presents information that you know to be obsolete and not consistent with current evidence-based guidelines.

CASE ANALYSIS

1. You have several advocacy options that you might consider for yourself and patients with diabetes. List them.

2. Given Meecham's characteristics of advocacy (saying what you think and believe, taking responsibility for yourself, trying to change the way things are done, and being willing to take risks), assess your own characteristics to execute the options you've identified in the first question.

3. List each option and the possible consequences of your actions for each.

Nurse Advocacy

Nurse advocates are those nurses who address their individual responsibilities to be informed about issues, to educate colleagues and the public about those issues, to collaborate with those who can offer solutions to identified problems, and to effect change in nursing practice that delivers better outcomes (Hilton, 2007).

Nurse advocates extend and expand their skills in self- and patient-advocacy to the role of advocating for other nurses and nursing in general. The Office of the National Nurse (http://www.nationalnurse.org) is one such initiative. Begun in 2005 with an opinion article in the *New York Times,* this initiative is a grassroots effort to elevate the chief nurse position in the U.S. Public Health Service to become the nation's nurse or National Nurse. Congressman Lois Capps (D-CA), a nurse herself, introduced legislation in the 2006 Congress that would create an office of the National Nurse. While the bill failed to pass, the grassroots efforts continue and grow, despite formal opposition from national nursing organizations, such as the American Nurses Association, the American Organization of Nurse Executives, and the National League for Nursing. The initiative's Web site chronicles the efforts to date and lays a case for advocating not only for nurses, but for the health of America's citizens (Nowlin, 2008).

Electronic Advocacy or e-Advocacy

The Internet provides an excellent tool for nurses to hone their thoughts and beliefs related to advocacy. The Internet-based approach to advocacy—electronic advocacy or **e-advocacy**—is a multifaceted process that uses an array of technology tools, tailored to specific advocacy goals. The Internet helps to inform "hard-to-reach" communities, organize nurses (and patients) for mass mobilization, strengthen offline tactics (such as holding rallies or protest marches), reach out to media, connect to more supporters for online donations, and target policymakers to pass or defeat proposed legislation (see Chapter 10). As a complement to traditional strategies, e-advocacy expands the possibilities for framing policy problems for a wide audience. In addition, e-advocacy facilitates audience engagement around policy solutions and builds a base of online support. The e-discussion formats promote interaction among advocacy supporters and mobilize supporters to take action on behalf of a campaign. When used effectively, e-advocacy can increase pressure on the public to make change happen (Chandler, n.d.).

E-advocacy has the following advantages in public advocacy campaigns:

- Online strategies reduce cost and increase speed and efficiency. A well-conducted e-mail campaign, for example, can replace the need for paper, envelopes, and postage, along with the staff or volunteer time needed to prepare and send letters to policymakers.
- Using various technology tools, such as a Web site or bulk e-mail lists, e-advocacy allows organizations to contact their audiences with targeted messages to build and strengthen their supporter base. When potential supporters are not directly connected with an advocacy campaign, they can be reached by receiving an e-mail message forwarded to them by a friend or colleague.
- Online strategies are an effective way for potential supporters to learn about a campaign, twenty-four hours a day, and find answers to their questions. Further, technology tools allow potential supporters to sign up for information updates and make it possible for the host organization to collect e-mail addresses and build e-mail lists.
- E-advocacy provides the means to target communications with content that is specific to supporter concerns, monitor supporter feedback, and track online activity to identify strong supporters. It has the capacity to monitor the number of times a campaign Web site is visited and the actions taken by its visitors, thus increasing the efficiency and effectiveness of online messages and content.
- E-advocacy keeps supporters informed of breaking news and developments that are central to an advocacy campaign. The power of e-mail is unmatched for turning around a quick response to breaking news and developments.
- By using a blog format, e-advocacy permits bloggers to post information immediately and encourages audiences/supporters to participate in shaping the discourse around an advocacy issue (Chandler, 2007).

Internet Exercise 22-1

Locate the Center for Nursing Advocacy at http://www.nursingadvocacy.org and Nursing Advocacy at http://medi-smart.com/advorgs.htm.

1. What types of information do these sites provide? Who is the audience?

2. If you were to become an active participant in the work of the Center for Nursing Advocacy, what would you hope to be the intended outcome?

3. What types of participation are fostered by the Center for Nursing Advocacy and the Nursing Advocacy sites, and what skills do participants need?

Workplace Advocacy

Workplace advocacy, in its broadest sense, consists of the means by which nurses' work-related concerns are addressed. These concerns consist of employment benefits such as salary/wages, fringe and retirement benefits, employer-sponsored health insurance, job security, and so forth, as well as work conditions and the degree of control that nurses have over their practice.

There are two types of workplace advocacy—through unions and through individual nurse advocacy. State laws give workers the right to organize for the purposes of collective bargaining by labor unions. In "union" states, where unions exist for the purposes of collective bargaining, nurses must become members *or* pay a fair-share membership fee to support the union's collective bargaining work. Laws in right-to-work states (see Chapter 10) specify that where unions exist, they must represent *all* the workers regardless of whether they belong to the union or not. These laws serve as a disincentive to organizing. All nurses have the right to unionize, whether they work in a union or right-to-work state (United American Nurses, n.d.).

Labor unions function as advocates for their members. Local union leaders serve as members of collective bargaining units, which negotiate on behalf of the union members with management in order to arrive at mutually acceptable wages and working conditions for employees (Boone & Kurtz, 1999). They also serve as advocates for union members in grievance procedures. A characteristic of union membership is that the union addresses advocacy needs of nurses, both collectively and individually.

Union membership accounts for 12.1% of employed wage and salary workers (U.S. Department of Labor, 2008) of the American workforce. However, the reach of unions has been broad. In health care, unions have bargained for improvements in working conditions, staffing policies, latex-free environments, policies banning certain chemicals, no-lift policies, and so forth (Encyclopedia of Public Health, n.d.). Registered nurses are organized by the United American Nurses, an affiliate of the American Federation of Labor and Congress of Industrial Organizations (AFL-CIO); the Service Employees International Union (SEIU); and a variety of other unions.

Workforce Advocacy

Nursing specialty organizations such as the American Association for Critical Care Nurses (http://www.aacn.org) and the Center for American Nurses (http://www.centerforamerican-nurses.org) develop and disseminate tools for nurses to employ to enhance their individual **workforce advocacy** skills, such as crucial conversations (to be described later), developing skills to confront and change bullying behavior in the workplace, and becoming versatile with the legal basics for nursing practice. These strategies focus on strengthening the individual nurse's voice and aiming for increased nurse involvement in workplace decisions that affect nursing care (Green & Jordan, 2002).

Shared governance is also an effective means by which nurses gain control over their practice. Shared governance is an organizational model that drives the control over nursing practice down to the level of the direct care providers. It ensures that the practicing nurse has the right *and* the power to make practice decisions. While shared governance consists of different structures, the models all possess the following concepts: (1) nurses have access to information necessary to make governance decisions, such as financial statements; (2) all staff nurses are able to be considered for membership in the governance structure; (3) decision-making is a process that heavily depends on consensus and conflict resolution; and (4) some administrative areas may continue to be the exclusive domain of administration. For shared governance to be effective, nursing leadership and agency administration must be fully supportive (Hess, 2004). Nurses involved in shared governance are advocates for themselves, their patients, and the profession.

Internet Exercise 22-2

Compare and contrast two Internet sites that employ workplace and workforce advocacy strategies: the United American Nurses (http://www.uannurse.org) and the Center for American Nurses (http://centerforamericannurses.org).

1. Analyze their home pages. What approaches do they appear to take toward workplace/workforce advocacy?

2. Search both sites for "advocacy" and compare the search results. Are they consistent with your assessment of the home page differences? What additional differences do you notice?

3. Compare and contrast their sites for information that will help you hone your advocacy skills. What tools are available on each site, and how could you use them?

Public Advocacy

Public advocacy consists of speaking out on behalf of an issue, a population group, or a concern in an effort to influence changes in public policy, laws, regulations, and/or practices. The advocacy process generally involves:

- Identifying problems that require a policy change or intervention.
- Establishing principles to guide a proposed remedy.
- Understanding the related issues and clarifying the policy needed to address those issues.
- Developing a policy strategy with related data and required resources.
- Building coalitions and gaining power to win the policy change or intervention sought (Bowers-Lanier, 2007).

Nurses serve in public advocacy roles when they are engaged in seeking changes within the public arena. Many of these activities are captured in chapter ten. For the purposes of this chapter, readers should bear in mind that the skills of advocacy remain similar, whether they be in the self-, patient-, nurse-, workplace/workforce, professional, or public arena. What is different, however, in public advocacy is the size of the targeted population, the strategies utilized to effect change, the types of changes proposed in the advocacy effort, and the potential outcomes. For example, the targeted population may be all patients with type 2 diabetes in a region, state, or the nation, instead of one patient with diabetes. Instead of one person or a team of individuals working to effect change through mostly interpersonal efforts, the strategies in public advocacy may depend on media campaigns, e-advocacy grassroots efforts with legislators, and other approaches involving larger investments of financial and human resources. Instead of seeking changes in patient care regimens, the changes in public advocacy are changes in policies, laws, and/or regulations. Finally, instead of the outcomes focused on one patient or a small group of patients, in public advocacy the outcomes are focused on population groups.

THE ETHICAL BASIS FOR ADVOCACY, OR THE DUTY TO ADVOCATE

Advocacy is essential for anyone working to ensure the nation's resources are shared by everyone. Whatever the issue may be, nurses have an obligation to take action when their patients' health is jeopardized and when their profession is threatened in such a way that quality nursing care is compromised.

Ends and Means

Advocacy has its roots in ethical and moral reasoning. The dictionary defines ethics as the study of moral standards and how they affect conduct or a system of moral principles governing the appropriate conduct of an individual or group (Soukhanov, 2001). When nurses speak of ethics, they are usually analyzing situations to find the answers to these questions: Do the means justify the ends? Or vice versa, do the ends justify the means? The answers are not always clear. And when nurses analyze the situations, they usually frame arguments in such situations as serving the public or patient good. For example, is limiting anthrax vaccine to the military (who provide protection for society) justifiable when the vast majority of the public is unprotected against anthrax (social inequity)? Is allowing a ventilator-dependent patient to die because she has no means to breathe for herself an evil act (murder) or a benevolent act (relief of suffering)?

Therefore, in examining the arguments of ends and means, nurses may be weighing "good ends" (relief of suffering) with "evil means," (causing the death of the quadriplegic), or "evil means" (rationing of vaccines) with "good ends" (protection of society). In balancing their assessment of ends and means, nurses generally look to the principle of **informed consent.** In the case of the ventilator patient, is there evidence that the patient chose a course of no assisted ventilation because she would not want to prolong her life in a state of dependent ventilation? In the case of the rationed vaccine, were policymakers acting in good faith that the military would be the first to experience a bioterrorist attack using anthrax?

Professional Ethics

In addition to analyzing ends and means, nursing practice is based on a code of ethics that govern the profession. Professional ethics is built on three components: purpose, conduct expected of the professional, and the skills and outcomes expected in professional practice (Curtin, 2007).

Purpose

The profession of nursing developed to meet a social need. Because the profession has its own set of knowledge from which nursing actions are derived, society expects that the profession aims to meet that need. Therefore, there exists (in legalistic terms) a contract between the nursing profession and society (Curtin, 2007).

The Conduct

Nursing's code of ethics describes the conduct that society has a right to expect from the profession. The conduct is not a list of procedures and acts, but rather a statement of values that outline the scope of practice and the relationships between nurses and patients. For example, patients have a right to expect that their nurses' primary commitments will be to them and their welfare (American Nurses Association, 2001).

The Skills and Outcomes Expected in Professional Practice

Nursing's standards of practice spell out the obligations that nurses have toward their patients. The specific practice components are dynamic and not forged in stone; however, the underlying components remain stable over time. For example, in demonstrating their commitment to patients, nurses assess patients' response to treatment, and the tools for assessment change with technological advances (Curtin, 2007).

Choices are not always easy for nurses in the role of advocates. Superimposed on professional ethics are nurses' individual beliefs about what constitute right and wrong and how and to what extent ends justify the means. These choices generally fall into the categories listed in Figure 22-2, which at any time may conflict with the nurse's individual beliefs.

Nurses engaged in moral dilemmas, therefore, weigh their own moral beliefs with the profession's code of ethics. Sometimes both are in congruence; at other times, they are not. For example, confronted with actions that will assist patients to die sooner than if life-saving measures are employed, nurses may find themselves in an ethical dilemma, especially if their religious beliefs are such that all life is precious and only God can determine when life should end. As advocates for patients, nurses may need to compromise their own religious beliefs for those of their patients.

Compromise, therefore, is one of the uncomfortable realities of ethical practice. The Microsoft Encarta College Dictionary defines compromise as a settlement of a dispute in which two or more sides agree to accept less than they originally wanted (Soukhanov, 2001). Therefore, compromise is considered a mutual win-lose method of conflict resolution that involves one party's giving up something and another party's gaining something, and vice versa. However, as a means of conflict resolution, in our culture the ability to compromise is seen as a virtue (Dixon, 2007).

Figure 22-2
Ethical choices in
nursing practice.

- The rights of the patient for health and medical decision making and the degree to which he or she is capable of exercising those rights.

- The choices about technical options available to the patients and the degree to which they want to reject or accept them.

- Choices about research on human beings and the subject's willingness to participate in such research.

- Choices about resource allocation, especially in situations of scarcity, such as disasters.

- Choices about care that appears to be futile and patient's autonomy to make decisions for himself.

- Choices about one's own self-interests and ability to make decisions about those interests, including one's decisions to engage in risky behavior.

- Questions of laws and regulations, including laws that are needed to assure the public's well-being and laws that support individuals' rights over the public's well-being (Curtin, 2007).

DELMAR/CENGAGE LEARNING

In situations involving patients and nurses, however, nurses may have to compromise their personal beliefs for the decisions of the patient, bearing in mind that patients expect nurses to adhere to a set of ethical norms that acknowledge the primacy of patient beliefs.

Various opinion polls reveal that the American public trusts nurses (Curtin, 2007). To the public, the registered nurse is the key indicator of quality care. Nurses, therefore, have an obligation to advocate for patients in the public arena, just as they are obligated to advocate for their own patients. To passively accept substandard conditions that negatively affect the quality of

Writing
Exercise
22-1

Hurricane Katrina's catastrophic reach in New Orleans was unspeakable. Hospitals were flooded and unable to care for their own patients or to admit storm victims. In one facility a physician and several nurses were charged with the deaths of untold numbers of patients following the storm. The physician's attorney released a statement that said in part:

The physicians and staff responsible for the care of patients, many of whom were gravely ill, faced loss of generator power, the absence of routine medical equipment to sustain life, lack of water and sanitation facilities, extreme heat in excess of one hundred degrees, all occurring in an environment of deteriorating security, apparent social unrest and the absence of governmental authority. Dr. Pou and other medical personnel at Memorial Hospital worked tirelessly for five days to save and evacuate patients, none of whom were abandoned (Griffin & Johnston, 2005).

Using Provisions 1 and 2 of the *ANA Code of Ethics* as a framework, write a brief summary of how the catastrophic consequences of Katrina may have compromised the ethical practice of nurses in the affected hospital.

patient care not only places patients at risk, but also demeans nurses' professional contributions. Moreover, passive acceptance abandons the public's trust. When nurses participate in changing laws, shaping health care policy, and improving their practice environments, they assure the public that they are willing to speak out and to provide the safe, dignified, expert care the public expects. Therefore, advocacy is a moral and ethical obligation that nurses assume as part of their professional practice (Curtin, 2007).

SKILLS FOR EFFECTIVE ADVOCACY

The following section discusses the skills necessary for effective advocacy, highlighted in Figure 22-3.

Intrapersonal Skills

Nurses involved in public advocacy should be well versed in **politics,** or the totality of interrelationships in the issues at hand, especially as they relate to power, authority, or influence. They must be systems thinkers, analyzing how proposed changes in one part of a system will affect changes in other parts of the system. They should determine the various stakeholders involved in the advocacy effort, seeking to include those who will support as well as those opposed to the effort. They must engage organizations and groups to form coalitions around issues to be changed. They must seek solutions that may not be completely the desired outcome, knowing that in this type of advocacy, compromise may have to occur. In order to be effective in the role, however, it requires a skill set that consists of intrapersonal and interpersonal competencies (Bowers-Lanier, 2007).

The critical intrapersonal competencies for effective advocacy consist of self-knowledge and understanding, critical thinking, and risk-taking. The critical interpersonal skill that translates intrapersonal competencies is communication.

Figure 22-3
Advocacy Skills
Check List.

Advocacy Skills Check List:
What you need for successful advocacy
√ Self-knowledge and understanding
√ Critical thinking
√ Risk-taking
√ Communication
√ Working with others in coalitions

DELMAR/CENGAGE LEARNING

Self-Knowledge and Understanding

Self-knowledge is commonly used in philosophy to refer to knowledge of one's particular mental states, including one's beliefs, desires, and sensations. Self-knowledge is built upon the messages one receives as a child and how one internalizes those messages into belief about self as an adult, about what is right and wrong, and about how one responds to situations. The role of self-understanding in choosing actions in situations is complex. However, in order to exercise the ability to decide on actions, knowledge of one's relatively stable traits and dispositions is crucial (Gertler, 2003).

A person who lacks self-knowledge may simply be ignorant about some aspect or state of the self, perhaps because he or she has not formed any relevant belief. But in extreme cases, an absence of accurate self-reflection, or ignorance about what is guiding one's reasoning, may allow one's interests, rather than one's stable traits and dispositions, to shape one's beliefs (Gertler, 2003).

An effective advocate, therefore, possesses a holistic self-knowledge that forms the basis for individuals to determine their role in advancing the cause under consideration. Self-understanding is formed early, and it can be modified if individuals weigh their actions in response to certain situations that test their abilities to respond (Gertler, 2003).

For example, a first-semester nursing student observes that a patient is forming a reddened area on his coccyx. The student knows the causes of pressure sores and believes that the patient's position or the bed should be changed to prevent skin deterioration. The student also knows she is in a very early stage of her education, and past experience has taught her to tread carefully in areas in which she is not totally comfortable. However, the student also knows that to remain silent may lead to a deteriorating situation with the patient. She weighs the consequences of remaining silent with speaking out and possibly suffering some embarrassment for her lack of experience. She decides to talk with her instructor about the situation. Her instructor coaches her through the possible courses of action and confirms that speaking out is the preferred action to take. She helps the student compose her presentation to the charge nurse and stays with the student as the student presents her case. Self-knowledge underpins the student's thought processes and positive course of action in this case.

Critical Thinking

Critical thinking is self-directed, self-disciplined, self-monitored, and self-corrective thinking. It presupposes the desire to achieve rigorous standards of excellence and mindful command of their use. It entails effective communication and problem-solving abilities and a commitment to overcome one's nature toward egocentrism (Scriven & Paul, 2007). People who think critically are keenly aware of the inherently flawed nature of human thinking when left unchecked. They use the intellectual tools that critical thinking offers—concepts and principles that enable them to analyze, assess, and improve thinking. They realize that no matter how skilled they are as thinkers, they can always improve their reasoning abilities and they will at times fall prey to mistakes in reasoning, human irrationality, prejudices, biases, distortions, uncritically accepted social rules and taboos, self-interest, and vested interest. They strive never to think simplistically about complicated issues and always consider the rights and needs of relevant others (Elder, n.d.).

Critical thinking is a process that takes place irrespective of the *content* required for the critical-thinking process. It consists of the examination of those structures or elements of thought implicit in all reasoning: purpose, problem or question-at-issue; assumptions; concepts; empirical grounding; reasoning leading to conclusions; implications and consequences; objections from alternative viewpoints; and frame of reference (Elder, 2007).

Effective advocates think critically (Figure 22-4). When presented with situations that require advocacy, the critical thinker assesses the components of the situation, determines the causes of the problem (as opposed to symptoms of the problem), considers possible conclusions with their intended or possible unintended consequences, and determines objections to solutions from opponents' perspectives (Elder, 2007).

Figure 22-4
Effective advocates think critically by assessing the situation, determining the causes of the problem, considering possible conclusions and consequences, and determining objections from opponents.

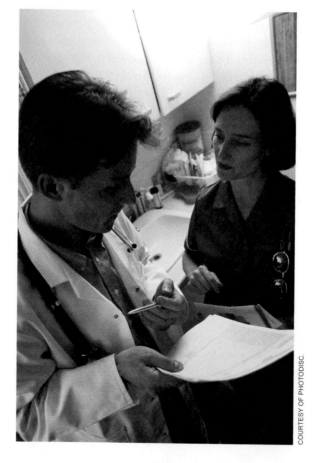

COURTESY OF PHOTODISC.

For example, a nursing student is caring for a patient with hypothyroid disease who is taking levothyroxine (Synthroid®) for replacement therapy. The patient's resting pulse is measured at 110/minute. The student correctly identifies this as tachycardia and consults a pharmacology text, where it says that tachycardia may be an early warning sign of hyperthyroidism. The student's assessment of the situation is that the patient may be experiencing an early sign of hyperthyroidism; however, tachycardia may be explained by other situations, such as fever, exercise, and so on. The instructor assists the student in assessing the alternative causes of tachycardia. They determine that the patient is afebrile and has not been exercising, nor has she experienced any recent stressor (as identified by the patient). Three courses of action are identified: (1) to wait and reassess the patient's pulse in two hours, (2) to consult with the physician, and (3) to do nothing. With the instructor, the student decides on the first two courses of action—to retake the vital signs and then decide on a subsequent course of action.

This situation required critical thinking that included identification of a potential problem, assessment of causes, determination of possible courses of action, and intended and unintended outcomes. Premature action in this case, i.e., consulting the physician without sufficient supporting data, could have led to a confrontation implicitly involving power and authority. The alternative course, i.e., no further action, could have ignored the possible significance of an early sign of levothyroxine overdose.

Risk-Taking

Risk-taking is defined as daring to try new approaches or ideas with no predictable control over the results or consequences (Gorkin, n.d.). Risk-taking is integral to human growth and development—just watch infants as they take their first steps, when crawling could accomplish the same thing. Risk-taking is integral to advocacy, because it involves situations in which individuals "go out on limb" for a cause, when one of the alternative solutions to the problem is to do nothing.

Risks have positive and negative aspects. The word itself, risk, has a negative connotation, similar to danger. And in fact, some risks are not very smart at all; as an example, a person who consistently J-walks on a busy street.

Florence Nightingale is the exemplar of risk-taking for nurses. In a time when the causes of disease were not well understood, she used her powers of observation and advocacy to change the environment in which wounded soldiers were being treated, and in the process, reduced mortality rates. On advocating for patients, she wrote in *Notes on Nursing*:

> For a long time an announcement something like the following has been going the round of the papers: —"More than 25,000 children die every year in London under 10 years of age; therefore we need a Children's Hospital."... The causes of the enormous child mortality are perfectly well known; they are chiefly want of cleanliness, want of ventilation, want of white-washing; in one word, defective *household* hygiene. The remedies are just as well known; and among them is certainly not the establishment of a Child's Hospital. (Nightingale, 1860, p.10).

Nightingale's voice, and her ability to wield power through her social status and use of the media, led to reforms that reduced mortality. However, her conclusions sound too familiar in our advanced technological age, where huge sums are invested in the *treatment* of disease rather than the *prevention* of disease. Nurses have been advocating for prevention for years, along with other stakeholder groups, such as public health officials, some physician groups, and increasingly, businesses faced with high health costs. Yet there is much work to be done in advocacy to change the care paradigm from treatment of disease to promotion of health.

Risk-taking can be relatively small, with few expected benefits, but rewarding and fulfilling, all the same. Or risk-taking can be large, based on the size of the problem, the stakes involved, and the potential outcomes. All of the examples provided in this chapter have involved a degree of risk-taking on the part of the advocate.

In situations that call for advocacy, the advocate must be prepared for negative personal consequences, even if the situation is resolved in the direction in which the advocate was aiming. For example, if in the situation of the patient on the verge of an overdose of levothyroxine, the nurse decides to consult with the physician about persistent tachycardia, the nurse is taking a risk that the situation with the physician may prove to be confrontational instead of constructive.

Writing Exercise 22-2	In this section, we have discussed three critical intrapersonal skills required for effective advocacy: self-knowledge and understanding, critical thinking, and risk-taking. Think about your own life experiences and identify a situation that involved your taking on the role of advocate. Write a summary of this experience, including the precipitating event that led you to become an advocate and how you employed each of the three intrapersonal skills. Then briefly analyze the outcome. How effective were you? What would, or did, you do differently under a similar circumstance the next time that you serve(d) as an advocate?

Interpersonal Skills

To advocate effectively, nurses must also possess the interpersonal skills of communication and forming coalitions. The importance of communication cannot be underestimated. Communication forms the link among the members of the health care team. And in health care, the ability to communicate effectively is critical in reducing errors. Approximately 98,000 deaths annually in health care can be attributed to human error, mostly involving dysfunctional systems, design flaws, and human error, some of which result from failure to communicate among members of the health care team (Kohn, Corrigan, & Donaldson, 2000). In a monograph titled *Silence Kills: The Seven Crucial Conversations for Healthcare* (Maxfield, Grenny, McMillan, Patterson, & Switzler, 2005), the authors found that there are seven **crucial conversations** that health care workers fail to hold that lead to errors. Defined, crucial conversations are those discussions between two or more people where stakes are high, opinions vary, and emotions run strong (Patterson, Grenny, McMillan, & Switzler, 2002). If health care institutions invest in teaching nurses and others how to hold crucial conversations, followed by adaptation of the techniques, it is likely that errors will be reduced. In addition, holding crucial conversations should be associated with increased staff morale, and job and patient satisfaction. The key is in the adoption of the crucial conversations tools.

In their research of over 1,700 nurses, physicians, clinical-care staff, and administrators, Maxfield, et al., (2005) found the following concerns in health care associated with error prone-ness: broken rules, mistakes, lack of support, incompetence, poor teamwork, disrespect, and micromanagement (Figure 22-5). Broken rules consisted of taking shortcuts from accepted protocols, such as not wearing gloves when performing phlebotomies. Outright mistakes included showing poor clinical judgment when making assessments that led to erroneous con-clusions and writing incorrect orders. Lack of support consisted of working with colleagues who were reluctant to help others or refuse to answer questions. Incompetence was character-ized as poor clinical judgment decisions. Poor teamwork was defined as working with others who refuse to work collaboratively; such as gossiping about others, bullying behavior, failing to do their fair share, or participating in cliques. Disrespect included working with individuals who were condescending, verbally abusive, and belittling of others. Micromanagement con-sisted of working with others who abuse their authority by pulling rank, threatening, or forcing their view on others (2005).

When asked why they did not speak up about these crucial concerns, respondents offered the following reasons: that it was difficult to do so, their belief that speaking up was "not their job," and low confidence that speaking up would do any good. Others stated that they feared retaliation. In order to deal with these situations, respondents offered the following strategies: talk about the problems with others, such as managers or coworkers, or work around the "problem people" and warn others about them. In each health care facility that participated in the study, the researchers found a small percent of respondents (5–15%) who were able to step up to the concerns and hold crucial conversations (Maxfield, Grenny, McMillan, Patterson, & Switzler, 2005).

The tools for holding crucial conversations are well established (Patterson, Grenny, McMillan, & Switzler, 2002). Because they are designed for conversations when the stakes are high, they are especially useful for advocates. Advocates who possess crucial conversation skills are able to elicit free flow of *meaning* between two or more people (p. 20). That is, they

Figure 22-5
Seven Concerns
in Health Care
Associated with
Error Proneness.
(Maxfield, et al., 2005.)

- Broken rules
- Mistakes
- Lack of support
- Incompetence
- Poor teamwork
- Disrespect
- Micromanagement

DELMAR/CENGAGE LEARNING

are skilled at making it safe for everyone to add their meaning to a shared pool that leads to greater exchange of ideas, strategies, courses of action, and so on.

The skills to conduct crucial conversations can be learned. They involve starting with self-knowledge of intent and purpose (in the conversation), observing and listening to the responses of others, and acting to create a safe, respectful environment. To conduct a crucial conversation, advocates must also know the stories that they create around difficult situations (such as jumping to a conclusion that may not be valid, based on the facts) and how to focus on the facts and what they may mean, while offering tentative alternatives. Crucial conversation users employ skills that help others explore their own stories through paraphrasing and mirroring their statements. Finally, crucial conversations carry on to actions and plans for next steps, with deadlines, deliverables, and identified responsible persons.

Why the emphasis on learning how to conduct crucial conversations? In addition to reducing errors, lifting morale, and increasing job satisfaction, the tools for conducting crucial conversations are useful in any situation that is emotional and where the stakes are high. Nurses who advocate for themselves, their patients, and the profession will frequently be involved in these types of situations; hence, if they have the ability to conduct crucial conversations, they will be that much more effective. Additional material on crucial conversations can be found at http://www.vitalsmarts.com/books_more.aspx and http://www.silencekills.com.

Internet Exercise 22-3

Conduct your own self-assessment of communication skills under stress (Style under Stress) at http://www.vitalsmarts.com/books_more.aspx. You'll need to click on "Join Now" (it's free) before you can take the test. The test is listed under "Access a self-scoring Style Under Stress" test.

1. What did you learn about your communication skills by taking this self-assessment?

2. Does knowing this information help inform areas that you may need to change in order to hold conversations that are more effective?

3. After assessing your skills under pressure once, imagine an interaction with a health care team member, such as a physician, a fellow student, or an instructor. Retake the survey. Does your score change?

The second interpersonal skill critical to effective advocacy is working through others in coalitions. A **coalition** is a group of individuals and/or organizations united around a common interest, working together to achieve a common goal (Bowers-Lanier, 2007). A coalition oftentimes can be more successful in advocating for a cause than an individual person or organization, because there is clout in numbers. For example, a nursing student organization might wish to take on a campaign to promote college students' health by eliminating unhealthy snack foods on campus. To increase the potential effectiveness of the campaign, the nursing students could invite other like-minded student organizations to join in the effort. These might include the nutrition/dietetic students, the health and physical education majors, the physical therapy students, and so on. Working together, the organizations are likely to increase the visibility of the campaign as well as its effectiveness.

Coalition building for the purposes of advocacy in the public arena occurred in conjunction with the launch of Michael Moore's film, "Sicko," which led to an organized effort among diverse stakeholder groups seeking universal health care (Adams, 2007).

The campaign, "Scrubs for SiCKO," highlights several characteristics that are associated with successful public advocacy; it was a well-organized coalition with a common mission that was effectively led, and which enlisted the support of multiple stakeholders from diverse perspectives. Additionally, the campaign was funded sufficiently to reach a large audience and have the capacity to sway public opinion. Let's look at each of these separately.

Mission

A well-defined mission or advocacy goal is essential and seems to go without saying. The "SiCKO" campaign planned to "urge support for a shift to a universal health care system" (http://www.newstarget.com/021921.html). If one parses out the key words in this goal statement, one can easily ascertain that a universal health care system was *not* what the campaign was aiming to accomplish; rather, to have people consider a shift to a universal health care system.

Leadership

Campaigns are not run without effective leadership. The leaders must be able to bring the advocates together, help them visualize a common goal, provide them with resources to achieve the goal, coach and cajole participation, make corrections in the course of work, and communicate regularly and openly with campaign participants. Without leadership the campaign will fizzle out (Bowers-Lanier, 2007).

Participation of Stakeholders

Public arena advocacy work is done best in groups working together. The "SiCKO" campaign consisted of nurses, physicians, patients and family members, and trade groups such as the California Nurses Association/National Nurses Organizing Committee, Physicians for a National Health Program, New York State Nurses Association, Massachusetts Nurses Association, United Steelworkers (USW) Health Care Workers Council, Pennsylvania Association of Staff Nurses and Allied Professionals, United Nurses and Allied Professionals (Rhode Island), Communications Workers of America, and the New England Nurses Association (Nurses, doctors announce "Scrubs For SiCKO" Campaign In Conjunction With Debut Of Michael Moore's Film To Spark Genuine Healthcare Debate, 2007). Ordinarily some of these groups would not work together to achieve a common goal. However, for a compelling cause, diverse stakeholder groups come together to achieve a goal of mutual interest (Bowers-Lanier, 2007).

The Work of the Advocacy Campaign

Advocacy campaigns should have well-defined work plans, consistent with the mission of the campaign. For example, the "Scrubs for SiCKO" campaign worked to recruit registered nurses, nursing students, and physicians to every theater in the nation where the movie was playing. Campaign participants wore scrubs and distributed information about the health care system and urged moviegoers to join them in calling for a fundamental overhaul of the nation's health care system. Their specific message was to help pass a single-payer, Medicare-type system, and to make it a focus of the 2008 presidential campaign (Nurses, doctors announce "Scrubs For SiCKO" Campaign In Conjunction With Debut Of Michael Moore's Film To Spark Genuine Healthcare Debate, 2007).

Funding

Adequate funding is essential for successful campaigns. Sometimes funds come from trade groups (such as those participating in the "SiCKO" campaign), dues, and donations; other times, donors are willing to give to campaigns. Often, participants work as volunteers.

Communications/Public Relations

Successful campaigns have compelling messages that resonate with people. Universal health care is a goal that is particularly poignant for those affected by catastrophic health care expenses, the uninsured, and those with prolonged, chronic diseases, especially those with experimental treatments. At any one time in the U.S. there are approximately 47 million Americans without health insurance (Center on Budget and Policy Priorities, 2006). Keeping the message before influential decision-makers is essential to achieving the mission of the campaign.

Measurement of Success of Advocacy Campaigns

Every campaign should be planned with optimal outcomes well defined. Were changes in policies made? Was legislation passed? How many people were informed of the need for change?

POWER AND ADVOCACY

No discussion of the skills needed for effective advocacy would be complete without an understanding of the role that **power** plays in advocacy. Savvy advocates understand power and know how to use it in its various forms.

Definitions of Power

Power is defined as the ability or capacity to do something; control and influence over other people and their actions; and the ability to influence people's judgment or emotions (Soukhanov, 2001). Nurses who are able to change policies in their work settings exercise power. Similarly, nurses serving in leadership positions who advance a platform adopted by the followers exercise power. Likewise, nurses exercise power when they persuade physicians to change treatment regimens so that they are more consistent with their patients' preferences. Power, therefore, is dependent upon the advocate's personal attributes in some cases, and in others upon the position that the advocate holds.

Types of Power

Social scientists describe power within the context of the situations in which power is used. In this manner, power can be described as expert, legitimate, reward, referent, information, connection, and coercive. Each is described in the next few paragraphs and summarized in Table 22-1.

Table 22-1 Types of Power

Type	Definition: Influence and Control Based on One's	The Person with This Type of Power
EXPERT	Specialized knowledge of a discipline/subject/skill.	Is seen as the "go to" person for information or assistance, such as a clinical nurse specialist.
LEGITIMATE	Position within an organization or based on one's credentials.	Uses one's position or credentials in influencing others, who grant that influence because of the person's position or credentials, such as a nurse-patient relationship.
REWARD	Ability to give others what they want.	Grants favors to others, such as a nurse manager giving a plum assignment to a staff nurse.
REFERENT	Perceived knowledge and expertise.	Holds power over others only if others perceive that the person has attained expertise and specialized knowledge. A novice nurse grants referent power to an experienced nurse.
INFORMATION	Knowledge/information possessed that others do not have.	May withhold information to maintain a power relationship or share information to help empower others. A nurse manager shares unit financial status with the staff, who are able to participate in fiscal decisions at the unit level.
CONNECTION	Business, religious, social, or any other type of network.	Knows individuals who can have recognized influence in a certain dimension. A nurse who attends church with the director of pharmacy may gain special favors from the pharmacy for the unit.
COERCIVE	Ability to exact punishment or create fear over others.	Uses punishment as a way to maintain a power relationship with others. A parent grounds his or her child.

Expert Power

Expert power is the ability to control and to influence people by virtue of holding special knowledge that others do not possess (Abood, 2007; Leavitt, Cohen, & Mason, 2007). Experts' power comes from their expertise. Nurses develop expertise as they gain experience and education. When people seek advice from nurses whom they believe possess unique knowledge, they are vesting expert power in the nurses.

Legitimate Power

Legitimate power is also known as positional power; that is, its basis is derived from the incumbent's position in an organization, such as a head nurse (Leavitt, Cohen, & Mason, 2007). In interpersonal relationships, persons holding legitimate power are expected to possess certain skills and competencies based on the position or the credentials that they possess.

Reward Power

Reward power is the ability to give other people what they want, such as rewards or favors. Reward power may also connote reciprocity; that is, a person may offer another a favor but expect something in return, perhaps not at the present time, but in the future. Rewards can also be used to punish, such as when they are withheld (Abood, 2007). For example, a head nurse may offer a staff nurse an influential committee assignment in recognition of excellent service. The savvy nurse should remember that this reward, while in recognition of excellence, may also mean that she/he will be expected to return a favor at a future time. This means, in the words of the vernacular, "There is no free lunch." This type of power is commonly used in political maneuvers.

Referent Power

Referent power is control and influence that is dependent upon others' respect in the person with whom they associate (Abood, 2007). For example, a novice nurse seeks out a well-respected nurse to serve as her mentor. The novice is vesting referent power in the well-respected nurse.

Information Power

Information power results when one holds (or is perceived to hold) knowledge/information that others do not possess. Sometimes the information power comes with the territory; for example, a head nurse (legitimate power) is more likely to have information that others do not have. Nurse advocates, however, should strive to stay abreast of information, through formal and informal associations in the work setting, belonging to the professional association, and reading journals and newsletters (Leavitt, Cohen, & Mason, 2007). Information should be shared, to the extent possible, with all who are involved in advocacy work. Sharing increases everyone's own information power.

Connection Power

Connection power is control or influence over others by others' perception that the incumbent has important connections that they do not possess (Leavitt, Cohen, & Mason, 2007). For example, a nurse who belongs to the same church or attends Sunday school with a legislator may have connection power, particularly if there is a legislative issue that will be coming before that committee. She can use her power to meet with the legislator (using the connection) to advocate for her cause. The effective use of connection power can be a crucial means for advancing important causes for nurses.

Coercive Power

Coercive power is control or influence over others through fear or the perception of fear (Abood, 2007). Abood states that coercion is the ultimate power of all governments (2007). Laws are created to be obeyed, and the consequences of breaking the laws are punishments by fines or imprisonment. We all understand this type of power, and it is appropriate for governments. However, coercive power has a negative connotation when applied from individuals to other individuals. Coercion is not an effective motivator in the work setting. Advocates are better served if they use reward power rather than coercion.

Empowerment

Empowerment is a related term and its understanding is pivotal for nurse advocates. Empowerment is the giving of power or authority to someone; it arises from shared power. Advocacy work is best accomplished by more than one person. For example, a nurse believes that a particular policy is outdated. She reviews the most recent research and evidence to support her belief. Prior to advancing her position, however, she enlists the aid of others on her unit by presenting them with the information, asking for their suggestions, and working with them to develop a course of action in which they are involved. By working together, the nurses are able to make a case for a policy change. Each person believes that he/she had an active role to play in advocating for the change. Each is empowered by the situation. Nurse advocates, therefore, should work to empower others to become advocates as well (Abood, 2007).

Nurse advocates employ many types of power in advocating for causes. For example, a projected severe nursing shortage served as the catalyst to bring together nurse leaders at the state level from diverse nursing organizations and specialty groups. Their aim was to bring awareness of the shortage to the level of public discourse in general, but specifically to the candidates for governor of the state. These leaders sought to involve influential nurses at the political level (referent power). Then they designated a nucleus of leaders (expert power) to create a plan that would advance the shortage issue as the priority policy issue in a gubernatorial campaign with three candidates. The nurses agreed that all three campaigns would have nurses in pivotal roles and that the nurses' political action committee would make generous donations to all candidates (reward power). They worked to find nurses who knew the candidates (connection power) and to involve these nurses in the campaigns. The professional association donated the time of its lobbyist to serve as a consultant to the group (information power). In addition, during the campaign, they worked to build the grassroots advocacy skills of other nurses to support the gubernatorial campaigns (empowerment). Their hard work was rewarded with the election of a governor who advanced the nursing shortage as a primary plank in his health policy platform. The governor's support subsequently led to a 10% raise for nurse faculty in all state-supported colleges and universities (successful application of coercive power of the state, because the governor's budget item restricted the funds for nursing faculty salary increases and forbade college presidents from diverting the funds to other budget items).

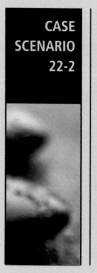

CASE SCENARIO 22-2

The nursing students' association has determined that its short-term policy initiative will be to increase nursing students' participation in student governance for the university. They believe that they can achieve greater participation within two years. You are the first vice-president of the association this year and will most likely become the president in your senior year.

CASE ANALYSIS

1. Review each of the types of power; which are most likely to achieve the intended results?

2. How useful might forming coalitions with other student organizations be as a strategy? Which student associations might be helpful in this capacity? How would you go about forming a coalition?

3. Aside from increased participation by nursing students in student governance, what other benefits might be had to nursing students and nursing, if this goal were to be achieved?

ON BECOMING AN ADVOCATE FOR THE PROFESSION IN THE PUBLIC ARENA

How do nurses become involved in public advocacy? The obvious answer is "one step at a time." Leavitt, Chaffee, and Vance (2007) describe a process of political development of nurses. The stages are summarized in Table 22-2. Leavitt, Chaffee, and Vance note that there are four stages: buy-in, self-interest, political sophistication, and leading the way.

In the first stage, "buy in," there is an "aha" moment when the individual nurse decides to get involved in a cause. This is a reactive stage; the perceived injustice or issue occurs, and the nurse begins to deliberate over it in reaction to the precipitating event. At some point, the nurse buys into the need for change.

In the second stage, "self-interest," the nurse perceives the causative issue as a problem related to her practice (such as her work with her patient). In this stage, the nurse begins to develop a plan to deal with the problem. This may involve seeking support from others or volunteering to serve on a work group designed to solve the problem.

Table 22-2 Stages of Advocacy Development

Stage	Description
BUY IN	A situation initiates in the individual a sense of outrage or perceived injustice. The individual begins to express a need for change.
SELF-INTEREST	The individual begins to develop a plan aimed at restoring balance or fixing the problem and engages others to help.
POLITICAL SOPHISTICATION	The individual and others learn how to negotiate solutions with policymakers and other stakeholder groups.
LEADING THE WAY	The individual becomes a leader in the advocacy cause.

In the third stage, "political sophistication," the nurse takes advocacy to a more public venue. She becomes involved in promoting nursing to legislators and other policymakers, participating in political coalitions around causes, and testifying before policymakers. She is seen as the expert about practice issues.

In the fourth stage, "leading the way," the nurse directs the dialogue and policy development for issues greater than the practice of a single nurse. In the example of "Scrubs for SiCKO," the nurses who led this effort were participating in this stage of advocacy development. Nurse leaders take on positions of leadership within state and national nursing organizations, run for political office, and serve in governmental positions.

The four stages of advocacy development are exemplified in the following example that describes the process of advocacy from identification of a problem through resolution achieved by legislation. It involves increasing access to maternity care by certified nurse midwives.

Until 2006, certified nurse midwives (CNMs) in Virginia, by law, worked in supervisory relationships with physicians. Obstetricians, burdened with increasingly high malpractice insurance, refused to "supervise" CNMs because of their fears of increased liability, even though CNMs carried their own malpractice insurance. The CNMs were placed in an untenable situation—needing physicians to serve as their "supervisors," while being unable to find physicians to serve in that capacity. The stage was set for decreased access to obstetric *and* midwifery care.

Seizing on the situation as an opportunity, the CNMs sought a statutory change to amend the law requiring physician supervision to physician "collaboration and consultation." Their advocacy strategy involved (1) working with their supervising physicians to help them understand how supervision had negatively affected their malpractice insurance rates, and (2) working with legislators to describe how midwifery services were decreasing in a time when women were also being denied access to other maternity providers, including obstetricians.

Through this advocacy strategy (that took place over two years), the CNMs were able to get a bill passed that changed "supervision" to "collaboration and consultation." What started out as a long journey of public advocacy for nurse midwives and their patients finally culminated in a law that serves to increase access to midwifery services. The ingredients used to achieve this outcome included a small group of committed CNM advocates, their patients, a lobbyist and several sympathetic legislators, perseverance, and public support created by the media reporting on decreased access to maternity care. It was not an easy journey, but it had a good outcome.

How can novice nurses become involved with public advocacy? The novice nurse starts with observing and working within the health care setting. Is there an "aha" moment when one must buy into a need for advocacy? Remember that this journey begins with a single step, and it doesn't have to develop all the way from self- and patient-advocacy to public advocacy overnight. The key is keeping one's mind open to possibilities and understanding that advocacy for patient care and nursing practice extends beyond the direct nurse-patient relationship.

SUMMARY

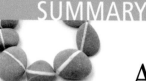

A critical competence for nurses is advocacy or the ability to speak up on behalf of themselves, their patients, the profession, and for causes that promote the health of the public. The intra- and interpersonal skills essential for successful advocacy involve excellent communication abilities, critical thinking, and working with and through others in coalitions. Advocacy is a journey that begins with self-knowledge and awareness, and an awareness of ethical principles as they apply to situations in which advocacy is needed. Related concepts include power and the effective and appropriate use of power in advocacy situations.

An individual has not started living until he can rise above the narrow confines of his individualistic concerns to the broader concerns of all humanity.

–Martin Luther King, Jr.

REFERENCES

ABOOD, S. (2007, January 31). Influencing health care in the legislative arena. *OJIN: The Online Journal of Issues in Nursing, 12*(1), Retrieved November 25, 2007, from http://www.nursing-world.org/ojin

ADAMS, M. (2007, July 2). Nurses launch national "Scrubs for SiCKO" campaign to endorse universal health care following Michael Moore's film.

NewsTarget.com. Retrieved December 1, 2007, from http://www.newstarget.com/021921.html

AMERICAN MEDICAL ASSOCIATION (n.d.). *Professional Resources*. Retrieved July 20, 2008, from http://www.ama-assn.org

AMERICAN NURSES ASSOCIATION. (2001). *Code of ethics for nurses with interpretive statements.* Washington, DC: Author.

BOONE, L., & Kurtz, D. (1999). *Contemporary business.* Fort Worth, TX: Dryden Press.

BOWERS-LANIER, R. (2007). Coalitions: A powerful political strategy. In D. Mason, J. Levitt, & M. Chaffee, (Eds.), *Policy and politics in nursing and health care* (pp. 135–144). St. Louis, MO: Saunders.

CENTER FOR AMERICAN NURSES HOME PAGE. (n.d.). Retrieved January 15, 2008, from http://www.centerforamericannurses.org/about

CENTER ON BUDGET AND POLICY PRIORITIES. (2006, August 29). *The number of uninsured Americans is at an all-time high.* Retrieved November 25, 2007, from http://www.cbpp.org/8-29-06health.htm

CHANDLER, A. (n.d.). *Click here for change: Your guide to e-advocacy revolution.* Retrieved November 24, 2007, from http://www.policylink.org/Projects/eAdvocacy/documents/final_report.pdf

CURTIN, L. (2007). Health policy, politics, and professional ethics. In D. Mason, J. Levitt, & M. Chaffee, (Eds.), *Policy and politics in nursing and health care* (pp. 243–255). St. Louis, MO: Saunders.

DIXON, A. Y. (2007). Conflict management: A critical part of politics. In D. Mason, J. Levitt, & M. Chaffee, *Policy and politics in nursing and health care* (pp. 221–226). St. Louis, MO: Saunders.

ELDER, L. (n.d.). Defining critical thinking. *The critical thinking community.* Retrieved November 25, 2007, from http://www.criticalthinking.org/aboutCT/define_critical_thinking.cfm

ENCYCLOPEDIA OF PUBLIC HEALTH. (n.d.). Retrieved January 10, 2008, from http://www.answers.com/topic/labor-union?cat=biz-fin

FOLEY, B. J. (2004). *Advocacy: A skill that must be nurtured.* Retrieved November 27, 2007, from http://nsweb.nursingspectrum.com/cfforms/GuestLecture/AdvocacySkill.cfm

GERTLER, B. (2003). Self-knowledge. In *Stanford encyclopedia of philosophy.* Retrieved December 28, 2007, from http://plato.stanford.edu/entries/self-knowledge/

GORKIN, M. (n.d.). *Creative risk taking.* Retrieved July 20, 2008, from http://www.stressdoc.com/creative_risk_taking.htm

GREEN, A., & Jordan, C. (2004, January 31). Common denominators: Shared governance and work place advocacy—Strategies for nurses to gain control over their practice. *OJIN: Online Journal of Issues in Nursing, 9*(1). Retrieved November 25, 2007, from http://www.nursingworld.org/ojin

GRIFFIN, D., & Johnston, K. (2005, December 22). Katrina investigation focuses on more than one person.*CNN.com.* Retrieved February 1, 2008, from http://www.cnn.com/2005/US/12/21/katrina.hospital/index.html

HESS, R. (2004, January). From bedside to boardroom—Nursing shared governance. *OJIN: The Online Journal of Issues in Nursing, 9*(1). Retrieved July 20, 2008, from http://www.nursingworld.org

HILTON, L. (2007, May 24). Patient advocacy and the oncology nurse. *Nursing spectrum.* Retrieved February 1, 2008, from http://include.nurse.com/apps/pbcs.dll/article?AID=/20070524/ONC/70410002

INDIANA CENTER FOR EVIDENCE BASED NURSING PRACTICE. (n.d.). *The Indiana Center for Evidence-Based Nursing Practice—Your online source for evidence-based nursing news, links, and resources.* Retrieved July 20, 2008, from http://www.ebnp.org

KOHN, L., Corrigan, J., &. Donaldson, M. (2000). *To err is human.* Washington, DC: National Academies Press.

LEAVITT, J., Chaffee, M. W., & Vance, C. (2007). Learning the ropes of policy, politics, and advocacy. In D. Mason, J. Levitt, & M. Chaffee (Eds.), *Policy and politics in nursing and health care.* St. Louis, MO: Saunders.

LEAVITT, J., Cohen, S., & Mason, D. (2007). Political analysis and strategies. In D. Mason, J. Levitt, & M. Chaffee (Eds.), *Policy and politics in nursing and health care* (pp. 84–108). St. Louis, MO: Saunders.

MAXFIELD, D., Grenny, J., McMillan, R., Patterson, K., & Swtizler, A. (2005). *Silence kills: The seven crucial conversations for healthcare.* Retrieved December 1, 2007, from http://www.aacn.org/aacn/pubpolcy.nsf/Files/SilenceKills/$file/SilenceKills.pdf

MEECHAM, D. (2003). *Understand self-advocacy.* Retrieved November 25, 2007, from http://www.edac.org.au/letmespeak/html/self advocacy.html

NIGHTINGALE, F. (1860). *Notes on nursing: What it is and what it is not.* (1969 Reprint). Mineola, NY: Dover Publications.

NOWLIN, A. (2008, June). National Nurse Debate. *Advance for nurse practitioners.* Retrieved July 20, 2008, from http://nurse-practitioners.advancweb.com

NURSES, DOCTORS ANNOUNCE "SCRUBS FOR SICKO" CAMPAIGN IN CONJUNCTION WITH DEBUT OF MICHAEL MOORE'S FILM TO SPARK GENUINE HEALTHCARE DEBATE. (2007, June 18). *PR News Wire.* Retrieved December 10, 2007, from http://www.prnewswire.com/cgi-bin/stories.pl?ACCT=109&STORY=/www/story/06-18-2007/0004610416&EDATE

NURSING ADVOCACY: WHERE DO YOU FIT IN? (2007, MARCH 21). Retrieved January 20, 2008, from http://www.emergiblog.com/2007/03/nursing-advocacy-where-do-you-fit-in.html

ONCOLOGY NURSING SOCIETY. (2007). *Oncology nurse practitioner competencies.* Retrieved January 30, 2008, from http://www.ons.org/clinical/Professional/QualityCancer/documents/NPCompentencies.pdf

PATTERSON, K., Grenny, J., McMillan, R., & Switzler, A. (2002). *Crucial conversations: Tools for talking when stakes are high.* New York: McGraw-Hill.

SAAD, L. (2006). Nursing tops the list of most honest and ethical professions. *The Gallup poll.* Retrieved November 25, 2007, from http://www.calnurses.org/media-center/in-the-news/2006/december/page.jsp?itemID=29117737

SCRIVEN, M., & Paul, R. (2007). Defining critical thinking. In *The critical thinking community.* Retrieved November 25, 2007, from http://www.criticalthinking.org/aboutCT/define_critical_thinking.cfm

SOUKHANOV, A. (Ed.). (2001). *Microsoft Encarta College Dictionary.* New York: St. Martins Press.

UNITED AMERICAN NURSES HOME PAGE. (n.d.). Retrieved November 25, 2007, from http://www.uannurse.org

UNIVERSITY OF MINNESOTA. (2007). *Evidence-based nursing.* Retrieved November 27, 2007, from http://evidence.ahc.umn.edu/ebn.htm

U.S. DEPARTMENT OF LABOR. (2008). *Labor statistics.* Retrieved November 30, 2007, from http://www.bls.gov/news.release/union2.nr0.htm

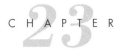

THE PRACTICE ENVIRONMENT: ANTICIPATING THE FUTURE

Kathleen M. White
PhD, RN, CEA-BC, Director, Master's and Doctor of Nursing Practice Programs,
The Johns Hopkins University School of Nursing

It is not necessary to be clairvoyant to know the future; it is only necessary to clearly interpret what has already happened and then project forward the likely consequences of those happenings.

–Peter Drucker

LEARNING OBJECTIVES

At the completion of the chapter, the learner should be able to do the following:

1. Describe the factors affecting the future of the nursing practice environment.
2. Identify specific actions that individual nurses can take to impact the future of the nursing practice environment.
3. Evaluate the chaos and complexity theory for prediction of the future practice environment for nursing.
4. Analyze the effect of the impact factors for safety and quality care.
5. Discuss the implications of future trends on the nursing profession.

KEY TERMS

Aging Population	Evidence-Based Practice	Quality
Chaos Theory	Future of Nursing	Safety
Communication	Health	Teamwork
Complexity	Health Disparities	Workforce Shortages
Consumer	Interdisciplinary Education	

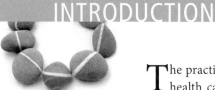

INTRODUCTION

The practice of nursing today continues to change at a rapid pace. The uncertainty of the health care environment and the continual advances in technology add other dimensions to that changing practice. The profession of nursing is challenged to keep pace with the changes and to strengthen the role for nursing in the future of health care. The literature abounds with descriptions of the future of nursing, for theory, research, education, and leadership. The prospect of describing the future practice environment for nursing is an exciting opportunity.

Lessons from other theories can help to shape our thoughts and discussions of the future of nursing practice. **Complexity** theory supports a holistic theory of health care and points to interconnectedness and the idea that the whole is more than a sum of its parts. Nursing has always embraced a holistic approach to direct care. As we think about the future of nursing practice, if significant changes are planned or foreseen, it is necessary that we look beyond nursing to the rest of health care, use the interconnectedness in the health care system, and assess the impact of each change, possible successes or failures, and be prepared for unpredicted outcomes. Enter chaos theory. The appeal of **chaos theory** is the view that organizations are complex adaptive systems with behaviors in different stages of stability that react to the chaos and constant change in the environment. In such an environment, goals for the future are not just a set of desired results but a series of contingency scenarios to which one can react in the short or long term. Nurses of the future must be flexible, willing to learn new things, prepared to question long-held assumptions, and recognize the profession can be blinded by its own prejudices and biases. Things that worked in the past will not work in the future, so we have to keep on learning and experimenting. As you consider your career and future employment, consider the many possibilities available to you by recognizing that a complex and chaotic health care environment exists, and plan for different opportunities and challenges, as the future is unpredictable (Figure 23-1).

Figure 23-1
Health care is, and will continue to be, a complex and chaotic environment. The different opportunities and challenges the future may hold should be taken into consideration when thinking about a nursing career.

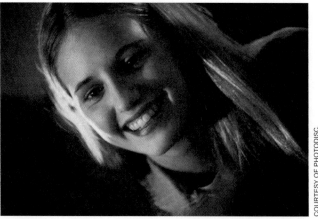

COURTESY OF PHOTODISC.

THE CHALLENGE

Nursing, medicine, and the other allied health professions have been challenged over the last decade by the Institute of Medicine (IOM), the Pew Commission, and other groups to better respond to the changing needs of the health care environment. Ten years ago, the Pew Commission released *Recreating Health Professional Practice for a New Century* (1998), the fourth and final report of the Pew Health Professions Commission, a group that had been asked to create a new vision of what health professionals ought to be doing in their practices. This report recommended changes to the professional education for all the health professions and detailed twenty-one competencies for the health professions in the 21st century that continue to be important for our practice (see Figure 23-2).

Figure 23-2
Twenty-one Competencies for the Health Professions in the 21st Century. *(Recreating Health Professional Practice for a New Century. The Fourth Report of the Pew Health Professions Commission.)*

1. Embrace a personal ethic of social responsibility and service.

2. Exhibit ethical behavior in all professional activities.

3. Provide evidence-based, clinically competent care.

4. Incorporate the multiple determinants of health in clinical care.

5. Apply knowledge of the new sciences.

6. Demonstrate critical thinking, reflection, and problem-solving skills.

7. Understand the role of primary care.

8. Rigorously practice preventive health care.

9. Integrate population-based care and services into practice.

10. Improve access to health care for those with unmet health needs.

11. Practice relationship-centered care with individuals and families.

12. Provide culturally sensitive care to a diverse society.

13. Partner with communities in health care decisions.

14. Use communication and information technology effectively and appropriately.

15. Work in interdisciplinary teams.

16. Ensure care that balances individual, professional, system and societal needs.

17. Practice leadership.

18. Take responsibility for quality of care and health outcomes at all levels.

19. Contribute to continuous improvement of the health care system.

20. Advocate for public policy that promotes and protects the health of the public.

21. Continue to learn and help others learn.

The IOM report *Health Professional Education: A Bridge to Quality* (IOM, 2003) called on the health professions to change the learning experiences of their students so that their graduates' professional identity formation would include the five competencies to deliver patient-centered care as a member of an interdisciplinary team, emphasizing evidence-based practice, quality improvement approaches, and informatics. These competencies shape the current and future practice environment for all health care practitioners, including nurses.

FACTORS THAT WILL IMPACT THE FUTURE OF NURSING PRACTICE

An uncertain and complex health care environment and new challenges to competency create a shifting practice milieu that is difficult to predict. However, there are important trends affecting the **future of nursing** practice that need to be monitored and evaluated. Nurses must be ready to respond to these factors and develop a preferred future so that the nursing profession can survive and thrive. Consider and reflect carefully on the following factors that will impact the future of nursing practice.

The U.S. Health Care System

The U.S. health care system, seen by many as the best in the world, is fraught with problems. Many say that it is not really a system at all, but episodic and illness-oriented, and that important and necessary linkages for quality health care are not easily available. There are also tremendous pressures to contain costs, increase access to health care for uninsured and underinsured persons, and to improve quality. Health care reform proposals abound at both the state and national level. Most of these proposals are aimed at providing insurance coverage for the uninsured. Several states have already passed legislation to make important reforms to health care in their state, but unfortunately, a single proposal that all are willing to accept does not exist. Nursing must be at the forefront of the development, implementation, and evaluation of these health care reform proposals and must be seen as part of the solution to a reformed health care system. Nurses need to stay informed about the initiatives and discuss what the reform proposal means for their practice. Advocacy at the local, state, and national level is more important now than ever before. It is important to engage support both within and outside the nursing community to endorse or oppose any health care reform proposals and to spread the word about the initiative and implications for health care practice.

Health Promotion

The definition of **health** in this illness-oriented health care system is slowly broadening to include wellness and risk reduction, with a focus on health promotion and illness prevention. The health of U.S. citizens continues to improve overall (National Center for Health Statistics, 2006). However, more Americans are living longer, and are consequently living with chronic disease and the associated disabilities and pain, as well as with other conditions associated with **aging**. This has caused a shift toward population-based care to improve health care. For example, disease management programs have been developed that specifically target populations of individuals with chronic illnesses such as diabetes or congestive heart failure. The programs provide regular and continual monitoring of their chronic illness, possible complications, treatment regimen, medication adherence, and lifestyle assistance. Nurses in population-based care are vital on both of these fronts. The role for nursing in health promotion and disease prevention is to create awareness of the multiple determinants of health, assist clients to make healthy choices, and reduce obstacles to health. On the other end of the continuum, nurses need to be in positions to champion the transformation of chronic care, emphasizing the need to support clients in treatment adherence and self-management of their condition.

Health Disparities

Improvements in the health of U.S. citizens have been made by race, ethnicity, income, education, and geography. However, **health disparities** by race and ethnicity still exist in both the provision of health care and for health care insurance coverage. Another IOM report (2003), *Unequal Treatment: Confronting Racial and Ethnic Disparities in Health Care*, is a good resource on this topic. Additionally, the Healthy People 2010 initiative calls for the elimination of long-standing disparities in health status that exist among segments of the population, including disparities that occur by race or ethnicity (U.S. Department of Health and Human Services, 2000). Both documents recommend the educational experience of health care practitioners be enhanced to include more emphasis on cultural competence, and that more research is conducted in order to change health policies that cause disparities in the provision of health care.

| Writing Exercise 23-1 | Reflect on your clinical practicum experiences. What barriers to health and wellness based on race and ethnicity have you seen? What cultural beliefs and attitudes of health care providers and clients contribute to health disparities? What is the impact of income and education on the health disparities across ethnic and racial groups? What role do nurses have in decreasing health disparities? |

Public Health

The public health of this nation is in critical need of attention. It affects every aspect of life in every part of the country, from local immunization programs to the national threat of bioterrorism. One of the most important problems to the public health of Americans is the fight to control obesity, especially among our children, who are more overweight than at any time in history.

Being obese puts a person at risk for many chronic health care problems. Equally important to the public health is the fight to stop tobacco use. Despite all of the efforts to decrease its use, one in five Americans is still smoking. Finally, the threat of pandemic and bioterrorism adds a whole new dimension to the need for public health. Emergency preparedness and disaster response programs are necessary for the U.S. population to be cared for effectively and immediately should a threat exist. Nurses understand the impact of health and disease at both the individual clinical level, and the population-wide level. Because nursing makes essential contributions to the population's health, it is paramount that the profession assures that there are adequately educated nurses that can function in public health settings and address the needs of the U.S. population.

Demographics of the Population

The shift in the demographics of the U.S. shows the population is growing older and more racially and ethnically diverse. Americans are living longer, with an average lifespan of eighty years for women and seventy-five years for men. Currently 12.5% of the population is sixty-five or older, but it is expected to be more that 20% of the population by 2020, and those over eighty-five years of age is the fastest growing segment of the population. Because of this longer life, as mentioned before, many Americans are living with one or more chronic condition and more are likely to need and seek health care and health care information. It is predicted by many that socioeconomic status, discrimination, lack of access, health practices, and cultural differences among minority racial and ethnic groups in the U.S. will likely continue to influence future patterns of disease, disability, and health care utilization. There is general agreement that the nursing profession must respond in two ways. First, the profession must aggressively increase the diversity of both students and faculty in order to increase the diversity of practicing nurses. The predicted majority-minority of the U.S. population will make this need even more important than ever before in order for nurses to provide culturally competent care and to sensitize the profession to health disparities based on race and ethnicity. The demographics of the nursing profession have remained fairly constant over the years. Ninety percent of all nurses are white, nonhispanic. Even though there has been an increase in minority registered nurses, the actual numbers remain small. African-American nurses make up only about 5% of all nurses, compared to 12% of the U.S. population. There are even fewer Hispanic nurses. The profession's second response to the shift in demographics of the U.S. population must be to increase the competency of all nurses in the care of the older adult.

Workforce Shortages

There will continue to be **workforce shortages** in many of the health care professions, including registered nurses, primary care physicians, physical therapists, and pharmacists, to name a few. The most recent data show a predicted shortage of 500,000 nurses by 2025 (Buerhaus, 2008). This prediction is an improvement of a once predicted 800,000-RN shortage, but is still a critical shortage of nurses. U.S. nursing schools have boosted enrollments and younger students are again entering nursing schools, which are all good trends, but the job turnover and retention of nurses is still a big issue. The nursing faculty shortage that has reached critical proportions will also limit the ability of schools of nursing to increase educational capacity. The nursing profession must continue to be innovative in ways to address these workforce shortages and enlist support from stakeholders and policymakers for creative solutions that benefit not only the profession, but also the health care system.

Internet Exercise 23-1

The National Sample Survey of Registered Nurses (NSSRN) is conducted every four years and represents an overview of the personal, professional, and employment characteristics of the 2.9 million registered nurses residing in the United States as of March 2004. It can be found online at the Health Resources Services Administration (HRSA) Web site: http://bhpr.hrsa.gov. Once you are on the HRSA home page, click on the "Bureau of Health Professions" found at the top of the page, and then click on "National Center for Health Workforce Analysis," found on the left side halfway down the Bureau of Health Professions Web page. This will take you to the latest NSSRN report. Look at the Web site and the report and answer the following questions:

1. Is the Web site helpful in finding information about the nursing profession?

2. Read the executive summary and discuss the difference in the findings from 2000 to 2004—what is improving for the nursing workforce and what is not?

3. What would you predict for the 2008 NSSRN and why?

Information Technology

The role of information technology in the health care environment continues to dominate. Health care organizations, in an effort to keep pace and to respond to growing quality and **safety** concerns, are adopting technological innovations at staggering rates. Smart equipment, bar code and scanning technology, integrated health information systems, wireless computer carts, voice-activated documentation systems, and advances in diagnostic and treatment technology, including genetics mapping, are a few examples. The predicted increased use of telehealth systems, as more health care is provided in the community, will challenge our current processes and demands. The vision that all nurses are computer savvy, understand the integration of technology in the health care environment, and have the skills necessary to access information and communicate that information must be the "big hairy audacious goal" as the profession strives to remain a major player in health care. It is impossible to predict the roles that will be available for nurses in health care information technology as the technology continues to advance.

Evidence-Based Practice

The emphasis on **evidence-based practice** (EBP) in health care settings today is fundamental to the clinical quality improvement that ensures the best quality care is provided to patients and families. In a study by the RAND corporation, McGlynn, et al., (2003) showed that, on average, Americans receive about half of the evidence-based recommended medical care processes. Another IOM report, *Crossing the Quality Chasm: A New Health System for the 21st Century* (2001), also clearly identifies a gap between knowledge of what is known to be "best practice" and what is actually practiced, and underscores the need to improve clinical performance and the quality of care. It is generally accepted in health care today that the "gap" between what we know works and what is actually done in health care practice is serious and poses a threat to the health of all Americans. Nurses must stay abreast of the best research and evidence, integrate it into practice, use the most appropriate information available to make clinical decisions for individual patients, based not only on the available evidence but also on patient characteristics, situations, and preferences, and be a leader in improving patient care. This requires that nurses have access, at the point of care, to the best evidence when making decisions about patient care, in order to optimize outcomes. There are many Web sites that provide evidence-based guidelines for care that can be accessed to assist in clinical decision making. The United States government, through the Agency for HealthCare Research and Quality (AHRQ), offers treatment guidelines based on EBP principles at the National Guideline Clearinghouse Web site http://www.guideline.gov. The Cochrane Collaboration sets standards for reviews of guidelines for care and offers "systematic reviews" of related research by disorder, and can be found at http://www.cochrane. org. The Virginia Henderson International Nursing Library through Sigma Theta Tau International offers online access to reliable nursing information that can be easily utilized and shared and is one of the most comprehensive resources for nursing information available. Through the library's complimentary *Registry of Nursing Research* database, access to search study abstracts and conference abstracts is available at http://www.nursinglibrary.org. The Cumulative Index of Nursing and Allied Health Literature (CINAHL) database can use evidence-based nursing filters as search strategies that filter your search for evidence-based practice resources when you combine them with your specific subject terms. The filters they use deal with diagnosis, etiology, prognosis, therapy, meta-analysis, and qualitative research. Finally, the Joanna Briggs Institute has a series of information sheets (or guidelines) that are produced specifically for practicing clinicians and are based on the best available research evidence as reported in systematic reviews. They are available both electronically and via the JBI Web site: http://www.joannabriggs.edu.au. The JBI home page will have tabs across the top, click on "EBP Resources and Services," and this will open a drop-down menu. Then click on "Best Practice Series Database" to view the best practice information on many important practice topics, such as smoking cessation, pressure ulcers, and dietary interventions in obese children. With all of this point-of-care access to research and best practices, every nurse must be able to ask three key questions before decision making: 1) Is the evidence from this study valid? 2) If it is valid, what is the strength of this evidence? 3) If valid and strong, is this evidence applicable to the care of patients in this setting?

Savvy Consumer

Today's educated **consumers** want information about their health care. Because of easy access to computer technology, consumers have information at their fingertips at all times, have a heightened demand for information, and expect to participate in health care decision making. Consumers who are more involved with their care tend to get better results and are more satisfied. They have been told that the single most important thing a patient can do to prevent a medical error in their health care is to be an active medical member of their health care team, which translates into taking part in decisions about their health care. In an effort to improve the quality and safety of the health care experience, there are many educational guides for the patient about taking responsibility in their health care. A good example of one of these information guides was designed by the Agency for Healthcare Research and Quality (AHRQ). It is called *Five Steps to Safer Health Care* (see Figure 23-3) and can be found on the AHRQ Web

Figure 23-3
Five Steps to Safer Health Care: A Patient Fact Sheet. *(Courtesy of Agency for Healthcare Research and Quality (2004). Five Steps to Safer Health Care: Patient Fact Sheet. AHRQ Publication Number 04-M005. Rockville, MD: Agency for Healthcare Research and Quality.)*

1. **Ask questions if you have doubts or concerns.** Ask questions and make sure you understand the answers. Choose a doctor you feel comfortable talking to. Take a relative or friend with you to help you ask questions and understand the answers.

2. **Keep and bring a list of ALL the medicines you take.** Give your doctor and pharmacist a list of all the medicines that you take, including non-prescription medicines. Tell them about any drug allergies you have. Ask about side effects and what to avoid while taking the medicine. Read the label when you get your medicine, including all warnings. Make sure your medicine is what the doctor ordered and know how to use it. Ask the pharmacist about your medicine if it looks different than you expected.

3. **Get the results of any test or procedure.** Ask when and how you will get the results of tests or procedures. Don't assume the results are fine if you do not get them when expected, be it in person, by phone, or by mail. Call your doctor and ask for your results. Ask what the results mean for your care.

4. **Talk to your doctor about which hospital is best for your health needs.** If you have more than one hospital to choose from, ask your doctor about which hospital has the best care and results for your condition. Be sure you understand the instructions you get about follow-up care when you leave the hospital.

5. **Make sure you understand what will happen if you need surgery.** Make sure you, your doctor, and your surgeon all agree on exactly what will be done during the operation. Ask your doctor, "Who will manage my care when I am in the hospital?" Ask your surgeon:

   • Exactly what will you be doing during the surgery?
   • About how long will the surgery take?
   • What will happen after the surgery?
   • How can I expect to feel during recovery?

   Tell the surgeon, anesthesiologist, and nurses about any allergies, bad reaction to anesthesia, and any medications you are taking.

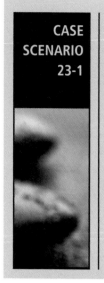

CASE SCENARIO 23-1

You are at your clinical rotation for the first day. The hospital has a "Hand Hygiene" campaign going on with posters around the hospital and targeted patient education to tell the patients to watch that their health professionals wash their hands before caring for them. You just received your assignment for the day and walked into your patient's room to get oriented to the patient and surroundings. Immediately, the patient says to you, wash your hands before you touch me.

CASE ANALYSIS

1. What do you do? You haven't even started your care yet and you are being criticized.

2. What is the evidence for this new initiative? Look for evidence about hand hygiene and patient safety, but also patient-centered care and patient engagement in health care.

3. Develop a few key phrases that you will use in your practice to involve patients in their care.

site: http://www.ahrq.gov. On the AHRQ home page, click on the "Consumer Health" tab on the left side of the page. This will take you to many informational guides for the consumer. You will need to scroll down this Web page to the heading "Quality Care" to find the *Five Steps to Safer Health Care*.

Finally, consumers also have many more choices about their health care than ever before. In addition to traditional western medicine, there is a wide variety of alternative and complementary medical approaches that are available. Research is ongoing to evaluate the efficacy and effectiveness of some of the treatments and approaches, and some insurance companies are paying for limited use of alternative approaches, and some academic medical centers have established centers for complementary and alternative medicine.

Health Care Teamwork

Most health care today is delivered by teams. The recent attention to **teamwork** is, in large part, a result of another IOM report, *To Err Is Human: Building a Safer Health System* (1999). One of the main findings of that report was that systemic failures in the delivery of health care account for more errors than does poor performance by individuals. And, because systemic successes and failures depend on the performance of teams, the IOM recommended interdisciplinary team training to increase patient safety and quality health care. This team approach to the practice environment requires teamwork behaviors and skills, the development of teamwork habits, and the creation of small work teams, all new skill sets for nurses, physicians, and other members of the health care team.

Paul M. Schyve, M.D., the senior vice president of the Joint Commission, was quoted saying, "Our challenge, therefore, is not whether we will deliver care in teams but rather how well we will deliver care in teams" (2005, p. 183). More recently, Allan S. Frankel, the Director of Patient Safety at Partners Health Care System of Boston, noted: "We can assure our patients that their care is always provided by a team of experts, but we cannot assure our patients that their care is always provided by expert teams" (2006, p. 1700). These two quotes seem to sum up the teamwork challenge facing health care today.

Teamwork depends on team member's ability to communicate effectively and efficiently, anticipate the needs of others on the team, adjust to the needs of the team, and to have a shared understanding of what is expected and what will happen. This is exemplified in the work of Dr. Peter Pronovost and his team at The Johns Hopkins Hospital Surgical Intensive Care Unit (ICU). Pronovost's team developed an ICU Daily Goals Worksheet to increase the care team's understanding of the daily goals for patients in the ICU; what work needs to happen for the patient that day; what is the greatest safety risk to the patient; what are the key processes for ventilator patients; what are the scheduled labs for the patient; catheter; what can be done to assist in facilitating **communication** with the family; and what needs to be put in place for the patient to leave the ICU. The tool was designed to facilitate communication among the team, empower nursing, and avoid duplicate work. The success of the goals sheet improved teamwork and reduced ICU length of stay.

Transforming Care at the Bedside (TCAB) is a Robert Wood Johnson Foundation-sponsored project in collaboration with the Institute for Healthcare Improvement designed to create, test, and spread hospital nursing-unit-level innovative strategies to improve the work environment and quality of care (see Figure 23-4). TCAB is now in its fifth year, and there are ten participating hospitals. The future of nursing practice will be created by these innovations and transformations to care. The four main themes of TCAB—Safe and Reliable Care, Vitality and Teamwork, Patient-Centered Care, and Value-Added Care Processes—are guided by the IOM's aims for care. These categories serve as a framework for organizing and focusing this work, but they are not mutually exclusive; working in one area can produce positive change in another. Hospitals have had success in testing, refining, and implementing change ideas within each category, many with very promising early results. Examples of these ideas include the following:

- Use of Rapid Response Teams to "rescue" patients before a crisis occurs.
- Specific communication models that support consistent and clear communication among caregivers.
- Professional support programs such as preceptorships and educational opportunities.
- Liberalized diet plans and meal schedules for patients.
- Redesigned workspace that enhances efficiency and reduces waste.

More information about the TCAB initiative can be found at the IHI Web site at http://www.ihi.org. From the IHI home page, click on "programs" on the left side of the page, then "strategic initiatives" should appear. Click on that, and then locate "Transforming Care at the Bedside."

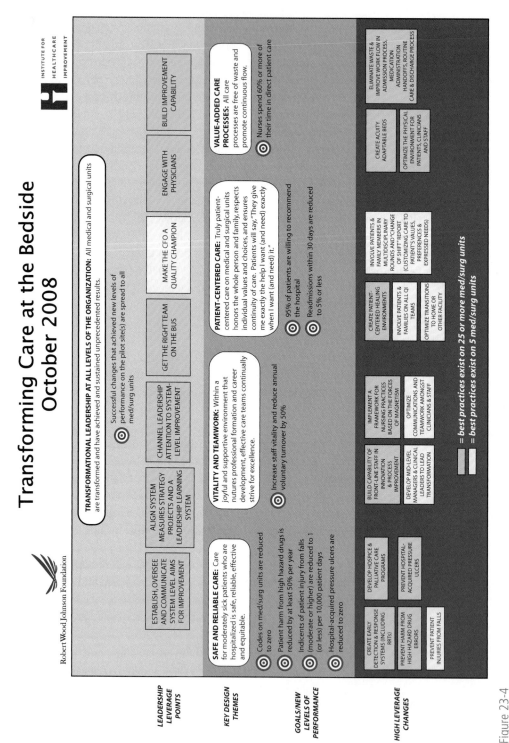

Figure 23-4
Transforming Care at the Bedside Framework. (©2008 Institute for Healthcare Improvement and the Robert Wood Johnson Foundation. Reprinted with permission.)

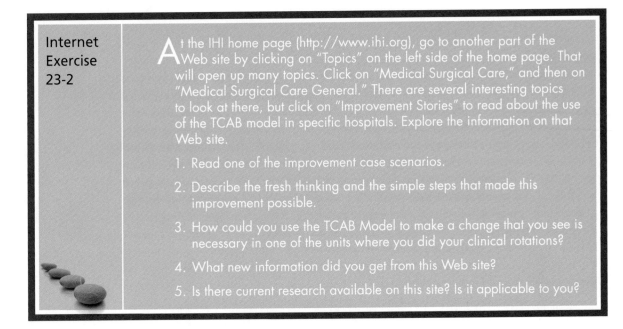

Internet Exercise 23-2

At the IHI home page (http://www.ihi.org), go to another part of the Web site by clicking on "Topics" on the left side of the home page. That will open up many topics. Click on "Medical Surgical Care," and then on "Medical Surgical Care General." There are several interesting topics to look at there, but click on "Improvement Stories" to read about the use of the TCAB model in specific hospitals. Explore the information on that Web site.

1. Read one of the improvement case scenarios.

2. Describe the fresh thinking and the simple steps that made this improvement possible.

3. How could you use the TCAB Model to make a change that you see is necessary in one of the units where you did your clinical rotations?

4. What new information did you get from this Web site?

5. Is there current research available on this site? Is it applicable to you?

Safety and Quality Movement

The 1999 IOM publication *To Err is Human* concluded that as many as 98,000 people die in any given year from preventable medical errors, and the era of patient **quality** and **safety** was born. The IOM and the Joint Commission on Accreditation of Healthcare Organizations (Joint Commission) acknowledged that most medical mistakes occur not because of negligence or carelessness, but because of complex system errors and the tremendous evolution in health care over the last decade. This includes the explosion of technology and critical personnel shortages.

The mission of the Joint Commission is to continuously improve the safety and quality of care provided to the public through the provision of health care accreditation and related services that support performance improvement in health care organizations. In 2002 they announced their first-time-ever National Patient Safety Goals, and we are in the seventh year of that continuing program. In addition, the Joint Commission has also specified patient safety standards that all accredited facilities must meet. In 2005 President George W. Bush signed the Patient Safety and Quality Improvement Act of 2005 (PSQIA). This legislation has helped to create a national patient safety database that encourages health care providers to report medical errors and near misses to patient safety organizations (Meushaw, White, & Walrath, 2006). The federal government has been very involved with patient quality and safety initiatives and, through the AHRQ and the National Quality Forum, has identified 30 Safe Practices for Better Health Care.

| Internet Exercise 23-3 | Access the Web site for AHRQ again (http://www.ahrq.gov). Once you are on the home page, click on the "Consumer Health" tab on the left side of the home page. Once you are on the "Consumer Health" page, scroll down to "Quality Care" and look for the "30 Safe Practices for Better Health Care Fact Sheet." These are 30 clinical practices that should be in place in every health care setting. The goal in the United States is to deliver safe, high-quality health care to patients in all clinical settings. Despite the best intentions, however, a high rate of largely preventable adverse events and medical errors occur that cause harm to patients. Adverse events and medical errors can occur in any health care setting and in any community in this country. The 30 safe practices have been endorsed by the National Quality Forum (NQF), which represents over 260 of the nation's leading health care providers, purchasers, and consumer organizations. These organizations strongly urge that these 30 safe practices be universally adopted by all applicable health care settings to reduce the risk of harm to patients. How many of these have you learned about or experienced in the clinical setting during your nursing program? Discuss the implications of numbers 7, 25, and 27 for patient safety with your clinical group. |

Pay for Quality

Because of mounting health care costs and misaligned reimbursement systems, employers, purchasers, insurance plans, and policymakers have begun to design and implement measurement and reporting systems, also called "pay for performance" or "pay for quality" programs, that will reward high-performing hospitals and other providers of health care. These programs are designed to increase accountability and achieve improvements in quality outcomes and safety initiatives. The current programs, implemented by the Center for Medicare and Medicaid Services (CMS) and a few other groups, have been aimed at hospitals and physicians, and much has been learned in implementing these voluntary programs. Nursing has not been a part of these measurement programs to date, and consequently, little is known about how a pay-for-performance system for quality nursing care should be structured. In the very near future, nurses will be responsible for contributing to and reporting measures of performance. Collecting nursing-care outcomes measures will allow nurses to continuously assess practice and make modifications to improve patient care.

Changes in Nursing Education

In October 2004, the members of the American Association of Colleges of Nursing (AACN) endorsed the *Position Statement on the Practice Doctorate in Nursing* (2006), which called for moving the level of preparation necessary for advanced nursing practice roles from the master's degree to the doctorate level by the year 2015. The AACN position statement calls for educating

Writing Exercise 23-2

There are currently many roles and settings for nurses. Think about how many of your nursing clinical experiences took place in ambulatory and community-based settings. In an essay, consider the following question: To what extent does the nursing curriculum reflect the realities of the changing world of health care and nursing practice? What suggestions would you have for the faculty for other educational experiences to prepare you for future practice?

advanced practice nurses (APNs), expert practitioners who can serve as clinical faculty, and other nurses seeking top clinical positions in Doctor of Nursing Practice (DNP) programs.

Nursing is moving in the direction of other health professions in the transition to the DNP. Medicine, dentistry, pharmacy, psychology, physical therapy, and audiology all offer practice doctorates. DNP curricula build on current master's programs by providing education in evidence-based practice, quality improvement, and systems thinking, among other key areas. Transitioning to the DNP will not alter the current scope of practice for APNs. State Nurse Practice Acts describe the scope of practice allowed, and these differ from state to state. (These requirements would likely remain unchanged.) The transition to the DNP will better prepare APNs for their current roles, given the calls for new models of education and the growing complexity of health care. This move to the DNP also coincides with recommendations by the IOM, Pew Commission, the Joint Commission, and other authorities who have called for the health professions to restructure their education to meet the needs of the changing health care delivery system. Nursing is answering that call by moving to prepare APNs for evolving practice. The other twelve trends discussed above demand a higher level of preparation for nursing leaders who can design and assess care for the complex health care environment.

WHAT IS THE FUTURE OF NURSING PRACTICE?

According to the 2006 Gallup poll that asks the public who they consider the most honest and ethical among twenty-three professional groups, nursing has topped the list, except for one year, since being added to the list of choices. Nurses, in a profession identified by 84% of the public as highly or very highly trusted, are valued for their knowledge, skills, and abilities to provide and coordinate health care. This is the future that nursing wants, to be a valued and knowledgeable provider of health care. The future is bright for nursing because nurses are pivotal to the health care system, and the future of the U.S. health care system depends on them.

The nursing practice of the future will be designed so that it is safe, timely, efficient, effective, equitable, and patient-centered. The six IOM recommendations have been deliberately ordered in this way to create an acronym, so that one could say that the road to quality care is "STEEEP." In order to accomplish the IOM recommendations for a safer health care system, significant changes to the nursing work environment will be made, and nurses will lead the design and

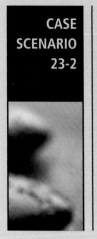

CASE SCENARIO 23-2

Your clinical group is assigned to the local middle school health suite for your community health clinical rotation this semester. You have been told to do a health-needs assessment for the school and develop a teaching plan to meet the health needs of the students. As you are doing your needs assessment, several of the middle school students want to know why you would want to be a nurse. Their perception of nursing is bedpans and injections. One student even asks: why don't you go to medical school?

CASE ANALYSIS

1. Develop a plan to assess the students' knowledge of the health professions.

2. Discuss the image of nursing, including the Gallup poll information above, with the students and determine what they really know about nursing.

3. Develop a teaching plan about nursing as a career.

implementation of new models of care delivery, examining work design, safety, quality practices, technology, decision making, staffing, and management practices. The importance of nurses' involvement in these practice and policy decisions will be paramount, and nursing leadership must be ready and able to take this on.

What will nursing practice look like in the future? Will nurses be touching patients? What will they be doing at the bedside? The essence of nursing care is a balance of caring and curing. The touching of patients is an integral part of this. Yes, nurses will always be touching and caring for patients at the bedside. But how nurses will care for patients will change, and nurses will be managers, coordinators, and engineers of that bedside care. They will be throughput experts, creating efficient environments where patients move from unit to unit and from one level of care to the next without delays. Nurses will be quality-control managers and they will identify threats to patient safety in the environment. Nurses will see an increase in importance of their advocacy role—advocacy for patients, families, other nurses, and other staff.

There will also be roles and positions for nurses that we can't even imagine or predict right now. Telehealth and telenursing will no doubt increase, especially with population-based care and in rural settings. Roles for nurses in safety and quality systems improvement will also increase. But what will the new strategic initiative of the future practice environment be? Whatever it is, nursing will be a part of it.

Teamwork will prevail in the future nursing practice environment, and **interdisciplinary** competence that values collaboration and the contribution of each health care professional will be the norm. Emphasis will be placed on educating nurses in teams with other health care providers, so that early appreciation of the value of each member's contribution to health care will be evident.

The information technology (IT) age will continue to explode, and the technological advances on the horizon that will assist and enable health care are beyond what we could predict or imagine today. The health care environment will be an early adopter of technology to deliver safe, high-quality care. Whatever this technology is, nursing will learn to use it. Nurses in all clinical settings and specialties will use and expand their core informatics competencies and will integrate IT into their daily practices to improve quality and safety of care. This enhanced IT practice environment will facilitate nurses' access to evidence-based knowledge at the point of care. The quality chasm will be bridged, and the health care that nurses provide will be the right care for the right patient in the right setting at the right time.

But how will nurses know that they are providing the right care? Nurses in the future will routinely collect nursing-sensitive outcomes measures that will allow them to continuously assess their practice. In all practice arenas, nurses will choose measurable outcomes that reflect the best evidence-based practice. They will regularly measure those outcomes, and make modifications to their practice to improve these outcomes. These outcomes will be publicly reported, and nurses will be rewarded for their performance and contributions to quality care.

Because nursing outcomes will be widely available and reported, nurses will finally be able to communicate what they do in health care to the public and, thereby, nursing's value to the health care system. This will enable nursing to quantify its contribution to the quality of patient care and the saving of health care dollars. The primary reason that patients are admitted to health care facilities is for nursing care, yet currently there is little evidence of nursing services on the hospital bill. With the availability of outcomes data, nursing will no longer be seen just as an expense, but will show its contribution to the saving of health care dollars and the revenue generation of the organization. Nursing will be a major player in the future health care organization.

The nursing profession will become more diverse, reflecting the cultural, ethnic, and gender diversity of the U.S. population. Nurses will also be a more culturally competent workforce, recognizing and being sensitive to different cultural practices and languages in the health care setting.

Finally, nursing will be the most sought-after career opportunity for both first and second career seekers. It will be recognized for what it is, a career with many options and opportunities for specialties, settings, roles, and positions. Nurses will have their choice of positions, and organizations will be creative and innovative in their efforts to attract and retain a sufficient workforce. Nurses will seek those workplaces that have high-performing teams that nursing is a part of. They will look for work environments that promote evidence-based practice and have the information technology to support that practice. Nurses will look for organizations that humanize their work environments and promote and reward their employees for professional development. Nurses will be highly valued for their contributions to the work environment.

SUMMARY

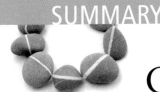

Chaos theory tells us to expect the unexpected and never assume that something will happen because it was predicted. There will definitely be a myriad of opportunities for nurses in the future health care practice environment. The future is there for nurses to determine. What will your practice be like? We will look to our nurse leaders to create new and evolving practice models that will take advantage of opportunities for improving the work environment for nurses, advancing technology, interdisciplinary collaboration, and the recognition of nursing's economic value to the health care system. However, every nurse must be a part of the profession's future. Will you be open to new opportunities, and will you be innovative and say yes to new and exciting challenges? The challenge is to ask yourself how you will impact the profession. The future will happen, one nurse at a time—don't you want to be one of them?

Think of a world without persons who know what nurses know; who believe as nurses believe; who do what nurses do; who have the effect that nurses have on the health of individuals, families, and the nation; who enjoy the trust that nurses enjoy from the American people. Imagine a world like that, a world without nurses.

–Margretta Madden Styles

REFERENCES

AGENCY FOR HEALTHCARE RESEARCH AND QUALITY. (2004). *Five steps to safer health care: Patient fact sheet.* AHRQ Publication Number 04-M005. Rockville, MD: Agency for Healthcare Research and Quality. Retrieved on August 22, 2008, from http://www.ahrq.gov/consumer/5steps.htm

AMERICAN ASSOCIATION OF COLLEGES OF NURSING. (2006). *Essentials of doctoral education for advanced practice nursing.* Washington, DC: Author.

BUERHAUS, P., STAIGER, D., & AUERBACH, D. (2008). *The future of the nursing workforce in the United States: Data, trends, and implications.* Boston: Jones & Bartlett Publishers.

FRANKEL, A. S., Leonard, M. W., & Denham, C. R. (2006). Fair and just culture, team behavior, and leadership engagement: The tools to achieve high reliability. *Health Services Research, 41*(4, Part II), 1690–1709.

GALLUP POLL. (2006). *Most honest and ethical professions survey.* Frank Newport, editor in chief. Retrieved on August 22, 2008, from http://www.gallup.com/video/25930/Honesty-Ethics.aspx

INSTITUTE OF MEDICINE. (1999). *To err is human: Building a safer health system.* Washington, DC: National Academy Press.

INSTITUTE OF MEDICINE. (2001). *Crossing the quality chasm: A new health system for the 21ˢᵗ century.* Washington, DC: National Academies of Science.

INSTITUTE OF MEDICINE. (2003). *Health professional education: A bridge to quality.* Washington, DC: National Academies of Science.

INSTITUTE OF MEDICINE. (2003). *Unequal Treatment: Confronting racial and ethnic disparities in health care.* Washington, DC: National Academies of Science.

MAXFIELD, D., Grenny, J., McMillan, R., Patterson, K., & Switzler, A. (2005). *Silence kills.* VitalSmarts.

McGLYNN, E., Asch, S., Adams, J., Keesey, J., Hicks, J., DeCristofaro, A., & Kerr, E. (2003). The quality of health care delivered to adults in the United States. *New England Journal of Medicine, 348*(26), 2635–2645.

MEUSHAW, M., White, K., & Walrath, J. (2006). Medical errors: Where are we now? *Nursing Management, 37*(10), 50–54.

NATIONAL CENTER FOR HEALTH STATISTICS. (2006). *Health, United States, 2006 with chartbook on trends in the health of Americans.* Hyattsville, MD: Author.

PEW COMMISSION. (1998, December). Recreating health professional practice for a new century. *The Fourth Report of the Pew Health Professions Commission.*

PRONOVOST, P., Berenholtz, S., Dorman, T., Lipsett, P. A., Simmonds, T., & Haraden, C. (2008). Improving communication in the ICU using daily goals. *Journal of Critical Care, 18*(2), 71–75.

SCHYVE, P. M. (2005). Editorial: The changing nature of professional competence. *Joint Commission Journal on Quality and Patient Safety, 31*(4), 183–184.

U.S. DEPARTMENT OF HEALTH AND HUMAN SERVICES. (2000). *Healthy people 2010: Understanding and improving health* (2nd edition). Washington, DC: U.S. Government Printing Office.

GLOSSARY

A

Accident (workplace): An unwanted event that results in injury or death.

Accreditation: Process to evaluate organizations and entities against established metrics that culminates in official recognition for a designated time period.

Accreditation Bodies: Organizational entities that evaluate against established metrics and confer accreditation status to the petitioner.

Acute Health Effect: An immediate untoward response to a single high dose of a chemical or other toxin.

Advanced Practice Registered Nurses: Registered nurses who have acquired advanced specialized clinical knowledge and skills to provide health care, are expected to hold a master's or doctoral degree, and are recognized by state boards of nursing to hold this title.

Advocacy: Pleading the cause of another.

Advocacy-Coalition Framework: Policy model based on the interaction of advocacy coalitions within a policy subsystem.

Aging Population: An increase in the median age of the population; people across the globe are living longer.

Allied Health: The fields of health care provision separate from nursing and medicine that contribute to the overall pursuit of health.

Allopathy: The traditional Western approach to medicine, treating medical conditions by treating their symptoms.

American Association of Colleges of Nursing: Begun in 1969 as the voice of baccalaureate and higher-degree nursing education. AACN became an accrediting agency for BSN and higher programs in 1996. The agency also provides strategies for faculty development, recruitment, and analyzing aggregate data gathered from students and faculty.

American Medical Association (AMA): An organization that democratically represents all professional doctors in the United States.

American Nurses Association (ANA): A national organization of registered nurses whose mission is to advance the nursing profession and promote health.

Antisepsis: The use of antiseptics, which kill germs and bacteria chemically.

Apothecary: Untrained purveyor of homemade remedies before pharmacy became a respected science.

Army Nurse Corps: Begun during the Spanish-American War, it admitted only graduates of nursing schools until demand superseded supply.

Asepsis: Preventive measures taken to stop harmful microbes from coming near sensitive patients who could succumb to infection.

Associate-Degree Nurse: First begun in 1952, these nurses had shorter program lengths but still sat for registered nurse licensure exams.

B

Baby Boomers: The generation born between the years 1946 and 1964, or directly after World War II.

Bad Debt: Unreimbursed care delivered to patients who can afford the care but who choose not to pay.

Beneficiary: The insured party.

Bibliographic Management Software: Various computer programs that allow the creation of electronic databases of citations of journal articles, books, Web sites, etc. Many are able to quickly change the style, i.e., APA, Chicago, MLA, etc. This tool is frequently used by authors to organize references.

Black Death: A pandemic of the Bubonic plague that swept Europe and Asia during the mid-1300s.

Brown Report: Issued in 1948, the report identified nursing education as a pivotal issue in the nursing shortage, calling for examination of every school and for periodic reexaminations to ensure standards remained intact.

Bullying: Interpersonal psychological violence motivated by the desire to have power over another person.

Bundled Charges: The grouping of individual procedure charges into one charge, with the impact of decreasing the overall charge.

C

Cadet Nurse Corps: The corps of nurses developed by the Nurse Training Act. Of 1,300 total, 1,125 nursing programs participated in the program, and men and minorities were actively recruited.

Capitation: The cap, or limit, on the money available in a given timeframe to pay out in insurance premiums, for example, to cover the cost of health care services. There is no incentive to over-provide care.

Carefronting: Confronting in a caring way to solve problems and provide quality care.

Care Management: The process of preventing or delaying disease progression through improved communication among practitioners and patients and through greater patient involvement and responsibility for their own health care decisions.

Care Networks: Those formal or informal structures that enable one to work. Care networks can be family members who watch children, as well as friends, day care, and school programs.

Case Report: A case report is a type of medical article that provides a detailed description of the symptoms, signs, treatment, diagnosis, or disease progression of a single patient that is often used for unusual cases or presentations.

Case Series: A type of medical publication similar to a case report that describes a small group of similar patients.

Centers for Medicare and Medicaid Services (CMS): The Federal Government offices that manage the Medicare and Medicaid programs.

Certification: A mechanism for verification of knowledge and experience beyond the educational degree.

Chaos Theory: A theory that describes the search for order in our disorderly and random systems.

Charity Care: Unreimbursed care to those patients who cannot afford the care, as distinct from bad debt.

Chronic Health Effect: A delayed reaction that may occur after prolonged, low-level exposure to a chemical or other toxin.

CINAHL: Cumulative Index to Nursing and Allied Health Literature is the primary database for the nursing and allied health literature. This database indexes journal articles, books, chapters, dissertations, continuing education material, patient education, computer programs, and more.

Clara Barton: Founder of the American Red Cross and a Civil War nurse.

Clayton Act: Federal act that prohibits price discrimination and mergers, acquisitions, and joint ventures that decrease competition.

Clean Indoor Air Laws: Federal, state, or local laws/ordinances enacted to protect citizens from secondhand smoke exposure.

Clinical Decision Making: The process of using sound critical-thinking skills and ethical reasoning to determine a course of action based on the best available evidence.

Clinical Practice Guidelines: Statements developed by a consensus of experts who systematically review the evidence to guide best practice.

Clinical Simulation: A contrived clinical scenario performed in a structured, safe learning environment that enables the student to participate in patient care decision-making and intervention.

Clinical Trials: Research studies used to determine safety, dosage, and effectiveness of medical therapies or interventions.

Coalition: A group of individuals and/or organizations united around a common interest, working together to achieve a common goal (Bowers-Lanier, 2007).

Cochrane Database of Systematic Reviews: A collection of systematic reviews done by international groups that follow a strict protocol. Each review examines a specific clinical question and examines the current knowledge base. Each Cochrane systematic review is periodically reviewed, and adjustments to the reviews are made as needed.

Coercive Power: Control or influence over others through fear or the perception of fear (Abood, 2007).

Coinsurance: The portion of covered health care costs that is due from the insured individual, usually according to a fixed percentage and after deductibles have been met.

Collaboration: The way one works with another on a joint project.

Communication: A process by which we exchange information and assign meaning to create shared understanding among individuals and groups.

Competencies: Expected levels of performance that integrate knowledge, skills, abilities, and judgment.

Complexity: The characterization of something with many parts in an elaborate arrangement; the degree of difficulty in predicting the properties of a system.

Compromise: Settlement of a dispute in which two or more sides agree to accept less than they originally wanted (Soukhanov, 2001).

Computer-Adaptive Examination: A computerized form of testing used for the NCLEX-RN®.

Connection Power: Control or influence over others by others' perception that the incumbent has important connections that they do not possess (Leavitt, Cohen, & Mason, 2007).

Constituent: One who lives in an elected person's district and has the authority to vote to keep that person in office.

Consumer: Individuals who use products or services provided by another.

Consumer Directed Health Plan (CDHP): Insurance plans that provide financial incentives for consumers to become involved in purchasing decisions regarding their health care. Generally these are high-deductible plans.

Co-Pay: A specified amount due per health care service from the patient, usually due at the time of service.

Co-Payment: Portion of cost of services paid by the insured.

Core Competencies: Curricular outcomes of an educational program that denote critical behaviors of a health care provider.

Core Measures: Program developed by the Joint Commission to promote standardized, quality care in hospitals.

Cost-Benefit: The analysis of cost of a procedure or product against the benefit derived from the procedure or product, with the goal of maximizing net benefits.

Critical Thinking: Self-directed, self-disciplined, self-monitered, and self-corrective thinking.

Crucial Conversations: Discussions between two or more people where stakes are high, opinions vary, and emotions run strong (Patterson, Grenny, McMillan, & Switzler, 2002).

Cultural Sensitivity: Application of background knowledge, values, and attitudes relative to the health traditions observed among the diverse cultural groups found in the setting.

D

Database: A database is a collection of records with fields that is organized, and so can be searched. Databases typically index a specific subject or type of material.

Dermatologists: Doctors who specialize in the diagnosis and treatment of skin ailments.

Diagnostic Related Group (DRG): Coding of hospital procedures in terms of cost and intensity, resulting in a flat rate per procedure regardless of the actual cost to deliver that care. This is the payment system used by Medicare for inpatient service.

Diagnostic Test: An examination, similar to a test such as the NCLEX-RN®, which determines the tester's strengths, weaknesses, and likelihood to pass the actual test.

Dichotomous Thinking: The belief that something is either good or bad and cannot be both good and bad at the same time.

Discipline: A body of knowledge embraced by a group of individuals.

Disease Management: See care management.

Disparities: Deficiencies in health care related to patients' personal characteristics such as gender, ethnicity, geographic location, and socioeconomic status.

Disproportionate Share: Amount added to government payment rates for providers, usually hospitals, which treat large numbers of patients unable to pay their bills.

Dorothea Dix: An early pioneer in mental health nursing and a Civil War nurse.

Dose: The actual amount of the chemical (or other hazard) received.

Doulas: Birth attendants who provide emotional and even physical support to mothers who are giving birth.

E

Educational Mobility: The ability of a student prepared at one educational level to enter a higher academic program. Includes movement of baccalaureate-prepared RNs into graduate programs, LPNs into RN programs, and associate-degree or diploma RNs into baccalaureate nursing programs.

Effectiveness: Care that is necessary and produces a desired outcome.

Electronic or E-Advocacy: The Internet-based approach to speaking up for oneself or one's beliefs (Chandler, n.d.).

Emergency Medical Treatment and Active Labor Act: Federal act that established the legal responsibility to screen patients and stabilize emergency medical conditions if the hospital has the capacity to do so.

Employee Health Nurse: An occupational and environmental health nurse who is employed by a health care facility, such as a hospital.

Employer-Sponsored Insurance (ESI): Insurance provided through employers with all or part of the premium cost paid for by the employer.

Empowerment: The giving of power or authority to someone; it arises from shared power (Abood, 2007).

Entry-Level Preparation: The education needed in order to sit for the registered nursing licensing examination.

Epidemiology: The study of the distribution and determinants of a disease or condition in a population.

Ergonomics: The science of fitting the job to the worker by reducing the risk factors associated with performing required tasks.

Essentials for Baccalaureate Nursing Education: An American Association of Colleges of Nursing (AACN) document that provides an educational framework for the preparation of the baccalaureate-prepared nurse by outlining expected curricular outcomes.

Evidence-Based Medicine (EBM): The integration of individual expertise with the best available external evidence from systematic research (Sackett and colleagues, 1996).

Evidence-Based Policy Process: Merging of the policy process with research to develop changes and improvements with a firm foundation of the best data that exist at the time.

Evidence-Based Practice: An approach to practice that uses explicit methods to ask practice questions, searching and critiquing current available evidence to answer those questions in order to create efficiency and effectiveness of practice.

Evidence Hierarchy: A system that rates the level of evidence according to rigor and causality, placing the randomized control trial at the pinnacle and expert opinion at the base.

Expert Power: The ability to control and influence people by virtue of a person's holding special knowledge that others do not possess (Abood, 2007; Leavitt, Cohen, & Mason, 2007).

Exposure: The opportunity to receive a dose.

Externships: Usually offered in the summer before the final year of nursing school. As an extern, the student nurse is assigned a preceptor and works with that nurse throughout the summer experience.

F

Fair Labor Standards Act: Established a national minimum wage, child labor standards, and overtime rules for both full-time and part-time workers.

False Claims Act: Federal act that establishes civil liability for knowingly presenting false or fraudulent claims to government payers, and for reckless disregard of the accuracy of the claims.

Family Medical Leave Act: An act that allows up to twelve weeks of unpaid leave during any twelve-month period for the birth or adoption of a child; the care of spouse, son, daughter, or parent of the employee who has a serious health condition; or a serious health condition of the employee that makes the employee unable to perform the essential functions of his or her position.

Family Medicine: The medical specialization in first-contact, continuous, comprehensive, personal, and family care.

Fast Track: A term that assumes one's career progression and achievement are in an accelerated fashion.

Federated Search Engine: A federated search engine is able to search multiple databases simultaneously. Due to the fact that databases are not created identically, there may be a loss of individual database features sacrificed for time and convenience.

Fee for Service: Model of insurance reimbursement in which the provider of health care is paid for each service that they provide.

First-Time Test Taker: A phrase used to formally describe a person who has graduated from a nursing program and is eligible to take the NCLEX® for the first time.

Fiscal Intermediary: An agent that has contracted with payers or providers to process claims for reimbursement. Fiscal Intermediaries may also be contracted for other services such as consulting, rules interpretation, and audit.

Florence Nightingale: The founder of modern nursing practice, education, and research.

Frontier Nursing Service: Founded by Mary Breckenridge, FNS provided public health services to the most rural areas of southeastern Kentucky. The documentation of these efforts established the positive impact of nursing care on health outcomes in poverty.

Future of Nursing: The scenario for tomorrow's profession of nursing and its work.

G

Galen: An ancient Roman physician who made great discoveries in anatomy and surgery.

Generation X: The generation of Americans born between the years 1963 and 1980.

Generation Y: The generation of Americans born between the years 1980 and 2000.

Girolamo Fracastoro: An Italian theorist who developed the foundation of modern germ theory.

Globalization: The process of cultural integration, education, tolerance, and acceptance.

Goldmark Report: Report issued in 1923, calling for higher educational standards and relocating professional nursing education into university settings.

Gross Domestic Product (GDP): The total spending on goods and services in the United States.

Gross National Product (GNP): The value of all goods and services produced in a nation.

Group-Model HMO: These HMOs hire physicians directly to provide care for their beneficiaries.

H

Harmony: A complementary balance of physical, psychosocial, and emotional elements of a person's life.

Harriet Tubman: Conductor on the Underground Railroad and Civil War nurse.

Health: A state of physical, mental, and social well-being.

Health Care Administrators: Managers of clinics, hospitals, nursing homes, and other medical facilities.

Health Care System: The totality of services offered by all health care disciplines within an organization or institution; relative to the structure of an agency, the health care system includes all the entities of health care services owned by a specific company.

Health Disparities: Racial and ethnic disparities in the provision of health care.

Health Hazard: "An agent or chemical substance for which there is scientific evidence to show that exposure may cause adverse health outcomes in susceptible employees who may be exposed" (Hatch, 2008, p. 168).

Health Indicators: Measurable behaviors, environmental factors, or health-system issues that affect health status.

Health Insurance Portability and Accountability Act (HIPAA): Legislation to improve the portability of health insurance from one job to another. The legislation also established privacy and security requirements regarding health information.

Health Literacy: The degree to which individuals can obtain, process, and understand basic health care information.

Health Maintenance Organization (HMO): A health care organization intended to promote wellness, shorten hospital stays, and move care to external settings. HMOs achieve these outcomes by paying physicians on a per-patient basis regardless of the extent of services required.

Health Policy: Collection of authoritative decisions made within any level of government that pertain to health and the pursuit of health.

Health Reimbursement Accounts (HRAs): Employer-funded and employer-owned accounts that are used to purchase health care services. Account funds can only be used for medical care, and unused funds revert to the employer if the employee leaves employment. Health Reimbursement Accounts are typically offered in conjunction with high deductibles.

Health Savings Accounts (HSAs): Designated accounts that can be used to buy health care. These accounts are owned by the employee, can be moved from employer to employer, and must be combined with a deductible of $1,000 for an individual or $2,000 for a family. Funds can be used for nonmedical purposes but are subject to tax if used in this manner.

Healthy People 2010: A federal initiative led by the Department of Health and Human Services to provide benchmarks for disease prevention and health promotion, and eliminate health disparities.

Healthy Work Environment: An environment that is a safe healing place where there is mutual respect for patients and health care professionals.

Hierarchy of Controls: A ranking of health and safety strategies by their degree of effectiveness.

High-Deductible Health Plans (HDHP): Health insurance plans with deductibles of at least $1,000 for individuals.

Hill-Burton Act: Provided funding to build hospitals and to plan public health care facilities based on assessed needs. These funds preceded a boom in building rural health services.

Hippocrates: An ancient Greek physician called the "Father of Medicine" for his contributions to the practice and philosophy of medicine.

History: The story of events, people, and ideas that shape a person, society, or profession.

HMO/PPO/IPA: Varieties of managed-care models.

Ignaz Semmelweis: Italian obstetrician who discovered the person-to-person transmission of infection due to physicians' unwashed hands and tools.

Imhotep: An ancient Egyptian chancellor, high priest, and court physician who pioneered and documented many early achievements in medicine and architecture.

Incivility: Low intensity deviant behavior with ambiguous intent to harm the target in violation of workplace norms for mutual respect.

Indemnity Plans: Pay a fixed, negotiated amount for a service, for example, a day in the hospital or a surgical procedure.

Industrial Hygienist: An occupational and environmental health professional with expertise in monitoring work environments for levels of hazardous chemicals and recommending ways to make sure the levels are reduced to safe limits.

Infection Control: How to keep infectious diseases from spreading.

Information Power: The ability to control and influence others by possessing knowledge or information that others do not possess (Leavitt, Cohen, & Mason, 2007).

Informed Consent: A process in which the risks, benefits, and alternatives are communicated and explained to patients so that they fully understand and then agree to participate. Informed consent is the term often used to obtain a patient's permission to proceed prior to surgery, treatment, or enrollment in a clinical trial.

Insider Strategies: A special interest group's strategy to influence policy by interacting with policy decision-makers.

Insurance: Protection from risk; usually a monetary payment if the holder of the insurance policy makes a claim after experiencing the event insurance protection is intended to cover.

Integrative Health Care: The holistic blending of the Western allopathic method of health care with traditional, nonwestern-based ideas and therapies.

Integrative Review: A method that identifies, analyzes, and synthesizes results from independent empirical studies, and summarizes conclusions on a particular topic.

Interdisciplinary Education: The provision of education that spans traditional boundaries and disciplines.

International Pharmaceutical Federation: The international organization for both professional and scientifically minded pharmacists.

Internists: Doctors who specialize in internal medicine.

Intervention Research: A research approach that involves development, implementation, and testing of an intervention.

Iowa Model of EBP: An EBP framework devised by Titler and colleagues (1994) that guides implementation of changes in clinical agencies and evaluates the impact of changes on the environment, staff, costs, patients, and families.

Isabel Hampton Robb: Director of the Johns Hopkins School of Nursing beginning in 1889, Robb promoted moving nursing education out of the hospital and into the academic setting. Robb founded the American Society of Superintendents of Training Schools for Nurses, the forerunner of the National League for Nursing.

J

JAMA: The *Journal of the American Medical Association,* a peer-reviewed periodical publishing modern medical developments.

James Derham: A nurse who worked in New Orleans, he used his earnings to buy his freedom as well as pay his way through medical school, becoming the first African-American physician in the United States.

Jane Woolsey: Nursing education activist, following her time as a Civil War nurse.

Joint Commission: The leading accrediting agency for health care organizations.

Joint Ventures: Business relationships among hospitals, insurance companies, doctors, and others developed to pool resources and allow expansion into new markets, increase price competitiveness, or achieve other business goals.

K

Knowledge Workers: Nurses who are at retirement age, but not ready to leave the work environment; these nurses add a dimension of experiential wisdom, knowledge, and skill that would cost several thousand dollars to replace through the orientation of an experienced, less knowledgeable nurse.

L

Lateral Violence: Hostility expressed between colleagues.

Lavinia Dock: Established the Henry Street Settlement House in New York City to provide health education, disease prevention, and primary care for infants. This project laid the foundation for Public Health practice in nursing.

Learning Organizations: Places that encourage employees to create their desired future and give them the tools to do so.

Legal Regulation: Responsible legal and regulatory bodies' oversight, monitoring, and control of designated professionals based on applicable laws and regulatory language, accompanied by the interpretation of those directives.

Legitimate Power: Influence and control that is derived from the incumbent's position in an organization (Leavitt, Cohen, & Mason, 2007).

Library at Alexandria: A former wonder of the world that is said to have contained volumes of Greek medical literature now lost.

Licensure Examination: A test that, for nurses, enables the person to become a licensed nurse under state law in the United States.

Life Transition: Predictable changes in our lives associated with a discontinuity with the past.

Lillian Wald: Worked in the House on Henry Street Settlement House in New York City, where she developed her theory on the correlation among poverty, squalor, and poor health. Wald published a nursing text and worked for women's right to vote.

Literacy: The ability to read, write, and comprehend written language.

Lobbying: The act of influencing policy decision-makers to obtain a desired outcome.

M

Macho Maternity: A slang term for leave that occurs when a woman only takes the absolute minimum time off to recover from childbirth in order to return to work earlier than scheduled, in order to show others that having a baby doesn't interfere with work.

Magazines: Magazines often contain more advertising than journals, articles are written by staff writers who are not experts, the editor, rather than peers, reviews the material, and they may contain more color photos. They do not contain original reports of research, but frequently interview the experts.

Magnet Status: Recognition that a health care facility has met the criteria established by the American Nurses Credentialing Center and is therefore a desirable place to work.

Maintenance Nap: Naps taken while on the job to improve productivity.

Managed Care: A system designed to constrain health care costs and improve quality and access to services.

Managed Care Organization (MCO): Collective term for a model of health insurance characterized by prepayment by a pool of beneficiaries for negotiated services by a selected group of providers; costs of services are set and providers share the risk and responsibility of giving service within the set financial parameters.

Mary Adelaide Nutting: Her 1918 testimony to the Rockefeller Foundation created the impetus for a closer examination of nursing education.

Mary Eliza Mahoney: First African-American graduate from the New England Hospital for Women and Children in 1879, inducted into ANA Hall of Fame.

Mary Seacole: A Jamaican-born nurse who traveled to Crimea to care for British soldiers. She was denied the ability to join Nightingale's nurses due to her biracial heritage.

Material Safety Data Sheet: A chemical manufacturer's full description of its product's health and safety hazards and control measures.

Medicaid: Health insurance program for eligible persons living in conditions of poverty; designed by the federal government but administered by states, so that there is variation in what coverage is provided according to state of residence.

Medicare: Federal program designed to provide medical care coverage primarily for all persons over the age of 65; also provides coverage for persons with certain disabilities and medical conditions for those persons under 65.

Medicare Prescription Drug, Improvement and Modernization Act: A federal law that assures citizens who receive Medicare benefits will also be eligible for some prescription drug benefits.

Medication Errors: Medication errors are all the mistakes involving the medications. It may be an error in the written prescription, an error in reading the prescription, an error in filling the prescription, an error in instructions about taking the medication, or a patient's failure to take the correct dosage and adhere to the correct schedule. These errors may involve prescription, over-the-counter, or alternative medications.

Medigap: Supplemental insurance coverage purchased by individuals to pay for medical services not covered by Medicare.

Mentee: A person who is guided by a mentor.

Mentor: A more experienced professional who can provide advice, instruction, or moral support to newer professionals as needed. More generally, a wise and trusted guide and advisor.

Mentoring: A fundamental form of human maturation where one person invests time, energy, and personal expertise to help another person in the process of their growth and development.

Mentoring Gap: A difference or disparity in attitudes, values, perceptions, character, and development, or a lack of confidence or understanding, perceived as creating a problem between more experienced, seasoned individuals and newer, more novice individuals.

Mentoring Relationship: A voluntary affiliation between two individuals, in which one individual (the mentor) guides the other (the mentee) through a period of change and towards an agreed-upon objective.

Meta-Analysis: A process that summarizes the results of multiple similar quantitative studies and provides a summary statistic that measures the single effect of an intervention across multiple studies.

Meta-Synthesis: Interpretive translations that are produced when findings are compared across qualitative studies. Sometimes referred to as integrative reviews.

Miasmatists: People in the 1700s through the 1900s who believed that medical maladies were caused by impure air.

Mommy Track: A woman who, usually in a white-collar career, willingly leaves the workforce in order to spend time with her children.

Moral Distress: The painful experience of knowing what is ethically right to do and not being allowed to do it, or being forced to act in a way that is inconsistent with your values.

Morbidity: Disease and disability.

Mortality: Death.

Multiple Streams Framework: Policy model describing how policies are formulated using three streams: the problem stream, policy stream, and politics stream.

N

National Institute for Nursing Research: A division of the U.S. Department of Health and Human Services, NINR offers training for fledgling nurse scientists and funds nursing research in strategic areas.

National Institute for Occupational Safety and Health (NIOSH): The federal agency that conducts research on occupational hazards and their prevention.

National League for Nursing (NLN): Developed from the American Society of Superintendents of Training Schools for Nurses in 1912, NLN advocated for standards of excellence among schools of nursing and has evolved into a political force on behalf of nurse educators and students. NLN continues to accredit schools of nursing of all levels.

National Quality Forum (NQF): A private, nonprofit organization that is working to improve the quality of health care through the development of standards and methods to measure quality care.

NCLEX® Test Plan: The blueprint for the NCLEX-RN®.

NCLEX-RN®: The licensure test to become a registered nurse in the U.S.

Negotiation/Compromise: Discussing and bargaining on a variety of issues so that everyone has to give up something for the good of the whole.

Networking: To develop contacts on an informal basis to further someone's agenda or career, a way of spreading the word or to help persuade legislators to consider and act upon a particular concern.

Nightingales: A special-interest group of nurses whose mission is to focus public attention on the behaviors of the tobacco industry and its involvement with tobacco-caused diseases and death.

Noise: Sound waves that are a physical hazard to hearing if they exceed a certain safe threshold.

North American Nursing Diagnosis Association (NANDA): Taxonomy containing diagnostic labels used to identify patient problems.

Novice: A person who is new to an occupation or activity.

Nurse Advocacy: The act of addressing one's individual responsibility to be informed about issues, to educate one's colleagues and the public about those issues, to collaborate with those who can offer solutions to identified problems, and to effect change in nursing practice that delivers better outcomes (Hilton, 2007).

Nurse Educator: A nurse who has obtained a graduate nursing degree and who is hired to an academic institution to teach nursing students.

Nurse Educator Shortage: An inadequate number of individuals to fill vacant nurse educator positions in nursing education programs.

Nurse Reinvestment Act: A federal policy enacted to combat the 21st-century nursing shortage.

Nurse Training Act: Sponsored by Francis Payne Bolton of Ohio, this legislation mandated an expedited education program for nurses. The program provided education and guaranteed employment at the end of the war.

Nursing Domains: General, high-level divisions of nursing practice most often defined to be practice, education, administration, and research.

Nursing Faculty: A collective group of nurse educators.

Nursing Informatics: A general term describing the technological advances in the computerization of patient-care information.

Nursing Interventions Classification (NIC): Listing of terms that describe nursing interventions.

Nursing Outcomes Classification (NOC): Listing of terms that describe nursing-specific patient outcomes.

Nursing Religious Orders: Religious cloisters, usually Catholic, where nuns offered health care, but the members also traveled to rural areas to ensure health care and teaching.

Nursing Role: "A cluster of prescribed actions; the behaviors we expect of those who occupy a particular social position" (Myers, 2005, p. 90).

Nursing Shortage: An inequity between supply and demand of nurses with the appropriate skill mix to fulfill job responsibilities in both the practice and academic settings.

Nursing Theory: The use of theory unique to the discipline of nursing, used to explain, guide, and direct nursing-care activities.

Nursing Workforce Centers: Entity within a state to develop long-term strategies to address the nursing supply and demand, to forecast changes, and to develop policies addressing the nursing workforce.

O

Obstetrician: A doctor who specializes in the care of pregnant women.

Occupational and Environmental Health Nurse: A nurse who focuses on preserving the health of worker populations through primary and secondary prevention interventions.

Occupational Safety and Health Act: Federal law that requires all employers to provide a safe and healthful workplace.

Occupational Safety and Health Administration (OSHA): The federal agency that is charged with protecting most employees from workplace hazards through regulation and inspection.

Online Learning: A form of distance instruction provided via the Internet.

Ophthalmologists: Doctors who specialize in the treatment of eyes.

Opticians: State-licensed professionals who specialize in supplying, fitting, and maintaining glasses and contact lenses.

Optometrists: Doctors of optometry who are qualified to diagnose eye abnormalities and prescribe and maintain corrective lenses.

Organizational Culture: Beliefs and values shared by all members of the organization. These shared values are reflected in the day-to-day operations of the organization.

Organization for Economic Cooperation and Development (OECD): An international agency that studies political and social policies and collects statistics that describe the health of the world's population.

Osteopathy: An approach to medical care that emphasizes a combination of mental and physical wellness as a key to health.

Otolaryngology: The medical specialization in care of the ears, nose, and throat.

Outcomes Research: A research approach that examines structures, processes, and outcomes of care to increase the effectiveness of health care services, improve point-of-care services, and health of populations. Outcomes research involves individuals and aggregates.

Outsider Strategies: A special interest group's strategy to influence policy by mobilizing the public to act.

P

Parity: Similar insurance coverage and reimbursement for services, regardless of the medical condition or disease that requires treatment.

Patient Advocacy: The ability to speak up for one's patients (Oncology Nursing Society, 2007).

Patient-Centered Care: Health care that is respectful of and responsive to individual patient preferences, needs, and values.

Patient Compliance: The degree to which patients follow instructions given by a health care professional related to a prescribed course of treatment or care.

Patient Education: Information and training provided by health care providers to patients and family to insure that they can understand and manage treatment and care.

Patients' Bill of Rights: A statement designed to ease communication between doctors and patients and to advocate nondiscriminatory provision of medical care and insurance.

Pay for Performance: Linkage between health care outcomes and payment for care.

Pediatricians: Doctors who specialize in the care of infants, children, and teenagers.

Peer Review: Review and evaluation of articles or book chapters by professional peers prior to publication.

Per Capita: Per person.

Personal Protective Equipment (PPE): Items designed to protect the wearer from a hazard, such as gloves, face masks, and lead aprons.

Pharmacist: A health professional who is trained in the preparation and distribution of medication.

PICO: Patient (or Population), Intervention, Comparison, and Outcome; a tool used to develop search statements to locate evidence-based practice information.

Podiatry: The medical field associated with the health and care of feet.

Policy: Described as both an entity (guidelines that direct human behavior toward specific goals) and a process (taking problems to government agents and obtaining a decision or reply in the form of a program, law, or regulation).

Policy Analysis: Step in the policy process that describes a particular policy or policy area, assessment of the impact, inquiry into the consequences, and evaluation of the policy's impact.

Policy Assessment: The first step of the policy process in which the problem, issue, or need is identified with initial data.

Policy Development: Step in the policy process in which data are collected and analyzed, research is reviewed, key stakeholders who will advocate for the plan are consulted, and the best plan of action is recommended.

Policy Evaluation: Step in the policy process where implementation, performance, and impact are evaluated to determine how well the policy has met its goals and objectives.

Political Action Committee: A special-interest group whose responsibility is to fund political campaigns and support elected officials.

Politics: The totality of interrelationships in areas of concern, especially as they relate to power, authority, or influence (Soukhanov, 2001). The art of the possible (Bismarck).

Population Trends: Data obtained by study of a certain population and its attributes, including projected trends for the future based on the current data.

Posology: A branch of medical science devoted to the study of dosage.

Power: The ability or capacity to do something; control and influence over other people and their actions; and the ability to influence people's judgment or emotions (Soukhanov, 2001).

Premiums/Group Premiums: The amount paid to the insurance company to provide selected coverage; can be paid by either a group or an individual.

Preventable Adverse Events: Medical errors.

Price Transparency: Availability to patients of cost or cost estimates of care to enable them to compare prices and/or determine the economic value of a health care product.

Profession: A group of individuals, educated in like manner, who are dedicated to a common cause and striving toward a common goal, guided by a prescribed code of ethics and behaviors.

Professionalism: The expected behavior of members of a particular profession.

Professional Journals: Journals publish the literature of a profession. They may be produced by professional societies or publishers. Authors are usually experts on the subject presented. They may contain reports of original research written by the investigators, news of the profession, or review articles on topics of interest.

Professional Nursing: The practice of nursing based in arts and sciences by those with collegiate education.

Professional Practice: The summative role of behaviors exhibited by a discipline.

Professional Regulation: A profession's oversight, monitoring, and control of its members based on principles, guidelines, and rules deemed important.

Prospective Payment System (PPS): Payment of health care providers according to rates of payment established in advance.

Protégé: A person who receives support and protection from an influential patron who furthers the protégé's career.

PsycInfo: PsycInfo is an electronic database of the literature of psychology that is produced by the American Psychological Association.

Public Advocacy: Speaking out on behalf of an issue, a population group, or a concern in an effort to influence changes in public policy, laws, regulations, and/or practices (Bowers-Lanier, 2007).

Public Health: A field of health care dedicated to the preservation of health in a society.

PubMed: PubMed is a free search engine to access MEDLINE, the premier database of the biomedical literature produced by the National Library of Medicine.

Q

Qualitative Research: A research approach that uses rich, descriptive, in-depth narratives to report the investigation of various phenomena, which may include lived experiences, cultural aspects, values, or generation and construction of theory.

Quality: A subjective term that describes the ability to satisfy needs or be free of deficiencies.

Quantitative Research: An empirical approach to collecting evidence that uses precise measurement of variables and statistical methods to arrive at conclusions.

R

Randomized Control Trial: A clinical experiment in which subjects are randomly assigned to various groups. Groups should be large enough to insure that they are statistically similar. Groups are treated differently and outcomes are measured and evaluated. One group may be the control; this group is given either the standard intervention or a placebo.

Rationing: A means of allocating goods and services.

Readability: The degree of ease or difficulty of a written text. Readability involves the reading level of the words, the size and font of the print, and other visual factors. It may be expressed as a grade-level equivalent.

Reality Shock: The role strain, conflict, and incongruity experienced by the new graduate nurse while transitioning from the ideal role of student to reality of staff nurse.

Recognition Criteria: Established metrics that must be met before official designation can be bestowed.

Refereed: Sometimes referred to as peer reviewed, they are journal articles or book chapters that have been reviewed by peer experts in the field. The process is intended to insure scholarly standards.

Referent Power: Control and influence over others that is dependent upon others' respect of the person with whom they associate (Abood, 2007).

Regional Health Information Organization (RHIO): Networks of care providers that are connected electronically for the rapid exchange of patient health information.

Regulations: Rules or laws by which conduct is regulated, and which define the scope of practice in specific terms.

Research Utilization: The synthesis and application of research results to solve clinical problems and change existing practice.

Residency: A learning period for new doctors in which they provide medical care under the supervision of more experienced staff members.

Resource Based Relative Value Scale (RSRVS): The scale used by Medicare to determine reimbursement to doctors based upon the amount of time and resources used, adjusted for overhead and geographic variation.

Respirator: A type of personal protective equipment that is designed to provide a barrier between the breathing zone and harmful agents that could be inhaled, such as *mycobacterium tuberculosis*.

Review: Review articles are not research reports. This publication type summarizes the literature on a particular topic or a specific aspect of a topic.

Reward Power: The ability to influence and control others by giving other people what they want, such as rewards or favors (Abood, 2007).

Right-to-Work States: One cannot be required to join a union or pay dues to a union as a condition of employment or continued employment. There are a few exceptions to this ruling, such as if one is employed by the airline or railroad industries.

Risk: Likelihood or chance of a certain event occurring.

Risk/Benefit Ratio: Relative costs versus benefits to individuals and/or societies of clinical, administrative, or policy interventions.

Risk-Taking: The willingness to make mistakes, advocate unconventional or unpopular positions, or tackle extremely challenging problems without obvious solutions, all without a predictable outcome.

Role: Predetermined expectations that others have toward one another.

Role Conflict: A situation that occurs when a person is expected to play the part of two different and incompatible roles simultaneously.

Role Overload: When there are multiple expectations, and the person may feel as if they are unable to devote enough time to any one role, only fulfilling several halfway.

Roles of the Professional Nurse: Traditional roles of the professional nurse include caregiver, communicator, teacher, client advocate, counselor, change agent, leader, manager, case manager, and research consumer (Berman, Snyder, Kozier, & Erb, 2008).

Role Specialty: Those advanced levels of nursing practice that intersect with another body of knowledge, have a direct influence on nursing practice, and support the delivery of direct care rendered to patients by other registered nurses.

Role Stress: The pressure or strain resulting from a variety of expectations that the multiple roles require.

Role Transition: Occurs when a person moves from one position to another and requires an individual to take on a new or modified set of role expectations.

Route of Exposure: Portal of entry into the body.

RSS Feeds: Really simple syndication is a Web tool to notify subscribers when new content is added to Web pages of interest.

S

Safety: Free of harm, hazards, error, or other adverse events.

Safety Professional: Someone with expertise in workplace accident prevention and investigation.

Sandwich Generation: Individuals who are simultaneously taking care of both their children and their aging parents.

Sanitary Commission: A government agency created during the Civil War to promote clean and healthy conditions in army camps.

Scope and Standards of Practice: Describes what constitutes the profession, what its members do, and those responsibilities for which they are accountable.

Scope of Nursing Practice: What a nurse can and cannot do within each individual state as defined by state law.

Search Engine: A Web page that searches and indexes Web content that is delivered in response to key words entered.

Search Statements: The concepts that are being searched, joined by Boolean operators.

Self-Advocacy: The ability to speak up for oneself (Meecham, 2003).

Self-Insured Plans: Insurance plans paid for by employers and contributions through premiums from the employees.

Self-Knowledge: Knowledge of one's particular mental states, including one's beliefs, desires, and sensations (Gertler, 2003).

Self-Regulation: An individual's demonstrated personal control based on principles, guidelines, and rules deemed important.

Service Plans: Insurance coverage for a specified set of medical services that are provided to those insured by the plan at a fixed rate, regardless of the number or cost of the claims made by those insured.

Sheppard-Towner Act: Federal funds to support women and children and welfare programs, used by public health service nurses to promote health in these populations.

Sherman Anti-Trust Act: Federal anti-trust act that prohibits collective restraint of trade and monopolies.

Sleep Debt: Consistent sleep deprivation.

Sleep Deprivation: Less than eight hours of sleep in a day.

Sojourner Truth: An abolitionist and Civil War nurse.

Special-Interest Groups: A group of individuals with a similar interest and who wish to influence public policy about their interest.

Specialty Hospital: A private hospital, usually for profit, that is established to provide treatment to a restricted group of diagnoses such as orthopedics.

Spillover: The extent to which family life interferes with work or vice versa.

Staff-Model HMO: Physicians are employees of the HMO.

Stakeholders: Individuals and groups that have power to influence policy development and enactment.

Stark: Federal law that prohibits physicians from referring patients to entities with which they have a financial interest.

State Boards of Nursing: Regulatory entities established by state government to protect the public's safety through the control, monitoring, and sanction of nurses.

State Children's Health Insurance Program (SCHIP): Joint federal and state program offering insurance coverage for children.

State Children's Health Insurance Program (SCHIP): A federal initiative that provides money to help states expand health care coverage to uninsured children.

Step/Stages Model: Policy model that divides policy into the stages of agenda setting, policy formulation, implementation, and evaluation.

Stetler Model: A conceptual map of research utilization that has evolved into a framework for EBP.

Susie King Taylor: Taught many African-American slaves to read and write despite laws forbidding them to do so; Civil War nurse.

Synergy Model for Patient Care: A needs-driven patient-care framework, developed originally for use in the critical-care setting, which stresses that nurse competencies should be based on the needs of the patient.

Systematic Review: A rigorous process conducted by experts who identify, analyze, and synthesize research studies on a specific question to draw conclusions about the worth of the data.

T

Teamwork: A group of team members working toward a shared goal; using diversity of background, education, and experience to enhance productivity, creativity, and innovation.

Temporary Permit: In the United States, some boards of nursing issue a permit that enables a new nursing graduate to practice nursing until the results of the NCLEX® are obtained.

Test Anxiety: A form of general anxiety; this refers to physiological, behavioral, and personal responses that result from concern about possibly failing a test.

Test Difficulty Levels: Techniques used by those who write test items to make the items at a certain difficulty level; the difficulty level is often expressed by a number value based on a statistical formula.

Test Preparation Plan: An organized sequence of test-taking strategies used to enhance success on test results; the plan is individualized to the learner.

Test Preparation Strategies: Activities that a leaner uses to become the best possible test taker.

Test Remediation Strategies: Activities used by testers to strengthen their abilities to take tests, especially after a test has been failed.

Test-Taking Skills: Essential techniques to enhance success in taking tests.**Textbooks**: Books used in school or college classes that deal with a subject or topic and are used in the presentation or teaching. They are a collection of the known knowledge on the subject.

Third Party Administrator: A company that manages benefits, claims, and administration of health insurance for self-insured companies and entities.

Tiered Health Plans: Plans that pay for care based upon the quality, cost, or satisfaction tier that the provider falls into. Tiered-premium pans require patients to pay more if they select a less restrictive network or better coverage, while tiered-provider plans pay better when the patient selects a provider that has been determined to provide higher-quality/lower-cost care.

Toxicity: The degree of potential harm of the hazard.

Traditionalists: The generation born between the years 1924 and 1945.

Trepanation: The use of a drill or other instrument to make a hole in the skull to expose a small part of the brain.

U

Unlicensed Assistive Personnel (UAP): Aides, orderlies, assistants, attendants, or technicians used to provide nursing-type patient care.

Usual and Customary: The charge for a service that is the predominant one in a particular medical specialty and geographic area.

V

Vaccines for Children Program (VFC): A Centers for Disease Control and Prevention vaccine program for children.

W

Ways of Knowing: A holist framework developed by Carper (1978), which includes empirical, ethical, esthetic, and personal ways of conceptualizing nursing knowledge.

Web sites: Information or documents stored on a Web server and accessed via the World Wide Web. It may be text, photos, graphics, or forms. Each page has a unique URL (uniform resource locator) and is accessed by using a Web browser such as Internet Explorer, Firefox, Netscape, or Opera.

Wiki: Wiki is the Hawaiian word for fast. A wiki is a collection of Web pages that allow readers to add, delete, or modify the contents. Wikipedia is one of the best known wikis.

Workers' Compensation Insurance: Employer-paid benefit that provides medical care and wage replacement after a workplace accident that arose out of or in the course of employment.

Work/Family Border Theory: A theory proposed by Clark that delineates the spheres of "work" and "family," stating that while both spheres influence one another, there are significant differences found that do not share the same space.

Work–Family Conflict: Conflict that occurs as the result of role pressures from the work and family domains being incongruent.

Workforce Advocacy: Individual nurses' efforts to advocate for improved working conditions and safe patient care (Green & Jordan, 2002).

Workforce Diversity Environment: The conditions, circumstances, influences, and differences encountered in a particular work environment that ultimately affect productivity and the outcomes of a particular work.

Workforce Shortages: Inefficiencies in supply or demand of a labor pool for the specific labor marketplace.

Workplace Advocacy: The means by which nurses' work-related concerns, such as employment benefits and job security, are addressed (Boone & Kurtz, 1999).

Workplace Violence: Physical attacks or threats of attack (verbal or behavioral) at work.

Workweek: Amount of time worked in a consecutive seven-day week.

INDEX